# FAMILY THERAPY REVIEW
## Preparing for Comprehensive and
## Licensing Examinations

# FAMILY THERAPY REVIEW
## Preparing for Comprehensive and Licensing Examinations

Edited by

Robert H. Coombs
*UCLA School of Medicine*

**LEA**

LAWRENCE ERLBAUM ASSOCIATES, PUBLISHERS

2005   Mahwah, New Jersey          London

| | |
|---|---|
| Senior Consulting Editor: | Susan Milmoe |
| Editorial Assistant: | Kristen Depken |
| Cover Design: | Kathryn Houghtaling Lacey |
| Textbook Production Manager: | Paul Smolenski |
| Full-Service Compositor: | TechBooks |
| Text and Cover Printer: | Hamilton Printing Company |

This book was typeset in 10/12 pt. Times New Roman, Bold, and Italic.
The heads were typeset in Sabon, Sabon Bold, and Sabon Bold Italic.

Lahaska Press, a unique collaboration between the Houghton Mifflin College Division and Lawrence Erlbaum Associates, is dedicated to publishing books and offering services for the academic and professional counseling communities. Houghton Mifflin and Lawrence Erlbaum will focus on becoming a major conduit for educational and academic materials in the psychological and educational counseling fields. The partnership of Lahaska Press was formed in late 1999. The name "Lahaska" is a Native American Lenape word meaning "source of much writing." It is also a small town in eastern Pennsylvania, named by the Lenape.

Lawrence Erlbaum Associates, Inc., Publishers
10 Industrial Avenue
Mahwah, New Jersey 07430
www.erlbaum.com

**Library of Congress Cataloging-in-Publication Data**

Family therapy : review preparing for comprehensive and licensing examinations / edited by Robert H. Coombs.
    p.  cm.
   Includes bibliographical references and index.
   ISBN 0-8058-4312-4 (case : alk. paper)—ISBN 0-8058-5175-5 (pbk : alk. paper)
   1. Family psychotherapy—Examinations, questions, etc.   I. Coombs, Robert H.
 RC488.5.F349   2005
 616.89′156′076—dc22

                                              2004010402

Books published by Lawrence Erlbaum Associates are printed on acid-free paper, and their bindings are chosen for strength and durability.

Printed in the United States of America
10  9  8  7  6  5  4  3  2  1

*for*

*David, Jeremy, and Kim*

# Contents

# Preface

Family therapy, an important component in today's healthcare system, offers affordable mental health care in the context of family circumstances. Family dynamics influence the physical health and emotional wellness of its members, present and future. Family therapists consider family circumstances an integral part of diagnosis and treatment, even when working with a single client. Individual problems are assessed within the context of family structure, boundaries, beliefs, roles, sentiments, activities, and interactions.

More than a collection of individuals, the family is a *living system,* an organic whole wherein a change in one member brings changes in the entire family system. Hospital psychiatrists noted in the 1950s that when certain patients improved another family member often got worse. Subsequent therapists learned that the most effective way to change the individual—the identified patient—is to alter the family dynamics (Nichols & Schwartz, 2001, p. 57). "The goal of family treatment," Glick and colleagues noted, "is the improved functioning of the family as an interlocking system and network of individuals" (Glick, Berman, Clarkin, & Rait, 2000, p. 21).

Like other schools of psychotherapy, family therapy includes the following elements (Glick et al., 2000):

1. An effective patient–therapist relationship
2. Release of emotional tension or development of emotional expression
3. Cognitive learning
4. Insight into the genesis of one's problems
5. Operant reconditioning of the client toward more adaptive behavior patterns using techniques such as behavioral desensitization
6. Suggestion and persuasion
7. Identification with the therapist
8. Repeated reality testing or practicing of new adaptive techniques in the context of implicit or explicit emotional therapeutic support
9. Construction of a more positive narrative about oneself and the world
10. Instillation of hope

Family therapy accomplishes each of these but "does so in the context of the whole family, with the goal of improving the entire group's overall functioning" (Glick et al., 2000, p. 240).

Research consistently shows that the more a client's family becomes appropriately involved in therapy, the greater the likelihood of treatment success. An edited book by Sprenkle (2002) analyzed hundreds of family therapy outcome studies—conduct disorder and delinquency, substance abuse, childhood behavioral and emotional disorders, alcohol abuse, marital problems, relationship enhancement, domestic violence, severe mental illness, affective disorders, physical disorders—revealing that family therapy is at least as effective as other therapies, and in many cases more so. With regard to family-based interventions for drug abuse problems, for example, Rowe and Liddle (2002, p. 76) note, "There is certainly cause for great excitement. . . . There is little doubt, given the existing empirical base, that the family-based treatment field is at the cutting edge of drug abuse intervention science."

Summarizing the outcome of more than five hundred family therapy evaluation studies, Glick and his colleagues (2000, p. 634) report:

1. Family treatment is more effective than no treatment at all. Studies that contrasted family and marital treatment with no-treatment control groups found statistically significant differences: roughly 67% of marital cases and 70% of family cases improved. These outcome results improved slightly when the identified patient was a child or an adolescent rather than an adult. No one method of therapy is clearly better than another.

2. The deterioration rate (i.e., the percentage of patients who become worse or experience negative effects of therapy) is about 10% lower than for individual therapy.

3. Family treatment is the preferred intervention strategy for several types of problems. Since 1970, outcome data suggest that couples therapy is superior to individual therapy for marital conflict situations, especially for increasing marital satisfaction and reducing couple conflict. However, both family therapy and individual therapy were tied for other problems, often in situations where the identified patient had a serious Axis I problem (i.e., any clinical disorder—except for mental retardation and personality disorders—as well as other conditions that may be at the center of clinical attention).

Family therapy clients represent a wide variety of problems including couples in crises, young children or adolescents with their parents, children and families in the foster care system, sexual abuse victims and perpetrators, individuals addicted to alcohol or other drugs and their families, other addicted people—compulsive gamblers, sex addicts, workaholics, compulsive buyers and eating extremists—and their families, juvenile offenders and others in the criminal justice system, families dealing with severe mental illnesses and emotional disorders, such as anxiety, depression, and grieving loved ones who have lost a family member.

Family therapists work in a wide variety of settings—private practice, schools and Head Start centers, businesses and consulting companies, employee assistance programs, social service agencies, government agencies, courts and prisons, county mental health departments, hospitals, community mental health centers and residential treatment facilities, universities and research centers (*Marriage and Family Therapists*).

Family therapists typically practice short-term therapy—twelve sessions on average—about one-half are one-on-one sessions with the other half divided between couple/family therapy, or a combination of treatments (*Marriage and Family Therapists*). Not only is family therapy usually relatively brief, it is also *solution-focused, specific,* with *attainable therapeutic goals,* and *designed with the "end in mind." (FAQs on MFTs).*

"Since the early 1970s," Guttman (in Glick et al., p. xxxiii) noted, "family therapy has developed exponentially, both as a philosophy and as a treatment modality." Since that time, the MFT profession has experienced a fifty-fold increase. At any given time, family therapists are currently treating over 1.8 million people.

The membership of the American Association for Marriage and Family Therapy (AAMFT), the professional association that serves family therapists, grew quickly, from 237 members in 1960, to 9,000 in 1982, and to more than 23,000 in 2002 (*A Career as an MFT*). And this number doubles when adding in members of the California Association of Marriage and Family Therapy (CAMFT)—more than 25,000 Californians, with few who hold joint memberships. The first state to license family therapists (in 1963), California has an extensive infrastructure of seventy-seven schools and universities that offer family therapy programs. Each year about one thousand California students take the family therapy examination. With twenty-nine regional chapters, CAMFT sponsors an annual conference, publishes the *California Therapist,* and has a strong voice in the state legislature. (Contact CAMFT at 7901 Raytheon Road, San Diego, CA 92111; telephone 619-292-2638; Web site: www.camft.org.)

Not surprisingly, states recognizing and regulating family therapists have grown steadily— from eleven in 1986 to forty-six in 2003. And other state legislatures are considering regulatory bills (*Directory of MFT Licensing Boards*). Of the states that license the family therapist, only four (10%) originated before 1980, and twenty-four of the forty (60%) were initiated after 1990.

Compared with psychiatry, clinical psychology, and social work, family therapy is clearly a newcomer. "Family therapy was born in the 1950s, grew up in the 1960s and came of age in the 1970s," noted Nichols and Schwartz (2001, p. 7). From "a radical new experiment" (p. 307), family therapy grew to be an established force in the 1960s and 70s, complete with its own association (the AAMFT) replete with state affiliates, a professional journal, and an annual national conference. Unlike other therapeutic movements organized around one major theory or innovator (e.g., psychoanalysis, behaviorism) or by professional degree (e.g., psychology, psychiatry, social work), family therapy uses a variety of theories and draws followers from many professional backgrounds (p. 307).

By the mid-1990s, the profession compared with other mental health professions in the following ways, as noted by a report of the U.S. Public Health Service's Center for Mental Health Services (Manderscheid & Sonnenchein, 1996):

• Family therapists comprised 11% of the clinically trained *mental health personnel in the U.S.* Counseling and psychology were at comparable rates (14% and 16%, respectively). Social work and psychosocial rehabilitation comprised the highest rates at 22% each, while the lowest rates were shared among psychiatry (8%), school psychology (5%) and psychiatry nursing (2%).

• Most people in the *mental health disciplines* were trained in social work or counseling with more than 30,000 trainees each. Psychology trainees followed with 18,000 trainees, with family therapy and psychiatry having between 6,000 and 7,000 trainees each. Psychiatric nursing had 2,000 trainees.

• The *distribution of family therapists* varied considerably across the states, ranging from fewer than 3 per 100,000 resident population in West Virginia, Delaware, Ohio, North Dakota, Louisiana, and Arkansas, to more than 20 per 100,000 in Oklahoma, Indiana, Texas, and Nevada, to more than 73 per 100,000 population in California. Generally, more states in the West and the Northeast had more than 10 family therapists per 100,000 than did states in the South and Central United States. The national average was 17.6 marriage and family therapists per 100,000 population.

- The *gender distribution* varied greatly by discipline. Family therapists and psychologists were the most balanced with 53% of family therapists female and 47% male. In psychology, 44% were female, 56% male. Psychiatrists were primarily male (75%), while psychiatric nurses (95%), social workers (77%) and counselors (78%) were mostly female.
- Psychiatrists and counselors were at opposite ends of the *age/experience* spectrum. Psychiatrists were primarily older males, 60% of whom had been in practice for over 20 years.
- Social workers, family therapists, and counselors were the primary clinical staff of *mental health and other health clinics*. Roughly 50,000 clinically trained professionals were employed in clinics, either as their primary or secondary work setting.
- Psychologists and family therapists predominated the approximately 140,000 clinically trained mental health personnel who worked in *private practice,* either as their primary or secondary work setting, followed by social workers and counselors. Psychiatrists and psychiatric nurses represented the lowest percentage of clinically trained mental health personnel who worked in private practice settings.
- Among the various work activities—patient care/direct service, research, teaching and administration—the *primary work activities* of mental health professionals usually involved direct patient care, ranging from 67% for school psychologists to 96% for psychosocial rehabilitation professionals. Almost nine of ten family therapists (88%) were involved in direct patient care.
- The disciplines involved in *research* were psychiatric nursing (25.1%), psychology (19.7%), psychiatry (17.4%), and MFT (16.5%). Counseling, social work, and school psychology have the lowest rates (0.1%, 1.3%, and 4.0%, respectively).
- *Teaching* was a very common activity among psychiatric nurses (59%), psychiatrists (49%), family therapists (47%), and psychologists (31%). Only 11% of social workers and 9% of counselors are involved in teaching activities.
- The majority of family therapists (56%), psychiatrists (52%), and psychiatric nurses (52%) were involved in *administrative activities,* followed by social workers (35%) and psychologists (27%).

AAMFT was originally called the American Association of Marriage Counselors (AAMC). Directed by David Mace, who later became my colleague at the Wake Forest University School of Medicine, AAMC was organized in 1942 as a professional organization to set standards for marriage counselors. In 1970 the AAMC changed its name to the AAMFT, emphasizing family therapy, yet retained a focus on couple relationships, and became the major credentialing body for the field. Through its requirements for membership, national family therapy standards have been set and are used by various states to regulate the profession. (Contact AAMFT at 1133 15th Street N. W., Suite 300 Washington DC 20005-2710, telephone: 202-452-0109.)

AAMFT's code of ethics addresses proper behavior with regard to the following: responsibility to clients; confidentiality, professional competence and integrity; responsibility to students, employees, supervisees, and research subjects; financial arrangements; and advertising. It also lobbies state and federal governments for the interests of family therapists, such as uniform state licensing. Because of its large membership, enough income is generated to make the AAMFT a powerful player in mental health politics and has aided recognition of family therapy as a distinct field by the government and the public alike (Nichols & Schwartz, 2001).

Though not as influential as AAMFT, other organizations provide conferences, publications, and networking opportunities. The American Family Therapy Academy (AFTA), for example, an organization not readily open to the rank-and-file family therapist, was organized in 1977 as a group whose membership presumably confers high status. Five categories of members are admitted: charter, clinical-teacher, research, distinguished, and international. To be considered for AFTA membership, applicants usually must obtain three enthusiastic support letters from existing members. Despite efforts to remain small, AFTAs membership doubled between 1983 and 2003—from 500 to over 1,000 (Nichols & Schwartz, 2001). AFTA holds an annual conference, a bi-annual clinical research conference, and publishes a newsletter three times a year for its members. (Contact AFTA at 1608 20th Street, NW, 4th Floor, Washington, DC 2009, telephone: 202-333-3690, fax: 202-333-3692, e-mail: afta@afta.org; Web site: www.afta.org.)

A world-wide family therapy organization, the International Family Therapy Association (IFTA), was organized in 1986 as a way for family therapists in different countries to interact. IFTA sponsors the World Family Therapy Congress in a different country each year, with past hosts including Finland, Greece, Holland, Ireland, Israel, Hungary, Mexico, Poland, and Turkey. In addition, IFTA publishes a biannual journal, the *Journal of Family Psychotherapy,* and a newsletter, *The International Connection.* (Contact IFTA at the Family Studies Center, Purdue University Calumet, Hammond, Indiana 46323-2094, telephone: 219-989-2027, fax: 219-989-2772, e-mail: trepper@calumet.purdue.edu, Web site: www.ift-familytherapy.org.)

National standards for the accreditation of family therapy training programs are set by a subsidiary organization of the AAMFT—the Commission on Accreditation for Marriage and Family Therapy Education (COAMFTE)—which accredits family therapy training programs at the master's, doctoral, and postgraduate levels. Recognized since 1978 by the U.S. Department of Education as the national accrediting body for family therapy, the COAMFTE works cooperatively with its parent organization (the AAMFT), state licensing and certification boards, and the Association of Marriage and Family Therapist Regulatory Boards (AMFTRB).

The COAMFTE accredits three types of programs:

- *Master's degree* programs designed to prepare individuals for beginning a career in MFT by providing basic didactic and clinical information, as well as professional development and socialization.
- *Doctoral degree* programs prepare students for academic careers, research, advanced clinical practice, and supervision. The doctoral curriculum includes advanced instruction in marriage and family therapy research, theory construction, and supervision.
- *Postgraduate degree clinical training* programs provide clinical education in family therapy to trainees with a master's or doctoral degree in family therapy, or in a closely related field. A program may allow for specialized training in a particular modality or treatment population (*About COAMFTE*).

The COAMFTE's accreditation process benefits the public, training programs, students, and the profession by:

- Providing assurance to the public and consumers that the accredited program has undergone extensive external evaluation and meets standards established by the profession.
- Providing a stimulus for self-evaluation and a cost-effective review mechanism that strengthens the reputation and credibility of a program because of the public regard for accreditation. Accredited programs become eligible for funding under several federal grant programs.
- Assuring students that the appropriate knowledge and skill areas necessary for entry into a chosen field are included in the course of study and that the training program is financially stable.

• Assuring prospective employers that the educational training of a job applicant with a degree from an accredited program indicates adequate professional preparation.

• Contributing to the family therapy professions' unity and creditability. The profession benefits by bringing together practitioners, teachers, and students in the vital activity of setting educational standards of entry level professionals, and of continually improving professional education, research, scholarship, and clinical skills.

What topics are mandated in family therapy training programs? According to national (COAMFTE) standards, students must complete 12 standard didactic units (SDUs) in the following areas (*Commission on Accreditation*):

• *Theoretical Foundations* (2 SDUs). The historical development, theoretical foundations, and contemporary conceptual directions of the field of family therapy. Students learn to conceptualize and distinguish the critical epistemological issues in marriage and family therapy. All teaching materials will be related to clinical concerns.

• *Clinical Practice* (4 SDUs). A comprehensive survey of the major models of family therapy, including methods and major mental health assessment methods and instruments.

• *Individual Development and Family Relations* (2 SDUs). Individual development, family development, family relationships, and issues of sexuality (including sexual dysfunctions and difficulties) as they relate to family therapy theory and practice. Courses also include significant material on issues of gender and sexual orientation as they relate to marriage and family theory and practice; issues of ethnicity, race, socioeconomic status and culture; and issues relevant to populations in the vicinity of the program.

• *Professional Identity and Ethics* (1 SDU). Professional identity, including professional socialization, professional organizations, licensure and certification. Content will also focus on ethical issues related to the practice and profession of family. The object is to inform students about legal responsibilities and liabilities of clinical practice and research, family law, confidentiality issues and the AAMFT Code of Ethics. Additionally, students learn about the interface between therapist responsibility and the professional, social and political context of treatment.

• *Research* (1 SDU). Research methodology, data analysis and the evaluation of research to include quantitative and qualitative research.

• *Additional Learning* (1 SDU). Students may choose the learning experience, or the program may mandate a course or other experience appropriate to students' specialized interest and background in family therapy.

All family therapists need certain basic skills, according to an AAMFT sponsored Core Competency Task Force that convened in September 2003. Within each of six domains—*admission to treatment*; *clinical assessment and diagnosis*; *treatment planning and case management*; *therapeutic interventions*; *legal issues, ethics, and standards*; and *research and program evaluation*—family therapists must master five sets of skills: *conceptual skills* (understand therapeutic principles), *perceptual skills* (be able to interpret relevant data through paradigmatic and conceptual lenses), *executive skills* (demonstrate appropriate behaviors, actions, and interventions in the therapy process), *evaluative skills* (be able to assess and appraise relevant aspects of therapeutic activities), and *professional skills* (be able to conduct therapy effectively) (personal correspondence from AAMFT, November 2003). These skills are elaborated as follows:

## Admission to Treatment

### Conceptual Skills

- Understand systems concepts, theories, and techniques that are foundational to the practice of marriage and family therapy
- Understand theories and techniques of individual, marital, family, and group psychotherapy
- Understand the mental health care delivery system
- Understand the risks and benefits of individual, couple, family, and group psychotherapy

### Perceptual Skills

- Recognize contextual and systemic issues (e.g., gender, age, socioeconomic status, culture/race/ethnicity, sexual orientation, spirituality, larger systems, social context)
- Consider health status, mental status, other therapy, and systems involved in the clients' lives (e.g., courts, social services)
- Recognize issues that might suggest referral for evaluation, assessment, or specialized care beyond clinical competence

### Executive Skills

- Gather and review intake information
- Determine who should attend therapy and in what configuration (i.e., individual, couple, family)
- Decide if, when, and how other professionals and significant others are needed to contribute to the clients' care
- Facilitate involvement of all necessary participants in treatment
- Explain practice setting rules, fees, rights and responsibilities of each party, including privacy and confidentiality policies and duty to care
- Establish and maintain appropriate and productive therapeutic alliances with the clients
- Solicit and use client feedback throughout the therapeutic process
- Develop and maintain collaborative working relationships with clients, referral resources, and payers
- Manage session dynamics with multiple persons
- Develop a workable therapeutic contract

### Evaluative Skills

- Evaluate case for appropriateness for treatment within professional competence
- Evaluate intake policies and procedures for completeness and contextual relevance

### Professional Skills

- Understand the legal requirements and limitations for working with minors and vulnerable populations
- Collaborate effectively with clients and allied professionals
- Complete case documentation in a timely manner and in accordance with relevant laws and policies

- Develop, establish, and maintain policies for setting and collecting fees
- Explain and discuss payment policies and other business procedures with clients, the appropriate subsystem in the family (e.g., parents), and payers

## Clinical Assessment and Diagnosis

### Conceptual Skills

- Know a systemic framework for assessment and diagnosis
- Understand principles of human development, human sexuality, gender development, psychopathology, couple processes, family development and processes (e.g., family dynamics, relational dynamics, systemic dynamics), issues related to health and illness, and diversity
- Comprehend the major mental health disorders, including the epidemiology, etiology, phenomenology, effective treatments, course, and prognosis
- Understand the clinical needs and implications of persons who suffer from co-occurring disorders (e.g., substance abuse and mental illness)
- Understand the theoretical concepts related to individual and systemic assessment and diagnostic instruments that pertain to mental health and relational functioning
- Comprehend individual, couple, and family assessment instruments appropriate to presenting problem and practice setting
- Understand the extant models used for assessment and diagnosis of mental health
- Understand the extant models used for assessment and diagnosis of relational functioning
- Understand the limitations of the extant models of assessment and diagnosis, especially as they relate to different cultural and ethnic groups
- Understand the concepts of *reliability* and *validity,* their relationship to assessment instruments, and how they influence therapeutic decision making

### Perceptual Skills

- Determine who is the client
- Assess each client's engagement in the change process
- Systematically integrate client reports, observations of client behaviors, client relationship patterns, reports from other professionals, and interactions with client to guide the assessment process
- Develop systemic hypotheses regarding relationship patterns and their bearing on the presenting problem
- Develop systemic hypotheses about the influence of treatment on extratherapeutic relationships and other client systems
- Connect assessment to interventions and expected outcomes

### Executive Skills

- Diagnose and assess client problems systemically and contextually
- Engage with multiple persons and manage multiple levels of information during the therapeutic process
- Provide assessments and deliver developmentally appropriate services to children
- Apply effective and systemic interviewing techniques and strategies
- Administer assessment instruments

- Screen and develop adequate safety plans for substance abuse, child and elder maltreatment, domestic violence, physical violence, suicide potential, and dangerousness to self and others
- Screen for physical/organic problems that can cause emotional/interpersonal symptoms
- Assess family history using genogram
- Elicit a relevant and accurate biopsychosocial history to understand the context of the clients' problems
- Make appropriate differential diagnoses
- Identify clients' strengths, resilience, and resources
- Elucidate presenting problem from the perspective of each member of the therapeutic system
- Communicate diagnostic information so clients understand its relationship to treatment goals and outcomes

### Evaluative Skills

- Evaluate assessment methods for relevance to clients' needs
- Assess ability to view issues and therapeutic processes systemically
- Evaluate the accuracy of differential and relational diagnoses
- Assess clients' acceptance of therapeutic goals and diagnosis

### Professional Skills

- Utilize peer consultation and supervision effectively

## Treatment Planning and Case Management

### Conceptual Skills

- Know which models, modalities, and techniques are most effective for the presenting problem
- Understand the liabilities incurred when billing third parties and the codes necessary for reimbursement

### Perceptual Skills

- Integrate client feedback, assessment, contextual information, and diagnosis with treatment goals and plan

### Executive Skills

- Develop measurable outcomes, treatment goals, treatment plans, and after-care plans with clients utilizing a systemic perspective
- Prioritize treatment goals
- Develop a clear plan of how sessions will be conducted
- Structure treatment to meet clients' needs and to facilitate systemic change
- Manage progression of therapy toward treatment goals
- Manage risks, crises, and emergencies

- Work collaboratively with other stake holders, including family members and professionals not present
- Assist clients in dealing with complex systems of care

## Evaluative Skills

- Evaluate progress of sessions toward treatment goals
- Recognize when treatment goals and plan require modification
- Evaluate management of risks, crises, and emergencies
- Assess session process for compliance with policies and procedures
- Assess self in terms of therapeutic behavior, relationship with clients, and the process for explaining procedures and outcomes

## Professional Skills

- Advocate for clients in obtaining quality care, appropriate resources, and services in their community
- Engage in forensic and legal processes on behalf of clients when appropriate
- Write plans and complete other case documentation in accordance with practice setting policies, professional standards, and state/provincial laws
- Utilize time management skills in therapy sessions and other professional meetings

# Therapeutic Interventions

## Conceptual Skills

- Comprehend a variety of individual and systemic therapeutic models and their applications, including evidence-based therapies
- Recognize strengths, limitations, and contraindications of specific therapy models
- Understand the risk of harm associated with models that incorporate assumptions of family dysfunction or pathogenesis

## Perceptual Skills

- Identify treatment most appropriate for presenting clinical problem or diagnosis based on current research and empirical findings
- Recognize how different techniques impact the treatment process
- Distinguish differences between content and process issues and their impact on therapy

## Executive Skills

- Match treatment to clients' needs, goals, and values
- Deliver interventions in a way that is sensitive to unique situations and dynamics (e.g., gender, age, socioeconomic status, culture/race/ethnicity, sexual orientation, disability, larger systems issues of the client)
- Reframe problems and recursive interaction patterns
- Generate relational questions and reflexive comments in the therapy room
- Engage each family member in the treatment process as appropriate

- Facilitate clients developing and integrating solutions to problems
- Defuse intense and chaotic situations appropriately
- Empower clients to establish effective familial organization, familial structures, and relationships with larger systems
- Provide psychoeducation to families with serious mental illness and other disorders
- Modify interventions that are not working to better fit treatment goals
- Move to constructive termination when treatment goals have been accomplished
- Integrate supervisor/team communications into treatment

## Evaluative Skills

- Evaluate interventions for consistency and congruency with model of therapy and theory of change
- Evaluate ability to deliver interventions effectively
- Evaluate treatment outcomes as treatment progresses
- Evaluate clients' reactions or responses to interventions
- Evaluate self as therapist (e.g., transference, family of origin, current stress level, current life situation) as enhancing or inhibiting effective interventions)

## Professional Skills

- Respect multiple perspectives (e.g., clients, team, supervisor)
- Set appropriate boundaries and manage issues of triangulation
- Articulate rationales for interventions related to treatment goals and plan, assessment information, and systemic understanding of clients' context and dynamics

# Legal Issues, Ethics, and Standards

## Conceptual Skills

- Know state, federal, and provincial laws that apply to the practice of marriage and family therapy
- Know professional ethics and standards of practice that apply to the practice of marriage and family therapy
- Know policies and procedures of practice setting
- Understand the process of making an ethical decision

## Perceptual Skills

- Recognize situations in which ethics, laws, professional liability, and standards of practice apply
- Recognize ethical dilemmas in practice setting
- Recognize when a legal consultation is necessary

## Executive Skills

- Monitor issues related to ethics, laws, and professional standards
- Develop policies, procedures, and forms to protect client confidentiality and to comply with relevant laws

- Inform clients of limitations to confidentiality and parameters of mandatory reporting
- Maintain client records with timely, appropriate, and accurate notes
- Develop safety plan for clients who present with potential abuse or violence
- Take appropriate action when ethical and legal dilemmas emerge
- Report information to appropriate authorities as required by law
- Practice within defined scope of practice and competence
- Stay current with MFT literature and advances in the field
- Maintain license(s) and specialty credentials
- Implement a personal program to maintain professional competence
- Consult with peers or supervisors if personal issues threaten to adversely impact clinical work

### Evaluative Skills

- Evaluate activities related to ethics, legal issues, and practice standards
- Monitor personal issues and problems to insure they do not impact the therapy process adversely or create vulnerability for misconduct

### Professional Skills

- Pursue professional development through self-supervision, collegial consultation, professional reading, and continuing educational activities

## Research and Program Evaluation

### Conceptual Skills

- Know the extant family therapy literature, research, and evidence-based practice
- Understand research and program evaluation methodologies relevant to MFT and mental health services
- Understand the application of quantitative and qualitative methods of inquiry in the practice of family therapy
- Understand the ethical issues involved in the conduct of clinical research and program evaluation

### Executive Skills

- Read current family therapy and other professional literature
- Use current family therapy and other research to inform clinical practice
- Critique professional research and assess the quality of research studies and program evaluation in the literature
- Determine the effectiveness of clinical practice and techniques

### Evaluative Skills

- Systematically evaluate self in terms of currency with literature and application

## Professional Skills

• Contribute to the development of new knowledge

***

After successfully completing graduate courses and passing a comprehensive examination, family therapy trainees typically must, as novice supervised clinicians (sometimes as unpaid volunteers), gain two years of clinical experience (equal to at least 3,000 hours in not less than 104 weeks, half of which must be done prior to qualifying for the master's degree).

The most stressful hurdle of all comes next—passing two occupationally oriented competency-based licensure tests. First, a *written exam* is given and then (in some states), an *oral exam* by a small group of experienced therapists. When family therapy candidates fail, they must retake these tests at least once a year to keep their files active.

Taking a licensure examination is like betting one's dream (plus several years of laborious time, energy, and financial investment) on a few hours' performance. And many fail! According to an online newsletter from the California Association of Marriage and Family Therapy, only 48% of Californians passed who took the family therapy oral exam in one year.

Understandably, most family therapy applicants grasp at whatever resources are available to give them an edge, though these aids are usually expensive. Preparing family therapy trainees to pass licensure examinations has become a thriving business in states like California where so many candidates pursue the family therapy license. One glance through *The California Therapist,* the state association's magazine, reveals the number of preparatory services and programs advertising preparatory courses offered to help licensure candidates pass these exams. Family therapy aspirants typically spend hundreds of dollars purchasing materials and attending workshops.

Although there is no lack of family therapy books for aspiring clinicians—an Internet search found more than 1,200 volumes on marriage and family therapy—few, if any, offer problem-based reviews specifically intended to help students prepare for school-based comprehensive and state licensure exams. By offering students and trainees a handy problem-oriented review guide, *Family Therapy Review* is designed *to* fill this gap.

This book can be utilized both as a professional handbook and a course textbook. Family therapy educators looking for up-to-date course outlines and accompanying textbooks will find the contents of this book attractive and useful, as will licensed therapists, clinical supervisors, and mental health professionals who want to update their knowledge and clinical skills. With well-organized and current content information, this comprehensive review book provides an up-to-date handbook of useful information.

Each written by leading experts, chapters cover the standard information usually tested on comprehensive and licensing exams. Organized into six sections, these topics include:

• *Individual and the Family*—family health and dysfunction, human lifespan development, human diversity, psychopathology and psychopharmacology
• *Therapeutic Skills and Tools*—theories and models, assessment, diagnoses and treatment planning, case management, and managing behavioral emergencies
• *Distressed Couples*—conflict and disenchantment, separation, divorce and remarriage, sexual problems, intimate partner violence
• *Child and Adolescent Issues*—developmental disabilities, behavioral and relationship problems, substance abuse, child abuse and neglect

- *Diminished Health and Well-Being*—care-giving and grief, alcohol and other drug dependencies, nonpharmacological addictions, depression and anxiety, HIV/AIDS
- *Professional Development*—ethical and legal issues, preparing for licensing examinations, and continuing professional growth.

Every chapter has a parallel format designed for a comprehensive and easy-to-follow review of family therapy information. Special features included in each chapter include:

- *Introductory Quiz*—true/false questions at chapter beginning
- *Insert Boxes*—four-item multiple-choice questions (formatted like those on licensing exams) that can be answered by reading the chapter
- *Discussion Questions*—provocative discussion questions at chapter end
- *Key Terms*—a list of key terms and their definitions
- *Suggested Further Reading*—an annotated list of leading content sources for additional study
- *References*—documentary information supporting chapter content, library references, and Internet sources for follow-up on chapter contents.

To get the maximum value from this book, I recommend that you follow these steps:

1. As a *pretest* before reading the chapter, write down your answers to the true/false questions given at chapter beginning and the multiple-choice questions placed throughout the chapter in insert boxes.
2. Carefully read the chapter, making *written notes* as you go along.
3. *Study your notes.*
4. Repeat Step 1 and *compare results* with your pretest and the correct answers provided in the answer key.
5. Note weak areas and *restudy* these sections.
6. Using your notes, *meet with another interested student*—someone with whom to discuss what you've learned and challenge you with questions. Then discuss the questions listed at chapter end.

To maximize your success with steps 2 and 3, I recommend you read Kelman and Straker's, *Study Without Stress: Mastering Medical Sciences* (Kelman & Straker, 2000). One of nine books in a book series I edited—*Book Series on Medical Student Survival*—this practical study guide teaches medical students how to master an overwhelming mountain of basic science materials. I guarantee you that the techniques explained there will help you.

If you follow these steps, I predict that you will confidently pass your examinations with flying colors the first time around!

# REFERENCES

*About COAMFTE.* (n.d.). Retrieved November, 2003, from www.aamft.org

*A career as an MFT.* (n.d.). Retrieved November, 2003, from www.aamft.org

*Commission on accreditation for marriage and family therapy education.* (n.d.). Retrieved November, 2003, from www.aamft.org

*Directory of MFT licensing boards.* (n.d.). Retrieved November, 2003, from www.aamft.org

*FAQs on MFTs.* (n.d.). Retrieved November, 2003, from www.aamft.org

Glick, I. D., Berman, E. M., Clarkin, J. F., & Rait, D. S. (2000). *Marital and Family Therapy* (4th ed.), Washington, DC: American Psychiatric Press.

Kelman, E. G., & Straker, K. C. (2000). *Study without stress: Mastering the medical sciences.* Thousand Oaks, California: Sage.

Manderscheid, R. W., & Sonnenchein, M. A., (Eds.). (1996). *Center for Mental Health Services.* Mental Health, U.S., 1996. (DHHS Publication No. SMA 96-3098). Washington DC: Superintendent of Documents, U.S. Government Printing Office.

*Marriage and family therapists: Commonly asked questions.* (n.d.). Retrieved November, 2003, from www.aamft.org

Nichols, M. P., & Schwartz, R. C. (2001). *Family therapy: Concepts and methods* (5th ed.). Boston: Allyn & Bacon.

Rowe, C. L., & Liddle, H. A. (2002). Substance abuse. In D. H. Sprenkle (ed.), *Effectiveness research in marriage and family therapy* (pp. 53–87). Alexandria, VA: Association for Marriage and Family Therapy.

Sprenkle, D. H. (Ed.). (2002). *Effectiveness research in marriage and family therapy.* Washington, DC: Association for Marriage and Family Therapy.

# Acknowledgments

I gratefully acknowledge *Carla Cronkhite Vera,* my esteemed assistant at UCLA, for her expert help with every aspect of this book. She assisted me in developing the book proposal, selecting authors, providing clear author guidelines, and effectively networking with all authors. She also suggested ways to improve chapter manuscripts, and handled myriad details and problems with characteristic efficiency and good cheer. *Carol Jean Coombs,* my life's partner, provided valued counsel and advice and suggested ways to effectively shorten lengthy chapter manuscripts without sacrificing important content.

# FAMILY THERAPY REVIEW
## Preparing for Comprehensive and Licensing Examinations

# BASIC CLINICAL KNOWLEDGE AND SKILLS

PART

# I

# INDIVIDUALS AND THE FAMILY

# 1

# Family Health and Dysfunction

John DeFrain
*University of Nebraska–Lincoln*

Richard Cook
*Bethlehem Institute of
Education, Tauranga,
New Zealand*

Gloria Gonzales-Kruger
*University of Nebraska–Lincoln*

## TRUTH OR FICTION?

___ 1. *Researchers have asked, "How do families succeed?" many more times than asking, "Why do families fail?"*

___ 2. *A problem-centered medical treatment model translates perfectly to the field of family therapy.*

___ 3. *Three decades ago, family therapists did not have clear models of family health to help guide them in their work.*

___ 4. *From a research standpoint, the judgment of professionals is the best perspective for understanding family strengths.*

___ 5. *Researchers use these terms to describe families who are doing well together: strong family, happy family, good family, healthy family, successful family, nuclear family, resilient family, balanced family, and optimally functioning family.*

___ 6. *The structure of a family tells a therapist a great deal about the emotional health of the family.*

___ 7. *Strong marriages are the center of strong families.*

___ 8. *When comparing strong families around the world, the differences from culture to culture are much more apparent than the similarities.*

___ 9. *In assessing the strengths of a family, a therapist will find family income a critical indicator of strength.*

___ 10. *The normative developmental transitions of the adolescent period of life are likely to disrupt healthy parent–child relationships for years to come.*

___ 11. *Most families around the world are dysfunctional.*

___ 12. *The strengths of families from culture to culture are much more similar than different.*

___ 13. *A positive emotional bond in a family is a very important foundation for effectively dealing with a crisis.*

___ 14. *After helping a family assess their strengths, a family therapist can then guide them in the process of developing plans that use their strengths to meet the challenges they face together in life.*

___ 15. *Talking with families about their cultural beliefs and values can serve to help them identify and acknowledge how they may be using these to be a strong family.*

A strengths-based approach to couples and families has more promise than one focused on failure and pathology. Looking to the future rather than the past, it focuses on where the family can go by working together, rather than assessing blame and how it got into the present predicament. "Nothing in the world could make human life happier than to increase greatly the number of strong families," said David R. Mace, a pioneer family counselor and marriage educator (Stinnett & DeFrain, 1985, dust jacket). What are the qualities that make a family strong? What do couples do for each other that makes their relationship work well?

When asking people from around the globe, "What makes your family strong?" the answers are remarkably similar from culture to culture. Studies focusing on successful families can be traced back nearly 75 years (Woodhouse, 1930). When Herbert Otto conducted a literature search on family strengths in the 1960s, he found that researchers used 515 terms to describe healthy family behaviors. Between the late-1940s and the early-1960s, however, the vast majority of the research projects focused on problems rather than health (Otto, 1962; Gabler & Otto, 1964), but the situation is steadily improving today.

1. The terms *health* and *dysfunction* as commonly defined today:
   a. are clear and concise.
   b. are well conceived by both conventional wisdom and professionals.
   c. help us understand strong families better.
   d. none of the above.

## HEALTH (THE ABSENCE OF DYSFUNCTION) AND DYSFUNCTION (THE ABSENCE OF HEALTH)

Medical texts typically focus on myriad maladies. One such volume has 2,900 pages of small print, yet offers no entry on *health* or *dysfunction*. This problems-oriented approach to medicine makes sense when talking about physical pain and suffering, but has limited value for you, the family therapist. Focusing on individual problems is not enough. Everything that happens to one family member impacts everyone else in the family because they are interconnected in one common "family system."

2. Family therapists had a variety of tools to use in the mid-1970s, including:
   a. various family systems theories.
   b. psychodynamic theories and behavioral therapies.
   c. non-directive client-centered therapies.
   d. all of the above.

By the early 1970s, **family systems theory** was receiving a great deal of attention and acceptance among professionals. The tools of a family therapist at that time included:

- A variety of family systems theories that suggested working with the entire family when possible to better understand its inherent complexities;
- Psychodynamic theories that focused on the past and how previous experiences influence personality development;
- Behavioral therapies that assessed present behaviors and implemented reinforcement procedures to foster positive and acceptable behaviors;
- Non-directive, client-centered therapies that emphasized the client's perspective and ability to find solutions to their problems (rather than the therapist's views and solutions).

The question remained, however, where do you go with these tools? What direction do you take with the entire family? Family therapists in the 1970s came up short in their search for a model of health. Instead, they fell back on clients' perceptions of their problems and helped them find appropriate solutions.

3. A strong family can be defined as:
   a. a family absent of problems.
   b. a nuclear family.
   c. a family that has fixed all its problems.
   d. none of the above.

## THE BASICS: WHAT IS A STRONG FAMILY?

Over the past 30 years, there has been growing interest in defining **family strengths**. Researchers began to measure family strengths, utilizing both quantitative and qualitative methods such as survey instruments, written qualitative testimony (i.e., "stories"), observations, interviews, and ethnographic methods. Some researchers relied on "outsider" perspectives, depending heavily on the judgment of professionals observing the family from a "nonmember" vantage point—somewhat removed from the daily workings of the family. Other researchers used "insider" perspectives, listening carefully to what family members themselves were saying about their internal dynamics. Because each perspective has advantages and disadvantages, the most compelling research utilizes a combination of approaches.

4. The best way to learn about family strengths is by conducting:
   a. quantitative studies.
   b. qualitative studies.
   c. ethnographic studies.
   d. a combination of the above.

Gathering multi-cultural perspectives on strong families and family strengths has proven useful over the years and added to the research base. Language and cultural barriers make the translation of family strengths concepts and methodologies from culture to culture very difficult—are we talking about the same thing in our different languages? How can we be sure? Can a data collection methodology that worked in a Western country work in another culture? Fortunately, these difficulties can be surmounted, and many meaningful studies have been conducted by linking researchers from outside a particular culture with cultural informants and researchers within that culture. By working together, the skills and knowledge of each of the participants in the research project complement each other.

A wide variety of terms have been used over the years to discuss families who are doing well together, including strong family, happy family, good family, healthy family, successful family, resilient family, balanced family, optimally functioning family, and so forth. Good arguments can be advanced in defense of many terms used, and it is also possible to quibble with each term. We use the term *strong family* here because it seems relatively simple and to the point. In short, it *works* for us. When engaged with families, however, it might be worthwhile to ask family members what terms they would use to describe their family today in this regard and what type of family they would like to work toward. Anything we can do as family therapists to tap into each unique family's culture and way of talking about themselves is likely to prove useful in advancing the process of growth.

> 5. Researchers use innumerable terms to define the various qualities that contribute to family strength. In reviewing many studies of this type, it becomes clear that:
>    a. the various models are impossible to synthesize.
>    b. there is considerable common ground and broad conceptual agreement among the various models.
>    c. the researchers all use precisely the same words to describe the various family strengths.
>    d. none of the above.

Table 1.1 outlines the conclusions of various researchers who have assessed family strengths in the United States and other countries. There are remarkable similarities among these investigators.

## AN INTERNATIONAL FAMILY STRENGTHS PERSPECTIVE

Research on strong families has not only resulted in models for better understanding the qualities of strong families; research has also suggested a number of propositions that influence how we look at families in general and how we can successfully live our own lives in families in particular.

Looking at families from a strengths-based perspective is not a Pollyannish approach, ignoring significant problems or sugarcoating one's view of families in the world. As seasoned family therapists, we are not naïve about the sometimes ghastly underside of family living. However, a family strengths perspective relegates problems to their proper place in life—as vehicles for testing our capacities as families and reaffirming our connections with each other.

The family strengths perspective evolves over time as our understanding of strong families increases. It is not a static set of ideas or rigorously testable hypotheses, but more like a family itself—a constantly growing and changing dialogue about the nature of strong families. The following may be considered elements of this evolving dialogue, or principles to keep in mind when counseling families (DeFrain & Stinnett, 2002):

• *Families in all their remarkable diversity are the basic foundation of human cultures.* Strong families are critical to the development of strong communities (and vice versa).

• *All families have strengths,* just as all families have challenges and areas of potential growth.

• *If one looks only for problems in a family, one will see only problems.* But if you look for strengths, you will find them.

**TABLE 1.1**

Dimensions of Family Strength as Delineated by Researchers

| *Theorists* | *Dimensions* |
| --- | --- |
| Beavers and Hampson (1990) | Centripetal/centrifugal interaction, closeness, parent coalitions, autonomy, adaptability, egalitarian power, goal-directed negotiation, ability to resolve conflict, clarity of expression, range of feelings, openness to others, empathic, understanding |
| Billingsley (1986) | Strong family ties, strong religious orientation, educational aspirations/achievements |
| Curran (1983) | Togetherness, respect and trust, shared leisure, privacy valued, shared mealtimes, shared responsibility, family rituals, communication, affirmation of each other, religious love, humor/play |
| Epstein, Bishop, Ryan, Miller, and Keitner (1993) | Affective involvement, behavior control, communication |
| Kantor and Lehr (1974) | Affect, power |
| Kryson, Moore, and Zill (1990) | Commitment to family, time together, encouragement of individuals, ability to adapt, clear roles, communication, religious orientation, social connectedness |
| Olson, McCubbin, Barnes, Larsen, Muxen, and Wilson (1989); Olson (1996) | Strong marriage, high family cohesion, good family flexibility, effective coping with stress and crisis, positive couple and family communication |
| Otto (1962, 1963) | Shared religious and moral values; love, consideration and understanding; common interests, goals and purposes; love and happiness of children; working and playing together; sharing specific recreational activities |
| D. Reiss (1981) | Coordination, closure |
| Stinnett, DeFrain, and colleagues (1977, 1985, 2002) | Appreciation and affection, commitment, positive communication, enjoyable time together, spiritual well-being, successful management of stress and crisis |

- *Our weaknesses do not help us solve problems, but our strengths do.* Thus, it is more important to delineate family strengths and how to use them to good advantage, than to blame and relentlessly focus on shortcomings.

6. Family structure:
   a. tells the investigator a great deal about a family's internal strengths.
   b. is a critical element of a family's strengths.
   c. is commonly focused on by researchers and society in general, though family functioning is more useful to look at from a family therapist's perspective.
   d. is a solid predictor of family functioning.

- *It's about function, not structure.* When talking about healthy families, researchers, and society in general, commonly make the mistake of focusing on external **family structure** rather than internal **family functioning**. For each family structure, there are countless representative strong families: there are strong single-parent families, strong stepfamilies, strong nuclear families, strong extended families, strong families with gay and lesbian members, and strong two-parent families. Likewise, for each type of family structure, there are also many families who are not currently functioning well. Simply knowing what type of family a client lives in tells us nothing about the strength of the family or its potential for future growth.

• *Knowing a family's ethnic or cultural or religious/spiritual group does not tell one a great deal either about the strengths of the the family.* Each ethnic, cultural, and religious/spiritual group has a host of wonderful families in it, and, of course, there are very troubled families in each group. An investigator has to dig deeper and gain a perspective on the internal dynamics of the family to really understand the family.

7. Strong marriages:
   a. are an essential element of strong families.
   b. are at the center of many strong families.
   c. are irrelevant in today's world.
   d. are an anachronism best left to the dustbin of history.

• *Strong marriages are the center of many strong families.* The couple relationship is an important source of strength in many families with children who are doing well. Two loving parents working together to nurture their children can be a powerful combination, and their modeling of a positive couple relationship can influence the child's life far into adulthood.

• *Strong families tend to produce great kids, and a good place to look for great kids is in strong families.* Nick Stinnett's research tells this story very well (Stinnett & O'Donnell, 1996). In a sense, Stinnett went backward in his study of more than 4,000 healthy adolescents and family strengths. Instead of looking at families who defined themselves as strong or healthy and then studying their children, he chose to enlist the help of professionals and laypersons in many communities to identify adolescents who were doing well in school, in religious organizations, and other social groups. In essence, Stinnett identified great kids in the words of adults in their community who worked with young people. Stinnett then worked back to these young people's families and found, to little surprise, that the vast majority came from strong families.

8. Individuals who grew up in a seriously troubled family:
   a. are doomed to pass the poison of their early years onto the next generation.
   b. are all seriously scarred.
   c. can create a strong family of their own as an adult.
   d. can quite easily create a strong family of their own as an adult.

• *If you grew up in a strong family as a child, it will probably be easier for you to create a strong family of your own.* But it's also quite possible to do so if you weren't so lucky and grew up in a troubled family (DeFrain, Jones, Skogrand, & DeFrain, 2003, pp.117–146).

• *The relationship between financial success and family strengths is tenuous, at best.* Once a family has adequate financial resources, more money is not likely to increase the quality of life, happiness, or the strength of their family relationships.

9. Strengths:
   a. develop over time.
   b. are genetically transmitted.
   c. come and go.
   d. are statistically related to income.

• *Strengths develop over time.* You may start out with a shaky marriage but end up with a healthy, vibrant family.

• *Strengths are tested through normative developmental transitions.* For example, couples commonly have many challenges to face when their children reach adolescence and young adulthood. These transitions are also quite predictable, and once the period has passed and the younger generation has gained relative independence from the parents, the family settles back into a more emotionally connected and comfortable mode.

10. Strengths:
    a. are often developed in response to challenges.
    b. are tested by life's everyday stressors.
    c. are tested by the significant crises that all families face sooner or later.
    d. all of the above.

• *Strengths are often developed in response to challenges.* A family's strengths are tested by life's everyday stressors and also by the significant crises that all families face sooner or later. For many couples and families, it takes several years before they believe they have become a strong family; and they know this because they have been tested over time by the significant challenging events that life inevitably bring.
• *Crises can tear families apart.* But crises can also be a catalyst for growth, helping to make family relationships stronger.
• *A family's strengths lay the foundation for positive growth and change in the future.* Families become stronger by capitalizing on their strengths, not their problems.
• *Most families in the world have considerable strength.* Human beings wouldn't have lasted through countless generations without these qualities.

11. Researchers have found that strong families:
    a. from culture to culture are remarkably different.
    b. are much more similar than different.
    c. have unique cultural ways of exhibiting their strengths.
    d. b and c.

• *People are people are people, and families are families are families.* From culture to culture, families share more similarities than differences. Though families in each culture have unique ways of exhibiting their strengths, the qualities that make families work well together are remarkably similar (DeFrain, DeFrain, & Lepard, 1994).

12. Strong families:
    a. are stress and crisis free.
    b. can have troubles getting along.
    c. are not perfect.
    d. b and c.

• *Strong families, like people, are not perfect.* Even the strongest families experience troubles.
• *Families are about emotion—strong emotion.* If family strengths could be reduced to a single quality, it would be a positive emotional connection and sense of belonging with each other. When this emotional bond exists, the family can endure almost any hardship.

13. Future research needs in the area of family strengths include:
    a. more and better research from multicultural perspectives.
    b. more investigations into how a family strengths perspective can be used in one's personal life and one's family.
    c. more investigations into how a family strengths perspective can be used by educators, policymakers, and family therapists.
    d. all of the above.

• *Future research needs in the area of family strengths include* the need for more and better research from multicultural perspectives and more investigations into how the family strengths perspective can be used in one's personal life, one's family, one's work as an educator, policymaker, and family therapist.

## QUALITIES OF STRONG FAMILIES

Over the past three decades, using both "insider" and "outsider" assessments, we have been developing a research based International Family Strengths Model. Our research has involved more than 21,000 family members from the United States and twenty-seven other countries. Regardless of culture, we learned that there are six major qualities of **strong families** and that each quality has sub-qualities. The six family strengths are:

• Appreciation and affection
• Commitment
• Positive communication
• Enjoyable time together
• Spiritual well-being
• Successful management of stress and crisis

These family strengths, interconnecting with one another, rest on an underlying sense of *positive emotional connection*. That is, people in strong families feel good about each other and work to ensure each other's well-being. Let's look more closely at these six family strengths.

### Appreciation and Affection

People in strong families deeply care for one another, and they let each other know this on a regular basis; they do not hesitate to express their love. Expressing appreciation and affection can be difficult for some individuals: "I don't want to be too positive because he'll get a swelled head," the thinking goes. And some cultures are more effective at expressing positive emotion than others. In some ethnic groups it is relatively easy to hug and kiss and compliment family members, while other groups have a more stoic, strong-and-silent, understated approach to living and family relationships.

14. In strong families, individuals:
    a. are not afraid to express appreciation and affection for each other.
    b. rarely directly express appreciation and affection.
    c. usually express appreciation and affection nonverbally.
    d. b and c.

As the classic family therapy story goes, a therapist is encouraging the husband to speak openly about his love for his wife. The husband tells the therapist that his wife knows perfectly well how much he cares: "I show her I love her by going to work, being a good provider, being faithful—by always being there." He then adds in a somewhat miffed way: "I told her twenty years ago when we got married that I loved her. If anything changes, I'll let her know."

Clear, unambiguous expression of appreciation and affection, is best done on a regular—at least daily—basis. We all need to hear how much our loved ones care. And not only in bed.

The following Appreciation and Affection Checklist will be useful for you in assessing this dimension of your family's strengths and can be used with families you are working with in therapy. After gaining a solid understanding of a family's strengths, the next step in the process of growth is to talk about how these strengths can be used to make positive changes, making it possible to deal effectively with challenges they face in life together.

All six checklists presented in this chapter were developed through our own 30 years of research on strong families. More information on the research and other family strengths resources is available at our University of Nebraska *NU For Families* Web site (http://nuforfamilies.unl.edu).

Have each person place an "S" (for strength) beside the qualities they feel their family has achieved, a "G" beside those qualities which are an area of potential growth, and "NA" if non-applicable.

In our family...

_____We appreciate each other, and let each other know this.
_____We enjoy helping each other.
_____We like keeping our promises to each other.
_____We like to show affection to each other.
_____We like to hug each other.
_____We enjoy being thoughtful of each other.
_____We wait for each other without complaining.
_____We give each other enough time to complete necessary tasks.
_____We are able to forgive each other.
_____We grow stronger because we love each other.
_____All things considered, we have appreciation and affection for each other.

## Commitment

Members of strong families are dedicated to one another's well-being, investing time and energy in family activities. They don't allow their work or other elements of their lives to take too much time or emotional energy away from couple and family interaction. Commitment to the marital relationship is part of this. When people were asked, "What are the strengths of your family?" we heard, "communication," "love", "fun times together," and "helping each other when we are down."

15. Elements of couple and family commitment include:
   a. emotional and sexual fidelity.
   b. investment in family activities.
   c. not letting work outside the home endanger family interactions in the home.
   d. all of the above.

This Commitment Checklist will help your clients assess their strengths and potential. Again, "S" indicates a strength, or quality the family has achieved, "G" is for those qualities that have potential for growth, and "NA" means not applicable.

In our family...

\_\_\_\_\_Responsibilities are shared fairly.
\_\_\_\_\_Everyone gets a say in making decisions.
\_\_\_\_\_Individuals are involved in making their own choices.
\_\_\_\_\_We find it easy to trust each other.
\_\_\_\_\_We like to do things for each other that make us feel good about ourselves.
\_\_\_\_\_We have reasonable expectations of each other.
\_\_\_\_\_We allow each other to be ourselves.
\_\_\_\_\_We have a high regard for each other.
\_\_\_\_\_We respect the roles each of us plays in the family.
\_\_\_\_\_We find it easy to be honest with each other.
\_\_\_\_\_We accept that each of us has a different ways of doing things.
\_\_\_\_\_We build each other's self-esteem.
\_\_\_\_\_All things considered, we value each other and are committed to our well-being as a family.

## Positive Communication

Successful couple and family relationships are not simply about solving problems and resolving conflicts. Members of strong families are good at task-oriented communication; they can identify difficulties, stay focused on them, and find solutions that work reasonably well for all family members. Strong families also spend time talking with and listening to one another just to stay connected. Some of the most important talk occurs when no one is working at it: open-ended, rambling, serendipitous, and fun conversations can reveal important information that helps smooth out the bumps of family living.

A favorite painting we have on an office wall shows a South Pacific islander family—in this case, a mom and two teenaged daughters in French Polynesia—lying on the front porch of their tiny house. We can imagine that it's a hot and muggy afternoon, the breeze is blowing off the lagoon, and the family members are relaxing together. They're all a little sleepy from the heat, but they are clearly enjoying being together, leaning on each other, not saying much, looking like a pride of lions after a big meal. Young Americans call this "hanging out"—it's a critical activity for strong families. When something important needs to be talked through, family members have a reservoir of good will and good feelings toward each other to build upon.

16. Elements of positive communication include:
    a. witty and sarcastic humor like on television.
    b. open-ended, rambling, serendipitous, and fun conversations.
    c. solving problems and resolving conflicts.
    d. b and c.

This Positive Communication Checklist can help your clients assess their strengths and potential.

In our family...

\_\_\_\_\_We like to share our feelings with each other.
\_\_\_\_\_It is easy to cue into each other's feelings.
\_\_\_\_\_We like talking openly with each other.

_____We listen to each other.
_____We respect each other's point of view.
_____Talking through issues is important to us.
_____We give each other a chance to explain ourselves.
_____We enjoy our family discussions.
_____We share jokes together.
_____Put-downs are rare.
_____Sarcasm is not generally used.
_____All things considered, our communication is effective.

## Enjoyable Time Together

A fascinating element of our research and educational activities has been asking respondents to take "A Journey of Happy Memories." We requested them to go back to their childhood memories and focus on their "happiest times." After giving them sufficient time, we asked them to describe one or two of the most pleasant. The vast majority replied that their most memorable times were spent with family. For those who grew up in unhappy circumstances, they were likely to describe good times with friends, favorite pets, or in solitude and communion with nature.

> 17. Researchers have found that "A Journey of Happy Memories" group exercise does not commonly include:
> a. a story about camping trips and time in nature.
> b. a story about pleasant mealtimes together.
> c. a story about money.
> d. a story about families.

Very few people in our investigations replied that money made an important contribution to their happy memories from childhood. Rarely, someone mentioned a trip to Disneyland or a memorable expensive meal out. More commonly, they talked about family gatherings at holiday times, games the family played together, working on fun projects together; camping trips and adventures in nature, or pleasant mealtimes at home. For most respondents, the happiest childhood memories are of the family being together and enjoying each other's presence. Arising spontaneously, out of family goodwill, these rarely cost lots of money and, most often, are not particularly carefully planned.

Use this Enjoyable Time Together Checklist to assess family strengths and potential. In our family...

_____We have a number of common interests.
_____We like to have fun together.
_____We feel comfortable with each other.
_____We like to give each other a chance to do new things.
_____We enjoy hearing our grandparents' stories about the past.
_____We enjoy simple, inexpensive family activities.
_____We like to have a place we call "home."
_____We feel strongly connected to each other.
_____Hanging out together builds strong relationships.
_____We have lots of good times together.
_____We often laugh with each other.
_____Observing family rituals and customs is important to us.
_____We enjoy sharing our memories with each other.

_____We enjoy having unplanned, spontaneous activities together

_____All things considered, we have adequate time for each other, and we enjoy the time we have together.

## Spiritual Well-Being

People in strong families describe spirituality in many ways: some talk about faith in God, hope, or a sense of optimism in life; some say they feel a oneness with the world. Others talk about their families in almost religious terms, describing the love they feel for one another with a great deal of reverence. Others express these kinds of feelings in terms of ethical values and commitment to important causes. Spiritual well-being can be seen as the caring center within each individual that promotes sharing, love, and compassion. It is a feeling or force that helps people transcend themselves and their petty day-to-day hassles and focus on that which is sacred to them.

Cultural differences make the investigation of spiritual well-being in families fascinating. Australian culture, for example, reflects a certain reticence toward discussing spiritual matters. While vigorous discussion about organized religion is common in the United States, Australians, deeming this a more private matter, regard it unseemly to bring up in polite conversation. But when discussed privately, it is clear how important shared values and a connection to something greater than self is important to many Australians.

Assess family strengths with this Spiritual Well-Being Checklist.

In our family...

_____We have a hopeful attitude toward life.

_____Our home feels like a sanctuary for all of us.

_____We have a strong sense of belonging.

_____We enjoy learning about our family history.

_____We feel strong connections with our ancestors.

_____There is a feeling of safety and security.

_____We feel a strong connection with the land.

_____We feel connected with nature and the world around us.

_____There is a sense of peace among us.

_____We believe love is a powerful force that keeps us together.

_____We benefit in many ways from our belief in a higher being.

_____It is easy to share our spiritual values and beliefs with one another.

_____Our personal religious beliefs are compatible with each other.

_____All things considered, we have strong connections that enhance our well-being.

## Successful Management of Stress and Crises

"Most of the problems in the world either begin or end up in families," noted David H. Olson (Olson & DeFrain, 2003, p. 576). Sometimes a family (or a family member) inadvertently creates a problem for itself; sometimes the world creates a problem for the family; and almost always, the family gets stuck with the problem no matter what the cause.

18. Families:
    a. create most of their own problems.
    b. create most of the problems in the world.
    c. have to deal with most of the problems in the world.
    d. are the root causes of most the problems children have in the world.

This Coping Ability Checklist assesses family strength and potential.
In our family...

\_\_\_\_\_A crisis has helped us to grow closer together.
\_\_\_\_\_It is easy to find solutions to our problems when we talk about them.
\_\_\_\_\_It is always important to to try change the things we can.
\_\_\_\_\_We work together to solve difficult family problems.
\_\_\_\_\_A crisis has helped make our relationships strong.
\_\_\_\_\_We try not to worry too much, because things usually work out okay.
\_\_\_\_\_We are able to face daily issues confidently.
\_\_\_\_\_We like to support each other.
\_\_\_\_\_Our friends are there when we need them.
\_\_\_\_\_A crisis makes us stick closer together.
\_\_\_\_\_We always find something good comes from a crisis.
\_\_\_\_\_We find it easy to make changes in our plans to meet changing circumstances.
\_\_\_\_\_We have the courage to take risks that will improve things for our family.
\_\_\_\_\_We feel it is important to accept the things we cannot change.
\_\_\_\_\_All things considered, we look at challenges as opportunities for growth.

Strong families are not immune to stress and crisis, but neither are they as crisis-prone as troubled families tend to be. Rather, they possess the ability to manage both daily stressors and difficult life crises creatively and effectively. They know how to prevent trouble before it happens, and how to work together to meet challenges which inevitably occur in life.

One tactic strong families use in difficult times is to search for new ways to define the situation. Therapists call this *reframing*. Basically, the family looks at the challenge from a different angle. For this reason, we have chosen not to talk about the opposite of family strengths—dysfunction or problems. Rather, we focus on family strengths and areas of potential growth. This is not simply playing with words, but a serious attempt at looking at families through a new, more discerning lens.

Traditional Chinese culture illustrates this principle. The Chinese pictographic writing system, going back several thousand years, uses a picture-like symbol for the word *crisis* that links two symbols: the pictograph for the word *danger*, and the pictograph for *opportunity*. For thousands of years, the Chinese have reframed difficult situations as opportunities for growth. A crisis is admittedly a difficult time in life, but, if viewed positively and creatively, it can be a catalyst for significant personal and family growth—a sign of better things to come.

19. Regarding love:
    a. A model of family strengths with the concept of love in the center works well for most of the cultures of the world.
    b. Love is both a feeling one has for others, and a series of loving actions we demonstrate regularly toward each other.
    c. A model of family strengths with the concept of love in the center works well for Western cultures.
    d. b and c.

Where does love fit in the family strengths model? In our earlier models we viewed all family strengths in a circular fashion—all intertwined, highly related, and essentially inseparable—and we placed the concept of love in the center. This model works well for Western cultures where love is a central concept. When we asked Americans about the strengths of their families, "love" was usually cited. We define love as both a feeling one has for others, and as loving actions that we demonstrate regularly toward each other. Loving actions toward others lead to warm and loving feelings, and these feelings lead to loving actions in a reciprocal process. An abusive spouse may say "I love you," but words without loving actions are meaningless.

20. In Chinese culture today:
   a. love is a central concept when talking about families.
   b. the concept of harmony resonates better than the concept of love.
   c. Western influences may be changing traditional views.
   d. b and c.

Research from the People's Republic of China, however, changed our thinking somewhat (Xie, DeFrain, Meredith, & Combs, 1996). When asked about their family strengths, the Chinese in Guangzhou, for example, indicated similar strengths to Westerners, with only minor differences. In traditional Chinese culture, "love" was not seen as central to family well-being; instead, the term *harmony*, dating back centuries to Confucian times, resonated better with them. To them, harmony meant a pleasing atmosphere of agreement and accord, a state of friendly relations—not much different from one way Westerners' use the word *love*. China is in a period of transition. Western influences abound—pop music, movies, and books—and the word *love* is becoming more common in Chinese language.

## ASSESSING AND IMPROVING FAMILY STRENGTHS

We have presented an 86-item family strengths inventory culturally specific to American families, divided into each of the six major family strengths.

21. A family strengths inventory is not:
   a. useful for seeing the similarities and differences among family members' perceptions of their strengths.
   b. to be used as a scientific clinical assessment tool for predicting future behavior in a family.
   c. useful for seeing how family perceptions of their past, present, and future are similar and different.
   d. useful for family therapy sessions.

The main purpose of the American Family Strengths Inventory is to spark discussion of family strengths. It could be used in family therapy sessions, for example, to get a better understanding of your clients' perceptions of their families' strengths and perceived areas of needed growth. Ask family members to each fill out these checklists and afterward discuss their perceptions of their family's strengths. You can then help clients reframe their problems, seeing them in more hopeful ways—as opportunities to build new family strengths.

The University of Nebraska's *NU for Families* Web site (http://nuforfamilies.unl.edu) also provides a wide variety of interesting and fun activities for family members to engage in together to strengthen their relationships with each other. These Web site materials suggest specific activities that will help your clients develop each of the six family strengths.

As a family therapist you can help your clients' families focus on and build their strengths in a number of ways:

- *Conduct initial assessments* that survey the strengths as well as the distress of a family.

22. A family's past is useful to explore from a strengths perspective:
    a. to see how the family has overcome past challenges together.
    b. to better understand what inspired family members to take helpful action in the face of past challenges.
    c. to help the family draw positive conclusions about themselves because of their past successes together.
    d. all of the above.

- *Take particular note of strengths* the family has demonstrated as they have overcome past challenges—big or small.
- *Survey family members' motivations for engaging in therapy* and write the positive motivations on a board or paper for all members to see.
- *Explore the strategies and skills being used when things go well* in the seemingly insignificant micro-moments and enlist the family's help to see if there are any patterns to these positive, strengths-based moments.
- *Use two-handed reflections and summaries*—the challenges on one hand and the strengths on the other. For example, a family with a teen who frequently becomes angry and walks out of the room may benefit from recalling other times someone has been very upset and how they tackled the challenge then.
- *Ask about any goodwill that is present from stronger aspects of the family's relationships* and how this has been built up.

23. Effective approaches to increasing one's positive influence as a marital and family therapist do not include:
    a. assessing a family's strengths as well as the family's area of distress.
    b. looking at effective approaches the family has used together in the past.
    c. finding the person who is at the heart of the problem and finding ways for her or him to live a more responsible life.
    d. using two-handed reflections and summaries, identifying challenges on one hand and strengths on the other.

- *Talk about the family's problems or challenges as an external dynamic that they can face together* rather than looking at the situation as one or more members of the family *being* the problem—or even having the problem inside themselves. Based on ideas developed by the originators of narrative therapeutic approaches, this makes the problem more tangible and recognizable (White, 1989).

**Narrative therapy**, developed out of social constructionist and post-modern thinking, involves therapists helping individuals and families develop a new story that works better than the old approach (White & Epston, 1990). The family, as storyteller, relates the current perspective on reality that it holds. The family therapist, in concert with the family members, helps develop a new narrative—or story—that makes it possible for the family to meet its goals in a more effective manner.

- *With your client's family, agree on a strength-building project and name it.* This technique invites family members to form a coalition, joining forces to develop appropriate strengths to change the problem dynamic. They might explore ways to use some of their existing strengths to confront specific micro-moments.

> 24. Micro-moments of strength in a family are useful:
>     a. in helping figure out where the family went wrong and why.
>     b. for exploring the specifics of an event that is more the way the family would like things to be.
>     c. for better understanding those small successes that can be used to solve problems and strengthen couples and families.
>     d. b and c.

• *Focus on small successes.* This makes the micro-moments of strength more noticeable and enables an exploration of how family members achieved success in that instance. Ask about what was said, done, thought, and chosen in the unnoticed minutes involved. Ask how that micro-moment might be part of the project of problem-beating and strength-building, and how it might be useful in future moments.

• *Explore the motivations for the micro-moments of strength and what these moments might mean about the family.* This line of inquiry helps family members to be more aware of the ideas that inspire their micro-moments of strength (Cook, 2000). It also helps them draw tentative new conclusions about their own ability to cope with the problem and develop strength together—conclusions strengthened over time as further micro-moments build on previous successes. For example, you might ask about the ideas that motivated the parent to sit and think, rather than jump up and react, or about what motivated the teenager to write a letter. You might ask what conclusion the family members draw about their ability to tackle "The Tug of War" dynamic and whether this represents a micro-moment of strength.

> 25. Cultural beliefs of many Latino families that can prove useful in family therapy include:
>     a. familism.
>     b. machismo.
>     c. respeto.
>     d. all of the above.

• *Finally, you can use beliefs, values, and other aspects of a client family's culture to help them focus on their strengths.* Talking with families about their cultural beliefs and values can help them identify and acknowledge how they may be using these to be a strong family. For example, the beliefs of many Latino families include familism, fatalism, *machismo, personalismo,* folk illness beliefs, *respeto,* and *simpatico* (see Cuéllar, Arnold, & Gónzalez, 1995 for a review of cultural beliefs). There is also a tendency, particularly among new and more traditional families, to support communalism or collectivism that is designed to keep the family connected (Keefe & Padilla, 1987).

> 26. Family rituals and proverbs:
>     a. can be very powerful tools for family therapists.
>     b. help highlight a family's strengths.
>     c. serve as useful reminders that a sense of connection and strength do exist.
>     d. all of the above.

There are family rituals and *dichos* (proverbs) that can be very powerful tools (Zuniga, 1992; Gónzalez & Ruiz, 1995). With people from any culture, talking about family rituals they have grown up with will highlight the family's strengths. It will also provide you an understanding of the strengths the family may have lost or repressed in the new culture, but can bring back into their life. Very often, families just need to be reminded that the connectedness and their strengths do exist—they just need to use them. Many aspects of a family's culture are designed, if used effectively, to support the development and maintenance of family strengths. To identify and discuss family strengths within a cultural context is one way for families to deal more effectively with life challenges.

---

A strengths-based perspective of family therapy, focusing on health rather than dysfunction, on capacities rather than catastrophes, reflects the words reputed to be written by Ralph Waldo Emerson many years ago: "What lies behind us and what lies before us are tiny matters compared to what lies within us."

## KEY TERMS

**family function:** The internal workings of a family, i.e., how family members behave toward each other. A strengths-based approach tends to focus on family function rather than structure.

**family strengths perspective:** A conceptual framework proposing family researchers and therapists focus on existing and potential strengths, because if they focus only on family problems, they will only find problems.

**family structure:** Refers to the various types of families in regard to membership, such as nuclear families, extended families, stepfamilies, and so forth.

**family systems theory:** Posits that because family members are interconnected, everything that happens to any one family member will have an impact on everyone else in the family.

**narrative therapy:** An approach in which the family therapist, in concert with family members, seeks to develop a new narrative, or story, that helps the family meet its goals more effectively.

**strong families:** Kinship groups who typically share these strengths: appreciation and affection, commitment to each other, positive communication, enjoyable time together, a sense of spiritual well-being, and the ability to effectively manage stress and crisis.

## DISCUSSION QUESTIONS

1. What value is there for a family therapist to consider the strengths of a client family?
2. How do healthy families deal with problems?
3. Families can be viewed from both an insider and an outsider perspective. What are the advantages and disadvantages of each?
4. Argue for or against Tolstoy's assertion that happy families are all alike.
5. "Most problems in the world either begin or end up in families." What does this mean?
6. How do family strengths vary from culture to culture?
7. What value is there in focusing on small successes in family therapy?
8. "People are people are people, and families are families are families." What does this mean?
9. Discuss how religious and spiritual foundations impact family health and well-being.
10. How can family therapists use Narrative Therapy to identify and build family strength?

## SUGGESTED FURTHER READING

Moore, K. A., Chalk, R., Scarpa, J., & Vandivere, S. (2002, August). Family strengths: Often overlooked but real. *Child Trends* [Research Brief]. From www.childtrends.org

> Data from two recent national surveys show levels of important family strengths are actually quite high in the United States.

Olson, D. H., & DeFrain, J. (2003). *Marriages and families: Intimacy, diversity, and strengths* (4th ed.). New York: McGraw-Hill.

> A comprehensive, 605-page family studies textbook looking at all major aspects of family relationships from an applied strengths-based perspective.

## REFERENCES

Beavers, W. R., & Hampson, R. B. (1990). *Successful families*. New York: Norton.

Billingsley, A. (1986). *Black families in White America*. Englewood Cliffs, NJ: Prentice Hall.

Cook, R. (2000). *Discourses inspiring the strengths of a selection of New Zealand families*. Unpublished master's thesis, University of Waikato, Hamilton, New Zealand.

Cuéllar, I., Arnold, B., & Gónzalez, G. (1995). Cognitive referents of acculturation: Assessment of cultural constructs in Mexican Americans. *Journal of Community Psychology, 23,* 339–356.

Curran, D. (1983). *Traits of a healthy family*. Minneapolis: Winston Press.

DeFrain, J., DeFrain, N., & Lepard, J. (1994). Family strengths and challenges in the South Pacific: An exploratory study. *International Journal of the Sociology of the Family, 24*(2), 25–47.

DeFrain, J., Jones, J. E., Skogrand, L., & DeFrain, N. (2003). Surviving and transcending a traumatic childhood: An exploratory study. *Marriage & Family Review, 35*(1/2), 117–146.

DeFrain, J., & Stinnett, N. (2002). Family strengths. In J. J. Ponzetti et al. (Eds.), *International encyclopedia of marriage and family* (2nd ed., pp. 637–642). New York: Macmillan Reference Group.

Epstein, N. B., Bishop, D. S., Ryan, C., Miller, L., & Keitner, G. (1993). The McMaster model of family functioning. In F. Walsh (Ed.), *Normal family processes* (pp. 138–160). New York: Guilford Press.

Gabler, J., & Otto, H. (1964). Conceptualization of family strengths in the family life and other professional literature. *Journal of Marriage and the Family, 26,* 221–223.

Gónzalez, R., & Ruiz, A. (1995). *My first book of proverbs/Mi primer libro de dichos*. Emeryville, CA: Children's Book Press.

Kantor, D., & Lehr, W. (1974). *Inside the family*. San Francisco: Jossey-Bass.

Keefe, S. E., & Padilla, A. M. (1987). *Chicano ethnicity*. Albuquerque: University of New Mexico Press.

Krysan, M., Moore, K. A., & Zill, N. (1990). *Identifying successful families: An overview of constructs and selected measures*. Washington, DC: Child Trends, Inc. [2100 M St., NW, Suite 610] and the U.S. Department of Health & Human Services, Office of the Assistant Secretary for Planning and Evaluation.

Olson, D. H. (1996). Clinical assessment and treatment using the Circumplex Model. In F. W. Kaslow (Ed.), *Handbook in relational diagnosis* (pp. 59–80). New York: Wiley.

Olson, D. H., & DeFrain, J. (2003). *Marriages and families: Intimacy, strengths, and diversity* (4th ed.). New York: McGraw-Hill.

Olson, D. H., McCubbin, H. I., Barnes, H., Larsen, A., Muxen, M., & Wilson, M. (1989). *Families: What makes them work* (2nd ed.). Los Angeles: Sage.

Otto, H. A. (1962). What is a strong family? *Marriage and Family Living, 24,* 77–81.

Otto, H. A. (1963). Criteria for assessing family strength. *Family Process, 2,* 329–339.

Reiss, D. (1981). *The family's construction of reality*. Cambridge, MA: Harvard University Press.

Stinnett, N., & O'Donnell, M. (1996). *Good kids*. New York: Doubleday.

Stinnett, N., & DeFrain, J. (1985). *Secrets of strong families*. Boston: Little, Brown.

Stinnett, N., & Sauer, K. (1977). Relationship characteristics of strong families. *Family Perspective, 11*(3), 3–11.

University of Nebraska. (2004). Cooperative Extension *NU For Families* Web site: http://nuforfamilies.unl.edu

White, M. (1989). *Selected papers*. Adelaide, South Australia: Dulwich Centre Publications.

White, M., & Epston, D. (1990). *Narrative means to therapeutic ends*. New York: Norton.

Woodhouse, C. G. (1930). A study of 250 successful families. *Social Forces, 8,* 511–532.

Xie, X., DeFrain, J., Meredith, W., & Combs, R. (1996). Family strengths in the People's Republic of China. *International Journal of the Sociology of the Family, 26*(2), 17–27.

Zuniga, M. E. (1992). Using metaphors in therapy: Dichos and Latino clients. *Social Work, 37*(1), 55–60.

# 2

# Human Lifespan Development

Joan M. Lucariello
Jacqueline V. Lerner
*Boston College*

## TRUTH OR FICTION?

___ 1. *Piaget is best known for his four-stage theory of child cognitive development.*

___ 2. *"Conservation" is the term that Piaget used to describe the child's understanding that objects continue to exist even when they are out of sight.*

___ 3. *Piaget's third stage of cognitive development, the "concrete operational" stage, is characterized by abstract reasoning and scientific thinking.*

___ 4. *Vygotsky, contrary to Piaget, believed that culture (e.g., language) plays a key role in children's cognitive functioning.*

___ 5. *The "zone of proximal development" or zpd was conceived by Vygotsky as a way to measure children's IQ.*

___ 6. *The information processing theory of cognitive development views the mind in terms of a computer.*

___ 7. *According to information processing theorists, younger children remember less well than older children because they are less likely to use memory strategies, such as rehearsal.*

___ 8. *Studies show that contrary to popular belief, young children's memory of events is actually as accurate as most adults and their "eyewitness accounts" are generally correct.*

___ 9. *If a child doesn't cry when her mother leaves the room, that child is insecurely attached.*

___ 10. *Associations have been found between parenting styles and certain behaviors in children.*

___ 11. *Gender roles are genetically determined.*

_____ 12. According to social learning theory gender roles are primarily a result of modeling others.
_____ 13. According to Erikson, one will not be successful in marriage if one has not resolved an identity crisis.
_____ 14. According to Erikson, one can resolve the identity crisis through achieving marital intimacy.

## THEORIES OF COGNITIVE DEVELOPMENT

### Piaget's Cognitive Developmental Theory

Jean Piaget (1896–1987) was the first person to advance a theory of children's cognitive development. Piaget believed that the goal of intelligence is to achieve a balanced, harmonious relation, known as *cognitive equilibrium,* between thought processes (cognitive structures) and the environment. Equilibration is the process of achieving this equilibrium. Cognitive disequilibrium refers to imbalances between children's thinking and the environment. Another key feature of Piaget's view of intelligence is its "active" nature. Children are not passive recipients of information. Rather, they actively construct and re-construct their knowledge of the world. These two factors—cognitive disequilibrium and the child's action and interaction with the physical environment—propel the cognitive system and lead to the development of more advanced psychological structures.

1. An approach to development that emphasizes how the child actively constructs mental structures to reason about the world is the _____ theory.
   a. psychoanalytic
   b. social learning
   c. cognitive-developmental
   d. mental-behavioral

### *The Processes of Intelligence*

Intelligence is influenced by biological factors in exhibiting two invariant functions: *organization* and *adaptation*. *Organization* refers to the fact that our psychological/cognitive structures are organized into coherent systems. Organization promotes *adaptation* to our environment. Adaptation consists of two complementary processes: *assimilation* and *accommodation*. In assimilation, current psychological structures are used to interpret the external world. Toddlers who overextend a known word (e.g., call the heretofore unknown cow a "dog") are using their current concept (of dog) to understand the world. Cognitive structures do not change during assimilation. Rather, the experiences and information encountered by the child are altered to fit existing psychological structures. In accommodation, new psychological structures are created or old ones are adjusted upon noticing aspects of the environment that current psychological structures do not capture. A child imitating a parent's gestures would be a classic case of accommodation. Assimilation and accommodation work together to help the child make sense of the world.

2. In Piaget's theory, assimilation and accommodation are part of _____.
   a. adaptation
   b. organization
   c. centration
   d. assimilation

## The Structures of Intelligence: Stages of Cognitive Development

Organization of thought and adaptation to the environment lead to the development of different psychological structures at different developmental periods throughout childhood. These psychological structures are represented in four stages.

**The Sensorimotor Stage (Birth–2 years).** Piaget believed that infants were not capable of mental thought—only overt actions. The psychological structures of the infancy period are sensorimotor action schemes, such as the reflexes of grasping or sucking. Schemes are organized action patterns. Hence, intelligence is built upon the basic reflexes of the infant. Piaget divides this stage into six substages of development over which these action schemes become more elaborate, related, and goal-directed.

Development in the sensorimotor stage culminates with the onset of mental representation. The toddler can now think mentally, not merely through action. That the infant has achieved mental representation is evident in a milestone of this stage—the development of *object permanence*. This is the understanding that objects continue to exist when the child is not seeing or acting upon them.

**The Preoperational Stage (2–7 years).** In this stage, mental representation (the symbolic function) emerges. The most obvious example of symbolic functioning is language. The child acquires words—and words, of course, symbolize or stand for their referents. There are other indications of symbolic functioning as well. We see the emergence of symbolic play. For example, the child may use a banana to stand for a phone in play.

3. As children move from the sensorimotor to the preoperational stage:
   a. the use of objects in play becomes more realistic.
   b. make-believe play diminishes.
   c. thinking becomes related to logical rules.
   d. symbolic mental activity increases.

While the preschooler is capable of thought, such thought has some significant limitations. One is **egocentrism**, or the inability to take another person's perspective. Indeed, children presume that others have the same viewpoint as themselves. Piaget considered young children's noncommunicative or egocentric speech evidence of their egocentric thought. Egocentric speech is speech that is spoken aloud but is noncommunicative or nonsocial. It is strikingly evident in what Piaget terms the *collective monologue*. Here the child speaks aloud with others present, but is actually speaking a soliloquy.

**The Concrete Operational Stage (7–11 years).** In this stage, children's thinking overcomes the logical deficiencies of the preoperational stage. Reasoning is now nonegocentric. However, despite cognitive accomplishments, thought in this stage has its limitations. This stage's label—concrete operational—denotes thought that is bound by concrete, physical reality. Children's reasoning is constrained to the content/material being reasoned about.

> 4. Andre is in Piaget's concrete operational stage. He can do all of the following EXCEPT:
>    a. conserve distance.
>    b. give verbal directions for getting from one location to another.
>    c. sort the stamps in his collection by class and sub-classes.
>    d. think abstractly about information he cannot observe directly.

*The Formal Operational Stage (11 yrs and onward).*   In this stage, reasoning becomes abstract. Now able to discriminate between thoughts about reality and actual reality, the child can have thoughts that may not actually represent the true nature of experience. Thus, the child's thoughts about reality can take on a hypothetical "if, then" characteristic: "*If* Dad can get off work tomorrow, *then* we can leave for Boston."

Adolescent and adult thinking is also scientific. As such, it is hypothetico-deductive and combinatorial. In considering a problem or situation, adolescents can begin with a general theory of all the possible factors or variables, and their combinations, that could influence an outcome. They also can deduce particular predictions or hypotheses.

Piaget originally proposed that everyone would achieve formal operational reasoning. He later thought, however, that such reasoning might only be attained when we reason about areas with which we are very familiar and highly knowledgeable.

> 5. Formal operational reasoning is:
>    a. used by all adolescents every time they solve a problem.
>    b. consists in scientific, abstract, logical thinking.
>    c. develops in the concrete operational stage.
>    d. part of long-term memory.

The ability to think hypothetically leads to a deficiency in reasoning that occurs most strongly at the beginning of this stage known as **adolescent egocentrism**. This refers to the heightened self-consciousness that adolescents experience. Adolescent egocentrism declines as progress in abstract reasoning is made during this stage. Due to their preoccupation about what others are thinking of them, adolescents fall prey to two distortions in reasoning. The **imaginary audience** concept refers to their sense that they are always "on stage," or at the center of everyone's attention. Hence, adolescents are extremely self-conscious. The second distortion in reasoning is known as the **personal fable**. This is an exalted sense of one's own importance and uniqueness. These sentiments can lead adolescents to think that others could not ever understand their experiences.

> 6. Young teenagers are convinced that they are the object of everyone else's attention and concern. This feature of adolescent thought is called _____.
>    a. propositional reasoning
>    b. the imaginary audience
>    c. rule assessment
>    d. theory of mind

*Critiques of Piaget's Theory.*   Piaget's theory of cognitive development is not one that predominates in the field today. It has been challenged from many quarters. One challenge, from theorists known as "neo-nativists," consists in showing that children develop many cognitive abilities much earlier in development than Piaget's theory predicted. Investigators have also shown that, contrary to Piaget's claims, children's development is not marked by a progression of stages. Finally, culture plays a large role in cognitive development, contrary to Piaget's view that it played little to no role. For example, schooling may play a role in attaining concrete and formal operational reasoning.

## Vygotsky's Sociocultural Theory of Cognitive Development

The theory of the Russian psychologist, Lev S. Vygotsky (1896–1934) has triggered an enormous amount of research on the study of child cognition.

*The Process of Internalization: The Role of Culture (Language) in Cognitive Functioning.*   Vygotksy believed in the social origins of cognitive functions as evident in his *process of internalization*. "Every function in the child's cultural development appears twice: first, on the social level, and later, on the individual level; first, between people (*interpsychological*), and then *inside* the child (*intrapsychological*)... All the higher functions originate as actual relations between human individuals" (Vygotsky, 1978, p. 57, emphasis in original). Hence, internalization is the process whereby cognitive functions and processes performed on an external plane between persons come to be performed internally, within the child.

Vygotsky (1962) studied the internalization of language because he believed that language, a cultural symbol-system, has a profound influence on cognitive functioning. Language helps children think, plan, and guide their actions. Vygotsky proposed that language is first used communicatively (the social level) between people. Of course, the social-communicative function of language continues to develop. However, language will also develop along a second line. It will become internalized as "inner speech" (individual/intrapersonal level) and serve an intraindividual-cognitive function. Egocentric speech marks the midpoint in this internalization process.

Accordingly, Vygotsky had a very different view of egocentric speech than did Piaget. Piaget saw egocentric speech as merely a reflection of the egocentric thinking of the preoperational child. He believed egocentric speech serves no function. It does not help or advance thinking. Nor does it guide the child's action. In contrast, Vygotsky believed that egocentric speech is very important to the child's functioning. Egocentric speech assists thinking and it guides the child's action. Indeed, Vygotsky demonstrated that children's amount of egocentric speech increases when they are trying to solve a problem. When we no longer hear the child using much egocentric speech, as they near 7 to 8 years of age, Vygotsky proposed that this speech has become internalized as inner speech. Inner speech, like egocentric speech, has the self-regulatory functions of guiding our thought and action.

7. Unlike Piaget, Vygotsky viewed cognitive development as a(n) _____ process.
   a. socially mediated
   b. active
   c. quantitative
   d. innate

8. According to Vygotsky, children speak to themselves:
   a. because they are egocentric.
   b. because they are lonely.
   c. for self-guidance.
   d. for the pleasure of hearing their own voice.

*The Zone of Proximal Development (zpd).*   The **zpd** is a second seminal concept in Vygotsky's theory. It is defined as the difference between the child's actual developmental level as determined by independent problem solving and the higher level of potential development, as determined through problem solving under adult guidance or in collaboration with more capable peers (Vygotsky, 1978, p. 86). The *zpd* has been applied to the assessment of intelligence. It is considered a *dynamic* assessment measure. Instead of measuring completed and independent development, as does an IQ test, the *zpd* measures the potential level of development that can be achieved with assistance from others. This potential developmental level may vary from the actual, independent developmental level. Vygotsky also applied the *zpd* concept to instruction. In contrast to Piaget, Vygotsky felt that learning or instruction leads development. Hence, good instruction is ahead of development.

9. According to Vygotsky, which of the following would be within a child's zone of proximal development?
   a. tasks that a child can accomplish alone or with the help of an adult
   b. tasks that a child has recently mastered independently following the assistance of an adult
   c. tasks that a child cannot yet handle on her own, but can do with the help of an adult
   d. tasks that a child accomplishes through her independent activity

10. A color matching activity is within Zelda's zone of proximal development (**zpd**). Hence, Zelda:
    a. can already master this task without assistance.
    b. will master this task on her own soon.
    c. needs direct teaching in order to learn this task.
    d. can complete this task with guidance from a more skilled person.

## Information Processing Theory of Cognitive Development

Information processing theorists adopt a computerlike view of the mind. This is evident in the multi-store model of memory (Atkinson & Shiffrin, 1968). This model has two features: structural and functional. The structural features are 3 stores—*sensory register, working* or *short-term memory,* and *long-term memory* (the knowledge base)—where information is stored or held. These stores are assumed to be universal and available for information processing by age two years, if not even earlier. The functional features are the *mental strategies* or *control processes* that operate on or process the information that flows through the stores. Development occurs with respect to mental strategies. Younger children are generally poor strategists, whereas older children and adults are more competent strategy users.

## Stores and Strategies

Information first enters the system through the sensory register. Only a very limited amount of information can be held by the sensory register and only very briefly. Sights and sounds are represented directly. Information in the sensory register can become transferred to the next store, short-term or working memory. In short-term memory, information is only held very briefly, unless strategies are performed on the information. Rehearsal, such as verbally repeating the information, is one important strategy to retain information. Young children are less likely to engage in strategies. They may know these strategies but fail to produce them thereby evidencing a production deficiency. For instance, if given a list of words to recall, younger children are not found to rehearse (e.g., whisper the names of) the words. Hence their recall is poorer than that of older children who engage in spontaneous rehearsal.

The longer we retain information in short-term memory, the greater the likelihood it will be transferred to long-term memory. This store is very durable; information can be retained for decades. Long-term memory also has a very large capacity. Given this large capacity, the retrieval of information from long-term memory can be problematic. However, the large amount of information held in long-term memory is organized. One can be strategic in retrieval by relying on such organization and thereby increase the likelihood of retrieval. For example, we can rely on taxonomic categories, such as animals and clothing, in recalling a categorized list of items.

11. In the information processing system, short-term memory:
    a. stores information permanently.
    b. is unlimited in capacity.
    c. the conscious part of our mental system.
    d. is the central processing resource pool.

12. In the information processing system, mental strategies are:
    a. conceptualized as the hardware of the system.
    b. inborn and universal.
    c. procedures that operate on and transform information.
    d. limited by the capacity and speed of information processing.

## Memory Is a "Constructive" Process

Memory is not thought to copy reality at storage nor faithfully reproduce it at retrieval. Rather, memory is a constructive activity, which is largely influenced by our current knowledge. We interpret, select, omit, add, and otherwise transform material in the memory process. For example, if given the sentence "The man dug a hole," when asked to retrieve this sentence some time later, we might remember it as "The man dug with a shovel," or "The man dug a ditch." Investigators have presented children with stories to recall and one can see the constructive nature of memory. Children often recall the more important features, while forgetting the less important ones. Also, they tend to reorder the story into a more logical sequence and add important, missing information.

## Kinds of Knowledge: Semantic and Episodic Memory

Long-term memory is thought to consist in at least two kinds of memory: semantic and episodic. **Semantic memory** refers to our general knowledge systems, such as our knowledge about words (e.g., definitions, antonyms, synonyms) and all other kinds of factual knowledge (e.g., geography, history, mathematics, science). **Episodic memory** refers to memory for a specific events that we have personally experienced (e.g., yesterday's lunch, our birthday parties, and vacations).

A salient form of semantic knowledge for young children is script knowledge. *Scripts* are mental representations (concepts) for expected, commonplace events. These include caretaking activities (e.g., having lunch, getting dressed) and what happens at the grocery store, or restaurants, or school. These representations specify the sequence of actions that occur in these events, as well as the actors' roles, and objects that inhere in these events. Children's semantic knowledge about events grows in middle and later childhood to incorporate knowledge about unexpected events, such as ironic events (Lucariello & Mindolovich, 1995, 2002). These include events such as the "backfired plan." Mental representations for these kinds of unexpected events may be called *counterscripts*.

*Autobiographical Memory.* One type of episodic memory is **autobiographical memory**. This refers to our memory or mental representations for singular and important events in our lives. These might include our first day at school or our first trip to Disneyland. It is commonly the case that we cannot retrieve memory for experiences that happened to us prior to age 3 years. This failure to recall such early-experienced events is known as **infantile amnesia**. Several accounts have been offered to explain infantile amnesia. Autobiographical memory demands that children organize their personal experience into some kind of coherent story. Hence, children's ability to structure memories into stories may develop from talking about these experiences with others (Nelson, 1996). Or perhaps autobiographical memories are dependent on a strong sense of self, which may not emerge prior to age 3 (Howe & Courage, 1997).

13. Recent research suggests that for early memories of events to become autobiographical, the child may need to:
   a. have a well-developed language system and a repertoire of memory strategies.
   b. overcome production and utilization deficiencies.
   c. be attentive to routines and embed novel events in terms of those routines.
   d. have a well-developed image of the self and the ability to organize personal experience into narrative form.

*Metacognitive Knowledge.* **Metacognition** refers to children's knowledge of their own cognitive thoughts and processes. Children become increasingly more aware of their own cognitive processes with age. For example, older children are better able to determine how much time it will take them to learn something and what steps might help them. One kind of knowledge about the mind is termed *theory of mind* (ToM). This is an appreciation of people as mental beings. It is the understanding of mental and emotional states (own and others) and that such underlie behavior.

14. One's own awareness of one's own mental strategies is called _____.
   a. self-reflection
   b. reflective thought
   c. metacognition
   d. self-referencing

15. Children's ideas about the internal mental and emotional states of themselves and others are called _____.
    a. a theory of mind
    b. reflective thought
    c. cognitive understanding
    d. mind-brain cognition

*Children's Eyewitness Memory.* More and more often children are being called upon in courtrooms to deliver eyewitness testimony. Younger children's memory is generally much less reliable than that of older children's in this context. Younger children are less resistant to leading and misleading questions of the kind that attorneys might ask (Roebers & Schneider, 2001). Younger children are also weaker at source-monitoring (identifying where they got their information) (Poole & Lindsay, 2001). Also court cases can be lengthy. Memory for the event in question may fade. Furthermore, children may substitute memory for a script in place of the original event. The script may incorporate features that were not part of the original episode (Ornstein, Shapiro, Clubb, & Follmer, 1997). Finally, young children are more susceptible to suggestibility and can be led into giving false testimony (Leichtman & Ceci, 1995).

# THEORIES OF SOCIAL DEVELOPMENT

## Attachment to Others

Attachment can be defined as the emotional tie that exists between a child and those people who are significant in his or her life. Clearly evident by 12 months of age, attachment both furnishes the child with the sense of security necessary for exploring the environment, and provides a safe haven and source of comfort during times of distress. Although specific attachment behaviors change as we grow older, attachment as an emotional experience remains with us throughout our lives.

John Bowlby, a British psychiatrist, believed that attachment originates from the infant's need for security and safety, that it has its roots in our evolutionary past, and that parents play a key role in its development (1988, see pp. xii, 205). Children around the world form attachment relationships with their parents or other primary caretakers, but not all attachment relationships are equal in quality. Although the majority of infants appear able to use their parents as a secure base from which to explore the world and as a safe haven to return to in times of distress, some infants seem to have more trouble in this regard.

Mary Ainsworth, a research associate of Bowlby's, studied these individual differences in attachment behavior in the laboratory (Ainsworth, Blehar, Waters, & Wall, 1978). Based on her observations of infants both at home and in the laboratory, Ainsworth and her colleagues identified three major types or qualities of attachment relationships that infants have with their parents or other primary caretakers.

16. A 14-month-old who wanders to her aunt, returns to her mother, interacts briefly with an uncle, and then returns to her mother again is demonstrating the concept of _____.
    a. stranger anxiety
    b. self-consciousness
    c. a secure base
    d. emotional self-regulation

1. A *securely attached* infant is able to use the mother as a secure base from which to explore the world. When separated from the mother, a secure infant may or may not cry; if so, it is because the infant has a strong preference for the mother over a stranger. Upon the mothers return, if distressed, the securely attached infant seeks contact with the mother and is comforted by that contact. If not distressed, the securely attached infant greets the mother happily when she returns.
2. Infants who have an *avoidant attachment* relationship show little distress during separations, and when distressed they are easily comforted by others. When the mother returns, they turn away from her and avoid contact with her rather than either greeting her happily or seeking comfort.
3. Infants who have an *ambivalent attachment* relationship are extremely distressed by separations, and seem unable to gain comfort from the mother when she returns. They continue to cry and will also express anger towards the mother.

In addition to these three major types of attachment identified by Ainsworth, researchers have since recognized a fourth type which they call *disorganized attachment* (Main & Solomon, 1986). Infants with disorganized attachment relationships exhibit a diverse array of fearful, odd, or overtly conflicted behaviors during laboratory separations from their mothers. Its presence is often associated with maltreatment or other clinical concerns. The avoidant, ambivalent, and disorganized attachment relationships are all considered types of *insecure attachment*.

17. Juan has developed a strong, affectional tie to his grandmother. He feels great pleasure and comfort during their interaction. Juan is exhibiting _____.
    a. attachment
    b. a culturally specific emotion
    c. temperament
    d. a dysfunctional relationship

In the United States, researchers have generally found that 60% to 70% of infants in low-risk, middle-class families are securely attached to their parents. Ainsworth and her colleagues (1978) found that infants who are securely attached at one year have experienced sensitive, responsive caretaking throughout their first year of life. Avoidant infants have experienced parenting that is often rejecting or overly-intrusive, while the quality of care that ambivalent infants have received is inconsistent—that is, the parents may respond to the infant with either affection or indifference, depending on their mood. Disorganized infants have often experienced either abuse or parental psychopathology. When followed over time, children who have secure attachment histories are more confident, more empathic, more popular with their peers, and more cooperative with adults than children with insecure attachment histories.

18. Which mother is more likely to have a child who is advanced in emotional understanding?
    a. Mary, who has four children
    b. Marguerite, who has a secure attachment bond with her child
    c. Madeline, who refuses to discuss disagreements with her husband in front of the children
    d. Maureen, who only talks about factual subjects with her child, avoiding emotional topics

## PARENTING

The key function of a child's family is to raise the young person in as healthy a manner as possible. Although there is variation in different cultures in the family structures used to serve this function, a caregiver's role is always to provide the child with a safe, secure, nurturant, loving, and supportive environment, one that allows the child to have a happy and healthy youth. This sort of experience allows youth to develop the knowledge, values, attitudes, and behaviors necessary to become an adult who makes a productive contribution to self, family, community, and society.

What a parent does to fulfill these duties of his or her role is termed *parenting*. Parenting is a term that summarizes behaviors a person (usually, but not exclusively, the mother or father) uses to raise a child. Parenting involves bidirectional relationships between members of two or more generations and can extend through all or major parts of the respective life spans of these groups.

The classic research of Diana Baumrind (1971) resulted in the identification of three major types of child rearing styles, **authoritative**, **authoritarian**, and **permissive**. The **authoritative** style is marked by parental warmth, the use of rules and reasoning (induction) to promote obedience, nonpunitive discipline (e.g., using "time out" or "grounding" instead of physical punishment), and consistency between statements and actions and across time (Baumrind, 1971). **Authoritarian** parents are not warm, stress rigid adherence to the rules they set (e.g., "Obey— just because we, the parents, are setting the rules."), emphasize the power of their role, and use physical (corporal) punishment for transgressions (Baumrind, 1971). **Permissive** parents do not show consistency in their use of rules; they may have a "laissez-faire" attitude toward their child's behaviors.

19. A parent hears the garage window smash. Going outside, he sees his child with a baseball bat after being told to go to the park for such activities. An authoritarian parent would:
    a. tell the child to sweep up the glass and make plans for replacing the window.
    b. walk back inside, letting the event itself teach the child.
    c. demand immediate clean up, and make the punishment a memorable one.
    d. help the child with clean-up, and assure her so she doesn't become upset.

The use of different parenting styles is associated with differences in behavior and development. Children and adolescents with authoritative parents have more social competence and fewer psychological and behavioral problems than youth with authoritarian, indulgent, or neglectful parents. Youth with neglectful parents are the least socially competent and have the most psychological and behavioral problems of any group. In turn, youth with authoritarian parents are obedient and conform well to authority, but have poorer self-concepts than other children. Though youth with indulgent parents have high self-confidence, they more often abuse substances, misbehave in school, and are less engaged in school.

## GENDER INDIVIDUALITY

An important aspect of individuality has to do with those differences that are a result of one's biological sex. Some differences are related to physical and biological development—usually referred to as sex differences; others are influenced by society, culture, and experience— usually referred to as gender differences. Thus, gender differences have more to do with the differences in roles and behaviors between males and females than with biological and physiological differences.

At about age 2 or 3 children first acquire the foundation of sex identity—they can distinguish themselves as a boy or girl. At this point, however, they are not certain that one's sex is for life, and believe that they can change it at their whim. It is not until age 6 or 7 that they understand that changing appearances cannot change sex. This is known as *gender constancy* and it slowly develops until children realize that they cannot change their sex under any circumstances.

20. Joseph is an extremely shy child. What can his parents do to help him overcome his fear of novel experiences?
    a. Provide warm, supportive parenting and appropriate demands for Joseph to approach new experiences.
    b. Provide warm, supportive parenting and protect him from minor stresses.
    c. Avoid overly supportive parenting in order to encourage independence.
    d. Provide intensive monitoring, even if intrusive, while making Joseph assume responsibility for his actions.

As in all other areas of development, how gender roles and gender-role behaviors develop is influenced by many sources—the child, the family, others in the context, the culture. From a *biological* or *nature perspective*, gender differences in behaviors between males and females are accounted for by genes, hormones or other physiological or anatomical differences. As biology interacts with one's context, behavior and experience can affect hormone levels and brain development. Thus, while we need to carefully examine the genetic, hormonal, and physiological differences between males and females, we cannot assume that these differences directly affect behaviors and development.

From a *social learning perspective*, children learn what is appropriate for and expected of their sex by observing and modeling others in the environment and by direct reinforcement of behaviors. Stereotypical messages and expectations begin early with the first toys and clothes that adults pick out for their infants. The media is also a strong model of gender-role behaviors for children.

21. Katelyn puts on a necklace and sees herself as having feminine behaviors and characteristics. This self-perception is her _____.
    a. gender confusion
    b. gender stereotyping
    c. gender identity
    d. gender typing

From a *cognitive developmental* perspective, the intellectual abilities of the child provide him or her with the tools for gender-role development. Thus, the child's understanding emerges as part of general cognitive development. According to cognitive developmentalists, children begin to label themselves as a boy or girl by about age 3. But because preschoolers are limited in their thinking, they do not show gender constancy, as we noted above. Related to the cognitive developmental perspective, **gender-schema theories** propose that such schemas, which are networks of gender-related information, influence the child's perceptions and behavior. After they acquire gender constancy, children form schemas for each gender and process new information into these schemas. They include the behaviors that are appropriate for each sex. Not only do boys and girls then act according to the behaviors that they have processed as appropriate for their sex, they are also likely to transform behavior that they saw if it did not fit in with their schemas.

22. Bobby enjoys playing dress-up with his neighbor, Lizzie. His enjoyment of this activity:
    a. will continue through adolescence.
    b. is an indication of a hormonal imbalance.
    c. occurs in boys earlier than in girls.
    d. may indicate less traditional gender stereotyping in Bobby's family.

23. _____ is/are widely held beliefs in a culture about appropriate behaviors and characteristics for males and females.
    a. Gender identity
    b. Gender roles
    c. Gender stereotypes
    d. Sex differences

# PSYCHOSOCIAL DEVELOPMENT ACROSS LIFE: ERIK ERIKSON'S STAGE THEORY

Erik H. Erikson was a psychoanalytically-oriented theorist who, following Sigmund Freud (1954), proposed a stage theory of human psychosocial development. Erikson saw ego development as proceeding through eight stages, in each of which a different emotional crisis must be resolved and a different ego capability developed. Simply stated, a successful passage through each stage is critical for the final emergence of a fully integrated, whole ego.

## Stages of Psychosocial Development

As a follower of Freudian psychoanalysis, Erikson saw the stages of psychosocial development as complementary to Freud's own psychosexual stages. Accordingly, the id-based psychosexual stages exist, but they do so along with the ego-based psychosocial stages.

### Stage 1: The Oral-Sensory Stage

Freud's first stage of psychosexual development is termed the *oral* stage. In that stage, the infant is concerned with obtaining appropriate stimulation in the oral zone. Erikson believed, however, that when one's focus shifts to the ego, one sees that the newborn infant is concerned not merely with oral stimulation. Rather, the infant has newly entered the world, and therefore all its senses are being bombarded with stimulation. In order to begin to deal effectively with the social world, the infant must first be able to incorporate all this sensory information effectively.

If the infant has relatively pleasant sensory experiences, he or she will come to feel that the world is a relatively benign, supportive place. According to Erikson, then, the infant will develop a sense of *basic trust*. If, however, the infant experiences pain and discomfort, he or she will feel that the world is not supportive, and will develop a sense of *mistrust*. Thus, the conflict to be resolved at this stage is one of trust vs. mistrust. Erikson stressed the point that people do not, and should not, develop *either* complete basic trust or complete mistrust. Rather, a given person will develop a feeling that falls somewhere along this dimension.

24. According to cognitive developmental theory, gender role development:
    a. does not follow a developmental sequence.
    b. develops according to the cognitive advances of the child.
    c. it totally dependent on social models.
    d. will be difficult if there is a hormonal imbalance in the child.

## Stage 2: The Anal-Musculature Stage

Freud's second stage of psychosexual development is termed the *anal* stage. To Erikson, however, psychosocial development involves the other muscles of the body as well. Here, then, psychosocial development involves developing control over all of one's muscles, not just those involved in psychosexual development. The infant must learn when to hold on to and when to let go of all his or her bodily muscles (Erikson, 1963), and develop the capability of being able to control his or her overall bodily movements.

Accordingly, if the child feels that he or she is in control of his or her own body—that he *himself* or she *herself* can exert this control over himself or herself—the child will develop a sense of *autonomy*. On the other hand, if the child is unable to exert this independent control over his or her own bodily musculature, then the child will develop a sense of *shame* and *doubt*. In sum, the second bipolar psychosocial crisis is autonomy versus shame and doubt.

25. Erikson's autonomy versus shame and doubt stage corresponds to Freud's _____ stage.
    a. oral
    b. phallic
    c. anal
    d. latency

## Stage 3: The Genital-Locomotor Stage

This third psychosocial stage corresponds to Freud's psychosexual phallic stage. Children must begin to employ the previously developed self-control over their muscles, take their own steps into the world, and thereby break their oedipal ties. If the child can move in the world without a parent's guiding or prodding, he or she will develop a sense of *initiative*. If, on the other hand, the child does not do this, he or she will feel a sense of *guilt*. Thus, the third conflict to resolve is one of initiative versus guilt.

## Stage 4: Latency

Freud did not pay much attention to the psychosexual latency stage because of his belief that the libido is submerged. However, Erikson attached a great deal of psychosocial importance to the latency years. Erikson believed that in all societies children begin at this stage to learn the tasks requisite for being adult members of society. If the child learns these skills well—if he or she learns what to do and how to do it—he or she will develop a sense of *industry*. If the child feels that he or she has not learned to perform capably the requisite tasks of his or her society (while feeling that others around him or her *have* acquired this), he or she will feel a sense of *inferiority*. Thus, to the extent that children feel that they have or have not developed the requisite skills of their society, they will develop feelings toward either industry or inferiority.

26. Unlike Freud, Erikson's theory accounts for _____ influences on the individual.
    a. sexual
    b. cognitive
    c. emotional
    d. social

## Stage 5: Puberty and Adolescence

This stage of development corresponds to the genital stage of psychosexual development in Freud's theory. Erikson, too, was concerned with the implications of the emergence of a genital sex drive occurring at puberty. But, again, Erikson here looked at the broader, psychosocial implications of all the physical, physiological, and psychological changes that emerge at puberty.

Erikson saw all these changes occurring with puberty as presenting the adolescent with serious psychosocial problems. If the child has developed successfully, he or she will have developed more trust than mistrust, more autonomy than shame and doubt, more initiative than guilt, and more industry than inferiority. In any event, all the feelings the child has developed have gone into giving him or her a feeling about who he or she is and what he or she can do. Now, however, this knowledge is challenged. The adolescent now finds him- or herself in a body that looks and feels different, and further finds that he or she is thinking about these things in a new way.

Accordingly, the adolescent asks him- or herself a crucial psychosocial question: Who am I? Moreover, at precisely the time when the adolescent feels unsure about this, society begins to ask him or her related questions. Society wants to know what *socially prescribed set of behaviors*—behaviors functioning for the adaptive maintenance of society—will be adopted. If the adolescent finds his or her role in society, if he or she can show commitment to an ideology, he or she will have achieved a sense of identity. Alternatively, if the adolescent does not find a role to play in society, he or she will remain in the identity crisis. In an attempt to resolve this crisis, the adolescent may try one role one day and another the next, perhaps successfully—but only temporarily—investing the self in many different things. Accordingly, Erikson maintains that if the adolescent does not resolve the identity crisis, he or she will feel a sense of *role confusion* or *identity diffusion*. Thus, this conflict is termed *identity versus role confusion*.

27. A main challenge for adolescents is to reconcile _____ with their own understanding of who they are, in order to resolve their identity crisis.
    a. their emerging sexuality
    b. their parents expectations
    c. peer pressure
    d. societal roles

## Stage 6: Young Adulthood

In this and the last two psychosocial stages, Erikson departed from the psychosexual model and provided a description of the psychosocial stage changes involved with the rest of the human life span. In young adulthood, the person is oriented toward entering into a marital union. The person should by now have achieved an identity and should know who he or she is. The society now requires the person to enter into an institution that will allow the society to continue to exist. Accordingly, the formation of a new family unit must be established—for example, through marriage. This psychosocial directive, however, leads the person into another emotional crisis.

Erikson argued that to enter into and successfully maintain such a relationship, a person must be able to give of him- or herself totally. To give of oneself totally, all the facets of one person (e.g., feelings, ideas, goals, attitudes, and values) must be unconditionally available to the other; moreover, the person must be unconditionally receptive to these same things from the partner. To the extent that one can attain such interchange, one will feel a sense of intimacy.

If, however, one has not achieved an identity in Stage 5 and thus does not have a total sense of self (to give of completely), then of course one will not be able to achieve this sense of intimacy. Accordingly, there are limits to intimacy with another; if one cannot (for whatever reason) share and be shared, then one will feel a sense of isolation. Thus, this conflict is termed *intimacy versus isolation*.

> 28. Catherine and John have been married for three years. They spend all their free time together, and have many friends, but Catherine is feeling lonely. According to Erikson, she may not have successfully resolved her _____.
>     a. oedipal ties
>     b. autonomy issues
>     c. identity crisis
>     d. attachment issues

## Stage 7: Adulthood

If a successful, intimate union has been formed, however, the person can now attempt to meet the next set of psychosocial requirements in adulthood. In this stage, society requires the person to play the role of a productive, contributing member of society. Accordingly, if the person is successfully playing the role society expects, then the person will have a sense of generativity, a feeling that he or she is performing his or her role appropriately. On the other hand, if the person finds that he or she is not fulfilling the requirements of his or her role, if the person is not producing as he or she should, the person will feel a sense of stagnation. Thus, this conflict is termed *generativity versus stagnation*.

## Stage 8: Maturity

In this stage of psychosocial development, the person recognizes that he or she is reaching the end of his or her life span. If the person has successfully progressed through his or her previous stages of development—if he or she has experienced more trust than mistrust, more autonomy than shame and doubt, more initiative than guilt, more industry than inferiority, and if he or she has had an identity, had an intimate relationship, and been a productive, generative person—then the individual will face the final years of life with enthusiasm and eagerness. Thus, Erikson argued that he or she will feel a sense of ego integrity. The person will feel that he or she has led a full and complete life.

Alternatively, if the person has not experienced these events—if, for example, he or she has felt mistrustful, ashamed, guilty, and inferior, and has felt a sense of role confusion, isolation, and stagnation—then he or she will not be enthusiastic about these last years of his or her life. In this case, Erikson said, the person would feel a *sense of despair*. Thus, this conflict is termed *ego integrity versus despair*.

29. Claude was envied by many. He had inherited wealth, was happily married, and had three lovely children. Yet, in his later years, he was beset with depression and despair. Erikson would assume he was missing a _____.
    a. sense of generativity
    b. mature sense of morality
    c. sense of initiative
    d. sense of intimacy

30. A recognized strength of Erikson's theory is:
    a. his establishment of invariant stages which all humans progress through.
    b. the integration of social and psychological forces in development.
    c. his enlightened view of women in society.
    d. his emphasis on classical conditioning.

Erikson's theory of ego development involves changes encompassing the human life span. His theory represents a synthesis between psychoanalytically based, classical stage notions and an explicit differential orientation to development. Erikson's (1963) theory has, at least in the last three or more decades, led to more research in developmental psychology than has any other psychoanalytically oriented theory.

## KEY TERMS

**adolescent egocentrism:** In Piaget's theory, this is the heightened self-consciousness that adolescents experience, that represents a deficiency in their reasoning.

**ambivalent attachment:** When an infant is extremely distressed by the separation from the caregiver, but seems unable to gain comfort when that caregiver returns.

**authoritarian parenting:** A style of child rearing characterized by parents who are not warm, stress rigid adherence to the rules they set, emphasize the power of their role, and use physical (corporal) punishment for transgressions.

**authoritative parenting:** A style of child rearing that is marked by parental warmth, the use of rules and reasoning (induction) to promote obedience, and non-punitive discipline.

**autobiographical memory:** A type of episodic memory that refers to our mental representations for singular and important events in our lives.

**avoidant attachment:** An insecure infant/caregiver bond, characterized by the infant showing little distress during separation and a tendency to avoid or ignore the caregiver when stressed.

**biological or nature perspective:** Advances the notion that gender differences in behaviors between males and females are accounted for by genes, hormones, or other physiological or anatomical differences.

**cognitive developmental perspective:** Advances the idea that the intellectual abilities of the child provide him or her with the tools for gender role development. Thus, the child's understanding emerges as part of general cognitive development.

**disorganized attachment:** The infant exhibits a diverse array of fearful, odd, or overtly conflicted behaviors during separation from the caregiver.

**egocentric thinking/egocentrism:** In Piaget's theory, a logical deficiency in preoperational thinking which is the tendency to view the world in terms of one's own perspective while failing to realize that others may have different points of view.

**episodic memory:** In information processing theory, memory for specific events that we have experienced.

**gender-schema theory:** A theory proposing that schemas that are networks of gender-related information, influence the child's perceptions and behavior.

**imaginary audience:** In Piaget's theory, a symptom of adolescent egocentrism wherein the adolescent believes him- or herself to be at the center of everyone's attention, as if "on stage."

**infantile amnesia:** The inability of older children and adults to remember experiences that happened to them prior to about age 3 years.

**insecure attachment:** The types of attachment relationships that are in this category are *avoidant, ambivalent,* and *disorganized attachment.*

**metacognition:** In information processing theory, cognition or knowledge of one's own thoughts and mental processes.

**permissive parenting:** A style of child rearing characterized by parents who do not show consistency in their use of rules; they may have a "laissez-faire" attitude toward their child's behaviors and they may give the child anything he or she requests.

**personal fable:** In Piaget's theory, a symptom of adolescent egocentrism wherein the adolescent exhibits an exalted sense of his or her own importance and uniqueness.

**securely attached:** When the infant is able to use the caregiver as a secure base from which to explore the unfamiliar, especially if distressed.

**semantic memory:** Our general knowledge system.

**social learning perspective:** The perspective that children learn what is appropriate for and expected of their sex by observing and modeling others in the environment and by direct reinforcement of behaviors.

**zone of proximal development (zpd):** Vygotsky's term for the difference between the child's actual developmental level as determined by independent problem solving and the higher level of potential development, as determined through problem solving under adult guidance or in collaboration with more capable peers.

## DISCUSSION QUESTIONS

1. How does children's memory change with age? Are young children strong memorizers? How do children become better at memory?
2. What problems and strengths do preschool children show in their thinking (think about Piaget's theory and information processing theory in answering)?
3. How does the five-year-old differ from the eight-year-old in cognitive functioning (think about Piaget's theory, Vygotsky's theory, and information processing theory in answering)?
4. How do adolescents reason about problems? What are their strengths and weaknesses in reasoning?
5. How do cultural things—such as social interaction with other persons (especially capable adults), instruction, and language—affect the child's cognitive development and functioning? How do these things help the child's development and functioning?
6. How might the characteristics of parenting influence the child's successful resolution of conflicts during the first three stages of Erickson's theory?
7. How do families influence gender role development during childhood?
8. What are some of the adjustment problems that could result in childhood and adolescence from an insecure attachment bond during infancy and early childhood?
9. What are the life circumstances that are likely to be associated with the successful resolution of the conflicts associated with stages 6, 7, and 8 of Erickson's theory?

## SUGGESTED FURTHER READING

Baumeister, R. F. & Twenge, J. M. (2003). The social self. In M. Theodore & M. J. Lerner (Eds.), *Handbook of psychology: Personality and social psychology: Vol. 5* (pp. 327–352). New York: Wiley.

The authors state that it is difficult to think about the self without referring to other people. Although the very concept of the self seems to denote individualism, the self is incomplete without acknowledging our interactions with other people. Topics discussed in this chapter include: belongingness, social exclusion, and ostracism (theoretical background, aggressive behavior and prosocial behavior, self-defeating behavior, cognitive impairment, larger social trends in belongingness and negative outcomes); the self as an interpersonal actor (self-esteem and interpersonal relationships, narcissism and interpersonal relationships, reflected appraisals, influence of others' expectancies); self-presentation (favorability of self-presentation, cognition and self-presentation, harmful aspects of self-presentation); interpersonal consequences of self-views (self-views alter person perception, self-evaluation maintenance, self-monitoring, partner views of self, self-handicapping); emotions and the interpersonal self (shame and guilt, embarrassment, social anxiety, disclosing emotion and personal information); and cultural and historical variations in selfhood (culture and society, historical evolution of self, medieval times to the twentieth century, the 1960s to the present).

Marcia, J. E. (2002). Identity and psychosocial development in adulthood. *Identity: vol 2* (pp. 7–28). Mahwah, NJ: Erlbaum.

Discusses psychosocial development in adulthood from several perspectives. The author addresses stage-specific crises in ego growth associated with different life cycle periods in terms of status measures expanding on Erikson's polar alternative resolutions (E. H. Erikson, 1959). Using these status measures, the author discusses the developmental linkages between these stages and examines development from one status to another within a particular psychosocial stage. With respect to identity itself, the author also illustrates the cyclical process that might describe identity re-formulation through the adult psychosocial stages. Finally, the author presents case studies of a fifty-three-year-old man and thirty-seven-year-old woman, respectively, as examples of adult psychosocial development.

## REFERENCES

Ainsworth, M. D. S., Blehar, M. C., Waters, E., & Wall, S. (1978). *Patterns of attachment*. Hillsdale, NJ: Erlbaum.

Atkinson, R. C., & Shiffrin, R. M. (1968). Human memory: A proposed system and its control processes. In K. Spence & J. Spence (Eds.), *The Psychology of Learning and Motivation* (Vol. 2). New York: Academic Press.

Baumrind, D. (1971). Current patterns of parental authority. *Developmental Psychology Monographs, 4*, No. 1, Part 2, 1–103.

Bowlby, J. (1988). *A secure base: Parent-child attachment and healthy human development*. New York: Basic Books.

Erikson, E. (1963). *Childhood and society* (2nd ed.). New York: Norton.

Freud, S. (1954). *Collected works* (Standard edition). London: Hogarth.

Howe, M. L., & Courage, M. L. (1997). The emergence and development of autobiographical memory. *Psychological Review, 104*, 499–523.

Leichtman, M. D., & Ceci, S. J. (1995). The effect of stereotypes and suggestions on preschoolers' reports. *Developmental Psychology, 311*, 568–578.

Lucariello, J., & Mindolovich, C. (1995). The development of complex metarepresentational reasoning: The case of situational irony. *Cognitive Development, 10*, 551–576.

Lucariello, J., & Mindolovich, C. (2002). The best laid plans: Beyond scripts are counterscripts. *Journal of Cognition & Development, 3*(1), 91–115.

Main, M., & Solomon, J. (1986). Discovery of an insecure-disorganized/disoriented attachment pattern. In T. B. Brazelton & M. W. Yogman (Eds.), *Affective development in infancy* (pp. 95–124). Westport, CT: Ablex Publishing.

Nelson, K. (1996). *Language in cognitive development: Emergence of the mediated mind*. New York: Cambridge University Press.

Ornstein, P. A., Shapiro, L. R., Clubb, P. A., & Follmer, A. (1997). The influence of prior knowledge on children's memory for salient medical experiences. In N. Stein, P. A. Ornstein, C. J. Brainerd & B. Tversky (Eds.), *Memory for everyday and emotional events* (pp. 83–112). Hillsdale, NJ: Erlbaum.

Poole, D. A., & Lindsay, D. S. (2001). Children's eyewitness reports after exposure to misinformation from parents. *Journal of Experimental Psychology, Applied, 7,* 27–50.

Roebers, C. M., & Schneider, W. (2001). Individual differences in children's eyewitness recall: The influence of intelligence and shyness. *Applied Developmental Science, 5,* 9–20.

Vygotsky, L. S. (1962). *Thought and language.* Cambridge, MA: MIT Press.

Vygotsky, L. S. (1978). *Mind in society: The development of higher psychological processes.* Cambridge, MA: Harvard University Press.

# 3

# Human Diversity

Barbara F. Okun
*Northeastern University*

## TRUTH OR FICTION?

___ *1. A father who is perceived by his colleagues and subordinates to be a "tyrant" at work is likely to be perceived by his children at home to be a "bully."*

___ *2. Though families play a significant role in the development of their offspring's personalities and life styles, they are not the sole determinant.*

___ *3. Fathers can provide more nurturing than mothers.*

___ *4. Immigrant families who insist on retaining their own cultural beliefs and practices will cause their offspring to have emotional problems.*

___ *5. Family systems theories suggest a model of how families should be organized and how they should function.*

___ *6. Cultural variables do not apply to dominant culture families in the United States.*

___ *7. Intercultural and gay/lesbian couples who have children are creating a risk of emotional difficulties for these children.*

___ *8. American citizens have been raised in high context, collective cultures.*

___ *9. Our notions of families and family development are social constructs and, therefore, differ from culture to culture.*

___ *10. The goal of family therapists is to help people respect cultural and systems differences and effectively negotiate these differences.*

___ *11. Biological connection is the primary determinant of a healthy family.*

___ *12. In general, bi- or multi-cultural children do not want to choose one parent's culture over the other parent's culture.*

___ *13. Marginalization and oppression have psychological impact on one's development.*

___ *14. Clinicians need to understand dynamics of power and powerlessness.*

___ *15. Marriage and family therapists need to consider both cultural context and individual difficulties with regard to assessing family dysfunction and resiliency.*

The goals of this chapter are to:

1. Provide you with an ecological/systems model of human diversity emphasizing intra- and inter-group differences regarding gender, race, ethnicity, sexual orientation, religion, disability, class, and other sociopolitical contexts.
2. Apply this model to a variety of family system types, including traditional and non-traditional (or postmodern)—that is, same and transcultural adoptive; interracial and interethnic; gay and lesbian with biological, adopted, or previous children; single parent by choice, divorce, or widowhood; grandparent led; childless couples; cohabiting couples; families using reproductive technologies; families with disabilities, chronic or acute illnesses; and refugee and immigrant. (Due to space limitations, only grandparent, intercultural adoptive, and gay and lesbian family types are discussed in this chapter.)
3. Explore clinical and conceptual issues for couple and family therapists.
4. Consider how the major models of family therapy theory and practice do and do not apply to today's family system types.

These goals are interrelated and serve as a framework for our discussions; the organization of the chapter will be more circular than linear.

For the purposes of this chapter, the term *intercultural family* is used to describe families comprised of gay/lesbian/bisexual, multiracial, interracial (by marriage or adoption), interfaith, interethnic members. Interracial families include those from other countries as refugees or immigrants, first or second or third generation, and American people of color, African-American and Native-American, for example. The term **diverse family structure** refers to grandparent, adoptive, foster, single parents, cohabiting, etc.—any type of family that does not fit into the mainstream, traditional, same cultural, heterosexual, two parent family. Both intercultural and diverse family structure families share some common experiences due to being 'different"; they also experience unique issues.

In order to learn about human and family diversity, we need to consider our own identities and how they've been shaped by our family experiences, which, in turn, have been shaped by larger sociocultural systems. Some of the learning activities in this chapter will help you become more aware of your own self (self in relationship to others) and worldviews, which influence how you view and work with clients.

The mainstream traditional concept of a family included a father, a mother, and an average of 2.5 biological children. A more contemporary definition of family includes anyone living in a nuclear family, living with a spouse or same-gender partner, living with minor children, living with unrelated children and perhaps with older parents (Maney & Cain, 1997). In addition to composition, the traditional family typically had traditional or conventional roles: a provider father, a caretaking mother, and gendered role children. This began to change in the 1970s, after women began to return to the workforce. Though society has traditionally deemed mothers as the primary caretakers, dual worker/career families have created diverse roles, including shared co-parenting, primary caretaking fathers, nannies, and daycare or extended family services.

1. Intercultural and diverse families:
   a. require more therapy than dominant mainstream families.
   b. resist therapy more so than dominant mainstream families.
   c. are often wary of dominant culture mainstream clinicians.
   d. will only work with a clinician of their own cultural group.

Gender roles continue to change. More and more men and women are choosing to adjust their work lives in diverse types of families to co-parent, and more and more men are finding that they are just as willing and as capable as women to parent (albeit in different styles). The nation's family courts no longer assume that the mother is automatically the better parent (Okun, 1996) and fathers' rights groups are advocating gender-free custodial plans. This often results in contemporary two-parent families (both heterosexual and homosexual) sharing both domestic and economic power.

2. Though we are all vastly shaped by the families into which we are born, the next most powerful influence is:
   a. the parent(s) job(s).
   b. the neighborhood in which you reside.
   c. federal laws.
   d. peer groups.

## AN ECOLOGICAL/SYSTEMS MODEL

An **ecological/systems model** considers any individual as embedded in his or her actual family system, which is, in turn, embedded in larger sociocultural systems (Fig. 3.1). This model assumes that our self-awareness, comfort, and discomfort differ in each of these different contexts. We not only feel and behave differently in different relationships and settings, but each relationship and each setting influences other relationships and settings. Figure 3.2 delineates this model by showing how Louise, aged fourteen, is embedded in larger systems. Each system has its own functions and operating rules and roles. It is based on the adolescent identified patient of a conflictual family system. The purpose is to understand the individual and family in larger sociocultural contexts so as to provide a multilevel treatment.

Consider that our population and family types have changed dramatically in the past two decades, due to post World War II societal changes: increased immigration, changing civil rights, women's liberation and gay rights, increased mobility, and the urbanization and suburbanization of metropolitan areas. The 2000 census (U.S. Census Bureau, 2002) reports an increasing mix of races and ethnic groups within a family as well as an explosive growth of Asian and Hispanic populations. It is estimated that within the next decade, Caucasians, the dominant ethnic group in this country, will become a statistical minority (Okun, Fried, & Okun, 1999). The census report also attests to the largest increase of gay and lesbian families, along with significant increases of single parent families, grandparent led families and other alternative family forms.

3. The two fastest growing families are:
   a. transracial and domestic adoptive families.
   b. grandparent and adoptive families.
   c. intercultural and adoptive families.
   d. gay/lesbian and intercultural families.

Due to these demographic changes, we have learned more about the impact of larger sociocultural systems on individual and family functioning. The family systems notion of "embedded in context" has been expanded to incorporate the powerful influences of community, local, state, and federal social systems and global/universal variables on families and, in turn, on

**Universal**
- Sexual Orientation
- Generation
- Geographic Region
- Gender
- Race
- Ethnicity

**Larger Social Systems**

Federal
Government /
State
Government:

- Laws
- Policies
- Agencies
- Money

**Community**
- Education/Training
- Judicial
- Health
- Religion
- Legal
- Welfare
- Work
- Peers
- Kin
- Social Services
- Family/Friends

**Family**
- Parents/Siblings
- Values      - Rules
- Roles       - Boundaries

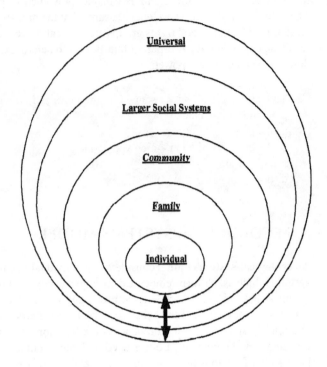

**FIG. 3.1.**   Individual in Contexts.

individuals. These powerful influences challenge our traditional assumptions about individuals and families. They also challenge traditional family therapy theories, resulting in newer post-modern paradigms, such as those underlying narrative and constructivist theories and emerging transcultural models (Khisty, 2001). In addition, the exploding knowledge from the fields of biology and neuropsychology challenges the traditional nature/nurture controversy, compelling us to reassess existing theories and models that ignore or minimize the influences of biology and neurology on an individual.

4. Most family therapy theories are based on:
   a. diverse family structure.
   b. universality about family functioning.
   c. dominant culture model of family.
   d. working class families.

Thus, the ecological/systems model allows us to better understand the importance of viewing people and events in their sociocultural contexts and to recognize that culture plays a significant

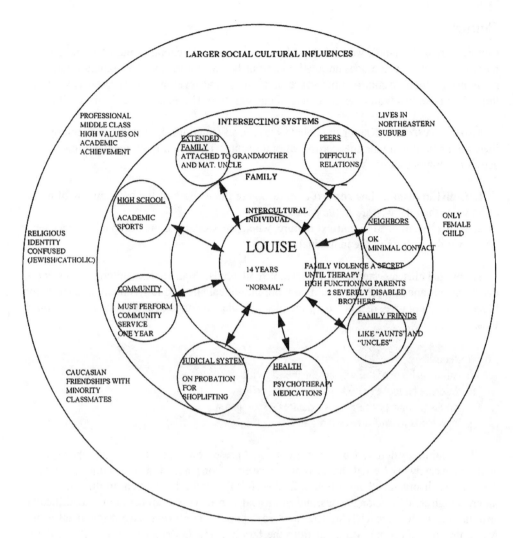

**FIG. 3.2.** Sample Ecogram.

role in determining how individuals make meaning or sense of themselves, their families, other relationships, and events in the world. In particular, we need to consider how culture influences families. How, for example does culture shape the composition of families, family rules regarding change, power distribution, emotional quality, and closeness and distance regulation?

5. The ecological/systems model:
   a. ignores individual accountability.
   b. emphasizes environment more than biology.
   c. considers the reciprocal relationships between individual, family, community, country, and larger sociocultural systems.
   d. is deterministic.

## Culture

Culture shapes a person's worldview—that is, one's basic perceptions and understandings of the world. Worldview includes notions about basic human nature, families, intimate and social relationships, locus of control, time, space, and activity and develops out of personal experience through interactions with other members of one's culture (Okun, Fried, & Okun, 1999).

*Family System.* Kantor and Lehr (1975) classify relationship systems, particularly families, on a continuum that cuts across cultural groups. Their family arrangement model cuts across two major cultural values:

1. **Individualism** or **low context** culture, where the welfare of the individual is of higher value than the welfare of the group, and
2. **Collectivism** or **high context** culture, where the welfare of the group takes precedence over the welfare of the individual (Fig. 3.3).

Traditional closed systems would resemble collectivist, high context cultural values; loose, disorganized random systems would be more individualistic and low context; open systems, based on collaborative, democratic principles provide a balance of individualism and collectivism.

6. Collectivism:
   a. values primarily the welfare of the individual.
   b. describes a low context system.
   c. values primarily the good or desires of the group.
   d. represents a random system.

Closed family systems are based on tradition—"preserve and ye shall prevail," open systems adapt more easily to external changes and are based on consensus and negotiation, and random systems are disorganized and value individual fulfillment in the moment to the utmost. The latter, though creative, spontaneous, and whimsical, can also become chaotic and are difficult to sustain when children reach school age and are required to conform to an outside social system where the rules are vastly different from the family rules. Different cultures value different systems types and many families change their style during the family life cycle. Kantor and Lehr's model is a descriptive model. There is value in each system type and there is usually a prevailing type despite variability. When a crisis occurs, a closed system initially becomes more rigid, an open system initially discusses endlessly, never reaching a solution, and a random system may collapse.

|        | Closed       | Open              | Random        |
|--------|--------------|-------------------|---------------|
| Space  | Fixed        | Movable           | Dispersed     |
| Time   | Regular      | Variable          | Random        |
| Energy | Steady       | Flexible          | Fluctuating   |
| Power  | Hierarchical | Shared/Consensual | Laissez-Faire |

**FIG. 3.3.** Kantor and Lehr's Family Arrangement Model.

7. Territoriality is likely to be a feature of:
   a. closed systems.
   b. random systems.
   c. open systems.
   d. collectivist society.

Let's consider that the husband was raised in and maintains a closed system view of time. If the invitation says 7:00 P.M., he expects to arrive at that very moment. The wife has a more open system view of time and to her an invitation saying 7:00 P.M. means around 7:30 P.M. So they argue over who is right and end up accusing each other of rigidity and inconsideration. Reframing this issue as a systems conflict rather than as a personal flaw attack enables the couple to detoxify their resentments and understand their differences from a new perspective.

*Intracultural Variations.*   Not only is each family shaped by their culture, but also within cultures, families have shared and nonshared experiences which lead to intracultural variations. So we can never assume that all families of a similar race, ethnicity, sexual orientation, religion, class, etc. share all of the same values to the same intensity. There are both similarities and great variation within cultural groups. Similarly, within each family system, members have shared and nonshared experiences and individuals may view the shared experiences quite differently. It is also important to remember that each of us has different identities in different contexts which may change over the life span due to experiences and changing contexts. Within some groups, for example, gender may be salient over race; in some groups, race may be salient over sexual orientation. Check this out in your own family by comparing your views of family members and events with those of your siblings.

When, therefore, you are working with a couple who seems to be similar in cultural experiences, there are still differences in their perceptions, experiences, and meaning-making. There may be cultural and intracultural differences about any number of variables: the meaning of family; gender roles and expectations; the meaning, use, and distribution of power; the meaning and process of parenting; relationships with extended family and friends; the meaning, purpose, and management of money; the meaning of a sexual relationship, lovemaking, expressiveness of emotions, and tolerable boundaries. Then there are differences in communication styles and processes (both verbal and nonverbal), energy levels, time management, etc. All of these differences require implicit and explicit negotiation for a mutually gratifying relationship to evolve.

8. Spouses who come from different systems orientations:
   a. are doomed to continuous strife and conflict.
   b. can be helped to negotiate their differences.
   c. will have difficulty accepting the value of other system types.
   d. inevitably will see their differences as flaws in each other.

*Marginality.*   Within major cultures, there is unequal distribution of power. There are some groups with high levels of power which guarantee higher degrees of privilege. Privilege provides access to resources and opportunities. Those with the least amount of power have little privilege and are not entitled to the same resources and opportunities as those with power—they are *marginalized*. Most of us who have been born into privilege take it for granted and do not even think about the life experiences of those without privilege. Until recently, for example, Caucasians never realized that white racial identity has developmental trajectories as do minority racial identities. It is important for family therapists to consider the impact of both privilege and marginalization on themselves and on other individuals and their families. Nondominant cultures internalize the values of the dominant culture, which can result in internalized racism, sexism, homophobia, and other biases and prejudices for both the dominant and nondominant cultures. Generational experiences of marginalization and oppression reinforce low self esteem and also result in marginalized populations being pathologized rather than respected for their differences.

In intercultural relationships, we need to consider the impact of marginalization on the individual and the couple and family systems. Have all members experienced it? Some more than others? How does this affect the functioning and development of the family unit?

9. Each of the sociocultural systems in local, regional, state, and federal communities:
   a. operates as a system with its own functions, system/subsystem roles, and rules.
   b. is influenced by its own political agenda.
   c. is caught in the middle between their constituencies and their funding systems.
   d. attempts to cooperate with other social systems.

## ALTERNATIVE FAMILY SYSTEMS

Many traditional as well as diverse family structures and intercultural families enter therapy through the problems of a child or marital conflict. It is not unusual for the problems to be attributed to unmet expectations regarding the spouse, the marriage, the child, or parenting. Intercultural and diverse family structures differ, however, not only in the influences from the family of origin, but also in the sociocultural background in which they have been socialized. So the differences in worldviews, values, and expectations may be sharper than the differences in same-culture and traditionally structured families. For example, the couple may differ in their expectations concerning gender roles, family rules, transactional styles, intimacy, expression of emotions, parenting style, financial management, and so forth. If clinicians can understand these differences, they are better able to focus on commonalities and strengths and enhance individual and family system levels of acceptance and negotiation of differences.

10. Disturbed children are likely to come from:
    a. closed family systems.
    b. open family systems.
    c. random family systems.
    d. any of the above.

### Gay and Lesbian Families

Gays, lesbians and bisexuals are a diverse group of men and women who acknowledge their same-gender sexual orientation at different times in their life cycle, in different ways, and to different degrees (Okun, 1996). It is important to keep this variability in mind: not all gays and lesbians are aware of or acknowledge and work though their sexual orientation identity at the same time, same pace, or in the same way. There are two predominant types of gay and lesbian families: children from previous heterosexual unions and gay/lesbian singles or couples who create their own family through biological or adoptive means.

In the past, most children of gays and lesbians were born into previous heterosexual marriages that later dissolved. For these families, the issues related to "coming out" are complex for the gay and lesbian parents who worry about the impact on their children, on custody decisions, as well as on how to help children understand the political, social, or legal ramifications of their choices.

11. Gay and lesbian parents:
  a. are more likely to have gay or lesbian children.
  b. isolate themselves from heterosexual families.
  c. are likely to be emotionally disturbed because of their own internalized homophobia.
  d. are a self selected, highly motivated minority of all gays and lesbians.

*Parenting.* In the past few years, child rearing has become a more viable option for openly gay and lesbian couples. There are a variety of ways this can occur: donor insemination for one member of a lesbian couple with subsequent two parent adoption; foster care; domestic or international adoption of an infant or older child with or without special needs; use of an egg donor or surrogate mother for gay couples; or arrangement with a lesbian couple for artificial insemination or actual insemination which might or might not include co-parenting. As with the heterosexual community, there may be blended families including biological and adopted children, split couples sharing or not sharing child rearing, single parent families, and interracial and interfaith families. The types of families and means for developing families depend on financial and social resources as well as geographical variables.

12. Children from alternative family systems will undoubtedly:
  a. suffer cruelty from being out of the mainstream.
  b. suffer from identity confusion.
  c. need parental support and discussion about differences.
  d. yearn to belong to a traditional family.

Franklin (2003) has reviewed the research on lesbian and gay parenting and noted that, though children raised in gay/lesbian families do not differ significantly in psychological, social, or sexual makeup from children raised in heterosexual households, current research is focusing on differences between gay and lesbian parents and heterosexual parents. Gay and lesbian parents are found to have some strengths in their more egalitarian and authoritative parenting styles, heightened emotional attunement, and advocacy of gender role flexibility. Franklin points out that lesbian and gay parents are a self selected, highly motivated minority of all gays and lesbians. In addition to coping with societal homophobia, they have had to contend with political ramifications of larger gay and lesbian communities who are just now beginning to accept this subset of their communities. Gay and lesbian families tend to affiliate with a larger, diverse parent community in place of or in addition to their associations with gay/lesbian/bisexual and heterosexual communities. Preliminary studies suggest that perhaps children should be told about their conception early in life. No clear data is available to date.

13. Children created via donor eggs or sperm:
    a. should be told about this early in life since it is not a secret.
    b. should be encouraged to look for their biological parent.
    c. should never be told about their biological origins.
    d. should be protected from becoming attached to the non-biological parent.

In addition to the issues all parents face, lesbian and gay parents are never able to forget that they are a minority among parents, and, like all minorities, they face certain prejudices and stereotypes. In the absence of institutional validation (i.e., domestic partnership and same-sex adoption legislation), lesbian and gay couples must develop extensive legal documentation to ensure protection of their families (Okun, 1996; Lev, 2000). This may include power of attorney papers that state both partners' legal rights to make medical decisions for the child(ren), as well as a will in which a parent's wishes for legal custody of the child(ren) are clearly outlined in the event of his or her death. Families of origin vary in their acceptance, support, and availability to their gay and lesbian family member.

*Legal Issues.* The "nexus" standard requires that there be a clear connection (or "nexus") between a parent's sexual identity and harm to the child before the parent's sexual orientation assumes any relevance in a custody, visitation, or adoption dispute (Lamda Legal Defense, 1997). Under this approach, the sexual orientation of the parent alone cannot form the basis of denying parenting rights unless it is demonstrated to cause harm to the child (currently about 60% of the states have adopted some variant of a nexus test.) As of April 1997, second-parent adoptions (adoption by the partner of a biological parent) by lesbian and gay couples has been approved by courts in the District of Columbia and twenty-one states (Lamda Legal Defense, 1997). Another legal issue concerns donor insemination. While laws governing this vary from state to state, most states' laws apply only to married women and exclude lesbians. The primary legal concern is whether the sperm donor will be recognized as the father of the child which is the reason that many lesbians choose anonymous donors through sperm banks (Lev, 2000). As more and more agencies are established to meet these new needs of prospective gay and lesbian parents, medical, legal, and emotional support will become more available and accessible.

14. Gay, lesbian, and cohabiting adoptive families:
    a. have difficulties in some states getting health benefits for their children.
    b. can only have two unmarried parent adoptions in a few states.
    c. are exposing their children to risks in getting into public schools.
    d. have no access to traditional community services.

## Adoptive Families

For adoptive families, straight or homosexual, there are psychological effects on the birth parents, the adoptive parents, the adoptee, siblings, and other members involved in the family. The birth parents deal with an unexpected or unwanted pregnancy, choices about whether or not to have the child as well as difficult choices about whether to keep the baby or give it to kin or put it up for adoption. If adoption is the choice, what type of adoption? Private? Through an agency? Open? Semi-open? Closed? Do the birth parents leave information for the child at a certain age or leave permission for a later search? The longer lasting effects on the birth parents have not been clarified, due to the paucity of studies about this particular sample. Each situation and set of circumstances is unique, which would complicate long-term study. In some cultures (e.g., African American and Latino), informal adoption of children within the community is prevalent.

15. Adoptees:
   a. have a biological imperative to seek out biological parents.
   b. are more compliant than biological children.
   c. create more marital stress for the adoptive parents.
   d. may have healthy, valid reasons for not wanting to seek biological parents.

Typically, the life cycle of the adoptive parents consists of coping with issues such as infertility, choosing to adopt, deciding between **domestic** adoption and **transcultural** adoption, coping with the frustrations of the placement process and with social stigma related to adoption, and developing family and social support for the adoption—all before the infant or child is adopted (Brodzinsky, Smith, & Brodzinsky, 1998). After the adoption, the adoptive parents take on their identity as adoptive parents and deal with their own, and later their child's, thoughts and feelings about the child's birth parents (Okun, 1996). It is important to remember that every adoption experience is different for each individual and for each family. Research on the prevalence of learning and emotional disabilities of adoptees is mixed (Miller, Fan, Christensen, Grotevant, & Van Dulmen, 2000; Sharma, Mc Gue, & Benson, 1998; Haugaard, 1998; Brand & Brinick, 1999; Okun, 1996). The differences depend on culture, race, ethnicity, class, birth parent history, prenatal history, genetic predisposition, the adoptive family history, and the environment in which the child is raised.

*Attachment Issues.* The *primal wound theory* is often associated with adoptees, suggesting that "Adoptees start life somewhat trust impaired and have to overcome the broken trust of being abandoned by their biological mother" (Groza & Rosenberg, 1998). Adoptees, because of their abandonment at birth, are thought to have attachment and separation issues resulting in being too trustful of others or, conversely, unable to trust or connect with others. Another theory is called *cumulative adoption trauma,* wherein the child continues to feel separation trauma when he or she understands that he or she was not born to the adoptive mother (Groza & Rosenberg, 1998, p. 9). Some adoptees might feel that because they were saved or rescued by their adoptive parents, they must be grateful to them and try to become who they perceive their adoptive parents want them to be. Others (Franklin & Ferber, 1998; Okun, 1996; and Groza & Rosenberg, 1998) suggest that children involved in open adoptions, where they may have varying degrees of information about or contact with their birth parents, are less likely to develop attachment difficulties.

*Identity Development.* Adoptees may have different identity experiences compared with nonadopted children. Not only may they experience divided loyalties and divided senses of self (the surface self, the hidden self), they struggle with two sets of mental parent images—one the imagined or real birth parents and the other the adoptive parents. Search and reunion are issues with which adoptees deal throughout their lives. There is no evidence that choosing to search is healthier than choosing not to search, although there are practitioners who are partial to a particular view. There are both psychological and health issues to be considered. The literature about search and reunion is now being applied to children from donor eggs or donor sperm. As I've stated elsewhere (Okun, 1996), until there is evidence suggesting that a search and possible reunion is necessary for healthy identity development, clinicians need to remain multipartial and help each individual come to terms with their genetic history in a way that makes sense and is meaningful to the individual.

16. Interracial and international adoptive families:
    a. should consider assimilation to be a major objective and ignore racial and ethnic differences.
    b. should acknowledge and expose the child to his or her race and culture.
    c. should expect their child to have learning and emotional disabilities.
    d. should avoid telling the child about his adoption until he is a teenager.

*Adjustment.* Acknowledging that adoption has psychological effects on all parties to the adoption triad—the birth parents, the adoptive parents, and the adoptees and other family members—is crucial. Recognizing and accepting racial, ethnic and physical appearance differences and integrating multiple family systems helps develop a healthy functioning family system. Families who only recognize the problematic information about the birth parents, particularly when an adopted child behaves or performs poorly, create "the bad seed theory" (Groza & Rosenberg, 1998.) Psychoeducation in the form of bibliotherapy and support groups are invaluable counseling interventions.

Current research on the psychological effects of adoption on children indicate that there is no clear evidence about the existence or degree of negative effects of adoption. It may be that adjustment difficulties in adopted children are overrated. It may be that adopted children are referred more frequently than nonadopted children for treatment due to more manifest problems, to adoptive parents' lower threshold for referral, or to biases in referral for mental health treatment by both parents, school personnel, and physicians. Most of the studies seem to indicate that the availability of pre-adoption education about resolving infertility issues and the possible risks of adoption as well as post-adoption long-term support are desirable.

## Intercultural Families

Increasingly, interfaith, interethnic, and interracial marriages are occurring. This can be attributed to the higher likelihood of meeting and developing relationships with diverse populations in school or college, at the work place, in more integrated neighborhoods, and at community and religious or spiritual centers. Though there is still a social stigma associated with these relationships, it has lessened and there are areas in this country (particularly major metropolitan areas) where little attention is paid to interracial families. Intercultural relationship development involves two major foci in addition to the usual individual, couple, and family development phases: (a) individual racial, ethnic, and religious identity development, and (b) couple/family multicultural identity development. Couple members find themselves in a paradoxical position of representing their own and their partner's cultural groups. In terms of racial awareness, each partner must understand his or her own, the partner's, their collective cultural groups, and the partner's cultural groups. They must learn to cope with social definitions or constructions of race and develop effective proactive and reactive strategies. Then, as their multicultural identities emerge, they can begin to develop self-sustaining strategies and see and accept themselves as "different," so that they can develop effective problem-solving skills.

17. Biracial children may:
    a. always feel they have to choose one race over the other.
    b. identify with the parent closest to them in physical appearance.
    c. attribute their parents' disagreements or fights to racial differences.
    d. learn to value multiculturalism.

Children of multicultural families need support for their multicultural identity development. Only recently, for example, have census and other forms allowed for "other' or "multicultural" classification. When children do not develop a firm sense of identity, their psychological development suffers and this suffering may be manifested in behavioral problems. Multicultural children struggle to merge their parents' different heritages without having to choose sides or compromise either one. Teachers, peers, peers' families, kin, and their neighborhoods and communities further influence these children's identity development, to say nothing of popular literature and the media. These external influences can foster multicultural identity or impinge upon it.

Much research (Okun, 1996; Kilpatrick & Holland, 2003; Franklin, 2003) points to the resilience and unique openness to and acceptance of different kinds of people and cultures demonstrated by children who are reared in gay/lesbian, adoptive, and multicultural families. However, these families experience heightened consciousness of racism, homophobia, prejudice and ignorance: strangers may stare and ask rude questions; peers may taunt children; family and former friends may disapprove and distance. Educational and health personnel also have biases and stereotypes, believing perhaps that there is genetic imperfections in some cultural groups, that multicultural children are inherently disadvantaged and are doomed to developmental difficulties and that adoptees and other multicultural children will be unable to conform to mainstream lifestyles and clearly establish self-identity. This marginalization is not helped by society's propensity to categorize people, thinking of non-dominant people as deviant and classifying any multicultural child with the non-dominant culture parents.

18. African American and Latino families typically:
    a. value intermarriage.
    b. accept readily homosexual and bisexual members.
    c. informally adopt children who need families.
    d. deny spirituality.

## Grandparent-Led Families

The 2000 census points out that the numbers of children in grandparent led households have increased 30% since 1990 and 105% since 1970 (U.S. Census Bureau 2002). The majority of grandparents raising grandchildren are ages 58 to 64, but 20% to 25% are over age 65. Although grandparent led families cross all socio-economic levels and all races, these grandparents are more likely to live in poverty than other grandparents. It is interesting to note that there are eight times more children in grandparent led homes than in the foster care system. Typically, these grandparents are responding to issues in the middle (parent) generation, such as illness, divorce, immaturity, incarceration of the parent, substance abuse, child abuse, or neglect. Drug and alcohol abuse account for 80% of grandparent families (Okun, 1996; U.S. Census Bureau 2002). Grandparents step in to fill a gap created by the problem as a result of the love they feel for their grandchildren, the shame they feel about their offspring, and a fierce determination to keep their grandchildren out of the foster system.

It is important for you, as a family therapist, to understand the additional challenges grandparent families face. There are complex legal issues around custody, guardianship, or adoption, and without legal status, grandparents may be unable to enroll their grandchildren in school or make medical decisions for them. Financial decisions may involve a grandparent's employment or applying for benefits like medical assistance, kinship care, foster care or Social Security. Appropriate childcare needs to be located, including day care, before and after school programs, and respite care. The grandparents' health, relationships with other offspring and kin, friends, and so forth create unique social and emotional needs related to parenting the second time around. Obviously, each family faces unique circumstances, dependent on financial, emotional, social, community, regional, legal, race, ethnicity, sexual orientation, and class variables.

19. Grandparent families:
    a. provide grandparents with the opportunity to repeat their parenting failures.
    b. provide grandparents with the opportunity to rectify their own parenting failures.
    c. exist largely in lower class minority families.
    d. put children at risk.

Family therapists can help grandparents grieve the difficulties of the middle generation and deal with shame and blame about the outcomes of their own parenting. They may also experience anger, embarrassment, guilt, and frustration and resentment at the disruption of their retirement dreams and the necessity to give up their own life plans. Grandparents may feel generational confusion, not understanding today's models of education, discipline, appropriate limits, and boundaries. The grandchildren may have special needs due to previous trauma, abuse, or neglect and may take their anger and resentment out on the grandparents, feeling divided loyalties and confusion about the temporariness or permanence of this situation. Understanding unique circumstances, kinship systems, and sociocultural contexts of each family is necessary for effective treatment.

## CLINICAL IMPLICATIONS

Regardless of discipline or specialization, clinicians need to be aware of their own cultural identities and biased assumptions and be open to multiple perspectives. These characteristics are essential to developing an effective helping relationship, no matter which theoretical model is utilized. Certain cultural groups distrust and resent both the concept and process of therapy and only by joining this resistance can the therapist patiently and empathically build trust. For example, a study by Crawford, McLeod, Zamboni, & Jordan (1999) found that psychologists are more likely to recommend adoption for a heterosexual couple than for a lesbian or gay couple. As reported by Franklin (2003), clinicians may not believe they are racist, sexist, or homophobic, but their decision-making may be influenced by unconscious prejudices. People raised in dominant cultures take privilege and power for granted and are often shocked when they learn about the routine harassment others experience. "Different than" does not mean "less than."

20. Clinicians need to:
    a. become aware of their own cultural identities and biased assumptions.
    b. understand that cultural identities underlie all presenting problems.
    c. understand that family theories are universal.
    d. apply the same treatment strategies to all clients.

However, therapists should not automatically assume that couple or family conflict is based on cultural differences. Conflicts may derive from temperament and personality differences; family system organization; or from a member's disabilities, health issues, substance abuse, poverty, unemployment, isolation, and so forth. Though we do not want to pathologize behavior that differs from mainstream norms, we need to find a balance between recognizing and acknowledging pathology if and when it does exist and difficulties due to cultural differences.

It is helpful to recognize that all families are part of two systems, namely, a dominant culture that is the source of power and economic resources and then their own nurturing system, the physical and social environment of the family and community (Kilpatrick & Holland, 2003). Whether these two systems are congruent or not may be a major issue. Khisty's (2001) model of **transcultural differentiation** helps families co-existing with both their culture of origin and their adoptive culture change and evolve into entities which transcend both the culture of origin and adoptive cultures.

21. Strategies for assessing cultural influences include:
    a. Rorschach
    b. MMPI
    c. Eco/genogram
    d. Family Assessment Instrument

Pinderhughes (1995, p. 266) suggested five areas of competence for clinicians:

1. Knowledge of specific values, beliefs, and cultural practices of clients.
2. Ability to respect and appreciate the values, beliefs, and practices of all clients, including those culturally different, and to perceive such individuals through their own cultural lenses instead of the practitioner's.
3. Ability to be comfortable with differences in others and not be trapped in anxiety about differences or defensive behaviors.
4. Ability to think flexibly and to recognize that one's own way of thinking and behaving is not the only way.
5. Ability to behave flexibly.

## Strategies for Exploring Cultural Differences

Some intercultural families resist discussing cultural differences, insisting that their difficulties are separate; others are willing and relieved to explore connections. However, when an intercultural family seeks or is referred to therapy, they need to experience a co-valuing, respectful working relationship in order to develop trust and make a commitment to doing their part of the therapeutic work.

22. A powerful strategy for working with intercultural and diverse family structure systems is:
    a. role playing.
    b. mirroring.
    c. empowerment.
    d. acculturation exercises.

There are many strategies that therapists can use to explore cultural differences. One is the **genogram** (McGoldrick, 1998), which can elicit different family patterns as well as cultural heritage influences (see Fig. 3.4). Another is an **ecogram** (see Fig. 3.2) which can be amplified to refine cultural differences. Congress (1994) has developed a **culturagram** which can be applied to immigrant populations or combined with the genogram into a cultural genogram. This family assessment tool assesses: (a) reasons for immigration; (b) length of time in community; (c) legal status; (d) age at time of immigration; (e) language spoken at home and in the community; (f) health beliefs; (g) celebrated holidays and special events; (h) impact of crisis events; (i) values regarding family, education, and work; and (j) contact with cultural institutions.

23. Family clinicians should:
    a. explain the rationale for their own assumptions.
    b. form an alliance with the most mainstream member of the family.
    c. be multipartial and flexible.
    d. minimize differences.

Narrative therapists suggest circular questioning, by asking a family member to answer the question, "What would your spouse's life have been like if he or she had lived life according to his or her family's and culture's expectations and prescriptions?" Would he or she have married you?" These questions can be developed ad lib and posed to other family members. Sanchez (1999) suggests that traditional structured questions and formal interviews are not designed to draw out families' authentic self-expression necessary for understanding families' experiences within their sociocultural contexts. He suggests that we let family members tell their own stories in their own ways.

Often, a family member who has discussed reasons for a consultation over the telephone prior to the first meeting comes to the session with an intercultural family. It has never occurred to them to mention these cultural differences; it is important for clinicians to raise these issues during the first session. On the other hand, when seeking therapy, family spokespeople may ask you over the phone about your experience with interracial, gay/lesbian, grandparent families, etc. The latter group is already expressing awareness about special issues their cultural group experiences.

Religious, racial, sexual orientation, alternative family structure, and ethnic differences can impact the balance of power in relationships and these can become particularly painful around weddings, holidays, gender roles, friendships, child-rearing, dress code, food, social responses—increasing as the children pass through the school years. Parents of intercultural families may take one of three positions: (a) ethnicity, sexual orientation are irrelevant, (b) children should be raised with the identity of the parent from the non-dominant group, or (c) children should be raised with inclusive identities of both parents. Clinicians can support the parents' choice of creating an intercultural family and provide suggestions for exposing children to multiple heritages. Clinicians can help parents and children talk openly to each other through teaching them the right words to use and by avoiding attributing problems to a mixed heritage. For example, multiracial children often hear the terms "oreo," "half-breed," "mutt," "hang black," "go white," "roll Asian," "fag," or "queer." Regardless of the presenting problem, helping families cope with societal oppression becomes an essential part of the therapeutic process.

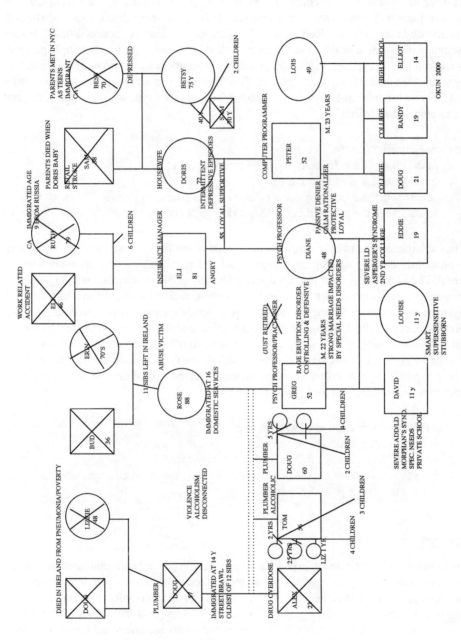

**FIG. 3.4.** Sample Genogram.

## Strengths and Resilience

Clinicians can emphasize strengths as a framework for family therapy while still acknowledging difficulties and obstacles. Many intercultural and diverse family structure families have given more thoughtful, careful consideration to marrying or partnering and having children than those from dominant, mainstream cultures. This can be considered a sign of strength and resilience in and of itself. Reframing difficulties experienced as "personal flaws" from a transcultural perspective enables the family to look at the same event from multiple perspectives and can lead to feelings of efficacy. Affirming diversity is an important therapeutic tool if communicated authentically and empathically. Therefore, it is incumbent on therapists who do not feel comfortable working with a particular family system type to acknowledge this and make an appropriate referral.

24. Family clinicians should:
    a. fit the client family to the clinician's preferred model.
    b. fit the theory to the client family.
    c. when using a theoretical model, utilize only the techniques derived from that model.
    d. be atheoretical when working with non dominant family types.

Thus, clinicians need to be sensitive to the special issues that diverse families face as well as continuously developing their awareness of self, of relationships, and of others who are different. The literature is clear that open acknowledgment of differences; encouragement of participation in multicultural activities; and open communication within subsystems, between subsystems, and with outside support systems help family systems adapt by redefining roles, enforcing rules and control, aiding subsystem disruption, and accommodating to developmental and sociocultural changes. For example, when a two-parent family is separated by divorce or death, the rules, roles, boundaries, and communications processes necessarily change and family therapists can work with the parents, the couple in the case of divorce, and the children to reappraise and reformulate systems operations.

25. The family into which one is born:
    a. is responsible for individual pathology.
    b. is shaped primarily by the family of origin systems.
    c. is a powerful but not the only major influence on their children's development.
    d. defines the lifescript for each child.

## Advocacy

It is helpful for you, as a clinician, to provide information on general and community resources, referrals to support groups, access to specialized services, and advocacy support. Empowerment is one of the most effective strategies family therapists can employ, focusing on family strengths and utilizing role-playing and other cognitive/behavioral techniques to move from "victimization" to "efficacy" stands on the part of the family members and family system as a whole. Many intercultural families are isolated and lack support services as well as updated information. They are afraid to be in contact with the schools, to ask questions, to advocate for services because they expect to be "put down" and rejected.

An example of advocacy with grandparent led families, is to include in your assessment the needs and issues of the grandparents, that is, increased financial difficulties, disruption in life expectations, increased demands on their physical health as well as pre-existing conditions, increased social isolation due to increasing demands of children, and impact on the marriage. These grandparents can be introduced to the more than 400 groups in the United States— Grandparents Rights Group, Grandparents Raising Grandchildren, Parents Again, United Grandparents Raising Grandchildren, Second-Timers Support group. Boston, for example, is the first city to construct public housing for grandparents with both handicap accessible and toddler-proofed facilities. These families also need access to legal clinics who will help them with the legal papers necessary for guardianship. In addition, clinicians need to be sensitive to generational differences and societal reactions. These reactions include both respect for the grandparents' sacrifice to keep the family together, but also blame toward the very same grandparents for the reasons their offspring (the grandchildren's parents) are unable to parent. Additional strategies include the use of bibliotherapy, Internet searches, specific suggestions or referrals to information sources, support groups, collateral professionals, etc.

26. Research:
   a. supports the use of constructivism with diverse family structures.
   b. supports the use of strategic interventions with diverse family structures.
   c. does not validate any one theoretical model for any one cultural group.
   d. does not attempt to measure outcomes.

Adoptive families, particularly transracial adoptive families, and foster families not only require support regarding issues associated with raising adopted children, but exposure to the birth parents' cultural group and culture-specific support. These parents often want to know when and what to tell their adoptees. Parents of children from donor eggs or donor sperms want to know what, if anything, to tell their children and what to attribute to biology and what to attribute to environment. As therapists, we must also be educators and advocates. We need to keep up with research findings and local resources.

The ecological/systems perspective requires clinicians to intervene and respond systemically both with families and the organizations with which they are involved as opposed to limiting their focus to family systems (Leitch, 1999; Okun, 1996). We need to empower the family to link with resources in the community, the state, and larger sociocultural systems. We need to establish collateral contact with the schools, health, or judicial personnel—whomever is part of the family's life. By advocacy, I mean clinicians making phone calls and collecting and disseminating information. Some clients do not know how to read very well or even how to collect information and need our tutelage and example to learn how to do so. Specifically, we need to acknowledge isolation—which contributes to the feelings of differences—financial realities, crises, and coping mechanisms of the family. We need to educate parents how to openly discuss differences, how to provide significant same culture models, and encourage participation in same cultural activities for each member of the family.

## APPLICATION OF THEORETICAL MODELS

The original family systems theorists and practitioners (Ackerman, Bowen, Haley, Minuchin, Satir, Whitaker, and others) based their models on the traditional dominant culture: white, married heterosexual parents, patriarchal, with middle class values. Their theories implied a dominant, preferred model of the family. To date, the research does not validate any one theoretical model for any one cultural group. Some cultural groups want directives from experts; some require a more relational friendly relationship. Most research focuses on the trusting, understanding relationship with the therapist as the main vehicle for change. Techniques may only be effective within the context of mutual trust and respectful understanding.

Though techniques from each theoretical model can be helpful, it is important to examine the theoretical model itself to understand whether the underlying premises are suitable to today's varied family systems. Remember, these theories were developed for the mainstream, nuclear family and they imply a model of the way families are "supposed to be." It is also important to keep in mind that many families are not seeking ongoing therapy; after the presenting issues are cleared up, they may want to keep the door open for further consultation, but the therapist's goal is not to foster dependency but to empower them to learn new problem solving skills. This does not mean that an individual family member may not require or benefit from individual or group therapy.

27. If each parent in a family comes from a different cultural or system type:
    a. one type has to prevail.
    b. a power struggle about whose view is the best will prevail.
    c. misunderstandings are inevitable.
    d. negotiation of differences is necessary.

There are aspects of each theoretical model that can be helpful to diverse families. The empathic joining with the family, using their language, positively reframing, and facilitating open communication can create the type of respectful context in which self and system esteem can rise. This type of relationship is compassionate and focuses on family strengths rather than problems, victimization, and blame. However, her notion of "open communications" and flexible family style may or may not conflict with the cultural values and beliefs of some members of the family.

Bowen's (1961) coaching to facilitate connection to current family members and family of origin systems can foster compassion and understanding of cultural and structural differences. By focusing on multigenerational influences, the client family may develop better understanding of current beliefs, values, and patterns of functioning. However, the theory's western culture focus on differentiation of self may not be in accord with the values and beliefs of families from high context cultural groups.

Strategic (Haley, 1971) and solution-focused strategies can provide the straight directives for which many families yearn. Many families come in because they want "to fix the problem," usually of the identified patient, and if these strategies resolve the presenting problem, it is likely that the secondary gain will involve family reorganization. These approaches may be effective because of the "expertise" of the therapist in assuming responsibility for the process of therapy. It is important to be cautious about the use of paradoxical directives, however, as they could breed distrust by not fitting into the family's type of meaning-making.

Structural therapy, which focuses on reorganizing the family system to resolve presenting difficulties, can also be helpful with diverse families even though this model assumes a hierarchical, traditional family structure. Minuchin (1974) is conscious of cultural differences and joins the family in such a way as to mime their language and patterns of interaction by observing their interactional patterns. His use of repetition of the interactional patterns creating and sustaining the "problem," can enable the family to "get it" and be amenable to alternatives.

28. A theoretical model that may be particularly suited to diverse family structures and intercultural families is:
    a. structural family theory.
    b. strategic family theory.
    c. experiential family theory.
    d. constructivism family theories.

The constructivist therapies (White & Epston, 1990) are particularly suited to diverse family structures and intercultural families by focusing on the family's meaning-making processes and the social constructions which they have assumed as "the truth." Relying on storytelling or narratives, this approach enables the therapist to collaboratively co-instruct alternative stories or narratives to bring about change. Families from high context cultures may have difficulties questioning their assumptions and accepting optional perspectives, but this approach allows for a respectful therapeutic stance which can create the context for growth and development.

29. Clinicians need to consider which of the following when working with single parent families:
    a. help children to seek role models of the parent's opposite gender.
    b. help children to accept doing a disproportionate amount of chores.
    c. expect the single parent to use a child as a replacement partner.
    d. help the family to restructure their system with developmentally appropriate rules and roles.

Table 3.1 summarizes the theoretical applications to intercultural and diverse family structures. When working with families, it is important to assess and formulate treatment plans that most effectively meet the needs of the client system, rather than adapting your own treatment preferences to families you treat. Considering intra- and intersystem variables is critical.

30. Table 3.1 indicates:
    a. there is one preferred theoretical model for alternative families.
    b. there is one theoretical model that is better than other models.
    c. each theory has something of value to contribute.
    d. clinicians should be trained thoroughly in one model.

# KEY TERMS

**collectivism:** Cultural value is on the welfare of the group over the welfare of the individual.

**culturagram:** A transgenerational family systems mapping of cultural identities and affiliations, including times and patterns of immigration.

**diverse family structure:** Nonmainstream family systems, i.e., grandparent led, adoptive, foster, single parent, cohabitating groupings. May or may not be biologically related.

**domestic adoption:** Refers to adoption that takes place within the United States of America.

**ecogram:** Mapping of multiple contexts that shape one's identity, i.e., primarily family, school, work, communities, cultural attitudes, ideologies, race, class, ethnicity, etc.

**ecological/systems model:** Consideration of individual as embedded in his or her family system, which is, in turn, embedded in larger sociocultural systems, i.e., neighborhood, community, state, federal, universal systems.

**TABLE 3.1**

Highlighted Application of Different Theoretical Models to Family Types

| Family Type | Experiential/ Communication | Structural | Strategic | Bowenian | Constructivism |
|---|---|---|---|---|---|
| GAY/LESBIAN | Relational joining Positive reframing Focus on strengths and make implicit rules and operations clear | Focus on boundaries and organization Miming language and patterns of interaction | Focus on resolving presenting problems by straight & paradoxical directives May use behavioral strategies | Focus on self differentiation levels and detriangulation May include outside social systems and families of origin | Focus on ways family members have experienced and interpreted oppression using questions encouraging each member to tell own story: help family work together to cope with externalized problems rather then blame selves/each other. |
| ADOPTIVE | Relational joining Open secrets for honest communications—adoption story Acknowledge differences Make implicit rules clear | Focus on boundaries and parental hierarchy | Focus on resolving presenting problems by straight and paradoxical interventions May use behavioral strategies | Focus on genogram and, if available, birth parent information to relieve anxieties about these issues and repair boundaries | Family "adoption" story, story about birth parents, story about adoptive parents and interpretation of adoption experiences; help them to examine effects of these stories on family problems and broaden scope of stories. |
| INTERCULTURAL | Model respect for differences Focus on clear expressions of experiences of marginalization Help family to negotiate differences effectively | Balanced organization Attends to coalitions along cultural lines | Focus on resolving presenting problems by straight and paradoxical directives May use behavioral strategies | Uses genograms to clarify transgeneral issues in different cultures and adjust boundaries | Focus on each member telling personal and cultural story, focusing on how racism or oppression influences these stories; help family respectfully develop transracial/cultural story as way of being together. |
| GRANDPARENT | Empathic support and appreciation of grandparents Psychoeducation and family sculpting to heal generational gaps Foster development of effective roles and rules | Emphasizes grandparental hierarchy and appropriate boundaries for absent parents | Focus on resolving presenting problems by straight and paradoxical directives May use behavioral strategies | Uses genograms to illustrate family patterns and develop appropriate individuation boundaries and rules. | Focus on stories of family members about parents, grandparents, grandchildren and how circumstances led to this type of family structure; help family to construct story that is sensitive to generational issues. |

**genogram:** Multi-generational mapping of family to elicit family patterns and cultural heritage influences.

**high context:** Refers to a culture that is collectivist, where the individual's group membership supercedes individual identity.

**individualism:** Refers to the value of individual autonomy superceding the needs and interests of the groups of which the individual is a member.

**low context:** Refers to a culture where individualism is valued more highly than group membership.

**marginality:** Occurs when dominant groups withhold access to power and privileges from nondominant groups.

**transcultural adoption:** Refers to adoption of a child of another race or ethnic culture.

**transcultural differentiation:** Occurs when families are able to co-exist with both their cultures of origin and adoptive cultures and form an integrated cultural identity.

## DISCUSSION QUESTIONS—GENERAL ISSUES

Answer these questions individually and then compare your answers with one to five other people—classmates, peers, friends, colleagues. Try to include some people who you think come from a different culture than you do. By different culture, I refer to race, ethnicity, gender, religion, sexual orientation, disability, generation, class, region, etc. The purpose of this exercise is to become aware of your definition of a family and how it compares to or differs from others' definitions.

1. Define a family from your point of view.
2. How did you decide whom to include and exclude in this definition?
3. Write down ten characteristics that you believe describes an "OK" family. (You decide what "OK" means to you.)
4. Describe what you consider to be the boundaries, operating rules, and roles of family members in your definition of an "OK" family.
5. How similar or dissimilar are your answers to these questions to the family system in which you were raised?
6. While there are great variations within cultural groupings, consider what variables might influence responses of families in the following situations?
   - How might an American family and an Asian American family view paternal involvement differently?
   - How might a small southern town respond to a lesbian family as opposed to a suburb of a midwestern metropolitan area?
   - How do you think a rural African American family might respond to their son dating a Caucasian woman?
   - How might a Mormon family deal with a lesbian daughter's *in vitro* pregnancy?
   - How might a Caucasian middle class family deal with their daughter leaving her husband and children to pursue her career?

## DISCUSSION QUESTIONS—CASES

1. Aimee, thirty-two, a Japanese American music teacher, and Lance, thirty-one, a Caucasian computer worker came for couples therapy because of incessant fighting. They argued

over money (she liked to plan and save and he liked to live from check to check), when to have children (she wanted to begin a family and be a stay-at-home mom like her mother and he wanted to wait until the economy recovered more), and whether they spent too much time with Aimee's family on holidays rather than being alone or with friends. Aimee's style of fighting was to verbally express her concerns in a pleading manner and Lance's style of fighting was to change the subject and walk out of the room. They could go for two to three days avoiding any kind of contact. What are your thoughts and feelings about this case example? With whom do you identify? What kinds of information do you want and what are the systems variables you want to consider? What cultural variables may be affecting this couple's relationship? How would you devise a treatment plan? What would your goals be?

2. Ginny is a forty-two-year-old Caucasian who has been married to a forty-four-year-old Kenyan professor, Mark, for sixteen years. They have a five-year-old son who is having difficulty in pre-kindergarten in an all-white private school. Ginny gave up her career to raise her child and her husband, a driven workaholic, is only now engaging with the son around school issues. The parents are upset about their son's "immaturity" and distraction by peers. The family has no social life and Ginny is beginning to wonder about her son's racial identity. What questions might you ask Ginny about her experiences as part of an interracial couple in each of the countries in which she has lived? Discuss possible recommendations you might make for dealing with racial identity. What resources might you refer this family to?

3. John, thirty-seven, and Clark, thirty-five, have decided to have children. John wants to adopt a foreign child and Clark wants to use surrogacy to avoid adoption risks. They are coming to resolve this conflict. As a therapist, what issues would you want to raise with them? What information would you want them to learn? How would you help them to reach a mutually satisfying solution?

4. Ms. Smith brought her fifteen-year-old adopted daughter, Rosalie, to therapy. Rosalie has been oppositional at home, although a "delight" at school and Ms. Smith is desperate for help. The previous therapist told her that Rosalie needs to search for her biological mother in order to develop a whole identity. Ms. Smith is willing to help Rosalie do this, but Rosalie refuses and claims she is not interested in this search. Ms. Smith fears that Rosalie will be "damaged' if she does not pursue this. What are your thoughts and feelings about this? What would you say to this mother and daughter? How would you proceed?

## SUGGESTED FURTHER READING

Boyd-Franklin, N. (2003). *Black families in therapy: Understanding the African American experience* (2nd ed). New York: Guilford Press.

Utilizing case examples, this text addresses the problems and challenges facing African American families and communities of different socioeconomic class levels. The impact of racism on gender socialization and relationships is explored and multisystemic treatments are suggested utilizing spiritual and community resources for clinical change.

Degenova, M. K. (1997). *Families in cultural context: Strengths and challenges in diversity.* Mountain View, CA: Mayfield Publications.

This text includes chapters devoted to different ethnic American families, explaining their structures, lives, and experiences in a way that can help clinicians formulate effective culture sensitive theories.

McGoldrick, M. (Ed.). (1998). *Revisioning family therapy: Race, culture, and gender in clinical practice (2nd ed.).* New York: Guilford Press.

Distinguished authors broaden family systems theory and practice through cultural lenses. The chapters cover a wide range of diverse families and represent cutting edge perspectives integrating theories and practice.

Okun, B. F. (1996). *Working with diverse families: What practitioners need to know*. New York: Guilford Press.

This book discusses in depth the sociocultural contexts and developmental and psychological issues of adoptive families, gay and lesbian families, interracial families, grandparent and reproductive technology families. Attention is paid to family members' identities, supports, and obstacles, for example marginalization and theoretical and intervention implications for clinicians.

# REFERENCES

Bowen, M. (1961). Family psychotherapy. *American Journal of Orthopsychiatry, 31*, 40–60.

Brand, A. E., & Brinick, P. M. (1999). Behavior problems and mental health contacts in adopted, foster and non-adopted children. *Journal of Child Psychology and Psychiatry, 40*(1), 1221–1229.

Brodzinsky, D. M., Smith, D. W., & Brodzinsky, A. B. (1998). Children's adjustment to adoption: Development and clinical issues. *Developmental Clinical Psychology and Psychiatry, 38*, 1–142.

Congress, E. (1994). The use of culturagrams to assess and empower culturally diverse families. *Families in Society, 75*, 531–540.

Crawford, I., McLeod, A., Zamboni, B. D., & Jordan, M. B. (1999). Psychologists' attitudes towards gay and lesbian parenting. *Professional Psychology: Research and Practice, 30*(4), 394–401.

Franklin, K. (2003). Practice opportunities with an emerging family form: The planned lesbian and gay family. *Journal of Forensic Psychology Practice, 3*(3), 47–64.

Franklin, L. C. & Ferber, E. (1998). *May the circle be unbroken: An intimate journey into the heart of adoption*. New York: Harmony Books.

Groza, V., & Rosenberg, K. F. (1998). *Clinical and practical issues in adoption: Bridging the gap between adoptees placed as infants and as older children*. Westport, CT: Praeger.

Haley, J. (1971). *Changing families*. New York: Grune & Stratton.

Haugaard, J. J. (1998). Is adoption a risk factor for the development of adjustment problems? *Clinical Psychological Review, 18*(1), 47–69.

Kantor, D., & Lehr, W. (1975). *Inside the family*. San Francisco: Jossey-Bass.

Khisty, K. (2001). Transcultural differentiation: A model for therapy with ethno-culturally diverse families. *Australian and New Zealand Journal of Family Therapy, 22*(1), 17–24.

Kilpatrick, A. C. & Holland, T. P. (2003). *Working with families: An integrative model by level of need* (3rd ed.). New York: Pearson Education.

Lamda Legal Defense and Education Fund: Lesbian and Gay Parenting (1997). Retrieved September 29, 1997, from http://www.lamdalegal.org/cgi-bin/pages/documents/record/record=31

Leitch, M. (1999). The AMMFT Head Start training partnership project: Enhancing MFT capacities beyond the family system. *Journal of Marital and Family Therapy, 25*(2), 14–54.

Lev, A. I. (2000). Lesbian and gay parenting. Retrieved October 12, 2000, from http://www.lamdalegal.org/cgi-bin/pages/documents/record/record=31

Maney, D. W., & Cain, R. E. (1997). Preservice elementary teachers' attitudes toward gay and lesbian parents. *Journal of School Health, 67*, 236–245.

McGoldrick, M. (Ed.). (1998). *Revisioning family therapy: Race, culture and gender in clinical practice* (2nd ed.). New York: Guilford Press.

Miller, B. C., Fan, X., Christensen, M., Grotevant, H. D., & Van Dulmen, M. (2000). Comparisons of adopted and non-adopted adolescents in a large nationally representative sample. *Child Development, 71*(5), 1458–1473.

Minuchin, S. (1974). *Families and family therapy*. Cambridge, MA: Harvard University Press.

Okun, B. F. (1996). *Understanding diverse families: What practitioners need to know*. New York: Guilford Press.

Okun, B. F., Fried, H., & Okun, M. L. (1999). *Understanding diversity: A learning as practice primer*. Pacific Grove, CA: Brooks/Cole.

Pinderhughes, E. (1995). Empowering diverse populations: Family practice in the 21st century. *Families in Society, 76*(3), 131–140.

Sanchez, S. (1999). Learning from the stories of culturally and linguistically diverse families and communities: A sociohistorical lens. *Remediation and Special Education, 20*(6), 351–357.

Sharma, A. R., McGue, M. K., & Benson, P. L. (1998). The psychological adjustment of US adopted adolescents and their non-adopted siblings. *Child Development, 69*(3), 791–802.

U. S. Census Bureau. (2002). Current Population Reports. Washington, DC: Government Printing Office.

White, M., & Epston, D. (1990). *Narrative means to therapeutic ends*. New York: W. W. Norton.

# 4

# Psychopathology

Len Sperry
*Florida Atlantic University*

Maureen P. Duffy
Richard M. Tureen
Scott E. Gillig
*Barry University*

## TRUTH OR FICTION?

___ 1. *A delusion is a belief held despite evidence it is true.*

___ 2. *A personality trait is a personality pattern that is an inflexible and maladaptive pattern of inner experience and behavior that causes significant impairment, and is abnormal for the individual's culture.*

___ 3. *A dissociation is mental perplexity with respect to time, place or person.*

___ 4. *A borderline personality disorder is characterized by a pervasive pattern of instability of self-identity, interpersonal relationships, and moods.*

___ 5. *Schizophrenia is a* Cluster B Personality Disorder *and is characterized by dramatic, emotional, or erratic behavior.*

___ 6. *In describing dysthymic disorder by specifiers relating to age of onset and the pattern of symptoms, use the* Early Onset *specifier if symptoms start before the age of 21.*

___ 7. *GAF is the DSM's Axis V Global Assessment of Functioning.*

___ 8. *Generalized anxiety disorder is excessive anxiety, worry, or apprehension about having a panic attack.*

___ 9. *Women are two to three times more likely than men to be diagnosed with panic disorder.*

___ 10. *Dissociative identity disorder is associated with significant child abuse, usually of a sexual nature.*

___ 11. *You would diagnose autism instead of Asperger's when there is no clinically significant delay in language acquisition and use and fewer repetitive motor behaviors and rituals.*

___ 12. *Anorexia nervosa is the refusal to maintain body weight at a minimally normal level necessary for health and growth combined with a fear of weight loss and a misperception about one's weight.*

___ 13. *Current research has shown relational disorders to have a strong biological component as with major depression.*

___ 14. *A delusional disorder is diagnosed when a prominent nonbizarre delusion is present but when the main criteria for a diagnosis of schizophrenia are not met.*

___ 15. *Panic attacks are strictly psychological events and can be associated with any mental disorder.*

The relationship between individual pathology and systemic or relational pathology is far from clear. Family therapy has traditionally located problems within the relationship or context, while traditional models of psychopathology have located problems within the person. Assessment of psychopathology at either the individual or relational level relies on the development of a system of classification. The primary system of classification of psychopathology in use today is the *Diagnostic and Statistical Manual of Mental Disorders,* Fourth Edition, Text Revision (*DSM–IV–TR*; APA, 2000). This classification system focuses overwhelmingly on individual psychopathology, not on relational pathology. Though there is disagreement among family therapists about the need for a system for diagnosing psychopathology at either the individual or relational level, many family therapists have actively worked for the inclusion of more categories of relational pathology in the *DSM–IV–TR.*

## INDIVIDUAL DYNAMICS VERSUS SYSTEMS DYNAMICS

Understandings of individual dynamics and systems dynamics are based on different philosophical and theoretical foundations. *Individual dynamics* focus on the manifestation of affective, cognitive, and behavioral **symptoms** within the individual person. By contrast, *systems dynamics* focus on the network of relationships within which the person functions; symptoms within a person are seen as a reflection of problems within that contextual network. For instance, consider the case of a defiant and oppositional teenager. From the individual dynamics perspective, you would assess the teenager in terms of his or her individual behaviors, attitudes, affect, and overall problematic functioning. From the systems perspective, you would assess the teenager by observing the interactional patterns between the teenager and his or her parents. The individual therapist would be more likely to locate the problem within the teenager and treat the teenager individually. The systems therapist would most likely treat the teenager and the parents together and consider the nature of the relationship between the parents and teenager a primary focus.

## POSTMODERN CRITIQUE OF THE DSM-IV

Within the past fifteen years, a strong critique of the philosophical foundations and political and ethical implications of diagnosis has emerged. The essence of this critique is that the categories of the *DSM* are not "real" in the same way that diagnoses like a broken arm are "real," but rather that these categories are constructions in language reflecting the dominance of the medical, pathological model in the Western world. Additionally, the postmodern critique holds that it is unethical to specify and characterize persons in pathological ways because objectivity is regarded as not possible. Despite these concerns, *DSM–IV* remains a useful diagnostic tool in marital and family therapy.

1. The current status on relational disorders in the *DSM–IV* is:
   a. There has been significant progress in agreeing on inclusion of relational disorders.
   b. Relational disorders are already included in the *DSM–IV*.
   c. Some family therapists are working for inclusion of relational disorders.
   d. There is a clear link between disorders at the individual and relational level.

2. The postmodern critique of diagnostic categories in the *DSM–IV* is that:
   a. They meet the criteria of scientific objectivity.
   b. Much progress has been made in improving their scientific reliability.
   c. The categories are not "real" in the sense that a diagnosis of diabetes is "real."
   d. Postmodernists offer no opinion on the *DSM–IV*.

## UNDERSTANDING THE DSM-IV-TR

The *DSM* has been the official classification for mental disorders in the United States since it first appeared in 1952. The second edition was published in 1968, the third edition in 1978, with a revision in 1987. A fourth edition, *DSM–IV,* went into effect in 1994, and the current edition, *DSM–IV–TR,* was published in 2000 (APA, 2000). In *DSM–I* and *II* there was one axis to designate a diagnosis. In an attempt to account for biological, psychological, and social functioning as well as overall adaptability to life's stressors, starting with DSM-III, a five axis system was adopted.

### The Five Axes

*Axis I* is for reporting any clinical disorders, as well as other conditions that may be a focus of clinical attention. *Axis II* is for specifying personality disorders and mental retardation. *Axis III* specifies any general medical conditions that are relevant to understanding or managing the individual's mental disorder. *Axis IV* is for reporting psychosocial and environmental problems that could affect the diagnosis, treatment, or prognosis of Axes I or II. *Axis V* is for specifying the individual's overall level of functioning using the **Global Assessment of Functioning (GAF) Scale**. These five axes provide a succinct summary of the biopsychosocial factors that influence an individual's symptoms and functioning.

*Case Example.* Marian K. is a fifty-two-year-old married female who reports symptoms of suicidal ideation, trouble sleeping, some weight loss, difficulty with early morning awakening, depressed mood, and loss of interest in usual activities. Her husband of twenty years has moved out rather unexpectedly to be with a younger woman. She is unemployed and the mother of three grown children, the youngest one having recently enlisted in the U.S. Army. She has not been taking care of her chronic diabetic condition since her husband left, and it is getting worse. The five axes *DSM–IV–TR* diagnosis for Marian would be:

Axis I: 296.21 Major Depressive Disorder, single episode, mild
Axis II: 301.6 Dependent Personality Disorder
Axis III: Diabetes (by history; regulated by medication)
Axis IV: Psychosocial stressor: Marital dysfunction (separation)
Axis V: GAF—50.

3. Regarding the five axis system of the *DSM–IV–TR,* Axis II is for:
   a. reporting psychosocial and environmental problems that could affect the diagnosis, treatment, or prognosis.
   b. reporting any clinical disorders, as well as other conditions that may be a focus of clinical attention.
   c. specifying any general medical conditions that are relevant to understanding the individual's mental disorder.
   d. specifying personality disorders and/or mental retardation.

## DIAGNOSING PSYCHIATRIC DISORDERS

### Psychotic Thought Disorders

*Schizophrenia.*   Schizophrenia is a **psychosis** involving significant dysfunctions in a person's thought processes, speech patterns, behavior, **mood**, **affect**, motivation, and social and occupational functioning. This disorder includes both *positive* and *negative* symptoms that must be present for at least one month, or less, if successfully treated. The positive symptoms (meaning prominent or added symptoms) include **delusions**, which are cognitive distortions, and **hallucinations**, which are perceptual distortions. Delusions are false beliefs and misinterpretations of experience that can be either *bizarre* (highly improbable) or *nonbizarre* (realistic but highly unlikely). Hallucinations are perceptual distortions that can affect any of the sensory domains, but are most commonly auditory in nature. The negative symptoms (meaning absence of normal behavior) include disorganized speech, restriction or flattening of affect, deterioration in self-care, and reduced motivation to set and implement goal-directed behavior (avolition).

There are five sub types of schizophrenia, the diagnosis of which is based on the most recent clinical evaluation. The five sub-types are:

1. The *Paranoid Type*—delusions and auditory hallucinations organized around a central persecutory and/or grandiose theme.
2. The *Disorganized Type*—disturbances in speech, affect, behavioral organization, goal-directedness, and self-care.
3. The *Catatonic Type*—significant disturbances in motor behavior ranging from immobility and rigidity to agitation, restlessness, and echolalia (imitation of words or phrases).
4. The *Undifferentiated Type*—meets the criteria for schizophrenia; but not the criteria for above subtypes.
5. The *Residual Type*—meets the criteria for schizophrenia; has some negative symptoms but lacks current psychotic symptoms.

*Delusional Disorders.*   A delusional disorder is diagnosed when a nonbizarre delusion is present for at least one month but the main criteria for schizophrenia (auditory or visual hallucinations, bizarre delusions, and negative symptoms of disorganized speech, affect, and behavior) are not met. An example of a nonbizarre delusion is the client believes Tiger Woods is in love with her and is her secret admirer. The challenging aspect in diagnosing a delusional disorder is distinguishing nonbizarre from bizarre delusions. There are several sub types of delusional disorder including:

1. *Erotomanic Type*—belief that a celebrity or well-known person is in love with the client.
2. *Grandiose Type*—belief that the client possesses a superior talent or gift.
3. *Jealous Type*—belief that the client's spouse or lover is unfaithful; he or she gathers evidence from normal events like finding a hair on the lover's coat.
4. *Persecutory Type*—belief that others are out to get the client.
5. *Somatic Type*—belief that there is something wrong with the client's appearance or a part of his or her body; for example, that he has a foul smell coming from somewhere.
6. *Mixed Types*—combination of types.
7. *Unspecified Types*—absence of a central delusional theme or does not fit in any of the sub-type categories.

*Case Example.*   Joan T. was admitted to a psychiatric unit the day after her thirty-third birthday. For nine months her behavior was characterized by withdrawal, inappropriate moods, preoccupation with religious ideas, and the insistent belief that her husband and church elders were, as she stated, "Trying to do away with me on my thirty-third birthday like they did with Christ." For three weeks prior to that birthday she barricaded herself in her room to foil the plot. Her affect was flattened and at times she talked readily but inappropriately.
Diagnosis: Schizophrenia—Paranoid Type

4. In diagnosing the sub type *undifferentiated type* in the category of schizophrenia, the following item most accurately describes this condition:
   a. meets the criteria for paranoid, disorganized, or catatonic subtypes.
   b. only meets the criteria for the paranoid subtype.
   c. meets the criteria of the residual type.
   d. does not meet the criteria for paranoid, disorganized, or catatonic subtypes.

5. Which of the following descriptions of the sub types of delusional disorders is correct?
   a. The erotomanic type is the belief that one possesses a superior talent or gift.
   b. The persecutory type is the belief that one's spouse is being unfaithful.
   c. The mixed type is a combination of two of the seven sub types.
   d. The unspecified type is the absence of a central delusional theme or does not fit in the other sub type categories.

6. There are five sub types of schizophrenia, the diagnosis of which is based on the most recent clinical evaluation. The *disorganized type* is characterized by:
   a. delusions and/or auditory hallucinations organized around a central persecutory and/or grandiose theme.
   b. disturbances in motor behavior ranging from extreme immobility and rigidity to extreme agitation and restlessness and speech disturbances, notably echolalia (repeating words and phrases).
   c. disturbances that lack current prominent psychotic symptoms but include remaining evidence of negative symptoms like poverty of speech, reduced affect, and/or difficulties in goal-directed behavior.
   d. disturbances in speech, affect, and behavioral organization with significant impact on a person's ability to care for oneself and engage in goal-directed behavior.

7. Of the sub types of delusional disorders, the *grandiose type* is characterized by:
   a. the delusional belief that a person, often of higher status or a celebrity or well-known figure, is in love with the individual.
   b. the delusional belief that one possesses a superior, but often unrecognized, talent, gift, knowledge, idea, or discovery.
   c. the delusional belief that one's spouse, lover, or significant other is unfaithful. Evidence to justify the belief is gathered from normal events like the presence of a hair on a lover's coat or a phone number on a business card.
   d. the central delusional belief that others are out to get them. This belief includes being watched, followed, spied on, maligned, betrayed, obstructed, or otherwise prevented from achieving one's goals.

## Mood Disorders

*Major Depressive Disorder.*   Major depressive disorder (MDD) is characterized by either depressed mood or loss of interest and pleasure in daily life and the presence of four other symptoms from the following list: significant weight loss or gain; persistent sleep disturbances, in particular, awakening in the middle of the night and having difficulty returning to sleep and/or early morning awakening; increased agitation or restlessness or decreased movement and motor activity that is noticeable to others; chronic fatigue; inappropriate feelings of worthlessness, guilt, and self-doubt; difficulty concentrating and making decisions; and frequent thoughts of death and/or suicide with or without the formulation of a plan. These symptoms must be present for at least two weeks on a daily or almost daily basis.

MDD further distinguished by whether it is a single episode or recurrent and whether the symptoms are mild, moderate, or severe. If psychotic features are present the therapist must note and describe them.

*Dysthymic Disorder.*   Dysthymic disorder is diagnosed if a person has been chronically depressed for at least two years without meeting the criteria for MDD. In addition to depressed mood, two other of these symptoms must be present: disturbances of appetite and eating; sleep difficulties; chronic fatigue; difficulty concentrating and making decisions; feelings of hopelessness or worthlessness; and chronic self-doubt or self-reproach. Symptom-free periods may not last longer than two months. To make this diagnosis in children, you may see an irritable rather than a depressed mood and the symptoms need only be present for one year. Past history of mania excludes the diagnosis of dysthymia. Dysthymic disorder is further described by specifiers relating to age of onset and the pattern of symptoms; namely, *Early Onset* before the age of 21, and *Late Onset* at age 21 or older.

*Bipolar Disorder.*   The key diagnostic feature of bipolar disorder is the presence of a manic episode (Bipolar I) or *hypomanic* episode (Bipolar II). A manic episode is a period of expansive or irritable mood, lasting at least one week with three or more of the following symptoms: **grandiosity**; excessive energy and diminished need for sleep; talking more and faster than usual; racing thoughts and flight of ideas; distractibility; increase in goal-directed behavior; and high-risk activities such as overspending or bad judgment in business or sex. Untreated manic behavior causes significant family and occupational problems.

A hypomanic episode is a distinct period of at least four days of expansive or irritable mood during which the person feels exceptionally well or cheerful. Three other symptoms from the symptom list for mania must also be present (four if the mood is irritable only) and the mood changes must be noticeable to others.

Bipolar I can be associated with or without psychotic symptoms and is rated as mild, moderate, or severe. Bipolar II requires the presence of hypomania and MDD. Therapists can use other specifiers to make the diagnosis more precise and can also indicate the episodic pattern, such as seasonal pattern or rapid cycling.

*Case Example.*   A twenty-five-year-old male fourth-year medical school student, under pressure preparing for final exams and sleeping very little and irregularly, was at home visiting his parents during spring break. While at home, he attempted to strangle his father whom he thought was trying to hurt him. Prior to his visit home, his sister and local friends had commented on how many telephone calls they were getting from him at weird hours and how hard it was to get a word in edgewise when he was talking. His roommates had been humoring him during the past two weeks about his boasts that he was going to ace the finals and that he wasn't at all concerned about them.
Diagnosis: Bipolar I Disorder, Single Manic Episode, Severe with Psychotic Features.

8. In addition to either depressed mood or loss of interest and pleasure in daily life, major depression is *not* characterized by the presence of:
   a. weight Gain.
   b. sleep disturbance.
   c. belief that others are out to get them.
   d. feeling chronically fatigued.

9. The symptoms of major depression must be present for _____ for the diagnosis to be made:
   a. two months on a daily or almost daily basis
   b. one month on a daily or almost daily basis
   c. two weeks on a daily or almost daily basis
   d. six months on a daily or almost daily basis

10. Dysthymic disorder is characterized by which of the following:
    a. The symptoms may be due to the use of substances.
    b. The symptoms may occur during a manic episode.
    c. The symptoms last for at least two years in adults.
    d. There have been brief episodes of major depression.

11. Which of the following best describes bipolar I disorder, single manic episode?
    a. There has been a past major depressive episode.
    b. The has been only one manic episode.
    c. The episode is superimposed on a delusional disorder.
    d. There has been a two year interval without a manic episode.

12. Which of the following disorders is most likely to be associated with psychotic symptoms?
    a. bipolar disorder
    b. schizoid disorder
    c. dysthymic disorder
    d. posttraumatic stress disorder

13. The key diagnostic features of major depression include all of the following *except:*
    a. sudden onset of symptoms like, sweating, trembling, racing heart, chest pain, short-ness of breath, rapid breathing and pulse, along with dizziness or lightheadedness.
    b. loss of interest and pleasure in daily life along with significant weight loss or weight gain that is not purposeful.
    c. daily or almost daily sleep disturbances, in particular, awakening in the middle of the night and having difficulty returning to sleep and/or early morning awakening.
    d. feelings of worthlessness, guilt, and self-doubt that are not realistically appropriate along with difficulties concentrating and making decisions.

## Neuroses: Anxiety, Dissociative, and Somatoform Disorders

The term *neurosis* is now regarded as an artifact of psychoanalytic thought and refers to the clinical symptoms that are regarded as emerging from unresolved emotional conflict, usually in the form of **anxiety**. These symptoms are not as disabling as the symptoms of the psychotic disorders because they do not involve loss of touch with external reality or impairment of overall functioning as severely as in the psychotic disorders. As advances in biopsychiatry emerged, the physiological basis of anxiety symptoms was emphasized and terminology shifted away from the use of the psychoanalytic term *neurosis* and toward the *DSM–IV–TR* categories of anxiety disorders (panic disorders, agoraphophia, generalized anxiety disorder, and posttraumatic stress disorder), dissociative disorders, and somatoform disorders.

*Panic Disorders and Agoraphobia.*   One can only understand panic disorder in rela-tionship to *panic attacks*. Panic attacks are a constellation of physiological and psychological events and can be associated with any mental disorder and a number of medical disorders such as mitral valve prolapse. People who have panic attacks describe them as terrifying experiences. Therapists can make a diagnosis of panic disorder when panic attacks recur and are unexpected and when people ruminate and worry about them for a period of at least one month. A panic attack has a clearly identifiable sudden onset of physiological symptoms such as: sweating, trembling, racing heart, chest pain, shortness of breath, rapid breathing, dizziness, chills or hot flashes, and numbness or tingling. These physiological events build quickly, usually within ten minutes. Accompanying these physiological experiences are a range of psychological experi-ences including a fear of dying and losing control, a sense of dread, and a fear of going crazy. A panic attack is diagnosed when four or more of these symptoms are present.

Panic attacks can be unexpected, cued, or situationally predisposed. A cued panic attack occurs when triggered by exposure or in anticipation of a situational cue. For example, if a woman has had a previous panic attack at a crowded shopping mall, either crowds or the shopping mall could trigger future attacks, possibly resulting in a **phobia** of crowds or malls. Situationally predisposed panic attacks occur when in the presence of a trigger or cue, but a panic attack does not always follow. For example, the woman with a history of panic attacks at the mall could go to the mall on some occasions without experiencing a panic attack, although she would be predisposed by the trigger of being at the mall to have one there. Panic disorder may occur with or without *agoraphobia*. Agoraphobia is the learned avoidance of events or activities that may trigger a panic attack; for example, avoiding going to the mall or being in crowds.

*Generalized Anxiety Disorder.*   The key feature of generalized anxiety disorder is excessive worry about many things for at least six months. In spite of making efforts to do so, the person can't control the anxiety. Three or more other symptoms must also be present: restlessness, tiring easily, difficulties concentrating, irritability, muscle tension, or sleep problems.

*Posttraumatic Stress Disorder (PTSD).*   Witnessing or experiencing a traumatic event like rape, combat, a natural disaster, or a fire and responding with strong feelings of fear, shock, and helplessness set the stage for the development of PTSD. **Flashbacks**, recollecting the event, dreaming about it, reexperiencing it emotionally and physiologically, and having unwanted thoughts about the event are diagnostic, as are associated attempts to avoid thinking or talking about the event. Arousal symptoms like an overactive startle response and hyper-vigilance are also indicative. Symptoms must be present for at least one month. For example, a client developed PTSD after her daughter was involuntarily removed from her home in the middle of the night by child protective workers. The sound of a car slowing down in front of her house after dark triggered her PTSD symptoms.

*Dissociative Disorders.*   Disorders involving **dissociation** are controversial. Some therapists think there is a propensity in some dissociative states for the person to be exaggerating their symptoms or even faking. Others think that dissociative states result from a high level of suggestibility. People with dissociative **amnesia** can't remember their names or past traumas. People with dissociative **fugue** abruptly leave their homes and can't remember who they are. Dissociative identity disorder was previously called multiple personality disorder (MPD). It is characterized by the emergence of more than one personality and is associated with child sexual abuse. The movie *Sybil* portrays classic MPD. **Depersonalization** disorder is the experience of detachment from one's self.

*Somatoform Disorders.*   Somatoform disorders describe the presence of a physical symptom that cannot be fully explained by a medical problem. There are seven types of somatoform disorders: somatization disorder (many complaints before age 30), undifferentiated somatoform disorder, **conversion** disorder, pain disorder, hypochondriasis, body dysmorphic disorder, and somatoform disorder not otherwise specified. Individuals with fears of having a serious disease based on their misinterpretation of bodily symptoms or who overutilize medical services, have frequent doctor visits, lab tests, etc. could meet criteria for one these disorders.

*Case Example.*   A thirty-five-year-old male presented in therapy with fears of leaving his apartment, driving over bridges and through tunnels, and doing routine everyday tasks like grocery shopping. He stated that after a few minutes in the grocery store he would hyperventilate and feel his heart race. He would then leave his groceries in the cart and go home. He found that the only way he could manage in the grocery store was to purchase just a few items so that he could get in and out quickly. This caused more difficulties because he had to make more trips to the grocery store than usual which was stressful for him as he was avoiding going out. Diagnosis: Panic Disorder with Agoraphobia.

14. Which of the following best describes the time frame necessary for a diagnosis under the general category of panic attack?
    a. Peak symptoms develop abruptly and reach a peak within ten minutes.
    b. Peak symptoms develop slowly and reach a peak within ten minutes.
    c. Peak symptoms develop almost immediately.
    d. Peak symptoms reach a peak in thirty minutes.

15. Which of the following items is *not* descriptive of generalized anxiety disorder?
    a. excessive worry, anxiety, or apprehension
    b. occurring most days for at least two months
    c. The anxiety is not part of the symptom set for another Axis I diagnosis.
    d. The anxiety is not limited to one or two specific concerns.

16. Posttraumatic stress disorder is diagnosed when the duration of the disturbance is:
    a. more than six months.
    b. more than one month.
    c. more than two months.
    d. at least two weeks.

17. Which of these disorders is marked by the experience of feeling outside of one's self or detached from one's own self and life, as if in a dream?
    a. somatization disorder
    b. dissociative identity disorder
    c. conversion disorder
    d. depersonalization disorder

18. Which of the following dissociative disorders is characterized by a sudden, unexpected travel away home or work and an inability to recall one's past?
    a. depersonalization disorder
    b. dissociative fugue
    c. dissociative identity disorder
    d. amnesia

19. Somatization disorder is characterized by:
    a. a history of many physical complaints over a number of years beginning before age 30.
    b. at least two physical complaints beginning before the age of 25.
    c. four physical complaints beginning after the age of 30.
    d. one physical complaint that lasts at least three years.

## Disorders of Childhood and Adolescence

*Attention Deficit/Hyperactivity Disorder (ADHD).*  The key feature of ADHD is an ongoing pattern of inattention and/or hyperactivity or impulsivity, with some symptoms present before the age of seven. Symptoms are divided into two categories; namely, *inattention* and *hyperactivity–impulsivity*. A diagnosis of ADHD is made by observing six or more symptoms from either category that have been present for at least six months. The symptoms of inattention are: making careless mistakes, having poor attention, not listening, not following instructions, having poor organization, avoiding tasks that require concentration, losing things, being easily distracted, or being forgetful in daily activities. The symptoms of hyperactivity–impulsivity are: fighting, leaving one's seat in the classroom, running about and climbing excessively, having difficulty in playing quietly, talking excessively, blurting out answers, having difficulty awaiting one's turn, and interrupting or intruding on others. Some impairment in two settings such as school and home is necessary to make the diagnosis. Subtypes of ADHD are the combined type, the predominantly inattentive type, and the predominantly hyperactive–impulsive type.

*Autism and Asperger's Disorder.*  Autism and Asperger's are disorders of childhood within the spectrum of pervasive developmental disorders and are marked by striking and enduring impairment in interpersonal and social interactions. Causes of autism are hotly debated and include environmental pollution and childhood vaccines.

Autistic kids are usually easier to spot than Asperger's kids. To make a diagnosis of autism one must see six or more symptoms from the following list, with at least two from the *social interaction* category, one from the *communication* category and one from the *repetitive, stereotyped movements and interests* category. The social interaction category includes impairment in the use of nonverbal behavior such as eye contact, facial expression, posture, and gesture; no meaningful peer relationships or sharing with others; and lack of reciprocity. The communication category includes absence or delay of language development, odd and repetitive use of language in those with speech, and lack of imaginative and imitative play. The repetitive, stereotyped movements and interests category includes intense preoccupation with one thing; rituals; repetitive body movements like rocking, banging, or clapping; and preoccupation with parts of objects. Onset must be before age three. Asperger's would be diagnosed instead of autism when there is no clinically significant delay in language acquisition and less repetitive motor behaviors. A child with Asperger's would use language, probably in an eccentric way, but would miss social cues from others.

*Eating Disorders.*  Eating disorders include anorexia nervosa and bulimia nervosa. *Anorexia* is the refusal to maintain body weight at a minimally normal level necessary for health and growth (85% of minimal normal body weight) combined with an overwhelming fear of weight gain and a significant misperception about one's weight and shape. Like Karen Carpenter, young women with anorexia frequently deny the seriousness of their disorder. In girls who have started to menstruate, there will be an absence of at least three consecutive periods. Anorexia nervosa—restricting type is diagnosed when there is no history of binging or purging in the current episode. The binge-eating/purgingtype is diagnosed when there is a history of vomiting or inappropriate use of laxatives, diuretics, or enemas in the current episode. The key feature of *bulimia* is recurrent binge eating of inordinate amounts of food with a sense of loss of control and preoccupation with weight and shape. Compensatory behavior includes self-induced vomiting and the misuse of laxatives, enemas, diuretics, exercise, and fasting. The binge eating and compensatory behavior must occur an average of twice a week for at last three months. The purging type is characterized by regular self-induced vomiting or use of other purgatives. The nonpurging type involves excessive exercise or fasting.

*Case Example.*  Mark is an eight-year-old boy who was brought to family therapy by his single- parent mother because of his teacher's concerns. The teacher states that Mark is always getting out of his seat to talk to other kids and she adds that during study time he is always looking around whenever he hears a noise in the room. Additionally, he interrupts other students and breaks into their games. Mark's mother and teacher are in agreement that there is a problem because at home he loses papers and forgets where he leaves his homework. Mark just cannot seem to sit still for any length of time, in spite of his promises to try harder. Diagnosis: Attention-Deficit/Hyperactivity Disorder, Combined Type.

20. For a diagnosis of attention-deficit/hyperactivity disorder to be made, the time frame criteria for a diagnosis to be made is:
    a. three months.
    b. one year.
    c. one Month.
    d. six months.

21. Which of the following is *not* a subtype of attention deficit/hyperactivity disorder?
    a. combined type
    b. predominantly inattentive type
    c. predominantly acting out type
    d. predominantly hyperactive-impulsive type

22. Which of the following is *not* a criterion for a diagnosis of inattention in attention-deficit/hyperactivity disorder?
    a. often fidgets with hands or feet or squirms in seat
    b. often does not seem to listen when spoken to directly
    c. is forgetful in daily activities
    d. makes careless mistakes

23. Which of the following is *not* characteristic of autistic disorder?
    a. lack of social or emotional reciprocity
    b. persistent preoccupation with parts of objects
    c. onset prior to age 8
    d. apparent inflexible adherence to specific, nonfunctional routines or rituals

24. Anorexia nervosa is characterized by a refusal to maintain body weight of what percent of that expected for normal weight for age and height?
    a. 95 percent
    b. 75 percent
    c. 80 percent
    d. 85 percent

25. Which of the following items is *not* a characteristic of anorexia nervosa?
    a. refusal to maintain body weight at a minimal level for health and growth
    b. an absence of at least two consecutive periods for girls who have passed menarche
    c. a significant misperception about one's weight and shape
    d. a denial of the seriousness of the disorder

## Personality Disorders

**Personality** can be described as the distinctive pattern of traits that characterizes an individual. A *personality disorder* is an inflexible and maladaptive pattern of inner experience and behavior that deviates markedly from expectations of the individual's culture and is manifest in at least two of the following areas—cognition, affectivity, interpersonal functioning, or impulse control—and leads to clinically significant distress or impairment. While not usually diagnosed until the individual is an adult, the presence of a personality disorder may be recognizable by adolescence, and these disorders continue throughout most or all of adult life.

In *DSM–IV–TR*, personality disorders are coded on Axis II. These disorders are classified in three clusters: A, B, and C. *Cluster A* includes paranoid, schizoid, and schizotypal personality disorders which are characterized by odd or eccentric behaviors. *Cluster B* includes antisocial, borderline, histrionic, and narcissistic personality disorders which are characterized by dramatic, emotional, or erratic behavior. *Cluster C* includes avoidant, dependent, and obsessive-compulsive personality disorders which are characterized by anxiety and fearfulness. Because of space limitations it is not possible to describe all ten Personality Disorders. Instead, we will highlight two rather common presentations in clinical practice.

*Borderline Personality Disorder.* This disorder is characterized by a pervasive pattern of instability of self-identity, interpersonal relationships, and moods. A marked, persistent disturbance of identity is noted in their uncertainty about their career, values, and even sexual orientation. Interpersonal relations tend to be intense and unstable and often involve the extremes of idealization or devaluation. Concerns about real or imagined abandonment can give rise to an nearly constant state of emotionality that is perceived by others to be inappropriate, for example, appearing jealous, suicidal, angry, or fearful. Marked mood instability and impulsivity are routine and often unpredictable.

*Narcissistic Personality Disorder.* This disorder is characterized by a pervasive pattern of grandiosity, lack of empathy, and hypersensitivity to others' evaluations and self-criticism. Despite their fantasies of brilliance, great success or beauty, reality tends to be quite different for individuals with this disorder. While they may attain significant achievements, they rarely derive genuine pleasure from them or accept them as sufficient. Similarly, feelings of grandiosity may alternate or lead to exaggerated feelings of failure. While outwardly appearing high, their self-esteem tends to be fragile and thus their need for constant admiration.

*Case Example.* Ralph T. inquires about psychotherapy, stating, "My wife is threatening to divorce me." He has been married for nearly two years to a wealthy socialite who was attracted to Ralph's handsome and confident demeanor. He wanted a "rich trophy wife" and pursued her relentlessly until she agreed to marry him. Because of his obsession with money and power, he spends most of his time putting together large commercial real estate deals. Not surprisingly, he has little time for his wife and when they are together they fight. She complains that he is inconsiderate and unempathic. He has extraordinary confidence in his ability to "read" people and succeed at business deals when others have failed. His self-image is grandiose while his manner is arrogant. Having the admiration of others is extremely important to him, but it never seems sufficient.
Diagnosis: Narcissistic Personality Disorder.

26. Which of the following is *not* an essential feature of a personality disorder?
    a. an enduring pattern of inner experience and behavior that deviates markedly from expectations of the individual's culture and is manifest in cognition, affectivity, interpersonal functioning, or impulse control
    b. the enduring pattern leads to clinically significant distress or impairment
    c. the enduring pattern is flexible and limited to specific personal and social situations
    d. the enduring pattern is stable, of long duration, and its onset is in adolescence or early adulthood

27. Which of the following personality disorders make up Cluster B?
    a. paranoid, schizoid, and schizotypal
    b. antisocial, borderline, histrionic, and narcissistic
    c. paranoid, antisocial, borderline, and histrionic
    d. avoidant, dependent, and obsessive-compulsive

28. Which of the following personality disorders make up Cluster C?
    a. paranoid, schizoid, and schizotypal
    b. antisocial, borderline, histrionic, and narcissistic
    c. paranoid, antisocial, borderline, and histrionic
    d. avoidant, dependent, and obsessive-compulsive

29. Which of the following criteria is *not* associated with borderline personality disorder?
    a. a pattern of instability in interpersonal relationships
    b. a pattern of marked impulsivity
    c. a pattern of distrust and suspiciousness
    d. frantic efforts to avoid abandonment

## Cognitive Disorders: Delirium and Dementia

This *DSM–IV–TR* category was previously called *Organic Mental Syndromes*. The term *organic* is no longer used in the *DSM* because it implies that other mental disorders have no biological or organic basis. The shared clinical features of disorders in this category is brain dysfunction, which is manifest primarily through cognitive deficits.

*Delirium.* A key feature of delirium is a disturbance in consciousness which involves widespread brain dysfunction. Individuals with this disorder have difficulty maintaining attention and are easily distracted. Symptom onset is rapid, that is, hours to days, and severity of dysfunction can fluctuate widely over the course of waking hours. Cognitive changes are also noted in perception (e.g., hallucinations or illusions), memory (e.g., **disorientation**), or in language dysfunction. Delirium can result from a general medical condition, trauma (e.g., head injury), medications; substance use, (e.g., intoxication or withdrawal), or from a combination of these factors. Delirium can begin rapidly, as with a head injury, and the resolution depends on how rapidly the underlying causal factors can be identified and corrected. Complete recovery is common, although residual deficits may occur.

*Dementia.* Individuals with this disorder exhibit signs and symptoms of global brain dysfunction. This includes impairment of both short-term and long-term memory, as well as impairment of at least one other brain function, such as *agnosia*—the inability to recognize and name objects; *apraxia*—loss of a purposeful, voluntary motor skill; *aphasia*—the inability to understand or produce language; or *anomia*—the inability to speak or produce normal speech sounds. The cumulative impact of these impairments on work, close relationships, and social activities is significant. Visual hallucinations are not uncommon and neither is delirium.

There are many forms of dementia, including Dementia of the Alzheimer's Type (DAT). The deterioration of cognitive deficits in DAT develop slowly and are progressive. Although it varies greatly, the average life expectancy from onset to death is about 10 years. Memory and cognitive deficits such as aphasia, apraxia, and agnosia occur early, while motor dysfunction such as *ataxia* (muscle incoordination, particularly of gait) occur later.

*Case Example.* Jay R. is a sixty-eight-year-old male who is brought for an evaluation because of increased difficulty in caring for himself. His memory is worsening to the degree that he now gets lost when taking a walk in his neighborhood. Mr. R. believes that his neighbors are stealing tools from his garage and he has become combative when seeing people walk on the sidewalk in front of the family home. He has become increasingly suspicious over the past year, and his wife complains that, "He seems to be a different person from the man I married." He is alert but uncooperative with the mental status exam and cannot perform simple memory tasks. He is in relatively good health, does not use alcohol or recreational drugs, and is not being prescribed any medications.
Diagnosis: Dementia of the Alzheimer's Type.

30. Which of the following involves a disturbance in consciousness which involves widespread brain dysfunction with a sudden onset?
    a. delirium
    b. dementia
    c. somatoform disorder
    d. schizophrenia

## DSM-IV Relational Disorders and GARF

*Relational Disorders—V-codes.* V-codes are used to indicate a clinical focus on particular relational problems. In clinical practice, relational problems are a frequent focus of attention. Relational problems describe patterns of interaction between members of a relational unit that result in impairment in the functioning of one or more members of the unit or of the relational unit as a whole. Relational problems can be a significant source of individual dissatisfaction and symptomatology and should therefore not be minimized because third-party reimbursement for their treatment is less likely. Relational codes should be listed on Axis I when they are the principal focus of clinical attention; otherwise they are listed on Axis IV. Three commonly used relational codes are Parent–Child Relational Problems (for interaction problems between parent and children), Partner Relational Problems (for problems in interaction between spouses or partners) and Sibling Relational Problems (for impaired patterns of interaction between siblings).

*GARF and Family Assessment of Functioning.* **GARF** is the Global Assessment of Relational Functioning Scale and parallels the DSM's Axis V Global Assessment of Functioning Scale (GAF). The development of the GARF came out of the work of the Coalition on Family Diagnosis a group of mental health professionals who felt that the DSM's set of individual diagnostic categories was inadequate for clinical work with couples and families.

The GARF, like the GAF, uses a hypothetical continuum ranging from 100 (optimal, effective functioning) to 1 (severely impaired functioning). Therapists assess relational or family functioning in the areas of problem-solving, organization, and emotional climate according to how well or poorly the family meets the affective or basic needs of its members. *Problem-solving* includes dimensions like setting and accomplishing goals, completing tasks, flexibility and adaptability, communication, and conflict-resolution skills. *Organization* refers to concepts from structural and strategic family therapy like rules, hierarchy, boundaries, and subsystems. *Emotional climate* refers to the variety and tone of emotional exchanges, how attached and involved family members are with one another, their level of emotional supportiveness and respect, their sharing of values and beliefs, their depth of caring and commitment, and sexual intimacy. Typically, current rather than past levels of family functioning are assessed.

31. Generally, the category of Relational Disorders—V-codes is listed on Axis IV. On which of the other axes should psychosocial or environmental problems be recorded if they are the primary focus of clinical attention?
    a. Axis I
    b. Axis II
    c. Axis III
    d. Axis V

**TABLE 4.1**

Summary Table of *DSM–IV–TR* Disorders

| *Disorder* | *Essential Feature* |
|---|---|
| **Personality Disorders: A** | Cluster of personality disorders that is characterized by odd or eccentric thinking and behavior |
| **Personality Disorders: B** | Cluster of personality disorders that is characterized by dramatic, emotional, or erratic behavior |
| **Personality Disorders: C** | Cluster of personality disorders that is characterized by anxious or fearful behavior |
| **Cognitive Disorders** | Clinically significant deficits in cognition that are markedly different from previous functioning |
| Delirium | Disturbance of consciousness and cognitive changes that develop within a short time frame |
| Dementia | Multiple cognitive deficits, including memory impairment |
| **Psychotic Disorders** | Significant dysfunctions in thought processes, speech, mood, motivation, and functioning |
| Schizophrenia | Prominent hallucinations, bizarre delusions, negative symptoms of disorganized speech and affect |
| Delusional Disorders | A prominent nonbizarre delusion not meeting the main criteria for a diagnosis of schizophrenia |
| **Mood Disorders** | Disorders with mood symptoms |
| Depression | Presence of either depressed mood or loss of interest and pleasure in daily life |
| Dysthymic Disorder | Chronic experience of depression for a period of at least two years without major depression |
| Bipolar Disorder | Manic or a hypomanic with problems with mood, functioning, grandiosity, and increased energy |
| **Anxiety Disorders** | Symptoms that are regarded as emerging from emotional conflict, or biological sources |
| Panic Disorders | Sudden onset of physiological symptoms like sweating, trembling, chest pain, and shortness of breath |
| Agoraphobia | Learned avoidance of events or activities that may trigger a panic attack |
| Generalized Anxiety Disorder | Excessive anxiety, worry, or apprehension about many things |
| Posttraumatic Stress Disorder | Unwanted recollection or reexperiencing of a traumatic event with arousal symptoms |
| **Dissociative Disorders** | Symptoms of disturbance in self, memory, or awareness |
| **Somatoform Disorders** | Physical symptoms unexplained by a medical problem, substance abuse, or mental disorder |
| **Childhood and Adolescence** | Disorders that typically become manifest during childhood or adolescence |
| Attention Deficit Disorder | Pattern of inattention and/or hyperactivity/impulsivity with some symptoms before the age of seven |
| Autism | Delay or abnormal functioning before age three in social interaction, communication, and play |
| Asperger's Disorder | No delay in language acquisition and use and fewer repetitive motor behaviors than with Autism |
| **Eating Disorders** | Difficulties with too much, too little, or unhealthy food intake |
| Bulimia Nervosa | Recurrent binge eating with loss of control over one's eating and compensation for overeating |
| Anorexia Nervosa | Refusal to maintain body weight at 85% of minimal normal body weight, with a fear of weight gain |
| **Relational Disorders** | Particular relational problems of clinical focus, i.e, Parent–Child, Partner Relational Problems |

## THE ASSESSMENT PROCESS IN PSYCHOPATHOLOGY

### Clinical Interviews and Structured Interviews

The clinical interview is the cornerstone of assessment and diagnosis in both individual and family therapy. It consists of a detailed psychosocial history, history of the presenting problem and symptoms, and clinical assessment of mood, affect, behavior, perception, and cognition through the *Mental Status Exam* or *Mini-Mental Status Exam*. Structured clinical interviews may also be used to facilitate assessment. The *Structured Clinical Interview for the DSM–IV, Axis I* (SCID-I) and *Axis II Disorders* (SCID-II) is a frequently used structured interview for adults available from the American Psychiatric Publishing Company. The *Children's Interview for Psychiatric Syndromes* (ChIPS) and *Children's Interview for Psychiatric Syndromes-Parent Version* (P-ChIPS) are structured clinical interviews for children and adolescents also available from the American Psychiatric Publishing Company. *The Personality Disorder Interview-IV* (PDI-IV) is a semi-structured interview that is used in the assessment of the ten *DSM–IV* personality disorders and the two proposed personality disorders included for further review and study. The PDI-IV is designed to enable assessment of these twelve personality disorders in a reliable and valid way. The interview consists of a series of questions and scoring guidelines for each of the personality disorders.

### Psychological Inventory

The *Millon Clinical Multiaxial Inventory-III* is an adult self-report measure designed for the assessment of both *DSM–IV* Axis I clinical **syndromes** and Axis II underlying personality disorders. It is a paper-and-pencil, audiocassette, or computer administered inventory written at the eighth grade level. The clinical scales include eleven clinical personality pattern scales, three severe personality pathology scales, seven clinical syndrome scales, three severe syndrome scales, three modifying indices, and one validity index. It is normed on adult inpatient and outpatient clinical samples and inmate correctional samples. Table 4.1 provides a capsule review description of the main disorders covered in this chapter.

> 32. Which of the following methods would be inappropriate for assessing personality disorders?
>     a. The Personality Disorder Interview-IV
>     b. Structured Clinical Interview for the *DSM–IV* (SCID-II)
>     c. Millon Clinical Multiaxial Inventory-III
>     d. Structured Clinical Interview for the *DSM–IV* (SCID-I)

## KEY TERMS

**affect:** How an individual's mood appears to others.

**amnesia:** Total or partial loss of memory.

**anxiety:** A feeling of general discomfort that does not have a well-defined cause.

**conversion symptom:** A deficit affecting voluntary motor or sensory function that is the result of psychological rather than organic pathology.

**delusion:** A belief held despite evidence that it is not true.

**dementia:** Development of multiple cognitive deficits including memory impairment.

**depersonalization:** Loss of sense of personal identity often with feelings of being detached from self or being an outside observer.

**disorientation:** Mental perplexity with respect to time, place, or person.

**dissociation:** Disruption in the usually integrated functions of consciousness, memory, identity, or perceptions.

**dissociative fugue:** Confusion of identity or assumption of a new identity following a sudden, unexpected travel away from home or work along with the inability to recall one's past.

**DSM-IV-TR:** Current diagnostic manual of the American Psychiatric Association.

**flashback:** The reexperiencing of a past event including illusions, hallucinations, and dissociative episodes.

**GAF:** The *DSM*'s Axis V Global Assessment of Functioning Scale.

**GARF:** The Global Assessment of Relational Functioning Scale that parallels the DSM's Axis V Global Assessment of Functioning Scale (GAF).

**grandiosity:** A symptom of mania; used to describe the pretension of superiority often experienced by those in a manic episode.

**hallucination:** A visual, auditory, or olfactory perception which is not based in reality.

**ideas of reference:** The belief that unrelated events or activities refer to oneself.

**mood:** An individual's perception of feelings.

**panic attack:** Sudden onset of physiological symptoms like, sweating, trembling, chest pain, and shortness of breath.

**paranoid ideation:** Suspicion of others such that their motives are perceived as malevolent.

**personality:** Distinctive pattern of traits that characterizes an individual.

**phobia:** Marked and unrelenting fear that is disproportionate or unreasonable brought about by the presence or anticipation of a specific object or situation.

**psychosis:** A condition that involves the loss of reality and includes the presence of delusions, hallucinations, disorganized speech, or grossly disorganized or catatonic behavior.

**symptom:** Apparent manifestation of a physical or a mental disorder.

**syndrome:** Pattern of symptoms that occur together and characterize a disorder.

## DISCUSSION QUESTIONS

1. In the case of Marian K., which of her issues would require the most immediate attention and why? Are there any issues that could be put on the back burner, so to speak, and dealt with at a later time? How might you rank her issues in terms of those needing immediate attention and those that are severe? Would these be the same or different and why?

2. In the case of Ralph T., how might this case differ if the client had other Cluster B personality traits in addition to his narcissistic personality disorder? How might the addition of antisocial, borderline, and histrionic traits augment this client's description? How would the addition of these other traits change the way you would treat this client?

3. In case of Jay R., can you pick out any personality traits that this client seems to possess? Do these traits fit the pattern in any of the personality disorder clusters in particular? How would you determine whether these traits were preexisting aspects of his personality or simply a by-product of his dementia?

4. What is your view of the use of diagnosis in the helping process? What do you see as the major costs and benefits of diagnosing client issues?

5. In your diagnostic work with clients, how will you make the determination that a particular client has schizophrenia or a delusional disorder as opposed to having involvement in culturally explicable phenomena? In other words, how will you know that a given client needs treatment

and possibly medical treatment or whether that client is responding in a natural manner given the cultural context? Can you provide examples of ways that a client could be engaged in a normal cultural phenomenon yet interact in ways that suggest pathology?

6. In working with a client who presents with depressive symptomatology, on what basis will you decide to treat that client with individual, family, or group therapy versus sending the client for a psychiatric evaluation for possible medical intervention? Are there any depressive symptoms that would suggest that a medical intervention may be warranted? Could there be any legal or ethical implications if you do not refer? What types of treatment would be most effective in helping a person with depression?

7. In the case of the med student, how would this example look different if he were suffering from schizophrenia, paranoid type instead of bipolar disorder? Could there be any similarities? What would be different if the client were experiencing bipolar II disorder instead of bipolar I disorder? Which would you be most concerned with and why?

8. Would there be any sense in referring a client suffering from panic attacks for a psychiatric or a medical evaluation? What purpose would this serve? Could there be any legal or ethical liability consequences if you did not do this? Could making such a referral backfire by making such a client less capable of responding to talking treatment? How could this occur?

9. Is there any point of similarity between the dissociative disorders and the somatoform disorders? How are they different? Which would more likely stem from trauma in a person's life? Would a woman's wish to be made into a Barbie doll look-alike be more characteristic of one or the other types of disorders?

10. Provide at least three examples of relational problems that you have noticed on television programs. Discuss the dysfunctional patterns that you have observed. How might you approach working with such patterns? What advice would you give to the players in each of the dysfunctional relationships to improve their functioning?

## SUGGESTED FURTHER READING

Dzieglielewski, S. (2002). *DSM–IV–TR in action.* New York: Wiley.

Provides an overview to assessment, diagnosis, and treatment planning using the *DSM–IV–TR* along with many case examples, a detailed glossary, and sample treatment plans.

Othmer, E., & Othmer, S. (2002). *The clinical interview using DSM–IV–TR* (Vol. 1). Washington, DC: American Psychiatric Press.

Helps practioners integrate the processes of making a tentative psychiatric diagnosis, begin to understand how the patient experiences his or her difficulties and inner world, and understand what events may have contributed to those difficulties.

Sperry, L. (2003). *Handbook of diagnosis and treatment of the DSM–IV–TR personality disorders* (Rev. ed.). New York: Brunner-Routledge.

This revised edition highlights the many significant clinical and research advances in the diagnosis and treatment of personality disorders since the publication of the *DSM–IV*.

## REFERENCES

American Psychiatric Association. (2000). *Diagnostic and statistical manual of mental disorders* (4th ed., text revision). Washington, DC: Author.

# 5

# PSYCHOPHARMACOLOGY

Roy Resnikoff

*University of California, San Diego*

## TRUTH OR FICTION?

___ 1. *Combined psychotherapy and psychopharmacology are more effective for depression and panic than either alone.*

___ 2. *Psychopharmacology can be over used to find quick fixes for complicated interpersonal problems.*

___ 3. *Medication can be used to modify long-term temperaments as well as immediate target symptoms.*

___ 4. *Family therapy has been polarized into directive, "instrumental," problem solving versus nondirective, "expressive/relational," narrative camps.*

___ 5. *Personality disorders develop from a combination of biological and environmental factors.*

___ 6. *It is important for compliance to present the recommendation of medication in a style consistent with the style of the recipient.*

___ 7. *Family therapists need to be aware of their own biases toward medication and how they compare to those of the treatment family.*

___ 8. *Ideal attachment includes a flexible alternation of closeness and distance and can be enhanced by psychopharmacology.*

___ 9. *Biological temperaments vary in genetic vulnerability to stress.*

___ 10. *Posttraumatic stress disorder includes a combination of hypersensitivity and numbness.*

___ 11. *Medications for depression can sometimes stimulate a manic reaction.*

___ 12. *In comparison to conventional anti-psychotics, atypical anti-psychotics have fewer muscular side effects and correct negative (lethargy) symptoms.*

___ 13. *Parents often take polarized pro and con points of view regarding treatment for attention deficit disorder (ADD or ADHD).*

___ 14. *The eleven categorical personality disorders are grouped into three clusters: odd/eccentric, dramatic/erratic, and anxious/fearful.*

___ 15. *The multidimensional approach for personality disorders includes consideration of biological temperaments.*

## INTRODUCTION

Both family therapists and psychiatrists have long recognized that personality formation involves a complex mixture of environmental and inborn biological influences. In their work with patients, however, family therapists have traditionally used environmental methods while psychiatrists have emphasized biological methods.

Currently, an explosion of information about neurophysiology and psychopharmacology has helped family therapists more routinely consider psychotropic medications for families in treatment. And, after a period of excessive preoccupation with psychopharmacology, psychiatrists are again becoming more interested in psychotherapy (Luhrman, 2000; Gabbard & Kay, 2001).

Recent research for the treatment of depression (Keller et al., 2000; Thase, Greenhouse, & Frank, 1997) and for the treatment of panic disorder (Barlow, Gorman, Shear, & Woods, 2000) has demonstrated that a combination of psychotherapy and pharmacotherapy is better than using either alone. Similar combined therapy research for personality disorders is expected in the near future.

Yet the environmental-biological connection goes even deeper. Although not obvious in daily practice, relational (couples and family) therapy, though primarily an environmental therapy, can change not only psychological interactions but also brain biology. For example, it has now been demonstrated that human attachments and relationship experience are needed for the development of the orbito-frontal gyrus area of the brain and the subsequent ability to have intimate relationships (Schore, 1997; Siegel, 1999). Research has also shown that psychological treatments, without medication, can control compulsions and lower the metabolism of the caudate nucleus in the brain stem (Baxter, Phelps, Mazziotta, Guze, Schwartz, & Selin, 1987; Schwartz, 1995). Calming meditation can shift brain activity away from the brain's right hemisphere and yoga breathing can dramatically increase brain oxygenation (Goleman, 2003).

Conversely, research indicates that medication also has an environmental effect: it changes the neurobiology and, as a consequence, the psychology and interpersonal interactions of the patient (LeDoux, 1996). For example, serotonin-enhancing medications relieve depression and anxiety and also increase interpersonal connections (Stahl, 2000). The neurotransmitters oxytocin and pitocin can induce exploratory attachment behaviors in animals (Young, Lim, Gingrich, & Insel, 2001).

But how can one use this biological–environmental interrelationship effectively in practice? In this chapter, I will discuss four dimensional approaches ("bridges") for combining relational therapy and psychopharmacology in clinical practice (Resnikoff, 2001). I will briefly present the four "bridges" and then introduce a clinical example of a family in therapy. Each dimensional bridge will then be discussed and applied to the clinical material.

1. Combined psychotherapy and pharmacotherapy:
   a. is NOT a more effective treatment (research demonstrated) for depression than either alone.
   b. is a more effective treatment (research demonstrated) for panic disorder than either alone.
   c. has been proven with research to be the most effective treatment for personality disorders.
   d. is NOT an increasingly popular treatment for OCD.

2. Treatment for OCD:
   a. includes pharmacology in the form of serotonin-enhancers but not behavioral de-conditioning.
   b. includes behavioral de-conditioning but not pharmacology.
   c. cannot be successful with behavioral methods alone.
   d. lowers the glucose metabolism of the caudate nucleus with either behavioral or psychopharmacological treatment.

## A Word of Caution

At the outset, I must offer a word of caution. Medications are frequently misused. For example, they may be prescribed merely to suppress anxiety and other emotions rather than help patients manage and effectively incorporate emotions. Medications are also frequently overused in an attempt to find quick and easy solutions to complex family interactional problems. And the enormous influence of pharmaceutical companies may lead to overmedication. Used appropriately, the combination of medication with relational therapy gives a broader range of effective tools for psychotherapy and family therapy.

3. Psychopharmacology can have serious negative impacts NOT including:
   a. being the tool of big pharmaceutical companies trying to overmedicalize the field of psychotherapy.
   b. being overused to suppress potentially useful anxiety and depression.
   c. being part of the culture's attempts to find overly quick and easy solutions to complex interpersonal problems.
   d. being partly dependent on placebo effects.
   e. all of the above.

## THE FOUR DIMENSIONAL BRIDGES

### Bridge 1: Working Through the Four Stages of Family Therapy (Foreground versus Background Stages of Therapy)

This bridge will help clarify how psychopharmacology can be useful for different purposes as you help families through the four stages of relational therapy:

- In stage 1, to help with symptom control.
- In stage 2, to help facilitate flexible attachments, boundaries, and communication.

- In stage 3, to help reduce long-term personality style rigidities.
- In stage 4, to help with natural and unnatural life transitions and trauma.

## Bridge 2: Integrating Instrumental and Expressive/Relational Methods (Instrumental versus Expressive/Relational Methods)

This bridge offers a model for integrating the directive/problem-solving uses of medication ("instrumental") with nondirective/communication-enhancing uses ("expressive/relational").

## Bridge 3: Blending Environmental and Biological Factors (Biological versus Environmental Causes)

This bridge explores how human behaviors and family interactions are a complex blend of environmental and biological factors. Although some situations and personality interactions are more clearly biological and some more clearly environmental, an astute evaluation of the nature versus nurture dimension is important for the proper use of medication in family therapy.

## Bridge 4: Becoming Aware of Therapist–Family Interaction

This bridge helps the therapist consider his or her own preferences as they interact with the family members' preferences on issues such as:

- Using medication appropriately for each stage of therapy.
- Using directive problem-solving approaches that include medication and using nondirective, narrative approaches that include medication.
- Understanding the bases of family problems in both nature and nurture dimensions.

Figure 5.1 summarizes the four "bridges."

## CLINICAL EXAMPLE: DOUGLAS, JOYCE, AND JAY

The following composite example of family therapy that lasted one year illustrates the psychopharmacology integration model. In my practice, approximately half the treatment families do not use medications. For the purpose of this teaching example, however, all three members used medication.

A seventeen-year-old high school student, Jay, was referred to the principal after knocking down a locker in a fit of irritation. His school grades had been dropping and increased marijuana usage had been reported. Interpersonally, Jay had become more isolated and cynical. The principal recommended a psychiatric evaluation to the mother, Joyce, who is a physical therapist and is married to Douglas, a salesman for a biotech company.

The first session started with me outlining four areas of concern (the four stages of therapy):

- Immediate problems and family interactions
- Communication, attachment, and family organization
- Long-term personality styles and temperament polarities
- The current family and life transition

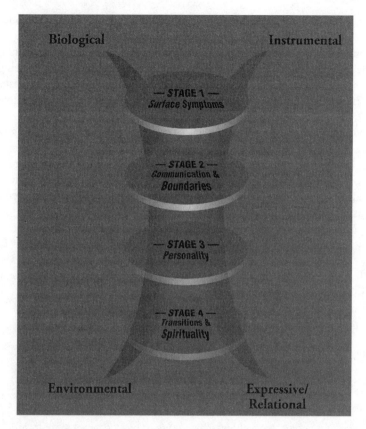

**FIG. 5.1.** Four main dimensions ("bridges") are considered for integrating pharmacotherapy with family treatment (Resnikoff, 2001): (1) foreground versus background stages of therapy; (2) instrumental versus expressive/relational methods (change oriented versus understanding); (3) biological versus environmental causes (nature versus nurture); (4) therapist–family interaction (therapist personal issues that resonate with family therapy treatment issues).

## Stage 1: Immediate Problems and Family Interactions

Although the personality styles and temperaments were apparent in the first interview with all three family members, the initial focus was the school episode and the family's responses.

The mother was the first to hear about the problem and, as usual, became worried and overreactive. Her "maximizing" reaction was to create excessive consequences for Jay's "inappropriate behavior." The father was on an out-of-town sales trip and heard about the locker incident by telephone. His "minimizing" reaction was to state that Jay was "just being a boy" and that there was nothing to worry about.

In the session, Jay explained that he was angry after being reprimanded by the gym coach for walking the one-mile run. In an individual session, he also described worries after being accepted at college. He worried about being separated from his girlfriend and not being able to handle the workload.

In this sequence, the son had an irritable/depressed mood and a violent outburst. The mother became overcontrolling and overreactive following this behavior; the father seemed cavalier, generally impulsive, and underreactive in the family. To form a collaborative therapy, I had to initially be on the same level as the family—that is, concerned with what to do about Jay rather than trying to confront contextual communication or personality issues.

The beginning therapy helped clarify that Jay was under stress because of impending graduation and college. The parents were helped to see the problem clearly instead of being polarized into a strict parent/lenient parent escalating sequence. I supported both understanding and compassion (father) as well as limits on violence (mother) in their most positive reframed forms.

To help with immediate symptoms, I prescribed low doses of Zoloft, 50 mg per day, for Jay. (A low bedtime dose of Depakote, 250 mg, was also included to protect against a possible coexisting bipolar potential, especially in view of the father's impulsive temperament.) With Joyce, medication for Jay was presented as problem solving. With Douglas, medication for Jay was presented as enhancing Jay's comfort zone. For Jay, medication was presented as a way to support his expression of concerns about emancipating.

4. In the clinical example, Zoloft and Depakote were prescribed for the teenager, Jay. Which is true:
   a. Medications can be useful in stage 1 to reduce target symptoms, increase awareness regarding target symptoms, and prove that change is possible.
   b. Depakote was added to the Zoloft to prevent overactivation, in light of the father's cyclothymic (bipolar) temperament.
   c. Jay would have the final say in his agreement to take medication.
   d. All of the above.

5. Regarding stage 1 of family therapy, which is NOT true:
   a. Stage 1 emphasizes finding the sequence of events surrounding the presenting problem.
   b. In stage 1, you can use psychopharmacology to reduce target symptoms.
   c. In stage 1, usually one parent is more the "instrumental" problem solver and the other more the "expressive/relational" compassionate caretaker.
   d. Stage 1 usually does not have elements of all the subsequent stages of therapy.

## Stage 2: Communication, Attachment, and Family Organization Styles

As Jay's problem was being discussed, it became clear that Joyce and Jay were very close, with Douglas being more peripheral. It was also clear that neither parent communicated well with Jay. Instead, each made assumptions based on their personality styles.

The attachment between the parents was strained. Douglas felt "emotionally betrayed" and rejected by Joyce's preoccupation with her work and Jay. Joyce felt "emotionally betrayed" by Douglas's flirtatiousness, flamboyance, and constant need to seek new excitement.

In this second stage of therapy, the lack of listening skills and the attachment disruptions were clarified and corrected. The listening and closeness versus distancing dynamics were considered as part of long-term personality styles (disorders), but again, the family was more interested in the overt communication difficulties than in historical patterns or personality issues.

Joyce used her anxiety to intrude on Jay's life but also to distance herself from Douglas. Douglas felt rejected by Joyce and found outside substitute excitement—including an affair at work. After Joyce discovered this affair on Douglas' e-mail, Douglas agreed to suspend that relationship while the family discussed the family and marital issues. Medications for Douglas and Joyce were not introduced until later in the therapy, during stage 3.

6. In stage 2 of the clinical example:
   a. The structure of the family, with mother and son in one subgroup was clarified.
   b. The attachment disruptions between the parents, Joyce and Douglas, were clarified.
   c. It was important to suspend Douglas's affair to avoid excessive distraction from the therapy.
   d. All of the above.

## Stage 3: Long-Term Ways of Facing Adversity, Personality Styles, and Temperament Polarities

In this third stage of therapy, Joyce and Douglas expressed their grievances about each other's personality traits. Joyce's feeling of having to take care of everything and Douglas's feeling of being restricted by irrational emotions were traced back to childhood. In addition, biological (hereditary and stress-induced) temperaments, including a complete psychiatric family history were explored. Douglas grew up in a chaotic family with a bipolar father who spent more money than he earned, dressed and talked in a flamboyant style, and was unfaithful. Joyce grew up in a strict religious household and learned to follow rules and regulations. Her mother was extremely anxious and controlling and there was some physical abuse.

Conversations regarding childhood stories helped Joyce and Douglas become more aware of the two sides of their personalities: restricted versus expressive, controlling versus laissez-faire, anxious versus relaxed. I introduced cognitive and experiential exercises to help Joyce learn from Douglas and Douglas learn from Joyce.

It had been apparent from the first that Joyce had a biological anxious/obsessive-compulsive temperament (with lifelong sensitivity, worrying, and anxiety) and that Douglas, with a flamboyant flair and a need for excitement, had a biological impulsive/cyclothymic (bipolar) temperament. In stage 3 therapy, medication was prescribed to address these long-standing biological temperaments in both parents: Depakote, 500 mg, and Lithium, 300 mg per day, were used as "mood stabilizers" to control Douglas's impulsivity, and a serotonin-enhancing agent, Prozac, 10 mg per day, helped Joyce with her anxiety and worry.

Joyce was willing to take medication to help her "get through all of this." Douglas was willing to take medicine as a gift to Joyce and to help him tolerate his review of painful childhood stories. He considered and began taking medication several weeks after Joyce.

Jay, as mentioned above, had already been given medication for depressive temperament features, including irritability. The plan was to use medications for approximately six months to help with the family transition and the process of therapy.

## Stage 4: Current Family and Life Transition

With reduced symptoms, better communication, and less personality distortion, this family began to discuss the stress and complications of Jay's leaving for college. He no longer had to create a problem that might bring the parents together. His anxiety and sadness about leaving home was, instead, discussed directly.

The parents began to plan their life together and find ways to both be serious (like Joyce) and have fun (like Douglas). Joyce needed help in connecting with community supports. Douglas needed help in staying home more and being more concerned for others. The medications initiated earlier in the therapy would help the transition.

Regarding my clinical interaction with the family, I was able to be flexible as a therapist without imposing my own preferences about stage of therapy, medication, discipline, or emancipation. I could identify with both Joyce's seriousness and Douglas's fun-loving styles. My approach was primarily expressive/relational, but I also addressed the instrumental goals of correcting Jay's depression, restoring the marriage, and helping Jay successfully leave home.

7. In the case example:
   a. Joyce, the mother, demonstrated a biological impulsive cyclothymic (bipolar) temperament, and was eventually treated with Depakote.
   b. Douglas, the father, demonstrated a biological anxious obsessive-compulsive temperament with lifelong sensitivity, worrying, and anxiety, and was eventually treated with Prozac.
   c. In therapy the two parents became more insightful into how their personalities conflicted—Joyce being more restricted, controlling, and anxious, and Douglas being more expressive, laissez-faire, and relaxed.
   d. Their son, Jay, showed evidence of a schizophrenic illness.

8. Considering the four stages of family therapy, which is NOT true:
   a. Symptom resolution is usually foreground.
   b. It is usually wise to initially focus on personality issues.
   c. Medications are potentially beneficial for all stages of therapy.
   d. The family and therapist negotiate when to stop therapy, frequently before all four stages of therapy are completed.

9. In the "bridges for healing" four-dimensional model:
   a. Biological versus environmental causes are not relevant for all stages of family therapy.
   b. Instrumental versus expressive/relational approaches are not relevant for all stages of family therapy.
   c. The therapist's interaction with the treatment family is relevant regarding the therapist's biases (stage of therapy, medication, directiveness).
   d. Medications are only relevant for stage 1 target symptom resolution.

## BRIDGE 1: FOREGROUND VERSUS BACKGROUND STAGES OF THERAPY

When a therapist first begins to work with a family, he or she encounters surface symptoms. We know that Jay had knocked down a locker; he was angry and depressed. It turned out that he was preoccupied with going to college, worried about whether he could do the work, and worried about leaving his girlfriend. In stage 1 (Immediate Problems and Family Interactions), we typically look at the surface symptoms and try to find the sequence of events, in this case the parents' reactions to Jay's action.

In stage 1 therapy, which took about a month, I talked with Jay alone and then met with the whole family to discuss whether the family would be able to have a successful emancipation. After Jay's initial problem was dealt with, it became necessary to confront the parents' lack of connection. That required couples therapy.

In stage 2 of therapy (Communication, Attachment, and Family Organization), my goal was to get Douglas and Joyce to talk more effectively to each other. Should I use historical backgrounds and psychopharmacology to address attachment difficulties, or should I make a more interpersonal connection, using only current issues, as described by Susan Johnson (Johnson, Makinen, & Millikin, 2001)?

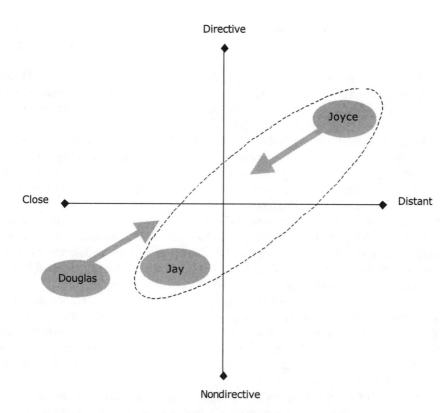

**FIG. 5.2.** Personality Trait Complementary Polarities. Using the (Olson) personality trait dimensions of close versus distant and directive versus non-directive, Douglas and Jay are in the expressive/relational quadrant and Joyce is in the instrumental quadrant. Using the (Benjamin) personality trait dimension of friendly versus unfriendly, Douglas is friendlier than Joyce. Joyce and Jay form a sub-group within the family.

In this case, because of the pronounced biological temperaments and long-term personality rigidities, I decided on a blending together of stage 2 and stage 3 therapy, including medication and historical therapy in addition to enhancing attachment. That is, I initially observed the way Douglas and Joyce communicated with each other while exploring patterns and core feelings that resonated with their family histories. The focus moved gradually from current issues toward historical patterns.

Figure 5.2 shows how Joyce was directive in the family while being a distancer. Douglas was in the complementary position of being expressive and "close" while maintaining a more passive role in the family. Jay was similar to his father in being passive and sensitive to feelings. Mother and son had formed a tight subgroup despite their polarized styles. Olson (1986), Millon (1991), and Benjamin (1996) have used similar diagrams.

A person becomes obsessive either because of biological temperament or because of training and culture. Joyce had both aspects and was repeating her family style.

Douglas had alcoholic parents and he, by both temperament and training, had a wild and hectic background. Douglas also could have become polarized, but he, too, reflected his family model.

During our sessions Joyce tended to scold Douglas. My objective was to have her, instead, express her emotion about being abandoned. In therapy, it is essential to experience and communicate core inner feelings, which in this case is the feeling of abandonment by her husband. So I asked her to be more specific. I prompted her with, "Joyce, please try saying, 'I feel like I'm all alone.' "

After Joyce accessed fundamental feelings of aloneness, the next question was, can Douglas empathize with her sense of betrayal and abandonment? So I asked him: "Douglas, can you connect with Joyce's emotions?" He needed therapeutic assistance to join and understand Joyce instead of reverting to his usual style of attacking her.

As it turned out, Douglas also felt abandoned because Joyce had been so involved with Jay; Douglas felt that there was nobody taking care of him. His was like a child feeling that "No one is taking care of me. I have to go out and take care of myself and entertain myself." Joyce also needed help with joining and empathy instead of attacking, even though both had potentially helpful criticisms of each other. This connection is essential to stage 2 therapy.

With Douglas and Joyce, the pronounced temperaments and long-term rigidities required continued therapy (stage 3) beyond enhancing attachment and communication. Medication helped Joyce, and later Douglas, review painful childhood experiences that resonated with their current emotions (see Scharff & Scharff, 1991). Historical therapy included both the benefits of heightened awareness as well as directed "corrective" exercises.

Once stage 1, 2, and 3 issues were addressed, in this case with the help of medication, it was possible to address stage 4 issues (Family and Life Transitions). Jay was going off to college, and Douglas and Joyce had to find out whether they could reattach and make a commitment toward their marriage. They will also need to consider what kind of community support will be available to them and what kind of spiritual support they are going to establish for new meaning in their lives.

Therapists tends to be more comfortable with one stage over another. For example, when I first began my professional life, I was especially interested in stage 1 problem solving. My goal was to be able to create action and make changes. With maturity, I have become more interested in stage 3 work—that is, how personality styles interrupt intimacy. As I grow older, I am also more concerned with spiritual issues, mortality, and the meaning of life (stage 4).

10. In the staging of family therapy, which is NOT true:
    a. Many families and family therapists prefer to end therapy after symptom resolution (stage 1) and improved communication and attachment (stage 2).
    b. Personality oriented therapy (stage 3), including medications for long-term temperaments, may be necessary to augment the connection enhancement therapy of stage 2.
    c. Life transitions are usually the backdrop (stage 4) for earlier stages of therapy.
    d. Directive ("instrumental") versus nondirective ("expressive/relational") approaches are not integrated in all stages of therapy.

## BRIDGE 2: INSTRUMENTAL VERSUS EXPRESSIVE/RELATIONAL METHODS

Families usually include one parent who favors active, problem-solving change ("instrumental") and another who favors clarification, understanding, and connection ("expressive/relational"). In this example, Joyce was more instrumental and Douglas more expressive/relational.

Professionals are also divided between directive "change" and nondirective "no-change" methods (Gurman & Fraenkel, 2002). Directive methods include problem-solving, cognitive-behavioral therapy, hypnotism, deconditioning, and desensitization (e.g., Linehan, 1993). Nondirective methods include psychodynamic, narrative, gestalt, emotion-focused, and existential therapy (e.g., Polster, 1995).

As a therapist one must be flexible enough to consider both points of view as needed in all stages of therapy (Edwards, 2002). Integrating instrumental and expressive/relational methods means considering the entire dimension, although the therapist may tend to favor one approach.

Medication can be considered and used from either point of view: It can be used in an instrumental model to change the brain, treat biological abnormalities, and control target symptoms. It can also be used in an expressive/relational model, to increase expression, understanding, and connection (Knutson, Wolkowitz, Cole, Chan, Moore, Johnson, et al., 1998), while also supporting the therapeutic process.

An instrumental person considers medication to create change; an expressive/relational person considers medication to facilitate expression and connection. An instrumental, practical partner may want a clear medication intervention early in the course of therapy; an expressive/relational partner may need a cautious, delayed introduction of medication. The couple's negotiations regarding medication help illuminate their personality polarities and help guide the introduction of medication. These negotiations about medications may be similar to discussions about food, money, sex, or in-laws.

To introduce medication the therapist should join the style of the person. In the clinical example, I had to speak a feeling language to Douglas and a problem-solving language to Joyce. Douglas understood how medication could help communication and attachment and how he could have better sex, better connection, and more fun. Joyce understood that medication helps sleep. She accepted a "medical" solution.

11. Psychotropic medication can be best introduced:
   a. by emphasizing medication as a symptom-reducing agent to families who favor a medical model.
   b. by emphasizing medication as an awareness- and communication-enhancing agent to families who favor narrative approaches.
   c. by describing inappropriate uses of medication such as the suppression of emotions.
   d. all of the above.

# BRIDGE 3: BIOLOGICAL VERSUS ENVIRONMENTAL CAUSES

## Robert Cloninger: Character verses Biological Temperament

In the case study, Jay had biological depression, the environmental stress of competing parents, and the stress of leaving home. Robert Cloninger (Cloninger & Svrakic, 1997) has stimulated much follow-up research and discussion with his research hypothesis that some personality factors are biological (novelty seeking, avoidance of harm, reward dependence, and persistence) and others are learned (accepting responsibility, the ability to be involved in relationships that are give and take, and the ability to look beyond one's self and think about the world).

My clinical experience tends to support Cloninger's belief that if the "environmental character traits" are not properly learned, then the likelihood of a personality disorder is increased. Cloninger's hypothesis is that self-esteem (which allows a person to accept and empathize with self, others, and the environment) is developed in childhood training rather than inborn. If both therapist and patient understand the combination of biological (including genetic, developmental, and post-traumatic) and learned/environmental factors in personality formation and personality disorders, they are in a better position to modify dysfunctional interpersonal patterns.

In the clinical example, medication for Jay, in addition to addressing his depressive symptoms, helped Jay's parents focus on his emotional needs rather than just defining him as a troublemaker.

12. In the work of Robert Cloninger:
  a. Reward-seeking, novelty-seeking, and persistence are viewed as learned personality factors.
  b. Concern for others is viewed as a biological personality factor.
  c. The dominance of nature in the development of personality, is emphasized.
  d. Although not yet proven, Cloninger's model has stimulated much follow-up research.

## Larry Siever and Paul Soloff: Biological Temperament Dimensions and Psychopharmacological Considerations

Another model integrating the biological and environmental components of personality temperaments is derived from the work of Larry Siever (1998) and Paul Soloff (1998). This model defines four main biological *temperament* dimensions:

- Schizoid
- Depressive
- Angry/violent/impulsive
- Anxious

Each dimension includes a range of biological influence from strong to mild. Strong biological influence is indicated by the early onset of symptoms, a strong family history, and severe diagnosable symptoms. Mild biological influence produces a personality-style expression of the biological temperament, mixed with environmental factors including gender, cultural, family, and developmental influences.

At the severe biological end of these dimensions, symptoms can be conceptualized as either separate diagnostic illnesses or as expressions of severe personality dimension difficulties (see Westin & Harnden-Fischer, 2001). I prefer the latter view that symptoms and categories should not be considered in isolation, but rather integrated into larger continuums.

*It is important to note that the psychopharmacology agents used at the severe end of a personality temperament dimension can also be effective, frequently in lower doses, when only a mild biological component is present, such as with Douglas, Joyce, and Jay.* However, the use of medications for such subclinical conditions is still considered "off label," that is, not officially approved by the Food and Drug Administration. Figure 5.3 summarizes the four temperament dimensions and the medications used for each.

### Schizoid Temperament Dimension

In the schizoid temperament dimension, the personality style ranges all the way from mild oddity and detachment to a flagrant schizophrenia or schizophrenic paranoia. For the schizoid

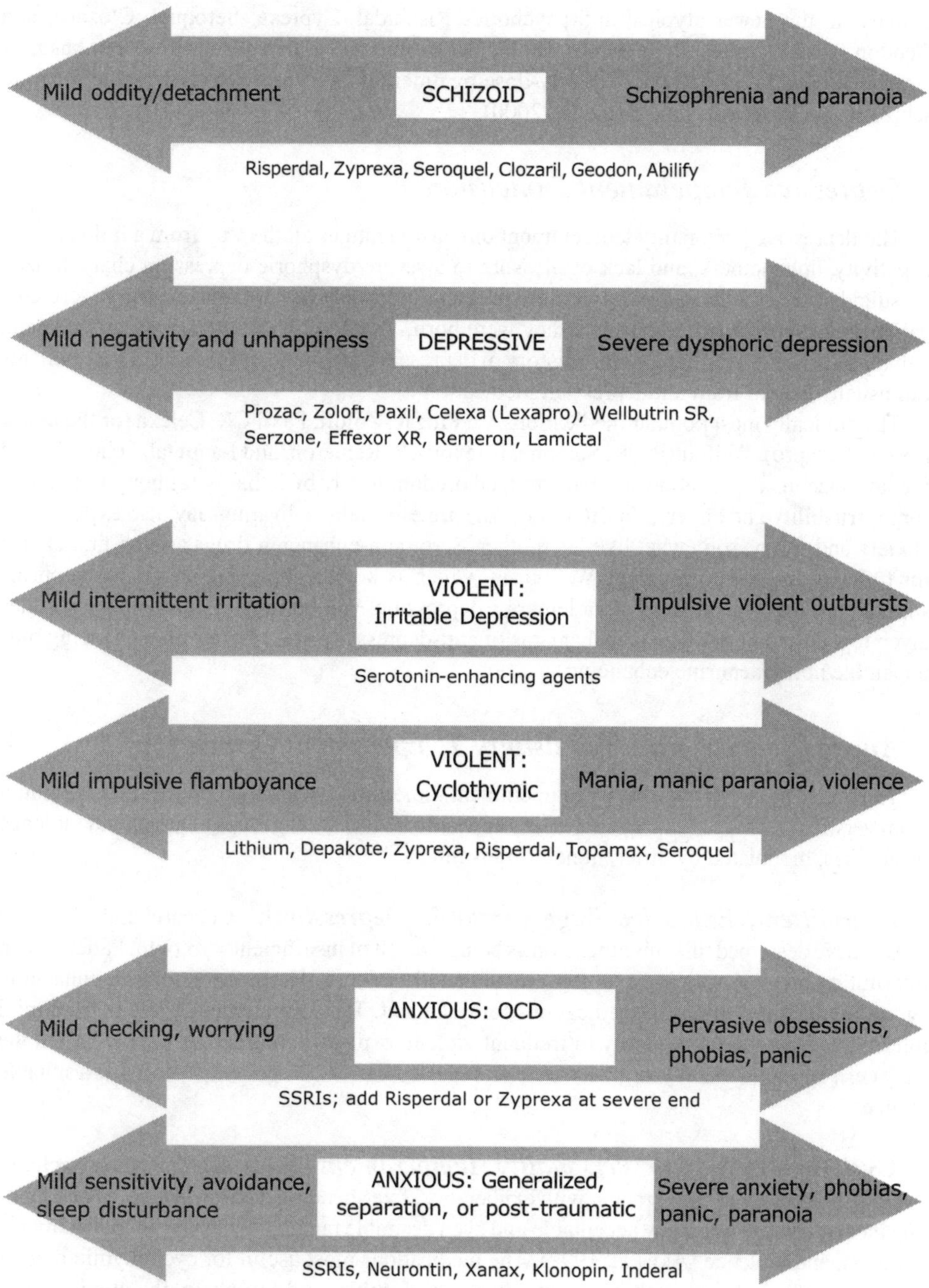

**FIG. 5.3.** Biological Temperament Dimensions (Siever, 1998; Soloff, 1998).

dimension, the newer atypical anti-psychotics Risperdal, Zyprexa, Seroquel, Clozaril, and Geodon are most clinically relevant. Abilify is a newcomer to this group. Research has now clearly demonstrated the benefit of low-dose treatment with Zyprexa and Risperdal for mild schizoid conditions (Kirrane & Siever, 2000).

### Depressive Temperament Dimension

The depressive personality temperament dimension ranges all the way from a mild style of negativity, unhappiness, and lack of pleasure to a severe dysphoric depression characterized by suicidal ideas, lethargy, negative thinking, and a depressive paranoia. At the severe end, patients have been "depressed since they were born," are beset with moodiness, anxiety, and unhappiness, and have a long family history of depression, suicides, and alcohol. These patients can usually benefit from antidepressant medication.

The clinically most popular medications are Prozac, Zoloft, Paxil CR, Celexa (or the newer isomer, Lexapro), Wellbutrin SR, Serzone, Effexor XR, Remeron, and Lamictal. I chose Zoloft for Jay since his depression was characterized predominantly by lethargy (although there was some irritability and anger). Zoloft and Prozac are especially activating. Jay also experienced anxiety and worry, somewhat like his mother. Serotonin-enhancing drugs are the first choice for treating obsessive worrying; Wellbutrin, which is both a dopamine and norepinephrine stimulant, is especially effective for lethargic depression. Wellbutrin and Zoloft are sometimes given together to provide two mechanisms of anti-depressant effect (serotonin enhancing plus dopamine/norepinephrine enhancing).

### Anger, Violence, and Impulsivity Temperament Dimension

The anger/violence/impulsivity temperament dimension occurs along a similar continuum from very mild to severe expression. There appear to be two main groups of anger and violence difficulties, modulated by different neurotransmitters.

#### Intermittent, Explosive Rage (Irritable Depression).
Coccaro and Kavoussi (1997) have described this subdimension as being a result of insufficient serotonin. Patients with intermittent explosive rage have non-premeditated violence. Here, the serotonin-enhancing agents are the most effective medications for treatment. The temperament range is from mild intermittent irritation all the way to frequent violent, explosive, murderous outbursts. On the surface, it appeared that Jay might have an irritable depression component; Zoloft was a suitable choice.

#### Cyclothymic/Bipolar Personality Temperament.
This subdimension includes symptoms from a very mild range, with exuberance, free spending, charm, sexuality, and flamboyance (all within a socially acceptable and even desirable range), all the way to mania, manic paranoia, and violence (Akiskal, 1999). The medications most useful for cyclothymic/bipolar difficulties are the mood stabilizers: in addition to Lithium and Depakote, the atypical anti-psychotics Zyprexa and Risperdal have been used. (Clozaril, also an atypical anti-psychotic, is used only at the severe end of the dimension because of white-cell suppression side effects. Seroquel may also be an effective mood stabilizer.) In addition, some newer anti-convulsants, including Topamax, appear to be effective for controlling bipolar aggression.

Douglas, in our clinical example, had a cyclothymic temperament. He got irritable, but his main style was moody and flamboyant. He had a bipolar II condition—he had frequently alternating, essentially simultaneous, experiences of exuberance and sadness. (Bipolar I patients have clear alternating periods, often weeks to months, of highs and lows. Bipolar III patients have drug-induced mania or hypomania [not fully manic]). Since many childhood depressions become more bipolar in adult life, and because Jay's father was bipolar, I added Depakote to "protect" him against this bipolar possibility.

It is important to differentiate between the two groups of anger/violence temperaments. An example of an individual with irritable depression would be the professional sports coach who, although generally serious, intermittently engages in explosive outbursts. This kind of patient responds best to serotonin-enhancing agents because people who are explosive are low in serotonin. But be aware that if the therapist misdiagnoses bipolar depression as irritable depression, a problem can be created because serotonin-enhancing agents can make bipolar conditions worse. It is, therefore, important to ask, "Is this person basically expansive and grandiose? Or is this person more violently depressed in a more explosive but intermittent way?"

## Anxious Temperament Dimension

The anxious biological temperament dimension describes mild avoidant anxiety and sensitivity at one end, all the way to major panic disorders and phobias at the other end. Most clinicians divide the anxiety spectrum into two major components.

### Obsessive-Compulsive Disorder (OCD) Spectrum.
This component involves obsessions and compulsions associated with anxiety. The mild end may include some minimal worry about dirt and contamination, while the severe end shows pervasive obsessions, phobias, and panic as well as obsessive-compulsive paranoia. The OCD biological spectrum should be distinguished from an obsessive-compulsive personality (OCP) disorder, which is characterized by a need for control and perfection driven by previous life experience. However, the two can occasionally overlap. The medications most effective for the OCD spectrum are, again, the serotonin-enhancing agents. If the syndrome is at the severe end, the atypical anti-psychotics, such as Risperdal or Zyprexa, can be effective in controlling delusional paranoid obsessions when combined with serotonin-enhancing agents.

The OCD subdivision implies biological/medical symptoms. That is, if the patient has compulsive hand washing, compulsive rituals to turn the lights on and off ten times before leaving the room, plus excessive worrying, and comes from a family of worriers, then there is a large biological OCD component to the anxiety.

Extensive work has examined how the caudate nucleus metabolism works excessively with obsessive-compulsive disorder as determined by proton emission tomography (PET) brain scans. As mentioned in the introduction, Lewis Baxter (Baxter et al., 1987) and Jeffrey Schwartz (1995) studied the use of behavioral treatments for OCD and have found that if treatment can get people to act less compulsively (or, by implication, less depressed) with behavioral or deconditioning methods, medication is not needed to create the corresponding lowered glucose metabolism in the caudate nucleus of the brain. Or, if medication is used to get patients started, it can then be omitted and the behavioral treatment continued to keep psychological and neurophysiological changes in place.

This is an important use of medication; it is a way to begin treatment with a small but clear improvement in symptoms. Once the door is opened, we can try to create more permanent cognitive changes, interpersonal changes, or broader lifestyle changes with relational and cognitive-behavioral psychotherapy.

In the last ten years, psychiatry has leaned toward medication only. Pharmaceutical companies supported psychiatric syndromes defined as medical illness needing medical treatment. Now the pendulum is swinging back the other way, to where we understand that nature and nurture have a complex interaction. We know that people are more obsessively anxious under periods of stress and we know that patients can control these anxieties by cognitive methods or deconditioning. An integration of medical and psychological approaches is usually the wisest course for OCD and OCP anxiety.

*Generalized Anxiety, Separation Anxiety, and Post Traumatic Anxiety (PTSD).* Again, this may be defined along a continuum all the way from mild sensitivity and sleep disturbance to major panic and diagnosable anxiety symptoms. If one has been terrorized, witnessed a murder, or experienced another unnatural catastrophe, then one may experience a posttraumatic reaction, usually including the extremes of hypersensitivity on the one hand, and emotional "numbing" on the other (Yehuda, 2002). For this anxiety temperament spectrum, medications that have been helpful include the serotonin-enhancing agents, the benzodiazapines, including Xanax and Klonopin (though these are not usually used for PTSD for fear of interrupting normal memory processes that are needed for recovery), and Neurontin (even though this anti-convulsive GABA-enhancing agent has not been formally approved for psychotropic use). Inderal, a beta-blocker, is also widely used for anxiety symptoms.

At times the posttraumatic consequences of early childhood sexual and physical abuse (and neglect) can be so severe that they create problems in all of the four temperament dimensions (Heim & Nemeroff 1999; Teicher, 2002): disrupted cognitions, unregulated affect, impulsive violence, and intense anxiety. Such a pervasive disruption of multiple temperament dimensions, in essence, describes the borderline personality (Gunderson, 2001; American Psychiatric Association, 2001). In addition to the medications listed above, monoamine oxidase inhibitors (MAOIs) have been successful agents for helping such borderline personality patients, but they have not been used generally because of diet induced tyrosine side effects.

## Attention Deficit Spectrum

An additional biological spectrum important for family therapy is the *attention deficit spectrum* (ADD or ADHD with hyperactivity). There is increasing evidence that ADD reflects a genetic defect in the dopamine vesicle production, release, and re-uptake needed by the brain for executive functioning and focusing (Faraone, Biederman, Weiffenbach, Keith, Chu, Weaver, et al., 1999). Stimulating drugs such as Ritalin or Adderall and their long-acting forms (Ritalin LA, lasting about 8 hours; Adderall XR, also lasting 7 or 8 hours; Concerta, lasting 12 hours) all increase dopamine and norepinephrine. Strattera is a new stimulant for ADD that works primarily on the cortex level of the brain (Spencer, Biederman, Wilens, & Faraone, 2002). A severe expression of the ADD severity spectrum is predicted by a strong family history and early onset, including excessive kicking during pregnancy. Girls tend to have less hyperactivity compared to boys, and during adult life hyperactivity frequently drops out, leaving the inattention.

It is difficult to place ADD in the four temperament spectrums described above. ADD could be considered within the cyclothymic/bipolar spectrum when there is hyperactivity. Others combine ADD, OCD, and Tourette's (tics) as part of a brain stem (globus pallidus) movement disorder spectrum (Walkup, 1999). ADD and bipolarity frequently co-exist; when they do, the distinction can be difficult. The bipolar condition usually shows more anger and mood difficulties and, generally, the overall functioning is worse. Both conditions have dopamine difficulties (ADD too little; bipolar too much). Some clinicians treat coexisting conditions with both stimulants and mood stabilizers, but add stimulants only after the bipolar condition is well under control.

As with any symptom, whether biological or not, frequently one parent wants more medication for ADD than the other. The art of family therapy is to respect and integrate both points of view. With ADD or ADHD the family can consider an "experiment" with certain days on medication and other days off, to compare results. Stimulant medications are suitable for such experiments because they produce immediate effects; most other psychopharmacology agents take days or weeks to become effective.

13. Regarding the temperament dimensions, the more severe end of the dimension spectrum is NOT characterized by:
    a. early age of onset.
    b. strong family history.
    c. severe target symptoms reflecting the temperament style.
    d. usually does not require the use of medication in stage 1 therapy.

14. Which is NOT true regarding atypical anti-psychotics:
    a. They have fewer muscular side effects compared to conventional anti-psychotics.
    b. They control negative symptoms but do not control positive symptoms.
    c. They can be used as mood stabilizers for bipolar conditions.
    d. They include Seroquel and Abilify, which are partial rather than complete dopamine blockers.

15. A bipolar (cyclothymic) temperament:
    a. is NOT characterized by excessive elation, sexuality, and impulsivity.
    b. can be modified with the help of "mood stabilizers" such as Lithium, Depakote, Zyprexa, and Risperdal.
    c. can be triggered by the use of antidepressant medication.
    d. is NOT in a continuum with the more severe manic-depressive illness that can include psychotic grandiose delusions.

16. Regarding anti-anxiety agents, which of the following is true:
    a. Serotonin-enhancing drugs such as Prozac are NOT effective for anxiety.
    b. Serotonin-enhancing drugs cannot help control OCD.
    c. Serotonin-enhancing drugs cannot help control the hypersensitivity and numbing of PTSD.
    d. Inderal (a beta blocker) and Neurontin (an anti-convulsant) are often used as anti-anxiety agents.

17. Medications for ADD:
    a. do NOT improve cognitive attention by augmenting deficient dopamine and nore-pinephrine.
    b. include long-acting forms of Ritalin and Adderall as well as the newer agent Strattera, all of which become effective almost immediately.
    c. are NOT frequently the focus of disagreement between parents (one pro, the other con, regarding usage).
    d. cannot be given in addition to medications for anxiety, depression, or bipolar conditions.

18. Intermittent explosive rage (Caccaro):
    a. is distinguished from sociopathic premeditated crime and is instead un-premeditated and impulsive.
    b. is characterized by a serotonin deficiency and treated with SSRIs such as Lexapro.
    c. is distinguished from bipolar violence, which is treated with mood stabilizers.
    d. all of the above.

19. In which of the four biological temperament concerns does Cloninger's *avoidance of harm* overlap?
    a. anxiety temperament spectrum (GABA and serotonin neurotransmitters).
    b. depression temperament spectrum (serotonin, norepinephrine, and dopamine neurotransmitters).
    c. bipolar temperament spectrum (norepinephrine and dopamine neurotransmitters).
    d. OCD spectrum (serotonin neurotransmitters).

## Personality Disorders

Mental health can be defined as a person's ability to cope with life's demands. This coping includes the ability to be able to enjoy work, play, and relationships. In addition, a healthy person can cope with daily stress as well as the stress of life transitions and adversity. Healthy functioning involves an awareness and respect for self, others, and the environment. Optimum mental health includes sensitivity and responsiveness to gender, cultural, and societal issues.

Traditionally, impediments to healthy living have been defined as falling into three main groups:

1. Immediate symptoms or preoccupations that interfere with facing life.
2. Communication difficulties that interfere with awareness of other people or the environment.
3. Long-standing pervasive rigid attitudes, internalized conflicts, and patterns of behavior that distort a person's awareness of and ability to cope with life's problems or relationships. This third group is the traditional *categorical* definition of a personality disorder.

### Traditional Categorical Definitions of Personality Disorders

Understanding the traditional categorical model of personality disorders is the first step toward applying the newer multidimensional model in clinical practice.

The eleven categories of personality disorders listed in the *Diagnostic and Statistical Manual of Mental Disorder* (American Psychiatric Association, 1994) are arranged into three clusters:

- Odd/Eccentric
- Dramatic/Erratic
- Anxious/Fearful

These groupings are based on lifelong internalized dysfunctional conflicts from one's childhood and one's "character defenses." For example, in the histrionic personality disorder, the patient repetitively tries to win love and acceptance by being highly seductive and overly dramatic. A typical family history would include a daughter trying desperately to win approval from her father. The character defenses would include excessive placating and "introjection" (extreme taking in) of what the child imagines the father would like.

In the traditional individually oriented categorical model, long-term distortions influence a person's cognitions, interactions, attitudes, and coping style. Understanding a patient's reaction to the suggestion of taking medication helps you diagnose personality traits and anticipate "resistance" based on personality distortions rather than realistic concerns (Benjamin, 1996). The list in Figure 5.4 provides a brief review. (These styles are now so well known that several patients have even given me humorous Internet versions.)

---

**Odd/Eccentric Cluster**

**Paranoid**—The patient might be very concerned about side effects that may be discovered over the next decade. He or she might point out the drug company's profit motivation. After taking the drug he or she might feel controlled and unnatural and might consider making a formal complaint.

**Schizoid**—The patient would be unlikely to consider medication, since there is no expectation that medication would help or that help is needed.

**Schizotypal**—The patient might object to a medication because the medication has a strange name. He or she may suspect hidden meanings, "energy," or telepathic powers coming from the therapist or medication.

---

**Dramatic/Erratic Cluster**

**Borderline**—The patient will probably consider the medication wrong or not enough. It is also likely that the patient will underdose or overdose with the medication.

**Narcissistic**—This patient might think that his or her depression is special and that an exotic medication is needed. He or she may expect free samples and think that his or her side effects are especially interesting. The patient may become angry if medication does not work and perhaps consider a lawsuit.

**Histrionic**—This patient typically jokes about being a medication poster child but gives vague descriptions of symptoms, symptom relief, or side effects. He or she mentions telling friends about the psychiatrist's special medication cocktails.

**Antisocial**—This patient might impulsively use medication to get "high" or as a manipulation to apply for disability. The patient might forge prescriptions or sell the drugs for profit, without remorse.

---

**Anxious/Fearful Cluster**

**Dependent**—The patient might tolerate extreme side effects without reporting them for fear of losing the nurturing and caring that the medication represents.

**Obsessive-Compulsive**—The patient might delay before taking medication, saying that he or she can control the symptoms. The patient might consider a medication after extensive Internet research but then alternate between thinking the medication is a wonderful "magic pill" and thinking it is "useless"

**Negativistic (Passive-Aggressive)**—The patient might reluctantly agree to medication as a last hope but be suspicious of side effects. He or she might take the wrong dosage and complain about results. The patient might try a series of medications with none "working."

**Avoidant**—The patient might avoid medication for fear of complications or having the medication indicate that there was "something profoundly wrong" with him or her. The patient might overdose rather than deal with problems of medication.

---

**FIG. 5.4.** Personality Style Reactions to Medications.

20. Following the typology of the eleven *categorical* personality styles, the patient who is most likely to impulsively use prescribed medication to get "high" or to forge prescriptions falls in which of the following groups?
    a. Odd/Eccentric Cluster: Paranoid
    b. Dramatic/Erratic Cluster: Histrionic
    c. Dramatic/Erratic Cluster: Antisocial
    d. Anxious/Fearful Cluster: Obsessive-Compulsive

## Modern Multidimensional Approach to Personality Disorders

Today, we understand that personality can be defined as a person's multidimensional and interpersonal approach to coping with life. Personality styles are affected by a combination of constitutional factors (biological influences) and external life circumstances, including development, gender, and culture (environmental influences).

Although a personality disorder occurs when there is excessive rigidity, excessive deviance from societal standards, or maladaptive interpersonal patterns, an ambiguous line exists between a personality style and a personality disorder (Kernberg, 2001).

In a multidimensional therapeutic approach, the therapist (and the treatment family) rapidly consider polarized points of view within each dimension (Polster & Polster, 1999). Even if one point of view is favored, integration takes place because the entire dimension is considered. This more inclusive, complex description of personality and relational personality therapy includes all stages of therapy in addition to the traditional categorical and historical perspective included as part of stage 3:

- Overt behavior and symptoms
- Style of interpersonal closeness and distance attachment (loving, nurturing, touching, and concern versus independent activities, emotional self-sufficiency, and non-self-disclosure) (Bowlby, 1988; Fonagy, Target, & Gergely, 2000)
- Maladaptive "character resistances" to intimacy (Scharf & Scharf, 1991)
- Interpersonal expression of inner childhood conflicts and core feelings (Benjamin, 1996)
- Expression of biological temperament dimensions (schizoid, depressive, impulsive, anxious)
- Regulation of mood and inner impulses such as sexuality, aggression, or hunger
- Numerous personality trait dimensions (such as extrovert versus introvert, thinking versus feeling, directive versus nondirective, and friendly versus unfriendly) (McCrae & Costa, 1999; Polster, 1995)
- Characteristic response to stress or perceived danger
- Style of coping with life transitions

In our clinical example, Joyce can be diagnosed categorically as an obsessive-compulsive personality (OCP). In a more multidimensional view, however, Joyce exhibits:

- Excessive behavioral anxiety symptoms and judgments
- Excessive closeness with her son, Jay, and excessive distance from her husband, Douglas (Joyce lacks accurate sensory and empathic awareness with both)
- Excessive domination of her son and attempted control of her husband
- Personality traits such as unfriendliness, judging, and high emotionality
- Biological temperament features of OCD-related anxiety
- A life-transition style characterized by a fear of change

| Antidepressants | Atypical Major Tranquilizers (Anti-psychotics) | Mood Stabilizers |
|---|---|---|
| Celexa (Citalopram)<br>Effexor XR (Venlafaxine)<br>Lamictal (Lamotrigine)<br>Lexapro (Escitalopram)<br>Paxil CR (Paroxetine)<br>Prozac (Fluoxetine)<br>Remeron (Mirtazapine)<br>Serzone (Nefazodone)<br>Wellbutrin (Buproprion)<br>Zoloft (Sertraline) | Abilify (Aripiprazole)<br>Clozaril (Clozapine)<br>Geodon (Ziprasidone)<br>Risperdal (Risperidone)<br>Seroquel (Quetiapine)<br>Zyprexa (Olanzapine) | Lithium (Lithium)<br>Depakote (Divalproex Sodium)<br>Topamax (Topiramate)<br>Zyprexa (Olanzapine)<br>Risperdal (Risperidone)<br>Seroquel (Quetiapine) |
| | **Anti-Anxiety Agents**<br>Buspar (Buspirone)<br>Inderal (Propranolol)<br>Klonopin (Clonazepam)<br>Neurontin (Gabapentin)<br>Xanax (Alprazolam) | **Stimulants**<br>Adderall (XR) (Dextroamphetamine and Amphetamine)<br>Dexedrine (Dexedrine)<br>Ritalin (LA) (Methylphenidate)<br>Strattera (Atomoxetine) |

**FIG. 5.5.** Medications: Brand and Chemical Names.

Similarly, Douglas can be diagnosed (categorically) as having a narcissistic personality with (dimensional) cyclothymic biological features and faulty attachment.

Family or couples therapy makes it easier for clients to see personality trait polarities and consider change (Resnikoff, 2002). For example, Douglas was preoccupied with the present tense. He thought: "How can I have sex, how can I have fun, and how can I have experiences?" Joyce was anxious and concerned about the future. I wanted to help Douglas become more concerned about details and think about the future; I wanted to help Joyce live more in the present and relax. In individual therapy, Douglas would focus only on the present tense and find it hard to consider future concerns; Joyce would do the opposite. In couples therapy, however, Douglas and Joyce learned from each other.

In a multidimensional approach to stage 3 personality therapy, we deal with the immediate personality trait conflicts and complaints, and then we trace those back to their long-standing (categorical) interpersonal styles. The new element that therapists may not be comfortable or familiar with is including the biological temperaments and medications (see Fig. 5.5) as they inform personality styles. In the clinical example, the low doses of medication prescribed helped Joyce be less anxious and helped Douglas be calmer as part of stage 3 treatment of personality style rigidities. This is different from the severe-end biological temperaments and medications for schizophrenia, major depression, mania, or panic that are utilized in stage 1 therapy.

21. Which of the following statements is correct?
    a. A dimensional approach to understanding personality disorders takes into consideration only genetic factors.
    b. Early onset of symptoms, a strong family history, and severe diagnosable symptomatology indicate strong biological loading in a patient's temperament spectrum.
    c. Emil Coccaro postulated that intermittent, explosive rage (irritable depression) is best managed with benzodiazepine medication.
    d. The cyclothymic bipolar personality temperament is best managed by electric convulsive treatments.

22. Categorical personality disorders diagnostic groupings:
   a. are NOT primarily based on historical psychodynamic experiences.
   b. overlap between categories, making research distinctions difficult.
   c. are NOT useful for understanding distorted reactions toward food, money, sex, and psychopharmacology.
   d. are MORE useful for research than dimensional definitions and approaches.

23. Multidimensional approaches and definitions of personality disorders:
   a. do NOT include an interpersonal emphasis.
   b. include biological temperaments.
   c. do NOT include personality traits that cut across categories.
   d. do NOT include all stages of therapy, including stage 1 symptoms being conceptualized as part of long-term dynamics.

24. In the work of Lorna Benjamin,
   a. The eleven categorical diagnostic groupings are given a dimensional dynamic by adding interpersonal dynamics.
   b. In addition to categorical considerations, diagrams including closeness and distance on one axis and expressiveness on the other axis are used for research.
   c. Closeness and distance can both be considered "friendly" (love) or "unfriendly" (hate).
   d. All of the above.

25. Which of the following statements is NOT correct?
   a. Lorna Benjamin created a link between categorical and dimensional personality diagnoses by redefining the eleven personality diagnoses in *interpersonal terms*.
   b. In general, couples frequently initially present with intense "transference" reactions to each other's personality.
   c. Therapists should immediately focus on long-term behavioral patterns or vulnerabilities.
   d. Therapeutic work with patients should begin with surface behaviors, proceed to attachment issues, then on to long-term personality issues, and finally to life stage transitional issues.

## BRIDGE 4: THERAPIST–FAMILY INTERACTION

Each of the dimensional personality traits mentioned above regarding treatment families will stimulate either the same trait or its opposite in the therapist.

In your clinical approach, you need to be aware of your own personality preferences and how they are similar to or different from those of the treatment family. These preferences all reflect the varied layers of your personality (symptoms, attachment, coping style, temperament, and life-transition approach) that parallel those of the treatment family.

For example, you should ask: What stage of therapy am I most comfortable with (problem solving, enhancing communication, historical patterning, or facing life's challenges)? Am I generally action-oriented with couples in solving problems or do I emphasize understanding and expression? Is my bias for or against medication? Do I have a particular personality transference message as I prescribe medications, such as "I can take care of you, I am powerful" or "I am weak and can't help without medication?" What transition am I experiencing in my own life (divorce, children leaving home, aging)? How do I cope with transitions and loss? Do I ask for help, or not?

With experience, you can use such awareness either openly or not, depending upon the clinical situation, to facilitate the therapy. With Joyce and Douglas, I joined both Joyce's problem-solving style and Douglas's live-in-the-moment style. Having recently had two sons of my own go to college, I could understand both the joy and the stress of their transition.

Once Jay leaves, Douglas and Joyce will face an empty nest. I remember facing that myself when my younger son left for college and even more so now that he has graduated. We all are, in fact, involved in a developmental transition, whatever that life transition may be. The question is, as therapists, should we impose our own ways of dealing with transitions on our clients? Of course the answer is "No." Douglas and Joyce may want Jay to come home every weekend. We have to honor what they want even if it is different from what we would want.

To be most effective in our work with families, we have to know ourselves as therapists: our problem-solving style, boundary style, personality style, and how we handle life transitions.

26. Therapists frequently have biases about psychopharmacology (pro or con):
    a. based on their preference for a particular stage of therapy (or school of therapy).
    b. based on their own style (or allegiance to a school of psychotherapy) of being directive or nondirective.
    c. based on their own personality style or personal family experience with psychotropics.
    d. all of the above.

27. A therapist experiencing a life transition similar to the treatment family might try to impose preferences regarding:
    a. managing stress.
    b. seeking help from outside resources, including spiritual and community supports.
    c. being expressive or stoical regarding emotions.
    d. all of the above.

28. In order to become more aware of their own therapy personality preferences, therapists should ask themselves which of the following questions?
    a. Am I generally action-oriented with couples in solving problems or do I emphasize understanding and expression?
    b. Am I biased for or against medication?
    c. What transition(s) am I experiencing in my own life, such as divorce, children leaving home, aging?
    d. All of the above.

29. In therapist–treatment family interactions:
    a. The therapist should control the family.
    b. The therapist should be loyal to his mentor and school of psychotherapy.
    c. The therapist should model the proper family development.
    d. The therapist needs to be aware of his or her own dynamics and how they are similar or complementary to the treatment family's dynamics.

30. A flexible multidimensional family therapy includes:
    a. sometimes controlling destructive symptoms and at other times emphasizing awareness of presenting problems.
    b. using medications both to control symptoms, at times, and also to enhance communication and awareness, at other times.
    c. having flexible boundaries with family members, depending on the situation.
    d. all of the above.

This chapter has presented an integrated multidimensional "bridges for healing" approach for helping families. Relational family therapy combined with psychopharmacology offers therapists and families an expanded potential for therapeutic growth and well-being. It is important and helpful to carefully utilize decades old psychotherapeutic wisdom together with contemporary neuropsychiatric scientific advances.

## KEY TERMS

**attachment:** Pattern of interpersonal closeness and distance that creates protection and comfort. According to John Bowlby, ideal attachment includes a flexible interpersonal alternation of closeness and distance. Pathological attachment includes rigid closeness in a continuum with rigid distance or an unpredictable chaotic attachment.

**atypical anti-psychotics:** A group of medications that block brain dopamine receptors. They are a newer anti-psychotic group that includes activating properties to control negative symptoms, such as lethargy, in addition to positive symptoms, such as delusions. This group also has fewer muscular side effects compared to "typical" older medications.

**character defense mechanism:** An interpersonal pattern of relating that protects against excessive stress that can be either functional or pathological. Includes "projection" of one's experience on to the other person and "introjection," or taking in, of the other persons style or cognitions.

**cyclothymic (bipolar) temperament:** A personality style with components of both depression and elation. The elation includes grandiose thinking, excessive spending, hyper sexuality, and impulsivity. This biological temperament is a mild version of manic-depressive illness.

**dimensional approaches:** Methods or cognitions that include a rapid alternation of consideration of opposing polarities, for example, parts versus whole. Even if one polarity is temporarily favored, integration of polarities takes place in the dimensional process.

**expressive/relational schools of therapy:** Methods that emphasize clarification and interpersonal connections. Using the paradoxical theory of change, awareness and connection by itself will lead to growth, healing, and change. Includes psychodynamic, narrative, gestalt, and emotionally focused methods.

**instrumental schools of therapy:** Methods that emphasize changing anxiety, depression, delusions, and interpersonal interactions by directive exercises. Includes de-conditioning, changing cognitive-behavioral patterns, blocking obsessions, hypnotic relaxation, and practicing corrective interpersonal communication.

**obsessive-compulsive disorder (OCD):** A biological condition with excessive metabolism of the caudate nucleus in the brain. Includes pathologically repetitive thoughts (obsessions) and actions (compulsions) to ward off dirt or contamination and to create a feeling of symmetry and safety.

**obsessive-compulsive personality (OCP):** An environmentally caused personality disturbance characterized by a need to excessively control interpersonal interactions. Usually based on a repetition of excessive childhood control or a counter position from excessive childhood chaos.

**panic attack:** An extreme expression of the anxiety spectrum characterized by catastrophic fears, fears of dying, and physiological reactions such as palpitations and sweating.

**personality disorder (categorical):** An individual's long-term pervasive and mal-adaptive rigid pattern of attitudes, cognitions, behavior, and interactions based primarily on childhood experiences and training.

**personality disorder (multi-dimensional):** A long-term pattern of mal-adaptive interpersonal interactions and attachments based on biological temperaments as well as childhood experiences. Includes extremes of various personality trait polarities such as expressive versus non-expressive.

**post traumatic stress disorder (PTSD):** A severe chronic reaction to psychological and physical trauma. Characterized by both excessive sensitivity and excessive numbing to life experiences. Ordinary life events or people can be triggers to re-experiencing flashbacks to the traumatic event.

**psychodynamic:** The use of historical interpersonal and internal emotional and behavioral patterns.

**relational therapy:** Therapy that emphasizes interpersonal interaction and dynamics such as couples and family therapy.

**serotonin-enhancing medications:** Medications that increase the neuro-transmitter serotonin in the brain. Useful in the treatment of depression, anxiety (and panic), social anxiety, violence, and eating disorders.

**temperament:** A life-long biological style of interpersonal relating based on both genetics and life experience. Examples are schizoid, depressive, violent, and anxious with a continuum of normal to pathological in each temperament.

## DISCUSSION QUESTIONS

1. If you had the opportunity to have a "magic pill" that would do anything you wished (e.g., regarding symptoms, connections, personality style, or spiritual issues), what would you ask for? Would you consider taking such a pill?

2. Do you believe that men are more "instrumental" and women more " expressive/re-lational"?

3. Are the differences in "instrumental' versus "expressive/relational" styles based on genetics or cultural training?

4. Do you believe the pharmaceutical companies have had a negative impact on the field of psychotherapy?

5. Do you feel that the field of family therapy has been overly dominated by cognitive-behavioral and other symptom-focused therapies including psychopharmacology (as opposed to narrative and other awareness-based therapies)?

6. What are your own personal strong and weak points as a psychotherapist? What would the complementary counter-position be?

7. Who is the main mentor in your training? Do you still primarily use that person's approach?

8. Although medications for symptom control have been officially approved (by the Federal Drug Administration), the use of medications for treating personality temperaments or for improving attachments is still considered "off label." What are your opinions about the "designer use" of such medications to alter personalities?

9. Some families object to taking unnatural pharmaceuticals but are willing to take natural substances such as Saint John's Wort. What would you advise such families?

10. Some therapists believe that attachment and connection patterns can be observed and improved in the current context without historical elaboration of the patterns and core feelings. What is your own belief and clinical practice?

## SUGGESTED FURTHER READING

Benjamin, L. (2003). *Interpersonal Reconstruction Therapy: Promoting Change In Non-Responders,* New York, Guilford Press.

Offers a multilayered approach integrating both medical and interpersonal methods.

Resnikoff R. (2001). *Bridges for Healing: Integrating Family Therapy and Psychopharmacology.* Philadelphia: Brunner-Routledge.

Offers numerous interesting clinical examples of when and how to include psychopharmacology.

Stahl S. *Essential Psychopharmacology.* (2000). 2nd ed. Cambridge/New York: Cambridge University Press.

Effectively uses cartoons to simplify how psychopharmacology works.

## REFERENCES

Akiskal, H. S. (1999). The evolving bipolar spectrum. *Psychiatric Clinics of North America, 22*(3), 517–534.

American Psychiatric Association. (1994). *Diagnostic and statistical manual of mental disorders* (4th ed.). Washington, DC.

American Psychiatric Association. (2001). Practice guideline for the treatment of patients with borderline personality disorder. *American Journal of Psychiatry, 158*(10), 1–52.

Barlow, D. H., Gorman, J. M., Shear, M. K., & Woods, S. W. (2000). Cognitive behavioral therapy, imipramine, or their combination for panic disorder: A randomized controlled trial. *Journal of the American Medical Association, 283,* 2529–2536.

Baxter, L. R., Phelps, M. E., Mazziotta, J. D., Guze, B. H., Schwartz, J. M., & Selin, C. E. (1987). Local cerebral glucose metabolic rates in obsessive-compulsive disorder. *Archives of General Psychiatry, 44,* 211–218.

Benjamin, L. S. (1996). *Interpersonal diagnosis and treatment of personality disorders* (2nd ed.). New York: Guilford Press.

Bowlby, J. (1988). *A secure base: Parent child attachment and healthy human development.* New York: Basic Books.

Cloninger, C. R., & Svrakic, D. M. (1997). Integrative psychobiological approach to psychiatric assessment and treatment. *Psychiatry, 60*(2), 120–41.

Coccaro, E. F., & Kavoussi, R. J. (1997). Fluoxetine and impulsive aggressive behavior in personality-disordered subjects. *Archives of General Psychiatry, 54,* 1081–1088.

Edwards, M. E., (2002). Attachment, mastery, and interdependence: a model of parenting processes. *Family Process, 41*(3), 389–404.

Faraone, S. V., Biederman, J., Weiffenbach, B., Keith, T., Chu, M. P., Weaver, A., et al. (1999). Dopamine D4 gene 7-repeat allele and attention deficit hyperactivity disorder. *American Journal of Psychiatry, 156,* 768–770.

Fonagy, P., Target, M., & Gergely, G., (2000). Attachment and borderline personality disorder: A theory and some evidence. *Psychiatric Clinics of North America, 23,* vii–viii, 103–122.

Gabbard, G. O., & Kay, J. (2001). The fate of integrated treatment: Whatever happened to the psychosocial psychiatrist? *American Journal of Psychiatry, 158*(12), 1956–1963.

Goleman, D. (2003). *Destructive emotions: A scientific dialogue with the dalai lama.* New York: Bantam Doubleday Dell.

Gunderson, J. G., (2001). *Borderline personality disorder: A clinical guide.* Washington, DC: American Psychiatric Press.

Gurman, A. S., Fraenkel, P. (2002). The history of couple therapy: A millennial review. *Family Process, 41*(2), 199–260.

Heim, C., & Nemeroff, C. B. (1999). The impact of early life experiences on brain systems involved with the pathophysiology of anxiety and affective disorders. *Biological Psychiatry, 46,* 1509–1522.

Johnson, S. M., Makinen, J. A., & Millikin, J. W. (2001). Attachment injuries in couple relationships: a new perspective on impasses in couples therapy. *Journal of Marital and Family Therapy, 27*(2), 145–55.

Keller, M., McCullough, J., Klein, D. N., Arnow, B., Dunner, D. L., Gelenberg, A. J. (2000). A comparison of Nefazodone, the cognitive behavioral analysis system of psychotherapy, and their combination for the treatment of chronic depression. *New England Journal of Medicine, 342,* 1462–1470.

Kernberg, O. (2001). The suicidal risk in severe personality disorders: differential diagnosis and treatment. *Journal of Personality Disorders, 15*(3), 195–208.

Kirrane, R. M., & Siever, L. J. (2000). New perspectives on schizotypal personality disorder. *Current Psychiatry Reports, 2,* 62–66.

Knutson, B., Wolkowitz, O., Cole, S., Chan, T., Moore, E., Johnson, R., et al. (1998). Selective alteration of personality and social behavior by serotonergic intervention. *American Journal of Psychiatry, 155*(3), 373–379.

LeDoux, J., (1996). *The emotional brain.* New York: Touchstone, Simon & Schuster.

Linehan, M. M. (1993). *Cognitive-behavioral treatment of borderline personality disorder.* New York: Guilford Press.

Luhrman, T. M. (2000). *Of two minds: The growing disorder in American psychiatry.* New York: Knopf.

McCrae, R. R., & Costa, P. T. (1999). A five-factor theory of personality. In L. A. Pervin & O. P. John (Eds.), *Handbook of Personality: Theory and Research* (2nd ed.) (pp. 139–153). New York: Guilford.

Millon, T. (1991). Classification in psychopathology: Rational, alternatives, and standards. *Journal of Abnormal Psychology. 100,* 245–261

Olson, D. H. (1986). Circumplex model VII: Validation studies and FACES III. *Family Process, 25,* 337–351.

Polster, E. (1995). *A population of selves.* San Francisco: Jossey-Bass.

Polster, E., & Polster, M. (1999). *From the radical center: The heart of Gestalt therapy (collected writings).* Cleveland, OH: Cleveland Gestalt Institute Press.

Resnikoff, R. (2001). *Bridges for healing: Integrating family therapy and psychopharmacology.* Philadelphia: Brunner-Routledge.

Resnikoff, R. (2002). Couples therapy and psychopharmacology. *Psychiatric Times, 19*(7), 29–30.

Scharff, D. E. & Scharff, J. S. (1991). *Object relations couples therapy.* New Jersey/London: Jason Aronson.

Schore, A. N. (1997). A century after Freud's project is a rapprochement between psychoanalysis and neurobiology at hand? *Journal of The American psychoanalytic Association, 45,* 807–840.

Schwartz, J. (1995). *Brain lock.* New York: Harper Collins.

Siegel, D. J. (1999). *The developing mind.* New York: Guilford Press.

Siever, L. (1998). New biological research strategies for personality disorders. In K. Silk (Ed.), *Biology of personality disorders* (pp. 27–61). Washington, DC: American Psychiatric Press.

Soloff, P. H. (1998). Algorithms for pharmacological treatment of personality dimensions—symptom specific treatments for cognitive-perceptual, affective, and impulsive dysregulation. *Bullitin of the Menniger Clinic, 62,* 195–214.

Spencer, T., Biederman, J., Wilens, T. E., & Faraone, S. V. (2002). Novel treatments for attention-deficit/hyperactivity disorder in children. *Journal of Clinical Psychiatry, 63*(Suppl. 12), 23–28.

Stahl, S. (2000). *Essential psychopharmacology* (2nd ed.). Cambridge/New York: Cambridge University Press.

Teicher, M. (2002). Scars that won't heal: Neuropsychiatry of child abuse. *Scintific American, Vol. 286* (Issue. 3), 68–75.

Thase, M. E., Greenhouse, J. B., & Frank, E. (1997). Treatment of major depression with psychotherapy or psychotherapy-pharmacotherapy combination. *Arch Gen Psychiatry, 154,* 1009–1015.

Walkup, J. T. (1999). Psychiatry of tourette syndrome. *CNS Spectrums, 4*(2), 54–61.

Westin, D., & Harnden-Fischer, J. (2001). Personality profiles in eating disorders: Rethinking the distinction between Axis I and Axis II. *American Journal of Psychiatry, 158*(4), 547–562.

Yehuda, R. (2002). Post traumatic stress disorder. *New England Journal of Medicine, 346,* 108–114.

Young, L. J., Lim, M. M., Gingrich, B., & Insel, T. R. (2001). Cellular mechanisms of social attachment. *Hormenes and Behavior, 40*(2), 133–138.

# THERAPEUTIC SKILLS AND TOOLS

# 6

# Theories of Family Therapy (Part I)

Kim Snow
*Northern Illinois University*

Hugh C. Crethar
Patricia Robey
Jon Carlson
*Governors State University*

## TRUTH OR FICTION?

___ 1. *Adlerian family therapists believe that all human beings have feelings of inferiority stemming from early childhood.*

___ 2. *Adlerian family therapy sees the past as having little influence on how people interact in their families today.*

___ 3. *Adlerians believe that it is important to have social interest or community feeling in order to be emotionally healthy.*

___ 4. *Genograms are messages that the family sends to the transgenerational therapist.*

___ 5. *Differentiation and triangulation are critical concepts in Bowenian or transgenerational family therapy.*

___ 6. *In transgenerational family therapy, the "I-position" is a model of communication in which a statement of opinion or belief is delivered clearly and fervently.*

___ 7. *Boszormenyi-Nagy's contextual family therapy addresses the ethical dimensions of family development.*

___ 8. *Fairness, decency, reciprocity, and accountability determine the healthy functioning of a family within contextual family therapy.*

___ 9. *In contextual family therapy, personal growth and symptomatic relief come as a result of facing emotional conflicts.*

___ 10. *Object relations family therapy views individuals as being more attached to objects than to people.*

___ 11. *Transference, interpretation, and insight play a vital role in object relations family therapy.*

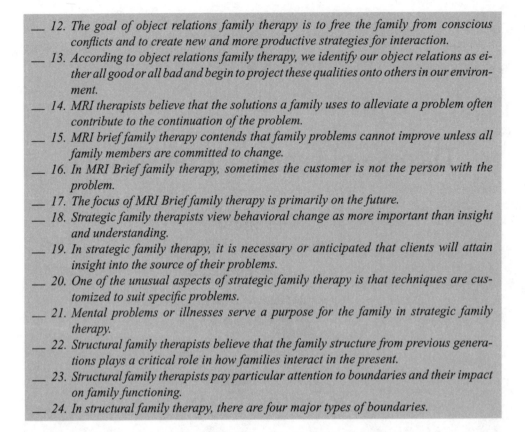

___ 12. *The goal of object relations family therapy is to free the family from conscious conflicts and to create new and more productive strategies for interaction.*

___ 13. *According to object relations family therapy, we identify our object relations as either all good or all bad and begin to project these qualities onto others in our environment.*

___ 14. *MRI therapists believe that the solutions a family uses to alleviate a problem often contribute to the continuation of the problem.*

___ 15. *MRI brief family therapy contends that family problems cannot improve unless all family members are committed to change.*

___ 16. *In MRI Brief family therapy, sometimes the customer is not the person with the problem.*

___ 17. *The focus of MRI Brief family therapy is primarily on the future.*

___ 18. *Strategic family therapists view behavioral change as more important than insight and understanding.*

___ 19. *In strategic family therapy, it is necessary or anticipated that clients will attain insight into the source of their problems.*

___ 20. *One of the unusual aspects of strategic family therapy is that techniques are customized to suit specific problems.*

___ 21. *Mental problems or illnesses serve a purpose for the family in strategic family therapy.*

___ 22. *Structural family therapists believe that the family structure from previous generations plays a critical role in how families interact in the present.*

___ 23. *Structural family therapists pay particular attention to boundaries and their impact on family functioning.*

___ 24. *In structural family therapy, there are four major types of boundaries.*

This chapter will introduce you to some of the most popular family theories and help you gain a basic understanding some of the terms and concepts used within these theories. Seven theories are covered in this chapter and additional theories will be covered in the subsequent chapter. Because we have included seven diverse theories in this chapter, we have broken them down into several uniform headings so that it will be easier for you to compare and contrast the various theories. We have also added a table (Table 6.1) at the end of the chapter so that you can see how these theories compare and contrast.

Though Alfred Adler is credited with working with families in Austria in the 1920s (Dreikurs, 1957), it was not until the 1950s that we saw family therapy emerge and become established in the United States. From the 1950s to the 1970s, numerous philosophies of family therapy materialized and family systems became the primary focus in working with families. Because there are so many divergent and important theories that play a role in the history and development of family therapy, we have highlighted some of the most significant theories that we believe are important for you to know.

## ADLERIAN FAMILY THERAPY

### Theory at a Glance

Alfred Adler is credited as the father of individual psychology and Adlerian family therapy. While working with families in Vienna, Austria, in the 1920s, Adler departed from his

**TABLE 6.1**

A Comparison and Contrast of Theories

| Theory | Key Figures | View of Human Functioning | View of Dysfunction | Therapist's Role | Client's Role | Therapeutic Goals |
|---|---|---|---|---|---|---|
| Adlerian | Alfred Adler, Rudolf Dreikurs, | Families are purposeful, social, and interpretive in their interactions, seen in a holistic systemic context. | Families are seen as discouraged with faulty private logic. | Educator, collaborator | Clients examine private logic and gain insight into faulty assumptions. | Encourage families, overcome inferiority feelings, reorientate families' thinking and interaction |
| Transgenerational | Murray Bowen | Family members are differentiated and able to maintain emotional connection with one another. | Families are unable to differentiate and often have triangulation. | Neutral guide, teacher, catalyst for change, self-monitor reactions | Clients differentiate from their family of origin and understand their patterns of emotional attachment and disengagement. | Decrease anxiety and increase differentiation from family of origin, improve family communication |
| Contextual | Ivan Boszormenyi-Nagy | Healthy families have a balance between rights and responsibilities of individual in a caring way. | Symptoms of dysfunction occur when there is injustice & lack of trust within family. | Active, engaged as advocate | Clients expected to engage in dialogues concerning rights and responsibilities | Balance the burdens of family, help members experience mutuality and autonomy |
| Object Relations | Nathan Ackerman | Human nature is based on innate drives; psychological adjustment is achieved by creating and maintaining good object relations. | Internalized problematic object relations cause unrealistic expectations and responses within family relations. | Neutral "good enough" parental figure, teacher, nondirective change catalyst | Clients confront resistances and explore parallels between past and present relationships through transference and insight. | Free family members from unconscious restrictions and help them gain new insights and awareness |
| MRI | Gregory Bateson | Successful communication results in families developing new solutions to problems. | Family dysfunction is affected by faulty communication patterns. | Active moderator of interactional patterns, often part of a team, focus on process over content | Clients are seen as customers expected to implement strategies for change. | Break ineffective patterns of behavior which is done through first and second order change. |
| Strategic | Jay Haley, Cloe Madanes | Functional families have clear boundaries and appropriate hierarchy of power. | Chronic problems are based on repeated ineffective solutions, flaws in family hierarchy, and efforts to protect or control through symptomology. | Active director | Clients are active participants | Identify problems in organization of family, change perceptions, and restructure family in hierarchy and boundaries |
| Structural | Salvador Minuchin | Families have leadership, hierarchical structure, and can set boundaries. | Dysfunctional family structures cause family members to be stuck in unhelpful patterns. | "Friendly uncle," initiator of change in family structure, stage manager | Clients are active participants | Map out family structure, alter the structure to allow it to solve its own problems |

psychoanalytic roots and developed his own philosophy called *individual psychology*. He worked with families in an open forum where parents, teachers, and communities could benefit from his psychoeducational model. Adler viewed people as social beings who are both creators and creations of their own lives. Of primary importance to Adler is the family because it is here that individuals search for significance and develop the behaviors, interactions, and perceptions that form their lifestyles. Individuals cannot be understood outside of the social context within which they live. Individuals seek significance by belonging to a social system. Adler believed that all human beings have **inferiority feelings** stemming from early childhood. In order to overcome these feelings of inferiority, individuals strive for mastery, success (superiority), and completion as they aspire toward an ideal self. This ideal self begins to form from our self-perceptions and interactions by age six and becomes the foundation and driving force towards an imagined central life goal, referred to as **fictional finalism**. Adlerians believe that people are motivated by **social interest** or a sense of belonging and a contributing member of society. Adlerians see all behavior as purposeful and goal oriented. Thus, all behavior can be understood in the context of this imagined, ideal, and often unconscious life goal. Adlerians seek to bring the beliefs about the ideal self and the fictional finalism into awareness.

Rudolf Dreikurs studied under Adler and is responsible for bringing these ideals to America. He refined and applied these Adlerian principles to education, child guidance, individual, family, and group psychotherapy.

## View of Human Functioning

Adlerians view family members as social, purposeful, subjective, and interpretive in their interactions with one another. Adlerian family therapists view individuals from a holistic and systemic context, therefore believing that individuals cannot be understood outside of the familial and social context within which they live. Family members are seen as interacting purposefully within an interactional social context that influences each member's perception, development, and worldview. These behaviors in turn shape the family as a whole.

1. Adlerian family therapists view individuals as _____.
   a. purposeful
   b. social
   c. subjective and interpretative in their interactions with one another
   d. all of the above

## View of Dysfunction

Adlerian family therapists perceive family problems and dysfunction to be the result of discouragement and faulty private logic within the family. Both parents and children become entrenched in negative patterns of interaction based upon mistaken goals that motivate all members of the family. These negative interactions between parents and their children are often seen as a product of either autocratic or permissive parenting styles.

## Therapist's Role

Adlerian therapists develop therapeutic relationships with families that are based upon mutual respect, equality, and cooperation. Guided by social interest, the therapist assumes the roles of educator and collaborator. Assessing and understanding the family structure comprise the primary focus. This is often achieved by gathering information on the **family constellation** (which includes birth order, sibling relationships, and parent relationships), unlocking the mistaken goals and interactional patterns of each family member, and reeducation.

2. Adlerian therapists develop therapeutic relationships with families that are based on _____.
   a. indebtedness and invisible loyalties
   b. mutual respect, equality, and cooperation
   c. coalitions and associations
   d. the individuation of all family members

## Client's Role

The family's role in therapy is to examine the mistaken goals that are the foundation of each family member's lifestyles. Family members complete a lifestyle assessment or family constellation which provides you with details of the family makeup, how family members perceive themselves and one another, and their own **private logic**. From the Adlerian stance, the therapists deems clients' private logic to be their worldview. Family members examine their private logic and gain insight into their faulty assumptions.

## Therapeutic Goals

An Adlerian family therapist's goals are to assess the family functioning, provide encouragement to the family, help family members understand and overcome feeling of inferiority, and challenge families to **reorient** their thinking. These goals are accomplished by examining the family constellation, each family member's private logic, and the motivation and mistaken goals behind interactional behaviors, and by exploring the family processes and interactions through a "**typical day**."

3. Which of the following is *not* a goal of Adlerian family therapy?
   a. assessing family functioning
   b. providing encouragement to the family
   c. helping family members to understand dysfunctional patterns of previous generations
   d. helping family members to understand and overcome feelings of inferiority

## Techniques Associated With This Theory

Adlerian family therapy techniques and interventions include encouragement, interpretation of the family constellation and **early recollections**, asking about the family's typical day, identifying adults' mistaken notions about children, and identifying the mistaken goals of children's misbehavior, reorientation, and logical consequences.

## Key Terms

**early recollections:** Childhood memories (before age 9) of a single event. These memories often present patterns or recurring themes that summarize their present philosophy on life.

**family constellation:** Social and psychological makeup of a family (system) that includes sibling relationships, parental relationships, birth order, and an individual's self-concept.

**fictional finalism:** An imagined life-goal that unifies a personality such that every behavior can be seen as a movement toward that life goal.

**individual psychology:** A term used by Adler to describe his approach to psychology.

**inferiority feelings:** Feelings that motivate a child's initial striving for success. Individuals constantly strive to overcome imagined and real inferiority feelings which help them to overcome handicaps.

**private logic:** Includes concepts about life, self, and others that form the philosophy upon which an individual's lifestyle is based.

**reorientation:** A process of refocusing the family that includes the following goals: ensuring safety and encouragement for family members, reframing and normalizing experiences, and unlocking repetitive patterns.

**social interest** (also called **Gemeinschaftsgefuhl**): Depicts a sense of being connected and giving back to one's community and humanity; an interest in the common good.

**typical day assessment:** Technique where by Adlerian family therapists ask families to describe a typical day. This enables the therapist to understand the needs, values, goals, and interactions of a family system.

## TRANSGENERATIONAL (BOWENIAN) FAMILY THERAPY

### Theory at a Glance

Transgenerational Family Therapy (TFT) originated as the result of Murray Bowen's work at the Menninger Clinic in Topeka, Kansas. Bowen was interested in the symbiotic relationship between schizophrenic children and their mothers. Further studies were performed at the National Institute of Mental Health (NIMH), where entire families were hospitalized. Researchers noticed that the presence of the father influenced the behaviors of both mother and child. As a result of this work, Bowen determined that family and individual clinical work should be considered in the context of multigenerational issues and anxiety.

In 1959, Bowen continued his research at Georgetown University School of Medicine, where he applied his theory to less dysfunctional populations. In his observation of family interactions, Bowen noticed that there were alternating cycles of closeness and distance between family members, particularly between mother and child. The anxiety produced by the cycles seemed to drive the relationship patterns automatically. Bowen hypothesized that the interdependent relationship between mother and child—and the anxiety regarding the attachment—limited the ability to distinguish and separate thoughts from feelings. Bowen used the term *differentiation* of self to describe the ability of the individual to withstand the anxiety in the relationship and to choose autonomous behaviors. He focused on the degree to which family members balanced emotional and intellectual functioning, and intimacy and autonomy in interpersonal relationships. Bowen found that anxiety among family members heightened as families transitioned through family-life cycles. These are development stages of family life that include: separation from one's family of origin, getting married, having children, growing older, retirement, and finally death.

4. In transgenerational family therapy, the stages of family life from separation from one's parent to marriage, having children, growing older, retirement, and finally death, are known as the _____.
   a. family developmental path
   b. family life-cycle
   c. family stage continuum
   d. function of the system

5. In transgenerational family therapy, the ability to behave flexibly in the face of anxiety and to respond with autonomy is known as _____.
   a. differentiation of self
   b. triangulation of self
   c. undifferentiation of self
   d. displacement of others

In TFT, the goal of therapy is to help the client decrease anxiety and increase differentiation of self. This is accomplished by changing the client's relationship with the significant others in his or her life. Change has occurred when anxiety is decreased. Understanding the family of origin and its influence is considered to be the vehicle through which changes are made.

## View of Human Functioning

In healthy families, each individual is able to maintain an emotional connection with other family members without anxiety determining behavior in relationships. Family members are differentiated and are therefore able to behave, feel, and think in response to their own principles, opinions, and beliefs, rather than react from their anxieties. In these families, anxiety is low. The parents are likely to have differentiated from their own families of origin and maintain good contact with them.

## View of Dysfunction

Bowen originally described dysfunction as the result of an individual's inability to deal with the anxiety felt as a result of the mother–child relationship cycles. The mother and child relationship sometimes becomes emotionally fused. **Emotional fusion** may be recognized by a need for excessive attachment and anxiety, or by isolating behavior, and is identifiable by two types of behavior. In the first, individuals demonstrate clinging behaviors and there is an inability to separate. This is called *symbiosis*. In the other, individuals engage in combative behaviors that result in the family experiencing **emotional cut off**, which is the only perceived way individuals can escape the anxious attachment.

The theory was later changed to include the concept of *triangulation*. When anxiety builds between two persons, a third person will automatically be involved—a **triangle** is formed. If the third person stays neutral, the anxiety will be lessened and symptoms will be decreased. If the third person becomes emotionally involved, the symptoms will likely increase.

Behavior disorders result from emotional fusion, which can be transmitted from generation to generation. In many families, children leave the home before differentiation is complete and maintain an emotional attachment to their parents. As a result, when they meet someone who behaves like their parents, they repeat dysfunctional patterns of behavior that they maintained with their own parents. Similarly, they may decide to marry someone who operates from nearly the same level of differentiation as themselves (a process known as *multigenerational transmission*). If not addressed, the conflicts remain unresolved and then resurface in new relationships where the patterns are often repeated.

6. In Transgenerational Family Therapy, an intense relationship between two individuals who are so dependent upon one another that their independent functioning is compromised is known as _____.
   a. Symbiosis
   b. Emotional fusion
   c. Assimilation
   d. Interdependence

## Therapist's Role

A TFT therapist acts as a coach and a catalyst for change. He or she uses techniques that encourage self-reflection and that are directed to individuals, rather than encouraging family dialogues, which often become emotional. TFT therapists should be aware of and control their own reactions and maintain a neutral position in counseling. Although the presence of all family members is not a requirement for therapy, an awareness of the family as a system must always be maintained.

## Client's Role

Family members play both an active learning and participant role in TFT. They learn how to differentiate from their families of origin, become better observers and listeners, control their emotional reactivity, and detriangulate from emotional family interactions.

## Therapeutic Goals

The goal of TFT is to help the client decrease anxiety and increase differentiation from the family of origin. Therapeutic change can be identified by the decrease in levels of anxiety and depression. Relationships should become less emotionally reactive. Individuals gain self-awareness and take personal responsibility for change rather than blaming the family system for their problems. Triangular relationships also become less intense. Communication is improved and individuals are able to discuss problems in a healthy manner.

## Techniques Associated With This Theory

Transgenerational family therapists believe that the most important facet of therapy is to understand how the family operates. However, there are some specific techniques used to facilitate the process:

- A *genogram* is a tool which helps organize and document the history and structure of a three-generation family system. The genogram (popularized by Monica McGoldrick) provides a framework for understanding the development of family stress over time. The genogram enables the therapist to collect comprehensive information regarding a family and sets the stage for the creation of a treatment plan.

- *Process questions* help the therapist gain information on how the family perceives the problem and what types of behavior are being used to maintain the problem. The questions are designed to decrease anxiety and help clients think more clearly. As a result, clients are able to create options for more effective interactions.
- *Relationship experiments* are behavioral tasks assigned to family members. The goal of these experiments is to help the family recognize and then change the dysfunctional behaviors and ineffective relationship patterns in the family system.
- *Neutralizing triangles* are a five-step process, developed by Philip Guerin. In this process, clients identify the triangle, define its structure and the flow of movement within it, reverse the flow of movement, and expose the emotional process. Finally, the therapist helps clients deal with the emotional process and develop more effective ways of communication.
- *Coaching* is used with families who are highly motivated and who are able to identify their own systemic and individual patterns of behavior. The therapist assumes the role of "supporter" and offers options for change. He or she then helps the family evaluate each option's potential and possible responses that may occur as a result of the change.
- Other techniques include the *"I-position"*—a model of communication in which a statement of opinion or belief is delivered neutrally and unemotionally without placing blame—and *displacement stories*—videotapes or stories that can be used to teach family processes without increasing defensiveness (Guerin & Guerin, 2002).

7. Which theory from this chapter has the most overt focus on process questions?
   a. strategic family therapy
   b. MRI brief family therapy
   c. contextual family therapy
   d. transgenerational family therapy

## Key Terms

**differentiation:** A developmental process in which an individual grows from complete dependence on another person to a position of individual autonomy.

**emotional cut-off:** The process in which an individual physically and emotionally separates from the parental family in order to reduce the anxiety associated by the lack of differentiation between generations.

**emotional fusion:** A state of emotional anxiety that results in an individual's inability to function autonomously.

**family projection:** A process in which the focus of the emotional energy of one or both parents is projected onto a child so that the adults can avoid confronting their own anxiety.

**multigenerational transmission process:** A pattern of behavior in which children grow up and marry partners whose level of differentiation is similar to their own.

**sibling position:** The birth order of an individual. It is believed that development of personality characteristics and the role that a child will play in the family are influenced by birth order.

**sibling rivalry:** The conflict between siblings that results from triangulation of the siblings' relationship with their parents.

**societal regression:** The influence of social anxiety on a family's ability to differentiate.

**symbiosis:** An intense relationship between two individuals who are so dependent upon one another that their independent functioning is compromised.

**triangle:** A three-person relationship that is considered by Bowen to be the smallest stable relationship system. It is likely to occur when two people in a relationship are in a cycle of distancing and a third person becomes involved as an ally or problem solver.

**undifferentiated ego mass:** A state of symbiosis that influences an entire system.

## CONTEXTUAL FAMILY THERAPY

### Theory at a Glance

Ivan Boszormenyi-Nagy was among the leading figures who contributed to the application of psychoanalytic theory to family therapy. Nagy's contextual therapy addresses the ethical dimensions of family development. *Relational ethics* focus on the long-term balance of fairness within a family and encompass what happens to the individual and within the family system. This includes the assignment of roles, power alignments, and patterns of communication. Ethical behavior in relationships is considered to be crucial to maintaining healthy families and communities. In this approach we are reminded of the importance of decency and fairness in our dealings with others.

8. In contextual family therapy, the concept of _____ refers to a focus on the long-term balance of fairness within a family.
   a. relational ethics
   b. paradoxical equilibrium
   c. invisible loyalty
   d. multigenerational accounting

9. Contextual family therapy addresses:
   a. the ethical dimensions of family development.
   b. the context in which family members relate to others within their community.
   c. the hierarchical nature of each family system.
   d. symptoms and pathology within families.

Conflict is a result of legacies of **invisible loyalties** and obligations from the past that are passed on through generations. Personal growth and symptomatic relief come as a result of facing the emotional conflicts. This growth cannot come at the expense of others in the relationship, however. Contextual therapy always includes consideration of the effect that a client's projections may have on others. This therapy attempts to build responsible and trustworthy behavior that takes the needs of all family members into account. As a result, family members develop a sense of fairness and accountability in their interactions with one another.

### View of Human Development

Healthy relationships balance between the rights of the individuals in the relationship and the responsibilities those individuals hold. Individuals are expected to behave in a caring and giving way. Family members trust one another and engage in behaviors that allow for all members to get their needs met. Collaboration and compromise are used to negotiate when there is a conflict among members. Fairness, decency, reciprocity, and accountability are among the characteristics that determine the healthy functioning of a family.

## View of Dysfunction

Symptoms of dysfunction appear when trust and caring break down in a family. When individuals experience what they perceive as an injustice, there is an expectation that some restitution will be forthcoming. If the restitution comes too slowly, or is not as great as expected, problems develop in the relationship.

## Therapist's Role

When using contextual family therapy, it is important to understand that patterns of behavior repeat themselves from generation to generation. However, therapists do not focus on symptoms or family pathology. Instead, they look for resources in the relationship that can be used as leverages for change. They view the relationship as a trustworthy one which will enable family members to be open to encouragement and engage in dialogues regarding issues of responsibility and personal rights. The therapist becomes personally engaged with the family and advocates for all members within the multigenerational context of the family.

## Client's Role

Clients are expected to engage in dialogues with the therapist and family members to discuss and explore issues regarding **family legacies, family loyalties**, and the assignment of responsibilities and personal rights.

## Therapeutic Goals

The goal of therapy is for each family member to balance the burdens imposed by the family system with the benefits that comes as a result of family membership. As a result, each member is able to experience both autonomy and mutuality. Conflicts are to be acknowledged and addressed. Individuals become self-fulfilled by asserting their rights and attending to their obligations. There is an improvement in the family's ability to relate to one another and in their ability to negotiate differences.

## Techniques Associated With This Theory

Symptom relief and personal growth come as a result of facing repressed emotional conflict, but healing cannot be facilitated at the expense of another individual. Therefore, therapy often makes renegotiation of relationships a necessary part of the process. Family members are encouraged to face their rational and irrational guilt. Irrational guilt is challenged so that it may be eliminated. Facing rational guilt, however, is an essential task in contextual family therapy and is seen as a means of creating accountability in families.

Problems in relationships occur when an individual perceives that he has been the target of an injustice and restitution is slow in coming or is too little to compensate for the injustice. To address this issue, the history of the problem must be examined, as well as the issue in the context of the multigenerational accounting system of injustices, **indebtedness**, and compensation.

For therapy to be successful, an environment of trustworthiness must be created. It is the primary condition that must be met to ensure that family members can address their family legacies and allow themselves to believe that they are **entitled** to better family relationships. Information must be gathered about family loyalty, understanding how the family is bound together, the expectations of members, how the family expresses its loyalty to its members, and what happens when members perceive that there is a deficit in the **family ledger** that tracks the behavioral expressions of loyalty.

## Key Terms

**entitlement:** A term used to describe what one has coming to him.

**family ledger:** A psychological accounting system that is maintained over generations and includes information about what has been given to whom and who still owes something to someone else.

**family legacy:** Refers to the expectations that are handed down from previous generations.

**family loyalty:** The allegiance children feel toward parents based on parental fairness.

**indebtedness:** A term that describes what one owes and to whom.

**invisible loyalty:** A state in which a child unconsciously tries to pay a debt to his parents, even to his own detriment.

**loyalty conflict:** Occurs when there is competition for loyalty between an individual's parents and his peer or spouse.

**split loyalty:** Occurs when parents create a situation in which a child must offer loyalty to only one parent at the cost of loyalty to the other parent.

10. In contextual family therapy, the term that describes what one owes and to whom is _____.
    a. cooperative balance
    b. entitlement
    c. indebtedness
    d. family loyalty

## OBJECT RELATIONS FAMILY THERAPY

### Theory at a Glance

Object Relations Family Therapy (ORFT) is based on the psychoanalytic work of Sigmund Freud. Although psychoanalysis is primarily concerned with individual processes, in the 1950s many psychoanalysts began to consider the influence of the family on individual dynamics. One of the leaders in the field was Nathan Ackerman, a child psychiatrist who became interested in families and the influence of the family on mental health and mental illness. He was especially interested in family dynamics and in applying psychoanalytic principles to the family members. Ackerman initiated a new way of thinking about families and individuals and encouraged practitioners to think of the individual's unconscious and its development in the context of family interactions.

ORFT bridges the gap between the study of individual drives and the study of individuals in the social context of the family system. ORFT suggests that, from birth, individuals have an innate desire to seek **objects** (people, usually mothers) with whom they can form an attachment and looks at relationships from a systemic viewpoint. This helps clients understand marital choices and patterns of family interactions. The unconscious and unresolved object relations are brought into the marriage and family relationships and can result in dysfunctional patterns of dependency. The goal of therapy is to free the family from unconscious conflicts and create new and more productive strategies for interaction.

## View of Human Functioning

Freud's theory proposed that human nature is based on innate drives such as sexuality and aggression. Internal conflict, in the form of anxiety or depression, arises when people begin to believe that the expression of these drives will lead to punishment. To resolve this conflict there must be either a strong defense against the conflicted wish or a relaxation of defenses to allow for some gratification of the wish. According to ORFT, psychological adjustment is achieved by creating and maintaining good object relations, resulting in a secure and successful **differentiation**.

## View of Dysfunction

As people grow, they begin to identify object relations as either all good or all bad and **project** these qualities onto other individuals in their environment—a process known as *splitting*. In this way they are able to make the people in their environment more predictable, which helps them control their anxiety. Eventually individuals begin to internalize—or *interject*—the good and bad objects within themselves. These interjects form the basis for how they interact and evaluate their relationships with others. A problem arises, however, when people fail to see the object realistically and repress the negative aspects of the object. Later, these negative aspects are projected onto their spouses or children.

## Therapist's Role

It is important to emphasize and encourage family interactions. To do this, therapists may take on several roles. In the role of teacher, the therapist helps families understand how unconscious past influences have an impact on the present. Also, the therapist may act as the "good enough parent" and provide the nurturing and encouragement that was absent at earlier developmental stages. And, although the therapist is nondirective, he or she acts as a catalyst for change by engaging the family, uncovering hidden emotions, and challenging, confronting, and interpreting the family process.

> 11. The role of ORFT therapists is _____.
>     a. teacher
>     b. the "good enough parent"
>     c. a catalyst for change
>     d. all of the above

## Client's Role

Clients tend to perceive therapists as parental figures. This creates a safe environment which allows for transference and countertransference. The client–therapist relationship tends to parallel the family-of-origin relationship. Clients are encouraged to confront their resistance and explore the parallels between past and present relationships. Ultimately it is hoped that the clients will gain new insights that will lead to individual and systemic change.

## Therapeutic Goals

The goal of therapy is to help the family free themselves from the unconscious restrictions that are influencing their relationships. This occurs when they interpret events and the family gains insight into the events. The challenge is that the events are at the preconscious level and the family may be barely aware of them. Once the family has achieved some insight, the therapist helps the family work through the issues and create new strategies for more effective behaviors and interactions. The family is then able to interact in a healthy way, based on reality rather than on the unconscious images from the past. Restructuring the personality and achieving differentiation is considered to be more important that just solving the immediate problem.

## Techniques Associated With This Therapy

The emphasis of ORFT is on the unconscious early memories and object relations. Awareness of the unconscious helps individuals realize how their internal repressed material may be bringing them closer to farther away from others. The therapist helps the family examine their basic defense mechanisms and how these mechanisms influence family relationships. Emphasis is placed on origins of dysfunction that relate to childhood experiences. In this way, the family is able to resolve current issues by exploring the ways the family reacted to difficult times in the past. There are several techniques associated with ORFT. These include:

- *Transference* helps clients work through feelings by viewing those feelings as unresolved issues. It is used to understand what emotions are directed to certain individuals. When a family–therapist bond is formed, and the client demonstrates actions toward the therapist that are similar to the actions they direct toward people with whom they are having difficulties, the family benefits from a release of emotion and gains new insights which lead to individual and systemic change.
- In *countertransference,* the therapist's own experiences and emotions are projected onto the family, which helps him or her to understand the family process and rely on your his or her self-knowledge and understanding in order to be effective. The therapist then uses the information from this countertransference to help the family understand their unconscious patterns.
- *Dream* and *daydream analysis* is used to analyze what needs in the family are not being met and to develop strategies for meeting those needs.
- *Confrontation* is a process in which the inconsistencies between the family's behavior and family members stated expectations are pointed out. This helps them become aware of their behaviors and create strategies for more effective functioning.
- **Interpretation** allows the therapist to draw conclusions about what may be going on with the family members and help them understand the meaning of their behavior and emotions.
- **Focusing on strengths** is used to help the family break through patterns of behavior by noting what the family is doing well and using that information to help them break the dysfunctional patterns, promote cooperation, and plan more effective behaviors.
- Taking a **life history** helps the family explore and assess their past and present interactions. The therapist takes the history, thereby facilitating the process so that the family recognizes the value of each member regardless of background. This process encourages trust between the therapist and the family and stimulates insight in family members.

12. The concept of _____ is used in object relations family therapy to understand what emotions are directed to what individuals.
    a. confrontation
    b. transference
    c. countertransference
    d. displacement

13. Techniques associated with ORFT include _____.
    a. transference and countertransference
    b. confrontation and interpretation
    c. paradox and imagery
    d. a and b

## Key Terms

**defense mechanisms:** Strategies individuals use to deal with anxiety and conflicts.
**denial:** The refusal to recognize that a problem exists.
**differentiation:** The ability to function autonomously.
**displacement:** The redirection of emotional response to a safe object.
**interlocking pathology:** The unconscious process in a family that keeps them connected.
**object:** Something that is loved, usually a person.
**projection:** Attributing unacceptable thoughts, feelings, or motives onto another person.
**rationalization:** Finding an intellectual rationale for justifying a behavior.
**reaction formation:** Choosing an action that is the direct opposite of how one is actually feeling.
**regression:** The immature behavior an individual may choose while under stress.
**repression:** The unconscious blocking of upsetting thoughts or memories.
**scapegoating:** The placing of blame for problems onto one individual.

## MENTAL RESEARCH INSTITUTE (MRI) BRIEF FAMILY THERAPY

### Theory at a Glance

The MRI approach to family therapy was greatly influenced by the work of Gregory Bateson and his ideas about **cybernetics** and communication. The MRI team was interested in how faulty patterns of communication influenced family dysfunction. They noticed that successful communication depended on the appropriate use of *semantics*, or the clarity of meaning between what is said and what is received (the speaker and listener agree on the meaning of the words used), *syntax*, or the way the message is delivered (the speaker and listener agree on the method of delivery), and *pragmatics*, or the consequences of the communication (the speaker and listener agree on the result of the interchange and how they are to realistically proceed from that point).

14. MRI therapists view successful communication as dependent upon the appropriate use of _____.
    a. respectful and empathic listening
    b. semantics, syntax, and context
    c. semantics, syntax, and pragmatics
    d. puns, paradox, and reframing

MRI therapists believe that the solutions that a family uses to alleviate a problem often contribute to the continuation of the problem. The continued repetition of a behavior that reinforces the problem is called a *positive feedback loop*. MRI therapists are particularly interested in exploring the unspoken family rules that govern the system. The goal of therapy is to create concrete strategies for behavioral change that will eliminate the presenting problem.

> 15. In MRI brief family therapy, the continued repetition of a behavior that reinforces the problem is called a _____.
>     a. positive feedback loop
>     b. cybernetic cycle
>     c. paradoxical symptom
>     d. cyclical reinforcer

This approach focuses on present behavior, is usually limited to no more than ten sessions, and is especially appropriate for families who want a solution to a current problem or who are looking for symptomatic relief.

## View of Human Functioning

MRI therapists resist defining a normative standard of human functioning. Instead, they believe that any way that people choose to live is all right unless they determine that they have a problem. However, they also believe that healthy families can be identified by their ability to recognize when solutions to problems are not working and their willingness to develop new solutions. Successful families react appropriately to problems and avoid creating problems where there are none.

## View of Dysfunction

Family problems arise and are prolonged when difficulties or conflicts are not resolved effectively. The problems become chronic when families continue to employ the same solutions to the problem, even though the solutions they have chosen are ineffective. This results in positive feedback escalations. The solutions eventually obscure the original problem and become the problem themselves. There are three ways in which problems are escalated: a) when some action is needed but not taken, b) when an action is initiated when there is no need to act, or c) when the action taken is at the wrong level of intervention.

## Therapist's Role

An MRI therapist's is an active one, in which clients are viewed as customers. The therapist responds to process rather than content, helping "customers" reshape their perspectives on current problems and **reframing** their perceptions of their previously ineffective behavior. Therapists may act as teams. Team members watch the sessions from behind a one-way mirror, and may interrupt the session to offer suggestions, advice, or feedback. This approach is designed to speed up the change in the family's pattern of interactions.

## Client's Role

It is not necessary for clients to gain insight or to become educated about past history that might have influenced present behavior. Clients are expected to agree to implement strategies for change that are different from the ones they are currently using. Sometimes the client is not the person with the problem. The therapist determines who has the most motivation for change and will work with that person, believing that the problem will improve if even only one person in the family is willing to change.

## Therapeutic Goals

The therapeutic goal is simple—to break the ineffective pattern of behavior so that the presenting problem is resolved to the client's satisfaction. There are two types of change that a family or individual may implement. *First order change*, which tends to be short-lived, is a superficial behavioral change in the system that does not change the structure of the system itself. *Second order change* is a fundamental revision of the system's structure and function. Once the problem is resolved, the therapy is considered to be completed, even if the therapist believes that there are other problems in the family that should be addressed.

16. A primary goal of MRI brief Family therapy is to _____.
    a. foster insight
    b. promote individuation of family members
    c. interrupt dysfunctional feedback loop
    d. reinforce symptoms

## Techniques Associated With This Theory

The MRI approach is designed to help clients find quick, inexpensive, alternative ways to facilitate effective changes in individuals and families. Its basic techniques can be defined in three simple steps:

1. Identify and define the problem and the feedback loops that maintain the problem.
2. Identify the rules that support the problem.
3. Define and implement a concrete plan for change. Specific techniques include the use of **directives**, **paradox**, puns, imagery, **reframing**, **prescribing the symptom**, and the use of the **therapeutic double bind**.

## Key Terms

**cybernetics:** The science of communication and control in men and machines. It explains how systems maintain stability and control through the feedback they receive.

**directives:** Therapeutic tasks assigned by the therapist that are designed to interrupt patterns of interaction and encourage second order change.

**paradox:** A statement that contradicts itself (e.g. saying the very last thing the client would expect) and therefore the therapist catches the client off guard, thus disarming him or her.

**paradoxical interventions:** Directives that seem to be in opposition to the goals of the client.

**prescribing the symptom:** A technique in which the therapist directs the family to continue their behavior in the hope that the rules that support the dysfunction will be revealed.

**reframing** (or **relabeling**): Changes a label from negative to positive so that the problem is perceived differently.

**therapeutic double bind:** A technique in which the therapist uses a variety of paradoxical interventions that force the family into a no-lose situation.

## STRATEGIC FAMILY THERAPY

### Theory at a Glance

Like the MRI approach, Strategic Family Therapy (SFT) has its roots in Bateson's study of family communication and cybernetics. Milton Erickson also influenced SFT with his shift to a more directive approach in which the focus was on the problem and its symptoms. Jay Haley built upon this foundation with his belief that the structural components of a family and the rules that govern the family are at the core of family problems. The focus of SFT is on the development of strategies for changing the patterns of family interaction that surround the presenting problem. Haley believed that change came in stages and encouraged therapists to develop strategies that could be implemented over the course of treatment. Therapeutic strategies are tailor made to suit the needs of the family. Treatment is short term, with an emphasis on discovering family rules and challenging the tendency for family homeostasis. The therapist is active and flexible and works to plan strategies that will result in quick resolution of the problem.

### View of Human Development

Functional family structures have clear boundaries and an appropriate hierarchy of power. Parents should have control over children and be at the top of the hierarchy. Healthy family development can be identified by the successful completion of critical transitional stages. These stages include courtship, early marriage, the birth of a first child, raising and launching children, retirement and old age.

17. According to Jay Hayley, functional family structures have _____ boundaries and an appropriate hierarchy of power.
    a. clear
    b. rigid
    c. transparent
    d. focused

### View of Dysfunction

This theory proposes three areas of potential family dysfunction:

1. Difficulties become chronic problems when ineffective solutions are attempted and repeated, forming a positive feedback loop that maintains the problem.
2. Problems come as a result of a flaw in the family's hierarchy.
3. Dysfunction arises when individuals try to protect or control one another indirectly through their symptoms.

The problem often serves a purpose for the family. Cloe Madanes proposed the idea of the *incongruous hierarchy*. This occurs when a child uses her symptom to control her parents. Problems arise from four basic intentions of the family members involved: to dominate and control, to be loved, to love and protect others, and to repent and forgive. Symptoms are considered to be ineffective strategies used by one person to try to deal with another.

18. According to Cloe Madanes in strategic family therapy, problems arise from four basic intentions of the family members involved. Which of the following is not one?
    a. to dominate and control
    b. to love and protect others
    c. to repent and forgive
    d. to feel needed

## Therapist's Role

A strategic family therapist, is more interested in helping a family change its behavior than in helping them understand it, but is still aware of the family's structure and hierarchy looking especially for triangulated relationships. They observe how the problem behavior might be helping the family in some way and guide the family in reframing the problem so that they believe they have power over it and that they can control it. The therapist is actively involved in the process and would be responsible for planning strategies to resolve family problems.

19. Strategic family therapists are interested in:
    a. helping families gain insight into their behavioral patterns.
    b. helping families change their behavior.
    c. helping families maintain homeostasis.
    d. helping families to attain incongruous hierarchy.

## Client's Role

Clients are active participants in this process. With the therapist's assistance, they explore the patterns of interactions they have chosen to deal with the problem and are expected to follow the directives prescribed by the therapist. It is not necessary or anticipated that clients will attain insight into the source of their problems.

## Therapeutic Goals

Strategic family therapy helps the family identify the problems in its organization by facilitating discussion so that the family's perception of those problems changes. Directives for behavioral change are prescribed so that the interaction of the family is improved. The ultimate goal is restructuring the family, particularly its hierarchy and the boundaries between generations.

20. The ultimate goal of strategic family therapy is:
    a. helping parents to learn more effective parenting techniques.
    b. helping family members to adapt to change.
    c. restructuring the family, particularly its hierarchy and boundaries between generations.
    d. teaching the family more strategies to use in their communication and interactions.

## Techniques Associated With This Theory

Strategic family therapists are concerned with four interrelated elements: symptoms, metaphors, hierarchy, and power. Symptoms help the family to maintain **homeostasis** in the system and are viewed as metaphors for communication. Family struggles often arise from a flawed hierarchy and a displacement of power in the system.

> 21. Strategic family therapists are concerned with four interrelated elements. These are:
> a. symptoms, mentaphors, hierarchy, and power.
> b. ordeal, positioning, pretending, and prescribing
> c. encouraging, understanding, insight, and reorientation.
> d. first order change, second order change, integration, and reorientation.

Although there are no specific techniques applied to all situations, Haley did create a procedure for the initial interview. First, a relationship with the family is created. Then, the therapist helps the family identify the problem, after which the family is then encouraged to discuss the problem. At this time, the therapist observes the family interactions, then helps the family members assess the solutions they have tried in the past and evaluate their effectiveness. Eventually, goals are defined and sometimes family directives are given that will initiate change.

One of the unusual aspects of this theory is that techniques are customized to suit specific problems. However, SFT therapists do make use of some general techniques, including the use of directives, reframing, and paradox. Other popular techniques used in SFT include:

- Assigning *ordeals*—using neutral behavior that must be performed before engaging in an undesirable behavior. The goal is to make the symptom more difficult to maintain than the benefits derived from this behavior.
- Asking the client to *pretend* to engage in the problematic behavior. This process helps individuals gain control over an action that they thought was involuntary.
- The act of *positioning,* which involves the therapist exaggerating what the family is saying so they can see that it is not as bad as it could be.
- *Homework* is prescribed to initiate behavioral change and to speed up the process of the therapy.

Paradoxical techniques are also used. Examples include:

- *Restraining*—you hold the family back from making change by advising them that they are incapable of doing anything differently.
- *Prescribing*—you instruct the family to recreate a problematic behavior so that you can observe the interaction.
- *Redefining*—you put a positive connotation on behavior that is usually considered to be undesirable.

## Key Terms

**circular causality:** Explains that behavior occurs in cycles and in a context, rather than as a result of cause and effect.
**double bind:** A communication that leaves the receiver in a no-win situation.
**homeostasis:** The tendency within a system to seek and maintain balance by maintaining the current situation and resisting change.

# STRUCTURAL FAMILY THERAPY

## Theory at a Glance

Structural Family Therapy was formed in the 1960s by Salvador Minuchin, a psychiatrist from Argentina. According to this theory, a client's symptoms are best understood when observed in the context of family interactional patterns. A change in the family's organization or structure must take place before symptoms can be relieved. Three constructs comprise the central components of structural family therapy: (a) **family structure**, (b) **subsystems**, and (c) boundaries. Structural family therapists focus on present behavior working with the entire family system, and address problematic symptoms through restructuring the family.

22. The three constructs central to structural family therapy are family structure, subsystems, and _____.
    a. interpretation
    b. boundaries
    c. differentiation
    d. reorientation

## View of Human Functioning

Structural family therapists view people's current experience in the context in which they struggle with life's challenges and from which they grow and define themselves. These struggles bring about stress for the family and its members. Families must restructure and reorganize in order to adapt to stressors. Treatment is needed when families hold rigidly to specific transactional patterns without adapting to life challenges. Boundaries play a large part in structural family therapy. There are three major types of boundaries. *Clear boundaries* are rules and habits that allow and encourage dialogue and thus help family members to enhance their communication and relationships with one another. They allow negotiation and accommodation to occur, which facilitate change but still maintain the family's stability. When boundaries are clear, each family member feels a sense of belonging and also the ability to individuate. *Rigid boundaries* are overly restrictive in that little contact with outside systems is permitted. Families with rigid boundaries have inflexible rules and habits that keep family members separated from each other. When boundaries are rigid, members experience difficulty relating in an intimate way and become emotionally detached. This results in disengagement, or psychological isolation, leaving individuals/subsystems independent but isolated. *Diffuse boundaries* are structural arrangements that do not allow enough separation between family members. This results in some members becoming fused and dependent on other members. Diffuse boundaries cause poorly delineated distinctions between systems or subsystems, bringing heightened feelings of mutual support, at the expense of autonomy and independence. These boundaries exist with enmeshed parents, who are loving and considerate, but simultaneously foster dependence and discomfort in being alone.

## View of Dysfunction

Structural family therapy focuses on the social context in which people's functioning becomes stuck in self-defeating and hurtful patterns of thinking and interacting. The therapist attempts to bring order to the family's structure so that family members can regain mobility and power to overcome the "stuckness" or impasse and be free to change.

## Therapist's Role

The therapist is to be an observer and expert. He or she takes an active role in producing interventions to modify and change the underlying structure of the family.

23. Loss of autonomy due to overinvolvement of family members with each other, either physically or psychologically is _____.
    a. familial accentuation
    b. interdependence
    c. homeostasis
    d. enmeshment

## Client's Role

The client's role is one of active participation. Clients need to be open and willing to engage in the enactment process. They should be able to examine their boundaries and roles in the family context and challenge themselves to allow reorientation and reorganization to occur. Family members are best served in this approach when the major players in the family structure are available for the therapeutic process.

## Therapeutic Goals

In structural family therapy, the therapist works actively and creatively, mapping out family structure and instructing the family to enact certain experiences. Problematic behaviors and patterns of thought are brought out in the open for the therapist and family to examine and help change them. Therapy's primary focus is to alter the family structure in order to allow the family to solve its own problems. Ultimately, structural changes such as organizational patterns, sequences, and hierarchies, should be made. There are generally three phases of treatment: (a) the therapist joins the family and takes a leadership position, (b) he or she mentally maps out the family's underlying structure, and (c) helps to transform the family structure.

## Techniques Associated With This Theory

*Joining* is the process of "coupling" that occurs between the therapist and the family, leading to the development of the therapeutic system. There are four basic ways that to accomplish joining the family: (a) tracking, (b) mimesis, (c) confirmation of a family member, and (d) accommodation. **Tracking** involves following the content of the family (i.e., the facts), gathering information using open-ended questions to inquire about the interests and concerns of family members, while making no overt judgments. **Mimesis** is becoming like the family in the manner or content of their communications, adjusting behavioral style to fit that of the family. The therapist does this by using similar interpersonal styles and language as the family, such as joking with a jovial family or using the same metaphors that family members use. **Confirming a family member** means verbally clarifying the feelings and existence of a family member, often a member who is either less empowered or more marginalized by other family members. **Accommodation** requires making personal adjustments in order to achieve a therapeutic alliance with a family, such as wearing less formal clothing, sitting differently, and so forth.

The core of structural family therapy is *structural change,* which is achieved through the technique of *restructuring.* Restructuring makes the family more functional by altering the existing hierarchy and interaction patterns so that problems are not maintained. This requires gaining a sound knowledge of the present family structure.

*Reframing* is a process in which a perception is changed by explaining a situation in a different context. In this way different meaning is attributed to events, behavior, and experience. The facts of an event do not change, but the meaning of the situation is examined from a new perspective.

In the technique of *unbalancing,* a therapeutic alliance is created with a subsystem, wherein the therapist supports an individual or subsystem against the rest of the family or the currently dominant subsystem. This creates a disequilibrium, which forces the family to find a new equilibrium.

The structural method of *changing maladaptive transactions* by using strong affect, repeated intervention, or prolonged pressure with a family is called *intensity.* In this technique tone, volume, pace, and choice of words are used in a direct and unapologetic manner that is goal specific.

When practicing the technique of *shaping competence,* the therapist helps the family and family members become more functional by highlighting positive behaviors and reinforcing them for doing things well and making their own appropriate decisions.

With the technique of *enactment,* family members act out the actions that show problematic behavioral sequences to therapists. For example, the family may be asked to have an argument instead of discussing one. In enactment, family members experience their own transactions with heightened awareness. By examining their roles, members often discover more functional ways of behaving.

## Key Terms

**coalitions:** Alliances between specific family members against a third member. There are two types of coalitions. *Stable coalitions* are fixed and inflexible unions (such as mother and son) that becomes a dominant part of the family's everyday functioning. *Detouring coalitions* are ones in which the pair hold a third family member responsible for their difficulties or conflicts with one another, thus reducing the stress on themselves or their relationship.

24. In structural family therapy, the therapist's role is to function as observer and _____.
    a. coach
    b. teammate
    c. historian
    d. expert

25. In structural family therapy, an alliance between specific family members against a third member is called a/an _____.
    a. coalition
    b. alliance
    c. association
    d. federation

**family structure:** An invisible set of functional demands, predictable sequences, and organized patterns by which family members associate with each other. Structure is only revealed through family interactions. Families with a hierarchical structure are generally seen as more functional.

**scapegoating:** Occurs when the wife and husband are incapable of resolving their conflicts between each other and redirect their focus of concern onto their child. In lieu of worrying about each other, they worry about the child. This diminishes the strain on the parents; however, it victimizes the child and is therefore dysfunctional.

**subsystems:** Smaller units of the system as a whole, usually composed of members in a family who because of age or function are logically grouped together, such as children or parents. Subsystems exist to carry out assorted family responsibilities from changing the oil to walking the dog, and vary in length of existence. Without subsystems, the family systems would not function. Three key subsystems are the *spousal subsystem,* the *parental subsystem,* and the *sibling subsystem.*

## DISCUSSION QUESTIONS

1. In structural family therapy, scapegoating plays a large role in the etiology of some presenting problems. What would be an example of such a problem and how does scapegoating contribute to its existence?
2. Within the viewpoint of Adlerian family therapy, how does purposeful behavior contribute to the correction of family dysfunction?
3. Within Adlerian family therapy, how would you explain interaction between the concepts of *inferiority feelings* and *social interest* when working with a family that has a depressed child?
4. In using transgenerational family therapy, how would you most effectively encourage the goal of *differentiation of self* with a couple complaining of having significant intimacy problems?
5. What is the difference between the transgenerational family therapy viewpoint of *triangles* and that of structural family therapy?
6. Within contextual family therapy, how do family patterns passed from parents to children differ from the way they are seen within transgenerational family therapy?
7. Of the theoretical approaches reviewed in this chapter, which are more amenable to *DSM* diagnosis and which are not?
8. Object relations family therapy focuses on origins of dysfunction that relate to childhood experiences while contextual family therapy focuses more on building on family resources to bring desired changes. What parts, if any, of these two theoretical approaches are compatible?
9. Some marriage and family therapists integrate principals from the MRI approach into family therapy with other theoretical approaches. What are your thoughts about this type of approach?
10. How do views of family hierarchy differ from strategic family therapy and structural family therapy viewpoints? Which is more appropriate to you and why?

## SUGGESTED FURTHER READING

Carlson, J., & Kjos, D. (2002). *Theories and strategies of family therapy*. Boston: Allyn & Bacon.
Gladding, S. (2002). *Family therapy: History, theory, and practice* (3rd ed.). New Jersey: Merrill Prentice Hall.

Goldenburg, I., & Goldenburg, H. (2000). *Family therapy: An overview* (5th ed.). Belmont, CA: Wadsworth/Thompson Learning.

Guerin, P. J. (2002). Family therapy: The first twenty-five years. In P. J. Guerin, Jr. (Ed.), *Family therapy, theory, and practice* (pp. ——). New York: Gardner.

Nichols, M., & Schwartz, R. (2003). *Family therapy: Concepts and methods* (6th ed.). Boston: Allyn & Bacon.

Piercy, F., Sprenkle, D., & Wetchler, J. (1996). *Family therapy sourcebook* (2nd ed.). New York: Guilford Publications.

# REFERENCES

Dreikurs, R. (1957). Our child guidance clinics in Chicago. *Collected papers of Rudolf Dreikurs* (pp. 70–89). Eugene, OR: University of Oregon Press.

Guerin, P., & Guerin, K. (2002). Bowenian family therapy. In J. Carlson & D. Kjos (Eds.), *Theories and strategies of family therapy* (pp. 126–157). Boston: Allyn & Bacon.

# 7

# Theories of Family Therapy (Part II)

Hugh C. Crethar
*Governors State University*

Kim Snow
*Northern Illinois University*

Jon Carlson
*Governors State University*

## TRUTH OR FICTION?

___ 1. *In experiential family therapy, emotional experiencing is valued above cognitive response.*

___ 2. *In experiential family therapy, harmonious communication is seen as key to healthy family functioning.*

___ 3. *Experiential family therapy developed out of the behaviorism movement.*

___ 4. *Narrative therapy is generally considered a value-free approach to family therapy.*

___ 5. *Narrative therapy developed out the humanistic movement.*

___ 6. *According to narrative therapy, an individual's personal experience is fundamentally ambiguous.*

___ 7. *In feminist family therapy the therapist, maintains an emotional distance from the client in order to protect the relationship from societal contamination.*

___ 8. *In feminist family therapy, responding to traditional societal values and structures are seen as more important to healthy family functioning than evaluating family structure.*

___ 9. *The collaborative approach of the "reflecting team" serves to help clients understand themselves better without having to get direct feedback from outside sources.*

___ 10. *A crucial part of the efficacy of the team approach in collaborative therapy is the establishment of a clear power hierarchy.*

___ 11. *Solution-oriented family therapy and collaborative therapy come from the same philosophical roots.*

___ 12. *A key issue in effectively implementing solution-oriented family therapy is to assess the category of client with whom you are working and engage appropriately.*

___ 13. *The regularity of a problem is more important than exceptions to the problem from a solution-oriented family therapy perspective.*
___ 14. *The cognitive-behavioral family therapy approach is generally nondirective.*
___ 15. *In behavioral family therapy the most effective way to help families to modify their behaviors is to alter the consequences.*

This chapter is a continuation of some of the most popular family theories and will assist you in gaining a basic understanding of some of the terms and concepts used within these theories. We have included six diverse theories in this chapter and we have broken them down into the same format and uniform headings that we used in the previous chapter so that it is easier for you to compare and contrast the various theories. We have also included a table summarizing the six theories (see Table 7.1) at the end of the chapter.

## COGNITIVE-BEHAVIORAL FAMILY THERAPY

### Theories at a Glance

Behavioral family therapy (BFT) first emerged in the 1970s when behavioral therapists began applying principles of learning to parent training, couples communication, problem-solving skills, and sex therapy. Although no one person is credited as being the founder of BFT, Gerald Patterson, Robert Lieberman, Helen Singer Kaplan, and Richard Stuart played key roles in the development of this approach. BFT has four basic forms: behavioral marital therapy, functional family therapy, behavioral treatment of sexual dysfunction, and behavioral parent training. Gerald Patterson developed behavioral parent training. Robert Lieberman focused on behavioral application with couples and families, Helen Singer Kaplan developed effective behavioral approaches to sexual dysfunction, and Richard Stuart initiated **contingency contracting** and the reciprocity of positive behavior exchanges with distressed couples. All of these approaches rely upon operant conditioning principles.

During the 1970s, theorists also began to acknowledge the importance of thoughts and attitudes in behavior modification. These views gave rise to cognitive behavioral family therapy (CBFT). Influenced by the work of Aaron Beck and Albert Ellis, CBFT can be defined as a hybrid of the BFT approach and a cognitive approach, with a particular focus on cognitive attributions made about the behaviors of others in the relationship. Some of the leaders of CBFT include Donald Baucom, Norman Epstein, and Frank Dattilio. James Alexander is also among the leaders of CBFT because he developed functional family therapy, which assesses the interactional sequences in which problems are embedded within the family. He contended that symptoms (or problems) within the family serve a function to create either closeness or distance among family members and educated families on learning new, more adaptive ways of functioning within the family. Due to the focus on measurable behavioral changes within individual members of the family (which is done separately from the family as a whole), this approach is not usually considered a systemic approach to family therapy.

### View of Human Functioning

The central premise of behavioral family therapy is that all behavior is learned and maintained by its consequences. BFT practitioners believe that learned behaviors will continue unchanged unless more rewarding consequences emerge or are presented. CBFT takes this assertion a step further by examining the interplay of cognitions, behavior, and emotions within family relationships and how each of these variables influence and maintain current patterns of relating and interacting within family systems.

## View of Dysfunction

Behavioral family therapists see problems as serving a function with the family and are maintained by the family's dysfunctional patterns of behavior and reinforcement. Dysfunctional interactions and behavior will remain resistant to change until the family has learned more adaptive and rewarding consequences. Thus, the most effective way to help families to modify their behaviors is to alter the consequences that maintain this dysfunction.

1. Behavioral family therapists see problems as:
   a. serving a function with the family and being maintained by the family's dysfunctional patterns of behavior and reinforcement.
   b. something that families have to learn how to adjust to.
   c. easily eliminated by using charts and homework.
   d. needing to be reframed so that family members can see the positive side of their family functioning.

From a CBFT perspective, the therapist views problems in a more complex manner and as being created and sustained by the interaction of cognitions, affect, and behaviors. Dysfunctional families tend to hold negative relationship-related beliefs that result in further distress and conflict. Family members who are having difficulties in their relationships hold faulty beliefs such as: they do not have to work at relationships, one family members' needs are more important and do not influence others within the family, and effective family functioning is conflict-free. In CBFT, the therapist works collaboratively with family members to adjust some of their irrational patterns of thinking and perceiving and help them learn more effective ways of thinking and interacting within their relationships.

## Therapist's Role

Both behavior family therapists and cognitive behavior family therapists function as models, experts—skillful and flexible coaches and teachers. There are many dimensions to the therapist's role because he or she builds a collaborative relationship, conducts a full assessment of family functioning, instructs and monitors family behaviors, and coaches and models problem solving and communication skills so that families can discover more adaptive ways of relating to each other. Therapists also help families understand and alter their cognitive distortions and understand the impact of their thoughts on their interactions and thus their family functioning. Family members who perceive another member in a positive light tend to interpret negative behaviors as situational. For example, a client might think, "My husband snapped at me because he had a long day and therefore is tired and cranky." Those family members who do not interact positively with one another tend to attribute negative behaviors as being an integral part of the person's character. Thus, such a person might think, "My husband snapped at me because he is cruel and mean-spirited." CBFT practitioners help family members see that the same behavior can have multiple interpretations and these interpretations play a significant role in the positive or negative interactions among family members.

> 2. Behavioral family therapists and cognitive-behavior family therapists function as _____.
>    a. models
>    b. coaches
>    c. teachers
>    d. all of the above

## Client's Role

Family members and their functioning are assessed and members are taught the principles of social learning and cognitive behavior to help them gain an understanding into the reciprocity and coercion of their own and other family members' interactions. Clients are seen as active students who collaborate in the therapeutic process and have the ability to learn new and more adaptive ways of relating with one another.

## Therapeutic Goals

A BFT therapist's therapeutic goals include increasing the rate of rewarding interactions in family relationships through clear rules, roles, and contingencies; decreasing the use of coercion and aversive exchanges; remediating undesired behaviors; and preventing future undesired behaviors. A CBFT therapist's goals would include the above, but would also focus on gaining an awareness and control of cognitive attributions made to behaviors of other family members as well as improved expectancies of what others will bring to the relationship. The therapist also evaluates the **family schema**, clarifying jointly held beliefs about the family, each other, and life in general and seeking out dysfunctional patterns of thought and interaction. As practitioners in both CBFT and BFT, therapists tend to emphasize actions taken by family members over insights made by them.

## Techniques Associated With These Theories

Behavioral family therapists use many techniques. They begin by assessing the contingencies that influence the problematic behavior and then create intervention strategies that will modify the contingencies, thereby eliminating the undesired behavior. Behavior techniques include teaching and modeling parent skills training, communication skills, assertion training, **systematic desensitization**, problem-solving strategies, coaching, **reciprocity, shaping, contingency contracting, quid pro quo**, cognitive restructuring, the **Premack Principle**, and implementing **token economies**. Homework, bibliotherapy, charting, and follow-up assessments are also used as means to promote, record, and measure the positive changes families make toward their stated goals.

CBFT practitioners move beyond these techniques because they help families understand that cognitions, emotions, and behavior all interact to affect relationship quality and family functioning. CBFT therapists collaborate with the family to tailor a variety of behavioral, cognitive, and affective techniques to help family members critically examine their beliefs, perceptions, and behavior and how these all interplay to affect the overall functioning of the family. Cognitive techniques include: disputing irrational beliefs, thought stopping, self-instruction training, cognitive restructuring, cognitive errors, self-talk, changing ones' language (from blaming to "I" statements), humor, role-playing, and imagery.

> 3. CBFT therapists collaboratively tailor a variety of behavioral, cognitive, and affective techniques with family members. Which of the following are examples of CBFT techniques?
>     a. disputing irrational beliefs
>     b. self-talk
>     c. role-playing
>     d. all of the above

## Key Terms

**aversive control:** Use of punishment or criticism to eliminate undesirable responses, commonly used in dysfunctional families.

**baseline:** Initial recorded observations of behavior that are expected change once treatment conditions are introduced.

**behavior modification:** The application of conditioning techniques to reduce or eliminate problematic behavior or to teach new responses.

**classical conditioning:** Respondent learning in which the unconditioned stimulus (UCS), such as food, which leads to an unconditioned response (UCR), such as salivation, is paired with a conditioned stimulus (CS), such as a bell. As a result, the CS begins to evoke the same response, salivation, as a conditioned response (CR).

$$UCS \rightarrow UCR$$

$$CS + UCS \rightarrow UCR$$

Stimulus generalization

$$CS \rightarrow CR$$

**contingency contracting:** A procedure wherein a contract is written describing the terms for the exchange of behaviors and reinforcers between individuals. In these agreements, each action is contingent upon another action.

**extinction:** In classical conditioning, the elimination of a conditioned response by the omission of the unconditioned stimulus. Also, the elimination of a conditioned response by repeated presentations of a conditioned stimulus without the unconditioned stimulus. In operant conditioning, the elimination of the conditioned response by the omission of reinforcement. Abolition of a learned behavior.

**family schema:** Jointly held beliefs about one's own family and about family life in general.

**modeling:** A form of observational learning wherein behaviors are learned by observing and imitating others, especially authority figures or those like oneself.

**negative reinforcement:** The strengthening of a tendency to exhibit desired behavior by virtue of the of the fact that previous responses in that situation have been rewarded by the removal of an aversive stimulus.

**operant conditioning:** A form of learning whereby a person or animal is rewarded (through positive reinforcement) for desired behaviors. This is the major approach of most forms of behavioral therapy.

**positive reinforcement:** The strengthening of a behavioral tendency by virtue of the fact that previous responses in that situation have been followed by presentation of a desired reward.

**Premack Principle:** An intervention wherein family members must do less pleasant tasks before they are allowed to engage in pleasurable activities.

**punishment:** A consequence that decreases the probability that a behavior will reappear. Any noxious stimulus imposed to reduce the probability of undesirable behavior.

**quid pro quo:** "Something for something" in Latin. This is often used in marital contracts, as a spouse agrees to do something as long as the other does something equivalent.

**reciprocity:** The likelihood that members of a couple will reinforce each other at approximately equitable rates over time.

**reinforcement:** An event, behavior, or object that, when applied, increases the rate of a particular response.

**reinforcement reciprocity:** The exchange of reinforcing behaviors between family members.

**shaping:** Reinforcing desired behavior in small steps that gradually approximate the desired behavior.

**systematic desensitization:** A behavioral therapy technique in which deep muscle relaxation is used to inhibit the effects of graded anxiety-evoking stimuli. Graduated immersion into the situation is used to decrease sensitivity to it.

**token economy:** A behavior therapy procedure based on operant conditioning principles in which tokens, such as poker chips, are given for socially constructive behavior, and are withheld when unwanted behaviors are exhibited. The tokens themselves can be exchanged for desirable items and activities such as time in the most popular chair or control of the television for an evening.

## COLLABORATIVE THERAPY

### Theory at a Glance

Collaborative theory developed from constructivist philosophy and metamorphosed into a more language-focused system, one which embraces a **linguistic paradigm**. The theory derived from problem determined systems therapy, and later evolved into a collaborative language systems approach. Leaders in the field were Harlane Anderson, Lynn Hoffman, Tom Andersen, and Harry Goolishian, who in the 80s and 90s, translated constructivism into an approach where the therapist and client engaged in more of a cooperative, egalitarian, and respectful relationship which sought to empower families. The theory was created out of an opposition to the cybernetic model and the traditional hierarchical therapist-client relationship. Rather than espouse techniques that manipulate the clients' language, collaborative therapy uses empathic conversations to promote new meanings. Collaborative therapy is seen as more of an attitude and process rather than a distinctive theory or a particular method.

4. Which of the following theories puts more emphasis on linguistics?
   a. solution-focused family therapy
   b. collaborative therapy
   c. experiential family therapy
   d. narrative therapy

Harlene Anderson and Harry Goolishian are the originators who moved collaborative therapy toward the postmodern approach to language. Lynn Hoffman departed from her strategic family therapy background and joined these pioneers in their new collaborative approach. Tom

Andersen, a Norwegian psychiatrist, took collaboration to a new level by developing the **reflecting team** approach. This reflecting process hides nothing from the clients and allows them to be present to view the team of therapists discussing the family and therapist via a one-way mirror. Thus, the family becomes an integral part of the discussion and a circular process of insight and feedback is shared among the family and the therapeutic team. The reflecting team approach has become a common characteristic of collaborative therapy. Collaboration has also been used in feminist, cognitive-behavioral, contemporary behavioral therapy, and narrative therapy.

> 5. Which of the following refers to a technique wherein the family becomes involved in being an integral part of the discussion and a circular process of insight and feedback is shared among the family and a group of therapists?
>     a. reflecting group
>     b. mirroring team
>     c. reflecting team
>     d. mirroring group

## View of Human Functioning

Collaborative therapists view the family as more of a team who has a considerable amount of expertise and knowledge about their particular family. This team just needs to be looking at their problems from a different perspective, which is the reason for the therapist to be there. The therapist–family team openly discusses what is happening leading to genuine conversations and discovering real human functioning within the family.

## View of Dysfunction

Collaborative therapists do not see the person as the problem, but instead the problem as the problem. The concept of dysfunction is rejected and replaced with the concept of *constraint*. Family members are viewed as constrained by numerous forces, including situations, interactions, and beliefs. In this manner, the family with dysfunction is viewed as a group in which some individuals view a particular person in a situation as a problem and miss the point that the real enemy is the problem itself.

## Therapist's Role

Collaborative therapists act as equal partners and co-explorers in the family collaboration. Attention and understanding is paid to the ways people relate to each other and what kinds of perspectives they have about the presenting problem. The therapist is interested in becoming a "member" of the family for the duration of therapy. The conversations that take place differ from the non-directive, empathic, Rogerian style because the therapist doesn't just reflect or rephrase but is also willing to offer ideas and suggestions in a respectful and tentative manner. The therapist takes a **not-knowing stance**, thereby allowing the family to be active participants in the process of finding solutions to their problems. Conversational questions are asked to inspire clients to view the problem from a new perspective. By being responsive, compassionate, and listening responsively, therapists provide opportunities for the clients to express their areas of concern. No specific hypothesis dominates the sessions, for fear of limiting more productive dialogue; instead the therapist remains open and learns from the family and their expertise. He or she joins in with the clients, using the expertise of all parties to dissolve the perceived problem.

6. In collaborative therapy, the therapist takes a(n) _____ stance, allowing family members to be active participants in the process of finding solutions to their problems.
   a. passive
   b. integrative
   c. not-knowing
   d. ambivalent

7. Collaborative therapists generally see themselves as _____ directive than the Rogerian approach to therapy.
   a. more
   b. less
   c. equivalent
   d. none of the above

## Client's Role

Collaborative therapists give family members the opportunity to comment on the process of helping and to share their expertise with the therapist and others. In this manner, clients elevate their status from passive needy recipients to active expert contributors. In this expert role, family members are invited to critique what has been going on, clarify what they appreciate, or coach the therapist towards what they need.

## Therapeutic Goals

Some of the goals of collaborative therapy are to empower families and help to co-create new meanings and solutions to problems *with* them. Your focus as a therapist is to actively understand and be involved in the clients' language, process, and interactions. The therapeutic conversation and dialogical process allow and encourage family members to generate meaning and take new actions to resolve their issues. Collaborative therapy is seen as a continuous process and termination is mutually and collectively determined.

## Techniques Associated With This Theory

There are no specific techniques in collaborative therapy; however, there is a focus on caring and empowerment. There is an emphasis on using a democratic style of communication and problem solving. Collaborative therapists use conversational questions which come from a "not knowing" stance and involve responsive listening and conversation. These questions evolve from really caring about, being involved in, and wanting to grasp the clients' stories. The therapist asks questions and formulates suppositions in a non-authoritarian manner, providing the client ample room and consent to disagree or correct the therapist. Collaborative therapists commonly acknowledge the validity of client-initiated stories of impossibility, blame, invalidation, and determinism and subtly and gently challenge them by introducing alternate possibilities.

## Key Terms

**collaborative:** All are equal participants in the therapeutic relationship.
**linguistic paradigm:** Describes the shift in the use of language used in therapy; the therapist is seen as "in language with the client" rather than using language as a hierarchical tool to "do therapy to" the client.

**not-knowing stance:** The position a therapist takes whereby he or she is an equal partner in a collaborative group and not the authority figure.

**reflecting team:** A team that discusses their reactions to what a family says—sometimes watches the therapy process from behind mirrors before coming out to join in the discussion.

## SOLUTION-ORIENTED FAMILY THERAPY

### Theory at a Glance

Solution-oriented family therapy (SOFT) is a brief, collaborative social constructivist approach that focuses on solutions rather than on problems. It assumes that the family is the expert but requires some consulting, empowerment, and guidance. Solution-oriented therapy is a brief therapy that focuses on the family's specific concern or complaint (rather than underlying dynamics and issues) and the strengths and resources of a family by helping the family to implement mutually agreeable and specific goals. It is much more present and future-oriented and does not focus on the past.

Though influenced by Milton Erikson, the late psychiatrist, Steven de Schazer and Insoo Kim Berg are credited with developing this approach. De Schazer's contributions include focusing on *ecosystemic epistemology* the theory—(that there is a reciprocal, mutual process of behavior, thinking, and deciding among the therapeutic team and family members; thus, a change in the family will impact the therapeutic process and vice versa). De Schazer also advocated the *binocular theory of change:* if the therapist presents the family with a slightly different pattern than their own, the family will recognize the similarities and accept the pattern of change including embracing the differences. This minute change can then cause shifts within the family process. Bill O'Hanlon took solution-oriented theory a step further by emphasizing solutions and created *possibility therapy* and Michele Weiner-Davis is known for her solution-oriented approach with couples.

> 8. _____ significantly influenced the solution-oriented family therapy approach.
>    a. Bandura
>    b. Erikson
>    c. Watson
>    d. Jung

### View of Human Functioning

The main focus of this approach is on increasing functioning by focusing on the strengths and resources within the family. Families are seen as growing and developing from their strengths toward their goals. Rather than addressing the past, underlying issues, and system dynamics, SOFT focuses on the presenting problems that bring the family or client into therapy at this time and what specific solutions they would like to see. For example, a family comes into counseling because their child has a problem with acting out behavior. A solution-oriented therapist would focus on the specific problem of misbehavior rather than looking at the acting out as a symptom of other things going on within the context of the family (such as problems in the marital dyad, lack of parenting skills, triangulation, etc.).

## Therapist's Role

A solution-oriented family therapist is an active consultant or "facilitator of change" who helps the family to access their strengths and resources. The category of client you are working with must be assessed—visitor, complainant, or customer (defined in following section)—and then engaged appropriately. All families are viewed as having the necessary skills to solve their own problems. The hopefulness, possibility, and encouragement the therapist provide are seen as crucial clinical skills in empowering families.

9. According to solution-oriented family therapy, clients tend to fall into *all but* which of the following categories?
   a. complainant
   b. visitor
   c. customer
   d. blamer

## Client's Role

Families play an active and involved role in the therapeutic process. They are active participants in setting the focus and direction of therapy and developing collaborative goals for the therapy and the entire family. Clients fall into three different categories. These include:

1. **Visitor**—a client who does not wish to participate in therapy, does not have a complaint, and does not wish to work on anything. The therapist's goal is to compliment the visitor and hope that a respectful stance and rapport will allow the relationship to progress towards a customer relationship.
2. **Complainant**—a client who describes a problem but is unwilling to resolve it. This relationship requires the therapist to engage in a solution-oriented conversation, compliment the client, and perhaps assign an activity whereby the client focuses on exceptions to the complaint. By respecting this relationship and not pushing for change, the likelihood is increased that the client will be more open to becoming a future customer.
3. **Customer**—a client who is actively involved in the therapeutic process. This client describes a problem and is motivated to change it. The therapist's role is to engage in solution-oriented conversation, compliment the client, and cocreate assignments to reproduce those behaviors that are exceptions to the problem.

## Therapeutic Goals

The therapeutic goals of SOFT are very specific—identifying the specific needs and desires the family has and finding a mutually agreeable direction and goal to work on. Solution-oriented family therapists do not emphasize the clinical understanding of the family situation nor do they emphasize understanding what is wrong. Instead, they focus on change. They help family members pinpoint what they see as solutions to their problems and then take action toward these solutions. They highlight exceptions to the problem and patterns of behavior in order to develop strengths from which to work. Small changes in behavior are encouraged and reinforced with the belief that this will lead to further change and solutions. SOFT therapists see all clients as capable of and wanting to change.

10. In solution-oriented family therapy, the therapist highlights _____ in order to develop strengths from which to work.
    a. solutions that have worked for others
    b. possible solutions from the therapist's perception
    c. exceptions to the problem
    d. problematic thought processes

## Techniques Associated With This Theory

*Acknowledging, tracking, and linking* are ways to coordinate complaints and goals. Each family member's perspective is recognized by the therapist restating it in the least inflammatory way possible but which still acknowledges and imparts its meaning and feeling. Therapists *connect* statements by using the words of each family member and building a common concern rather than opposing or competing with needs and goals. *Tracking* complaints, in addition to acknowledging and linking, help the therapist provide the family with descriptions of what actions or sequences of behaviors are occurring. The intent of these techniques is that the family can jump in and clarify any misperceptions or areas of discomfort until a mutually agreeable description emerges.

Other techniques a solution-oriented family therapist uses include:

*Asking the Miracle Question*—asking families for a hypothetical solution to their problem. For example, "If you were to wake up tomorrow and a miracle occurred and you no longer had this problem, how would your life be different? How would your behavior be different?"

*Focusing on Exceptions*—looking for the positive or the exception to the family's problem. For example, "Tell me about the one time that you didn't argue and fight, what caused the exception?"

*Scaling Questions*—asking clients questions using a scale to move them closer to their goal. For example, "On a scale of 1 to 10, where you do see your relationship as a couple? What would it take to make it higher?"

*Compliments*—are used to praise the family and focus on its strengths. Compliments are usually followed by a task or an assignment.

There are four main areas of intervention implemented in SOFT. These include

*experience, stories, actions,* and *context.* Experience covers all of the inner aspects of a person's life—his or her feelings, fantasies, sensations, and sense of self. Therapists should always start out by acknowledging what the client is experiencing. Change occurs within the other three interventions. Here the focus becomes changing the viewing (story) of a problem, changing the doing (action) of a problem, and changing the context of a problem:

11. Which of the following *is not* one of the four main areas of intervention used in implementing SOFT?
    a. experience
    b. stories
    c. actions
    d. content

*Changing the Viewing of the Problem*—When families enter therapy, they often have stories (ideas, beliefs, hypotheses) about each other or the problem. Some of these stories can be rigid and unhelpful for the family (such as **impossibility stories, blaming, invalidating**, and **deterministic stories**). SOFT therapists challenge or cast doubt on problematic stories so that more positive stories can emerge that can allow for growth and change to occur within the family. This is done by transforming and softening stories, by adding possibility, by finding counterevidence, or by finding stories or frames to fit the same evidence or facts.

*Changing the Doing of the Problem*—The therapist identifies and alters repetitive patterns of action and interaction involved in the problem or identifies and encourages the use of solution patterns of actions and interaction.

*Changing the Context of the Problem*—This involves identifying problematic patterns and influences (such as culture, gender, biochemical situations, etc.) that may hinder progress or change and finding new avenues that can be successful.

## Key Terms

**blaming stories:** Beliefs and stories which describe clients, therapists, or others as having bad intentions or traits.

**deterministic stories:** Stories that suggest that someone has no choices about what his or her body does (voluntary actions) or has no ability to make any difference in what happens to his or her life.

**impossibility stories:** Harmful or discouraging ideas that others impart on the family that suggest that change is impossible.

**invalidating stories:** Ideas or beliefs that a clients' personal experiences or knowledge is being undermined by others.

**theory countertransference:** The imposition of the therapist's beliefs and therapeutic values (and favorite diagnoses) on the client and her or his family.

12. A concept of SOFT, _____ is the imposition of beliefs and therapeutic values (and favorite diagnoses) on the family.
    a. belief compulsion
    b. *DSM* fever
    c. theoretical drift
    d. theory countertransference

## NARRATIVE THERAPY

### Theory at a Glance

Narrative therapy (NT) was born out of the postmodernist movement, wherein all knowledge is considered to be constructed. The focus of the approach is the manner in which individuals construct meaning rather than the way they behave. Narrative therapists believe that the narrative metaphor approach is incompatible with systems thinking. Assumptions basic to NT are that (a) an individual's personal experience is fundamentally ambiguous, (b) the manner in which people interpret their experience has a powerful influence on their lives, and (c) people have the ability to reauthor their life stories. Narrative therapists free clients from problems that are embedded in stories emanating from oppressive cultural practices.

13. From the narrative therapy perspective, dysfunction is a product of _____.
    a. behavioral patterns passed down generations
    b. conjoint constructs based on family narratives
    c. the family's shared emotional experience
    d. internalizing society and culture's dominant discourses

Michael White and David Epston are considered the codevelopers of narrative family therapy. Their pioneering work has grown to the point that the narrative approach is now considered one of the dominating forces in family therapy. White and Epston also credit the works of Gregory Bateson, Jerome Brunner, and Michel Foucault as playing instrumental roles in developing the narrative perspective. Other leading figures include Stephen Madigan, Kenneth Gergen, Karl Tomm, Jeffrey Zimmerson, Victoria Dickerson, Jill Freedman, and Gene Combs.

## View of Human Functioning

Narrative therapists view human behavior in terms of the narratives or stories with which human beings are involved. These stories about the clients' experiences and relationships are seen as central in their self-definition and understanding. People organize the understanding of their lives around specific meanings attached to stories of their experiences and existence. These stories function as guides to their upcoming interactions and preferences. In this way, the story an individual sees herself or himself living determines the meaning given to experience.

## View of Dysfunction

Dysfunction is the product of internalizing our culture's dominant discourses. Problems arise because people—influenced by the dominant culture—believe in restricted and self-defeating views of themselves and the world. The stories people tell themselves about reality based on these views cause them to construct their experience in unproductive ways. They see their experiences as problem oriented and become bogged down. Dysfunctions are due to the oppression brought about by individuals believing problem-saturated stories.

14. According to narrative therapy, dysfunctions are due to the oppression of problems through the maintenance of _____.
    a. ineffective family fables
    b. problematic family structure
    c. problem-saturated stories
    d. emotional deadness

## Therapist's Role

NT therapists function as facilitators, taking an active, collaborative, listening position with strong interest in the client's story. The therapist facilitates a sense of client agency such that family members become actively involved in the therapeutic relationship, redefining the key constructs behind their narrative en route to gaining greater influence in their own lives. NT therapists support a coauthoring of the narratives while honoring the clients' voices and perceptions. Further, they encourage and support clients in their efforts to pursue opportunity for agency within their own lives and context.

## Client's Role

The client's role is one of active participation as they are seen as experts, capable of developing alternative, empowering stories. Clients need to be open and willing to engage in the reauthoring process. Therapy is viewed as a process that occurs actively with the family.

## Therapeutic Goals

In NT, clients re-envision their histories and rewrite their potentialities. NT is a therapy of liberation, in that the main focus is on freeing clients from oppressive, culture-based assumptions and empowering them to become active mediators in charge of their own existences. NT therapists search for times in clients' histories when they were strong or resourceful, using questions to take a nonimposing, respectful approach to any new story put forth. People are never labeled, as they are seen as human beings with unique personal histories, and thus not readily categorized. The therapist helps people separate from the dominant cultural narratives they've internalized to open space for alternative life stories.

## Techniques Associated With This Theory

NT is not a very technique-driven approach to therapy, but is instead process-oriented with a set of types of questions used to help clients develop. The techniques of NT are seen as a three stage process. Stage one is the problem narrative stage. In this stage clients identify and separate themselves from problem-saturated stories by clarifying the stories' attachment to external phenomena, thus placing focus on the problem as an affliction by focusing on its effects instead of its causes.

In stage two, the finding exceptions stage, clients seek unique outcomes, or times when they have had some control over the problem. Clients, with the therapist's assistance, deconstruct their challenges, by seeing how they are socially constructed and problem saturated. In this stage, clients reauthor their stories and develop alternative and more constructive views of themselves. During this stage, clients are to speak of the problem as if it were a separate entity, existing outside the family or any family member.

15. As a part of narrative therapy, the therapist seeks unique outcomes, or times when clients have had some control over the problem. This process is known as the
    a. exceptions stage
    b. deconstruction stage
    c. fable stage
    d. myth undoing stage

Lastly, in stage three, move forward and recruit support. This final stage involves helping clients engage in some form of public ritual to reinforce newly developed stories and engage others in the process as well. Once family members no longer blame one another or themselves for a given problem, they begin working together to fight it.

NT uses a main series of questions, as nearly all interventions are delivered in question format.

16. Within narrative therapy, nearly all interventions are delivered in _____ format.
    a. question
    b. hyperbolic

> c. role-play
> d. didactic

The questions fall into a number of categories. *Deconstruction questions* externalize the client's problems and put them in their correct context. For example, "What does this problem tell you about your relationship?" *Opening space questions* function to map out unique outcomes or times that family members have had influence over the problem. Questions like this might include, "When is a time that you had more control over this issue?" *Rhetorical questions* are designed to elicit specific responses to help people see they are separate from and have power over the problem. Rhetorical questions come in the form of *preference questions* that make sure unique outcomes represent preferred experiences. For example, "Was the way you handled it more or less effective?" Rhetorical questions also come in the form of *story development questions* that build the story from the unique outcomes. For example, "How will you know when this new story has begun to play out for you?" *Reauthoring (or meaning) questions* are designed to challenge negative self images and emphasize positive agency. Questions such as this might include, "What does this tell you about yourself that is important for you to know?" *Questions that extend the story into the future* support growth and development. An example of this might include, "How do you see this working out for you during the next six months?"

## EXPERIENTIAL FAMILY THERAPY

### Theory at a Glance

Experiential family therapy (EFT) developed out of the humanistic psychology movement of the 1960s and primarily focuses on affect. Major underlying premises of EFT are that a climate of **emotional deadness** is created by family members' lack of awareness of their emotions and that this atmosphere causes family members to avoid engaging each other by engaging instead with activities outside the family. Another key premise is that all people have a natural tendency towards growth and **self-actualization** if allowed to develop. EFT considers expression of feelings to be the medium of shared experience and the means to personal and familial fulfillment. Experiential family therapists focus all energy on the present with greater focus on process issues than on theory. Key figures in the foundation of this approach include Virginia Satir, Carl Whitaker, Bernard Guerney, Louise Guerney, Walter Kempler, August Napier, Susan Johnson, David Keith, and Leslie Greenberg.

17. In experiential family therapy, _____ is created by family member's lack of awareness of their emotions.
    a. affective parallaxia
    b. experiential angst
    c. emotional deadness
    d. flatness of affect

18. Major underlying premises of EFT are:
    a. a climate of emotional deadness is created by family members' lack of awareness of their emotions.
    b. this atmosphere causes family members to avoid engaging each other with activities outside the family.
    c. all people have a natural tendency towards growth and actualization if allowed to develop.
    d. all of the above.

## View of Human Functioning

In EFT, symptoms in family members are seen as the result of suppression of feelings and denial of impulses, which rob members of their flexibility and strength. A result of this suppression is that family members are left incapable of autonomy or of experiencing real intimacy. The root cause of development of behavior disorders is **alienation from experience**. Healthy families foster a supportive environment wherein members can develop and individuate while maintaining a sense of family unity and support. EFT focuses beyond interactions between family members to also consider intrapsychic problems and "normal" problems (e.g., obesity, heavy smoking, overwork, etc.) in order to explain psychopathology. Mental health is viewed as a continuous process of growth and change, not a static or homeostatic state. A healthy family grows continuously, despite the challenges that come its way.

## Therapist's Role

The therapist's role is to serve as a facilitator and resource to clients. This is done by maintaining a stance that allows for flexibility and spontaneity, as this approach is not technique driven, but is driven by the therapist's personality. The therapist fosters authenticity and openness in clients, moving the family to become real, honest, and supportive of one another. The therapist is highly active as well as directive and may at some points take a very active role in setting examples for family members and at other points take a more detached role. The more detached role comes from the traditions of the less-structured approach, flowing with the natural direction of the therapeutic relationship without inserting direction. The therapist's role is more of an active participant though providing the family with him or herself as a whole person instead of an instructor or leader.

## Client's Role

Through engaging in EFT, clients learn to work out their own problems through rational and nonrational means. Clients are to use rational means to become more self-aware and gain a deeper level of self-understanding. They also use nonrational means such as spontaneous interactions with inventiveness and openness to try new and different things. It is believed that if clients allow themselves to let down their guards and become a little zany, they would also achieve deeper levels of passion and emotionality.

## Therapeutic Goals

The main focus of this approach is growth through increased personal integrity (feelings and behaviors becoming more congruent), increased sensitivity to others, increased freedom of choice, increased sharing of feelings with others, decreased dependence on others, and expanded emotional experiencing. Family relations are revitalized by authentic interactions among members struggling to be themselves. EF therapists strive to bring the family together emotionally, creating an environment where family members feel a sense of belongingness and freedom to individuate. They help individual family members become sensitive to their needs and feelings and to share these within the family. In this way, each family member gains a sense of belonging, while at the same time experiencing a sense of personal freedom to individuate.

## Techniques Associated With This Theory

As originally defined by Whitaker, this is not a very technique-driven approach, but is instead more focused on the relationship and interpersonal dynamics in session. Some techniques are incorporated into the therapeutic process. For example, the technique of *paradoxical intention* involves the therapist confronting the family in a paradoxical manner in order to break an impasse within the family, heighten the anxiety, and thereby promote growth and change. An EF therapist would likely focus on depathologizing symptoms and reframing how family members see them, a technique known as *redefining problematic symptoms*. An example of this might be redefining a child with conduct problems (who the family sees as the problem) into the savior because his behaviors brought the family into treatment at a time they were in need of help.

19. Experiential family therapists focus on depathologizing symptoms and reframing how family members see the problem, a technique known as _____.
    a. therapeutic reframe
    b. redefining problematic symptoms
    c. realigning the experiential plane
    d. flattening symptomatic parallaxia

A proponent of this therapeutic approach might use *choreography* in engaging clientele. In choreography, the counselor asks family members to enact a sequence or example of a pattern in their relationship. A specific family member is generally put in charge of the choreography. An example of this approach is *modeling fantasy alternatives* to real life stress. In this technique, the family member might be invited to discuss how she or he might act out a fantasy response to negative feelings instead of keeping them embittered inside. This technique is similar to that of *confrontation and provocation,* wherein the therapist encourages heightened emotional anxiety within the client leading to a deeper level of awareness and understanding.

Virgina Satir's approach included efforts in creating and modeling effective communication towards similar ends sought by Whitaker. Satir saw effective communication coming about by *leveling. Leveling* is creating "congruent communication" in which straight, genuine, and real expression of one's feelings and wishes are made in an appropriate context. When there is no leveling, people adopt four other roles: *blamer, placater, distractor,* or *computer.* The *blamer* places focus on others and takes no responsibility. The *placater* avoids of any conflict, even to the expense of his or her personal needs. The *distractor* tends to not focus on relevant issues or tasks, but instead actively tries to distract others from anything of any substance. The *computer* tends to be detached and unemotional, speaking intellectually about the problems, and avoiding commitment to having any specific feelings.

An important development from Satir is that of **"I" statements**. These are statements that express feelings in a personal and responsible manner and encourage others to express their feelings and thoughts. Family members are to use "I" statements when expressing their feelings. These are done with an emphasis on taking credit for one's own feelings and not giving blame to others.

Satir also developed a technique called **family reconstruction**, wherein new ways for family members to discover their personhood are set up through visual representations such as a visual representation of the structure of three generations of the clients family with adjectives to describe each family member's personality (*family maps*), chronologies of the more pertinent shared family experiences (*family life fact chronologies*), and diagrams clarifying key influential players and forces relevant to the family (*wheels of influence*) followed by enactments of these representations by family members.

Another technique is **sculpting**, wherein family members are molded during the session into positions symbolizing their current relationships to each other as seen by one or more members of the family. This is done in a process of five steps:

1. Setting the scene with the family based on a realistic scenario.
2. Selecting role players for each part in the scene, including a sculptor of the scene from among the family members.
3. Creating a living sculpture under the direction of the sculptor.
4. Processing the sculpture with the family members.
5. Resculpting the family to a desired design post the processing.

## Key Terms

**alienation (from experience):** This occurs when family members restrict their awareness of feelings—leads to restriction of family communication and corresponding separation/individuation difficulties.

**conjoint family drawing:** A technique in which family members are asked to draw their ideas about how the family is organized.

**emotional deadness:** A condition that exists when individuals in families either are not aware of or suppress their emotions.

**existential encounter:** The essential healing force in the psychotherapeutic process of experiential family therapy whereby the therapist establishes caring, person to person relationships with each family member while modeling openness, honesty, and spontaneity.

**family myth:** A set of beliefs based on a distortion of historical reality and shared by all family members that help shape the rules governing family function.

20. In experiential family therapy, a set of beliefs based on historical reality and shared by all family members is known as a(n) _____.
    a. family myth
    b. domestic construct
    c. experiential structure
    d. conjoint construct

**family reconstruction:** Satir's intervention designed to assist family members in discovering dysfunctional patterns in their lives resulting from dynamics in their families of origin.

**filial therapy:** A form of play therapy in which caregivers engage in play therapy with their own child in order to address the child's problem in the context of the relationship.

**"I" statements:** Statements that express feelings in a personal and responsible manner and encourage others to express their feelings and thoughts.

**leveling:** Harmonious communication in which straight, real, and genuine expressions of one's feelings and desires are made in an appropriate context.

**mystification:** R. D. Laing's concept that families distort their experience by denying or re-labeling it.

**sculpting:** A technique whereby family members are molded during the session into positions symbolizing their actual relationships to each other as seen by one or more members of the family.

**Self-actualization:** The process of developing and fulfilling one's innate, positive potentialities.

## FEMINIST FAMILY THERAPY

### Theory at a Glance

Feminist therapy grew out of criticisms of male-oriented gender bias in psychology and in existing approaches to therapy. First appearing in the 1960s in response to psychotherapy's failure to attend to the needs of women, it was originally developed as a means of helping women achieve political, economic, and social equality in western society. Feminist therapy developed primarily as a grass-roots movement through **consciousness-raising groups**, in which female therapists developed new norms for psychotherapeutic relationships. A focal issue in these new norms was developing *mutuality* in the therapeutic relationship, where therapy is seen as a partnership between equals. Feminist therapy is as much a philosophical orientation as it is a psychological theory as evidenced by its influence on nearly every other field—education, the humanitic business—all have critical analyses including feminist theory. It can be defined as a pattern of standpoints and notions that try to explain complex social phenomena at play in society, clarifying that women have been systematically denied opportunities and choices and treated with expectations that they have specific prescribed roles to fill in society and families. This viewpoint highlights the existence and effect of cultural forces on the individual. Feminist family therapy (FFT) focuses on shifting imbalances of power, clarifying that both men and women are victimized by gender socialization, countering the effects of power inequities on individual, couple, and family functioning, and focusing on change at the societal or collective level as well as at the individual level. Key figures in the development of this approach include Nancy Chodorow, Sandra Bem, Carol Gilligan, and Jean Baker Miller.

### View of Human Functioning

An FF therapist views family and individual functioning through the lens of acculturation. Many of the difficulties that families have are based on acceptance of cultural norms and expectations that are inherently unjust. The family is a core social unit within which socialization occurs, and thus an excellent place for resocialization to occur. As family members, we respond to experiences and information based on how we translate them via cultural and social templates. These templates are commonly fraught with stereotypes and inaccuracies that require adjustment prior to better functioning.

### Therapist's Role

In FFT, the therapist focuses on establishing an egalitarian, collaborative relationship with the clients in which each brings needs, responsibilities, and expertise to the table. A particular focus is placed on helping the family come to an understanding of how gender roles have played a part in the troubles they have been experiencing. Personal troubles are depathologized by placing them in a sociopolitical context. In this way, true positive regard is exhibited to the whole family, particularly the women in the family, who become increasingly **empowered** through active listening and helping them find their voice. Both external negative stereotypes as well as internal stereotypes are thus discouraged and diminished. In FFT, the therapist may often find it appropriate to use self-disclosure as a method of helping the clients move through this process.

21. The most appropriate role of a feminist family therapist is _____.
    a. expert
    b. teacher
    c. collaborator
    d. facilitator

22. In feminist family therapy, the therapist depathologizes personal troubles by placing them in a(n) _____ context.
    a. personal historical
    b. clinical
    c. enabled
    d. sociopolitical

## Client's Role

The role of the client in FFT is one of active responding. Clients need to be open to exploring and understanding the role that gender-role issues, values, messages, rules, and policies have on members of the family individually and as a whole. Family members are expected to explore the different ways in which these issues contribute to and preserve family dysfunction. From this perspective, the therapist works with family members with the expectation that they will take an active role in making changes in the manner in which such gender-role issues are played out in the family and societal setting. This is an issue of empowerment. Clients are empowered through increased awareness of social/cultural forces they confront, then helped to develop skills to respond more effectively to them while learning to see themselves in a more accurate light (i.e., less tainted by traditional views of them as women).

23. The role of the client in FFT is one of _____.
    a. vicarious learning
    b. active responding
    c. a student
    d. a visitor, complainant, or a customer

## Therapeutic Goals

The goal of feminist counseling is not only individual change and growth, but also social transformation. Specific therapeutic goals include clarifying social and cultural messages, particularly those revolving around gender, and their role in family dynamics; analyzing, understanding, and responding to power differentials between men and women; increasing awareness of divisive patterns that develop as women seek to increase their autonomy and power; affirming values and behaviors characteristic of females; recognizing and supporting possibilities for women beyond the roles of mother and spouse; and empowering family members to move toward their true potentialities and help other family members do the same.

## Techniques Associated With This Theory

The interventions of FFT for the most part have to do with the lens through which clients and their reality are viewed and how they respond to such a reality rather than particular techniques.

In FFT, the therapist views the process as equally important as product. This process should be nonoppressive, culture building, educational, democratic, nonjudgmental, dynamic, and developmental. The therapist cocreates goals with the family, based on the input of every member, putting particular emphasis on those family members who have been historically underrepresented in family goal-making processes.

One technique is to *demystify the therapeutic process* for the family. Feminist family therapists help the family understand the importance of using and developing their own power in the therapeutic relationship. The therapeutic relationship is geared to helping the family members, especially any women, see that they must be their own rescuers. Ultimately the power they long for is not in someone else, but in themselves.

A feminist family therapist helps clients *rename* and *reconstruct* their realities. In this way they become liberated through their own actions and self-reliance, learn to value "rugged collectivism," infuse consciousness and healthier values into the world, and view revolution as a process instead of an event. This process is often referred to as *relabeling*.

Feminist family therapists recognize *all* forms of oppression. They respect the inherent worth and dignity of all people and recognize that societal and political inequities are limiting and oppressive to *all* people. They place psychological distress within a socio-cultural context, clarifying the reality that experiences of oppression are based on gender, race, class, physical ability, age, religion, and affectional orientation. All are interrelated in complex ways. Feminist family therapists work to help family members come to this same realization and understand how such knowledge brings them new power.

A technique used to bring this about is **gender role analysis**, wherein the therapist works collaboratively with the family members to examine their values and how these values are reflected in role expectations within the family. The therapist puts particular effort into identifying implicit and explicit gender-role messages that the family members have experienced and internalized. Associated with this process is a **power analysis**, which is used to assist family members in understanding how power influences gender roles in the home and in society. In recent years, feminist family therapists have developed the **integrated analysis of oppression**, which focuses on the interconnectivity and overlap of devices of oppression in society.

## Key Terms

**androgyny:** The integration of traditional feminine and masculine characteristics as an ideal of mental health.

**consciousness raising groups:** Groups run in the 1960s that encouraged discussion and sharing of experiences of oppression and powerlessness.

**empowerment:** The process of change and development of a powerless entity (person or group) to become socially and politically aware and active.

24. In FFT, the process of change and development of a powerless entity (person or group) to become socially and politically aware and active is _____.
    a. enablement
    b. preventative politics
    c. social shaping
    d. empowerment

**feminism:** A collection of social and political philosophies aimed to end inequities based on patriarchy and gender through cultural transformation and radical social change.

**TABLE 7.1**

A Comparison and Contrast of Theories

| Theory | Key Figures | View of Human Functioning | View of Dysfunction | Therapist's Role | Client's Role | Therapeutic Goals |
|---|---|---|---|---|---|---|
| Cognitive-Behavioral | Gerald Patterson, Robert Lieberman, Richard Stuart, Donald Baucom, Norman Epstein, Frank Dattilio, and James Alexander | Behavior is learned and maintained by its consequences. Ways of thinking are also learned and can be unlearned. | Dysfunction is learned and maintained until more rewarding consequences are introduced. | Function as a coach and teacher, building open, collaborative relationships. | Function as active students and collaborators toward more adaptive thinking and behaving. | To increase rewarding interactions and better attributions and expectations. |
| Collaborative | Harlane Anderson, Lynn Hoffman, Tom Andersen, and Harry Goolishian | Families are "teams" with expertise and knowledge about themselves. | Dysfunction is seen as a misrepresentation of constraints placed on the family. Constraints, such as situations, interactions, and beliefs are more focal than work on dysfunction. | Become a "member" of the family for the duration of therapy. Act as an equal partner and co-explorer with the family, taking a "not-knowing stance," allowing family members to participate in the process of finding solutions. | Function as expert contributors in the therapeutic setting about their needs. They are invited to critique, clarify, and coach. | To empower families and help to cocreate new meanings and solutions. |
| Solution-Focused | Steven de Schazer and Insoo Kim Berg | Humans grow and develop from their strengths toward our goals. | Strengths and solutions are focal over weaknesses and dysfunctions. | Serve as an active consultant or a facilitator of change, building on already existing strengths and resources. | Active participants in setting the focus and direction of therapy, setting collaborative goals. | To change toward specific goals, built from strengths and resources. |

| Approach | Key Figures | View of Health/Normalcy | View of Difficulties | Role of Therapist | Role of Client | Goals |
|---|---|---|---|---|---|---|
| *Narrative* | Michael White and David Epston | Stories about experiences and relationships are central in self-definition and understanding. | Difficulties are due to the oppression brought about by maintaining problem-saturated stories. Dysfunction itself is a misnomer. | Facilitate client agency through active listening and co-authoring of helpful narratives. | Active participation in developing alternative, empowering stories. | To free clients from oppressive culture-based assumptions and empower them to become active mediators in charge of their own existences. |
| *Experiential* | Virginia Satir, Carl Whitaker, Bernard Guerney, Louise Guerney, Walter Kempler, August Napier, Susan Johnson, David Keith, and Leslie Greenberg | Mental health is viewed as a continuous process of growth and change, not a static or homeostatic state. | Difficulties are seen as the result of suppression of feelings and denial of impulses which are caused by incongruities between feelings and behaviors. | Facilitate and serve as a resource; foster authenticity and openness, moving the family to become real, honest, and supportive of one another. | Let down their guards and work out problems through rational and nonrational means. | To grow through increased personal integrity (feelings and behaviors becoming more congruent), increased sensitivity to others, increased freedom of choice, increased sharing of feelings with others, decreased dependence on others, and expanded emotional experiencing. |
| *Feminist* | Nancy Chodorow, Sandra Bem, Carol Gilligan, and Jean Baker Miller | Functioning is dependent on acculturation. | Many problems in families are based on inherently unjust cultural norms and expectations. | Establish egalitarian, collaborative relationship; depathologize personal troubles and assist in resocialization. | Need to respond actively, explore openly, and examine gender-role assumptions and other culture-based forms of oppression as applied to self and family. | To promote individual change and growth as well as societal transformation. |

**gender role analysis:** A collaborative examination of a family's values and the manner in which they reflect role expectations within the family.

**gender role socialization:** A multifaceted process of reinforcing specific beliefs and behaviors that a society considers appropriate based on sex. This process occurs across the life span.

**integrated analysis of oppression:** An expanded evaluation of issues from those of gender and power to include ethnicity, socioeconomic status, affectional orientation, age, ability, and religion.

**personal is political:** This is an ideal based on the understanding that personal problems and conditions have historical, material, and cultural dimensions. Also included are the concepts that in our connectedness with each other, there are no truly personal, private solutions; that failure to act is to act; that we achieve personal growth through political action; and that as we change ourselves, we change the world, which is an orientation toward fundamental structural change.

**power analysis:** An examination of the power differential between men and women in society and the home.

**resocialization:** A process wherein clients are encouraged to realize yet unseen value in themselves and other family members as well as learn to value the life experiences and viewpoints of all members, especially women.


## DISCUSSION QUESTIONS

1. Why does cognitive-Behavioral family therapy focus on behavior over understanding?
2. How are the values that underlie *contingency contracting* at odds with those that underlie *ecosystemic epistemology*?
3. How does the *reflecting team* approach of collaborative therapy function as a postmodern approach to therapy?
4. Can solution-oriented family therapy work well in the managed care environment? Why or why not?
5. Why are questions most focal in the solution-oriented family therapy approach?
6. What concepts lend to the ease of integrating narrative therapy with feminist family therapy and experiential family therapy?
7. If you were practicing experiential family therapy, what would you do to help your clients achieve increased sensitivity to others while developing increased personal integrity?
8. In experiential family therapy, how does the *existential encounter* relate to *emotional deadness*?
9. What therapeutic factor do you see as pivotal in the efficacy of feminist family therapeutic relationships?
10. In feminist family therapy, what role do you think the concept of *androgyny* might play in families renaming and reconstructing their realities?


## SUGGESTED FURTHER READING

Carlson, J., & Kjos, D. (2002). *Theories and strategies of family therapy*. Boston: Allyn & Bacon.

This is a basic overview of leading theories of marriage and family therapy. It is available with videotaped examples.

Dreikurs, R. (1957). Our child guidance clinics in Chicago. *Collected papers of Rudolf Dreikurs* (pp. 70–89). Eugene, OR: University of Oregon Press.

Freedman, J., & Combs, G. (1996). *Narrative therapy: The social construction of preferred realities.* New York: Norton.

This is a clear and comprehensive introduction to narrative therapy, recommended by leading proponents of the approach.

Gladding, S. (2002). *Family therapy: History, theory, and practice* (3rd ed.). Upper Saddle River, NJ: Merrill Prentice Hall.

This overview of family therapy lends itself well to integration of theoretical approaches in response to client needs.

Guerin, P., & Guerin, K. (2002). Bowenian family therapy. In J. Carlson & D. Kjos (Eds.), *Theories and Strategies of Family Therapy* (pp. 126–157). Boston: Allyn & Bacon.

Nichols, M., & Schwartz, R. (2003). *Family therapy: Concepts and methods* (6th ed.). Boston: Allyn & Bacon.

This is a comprehensive overview of family therapy theory and thought. The strength of this volume is the manner in which it is put together in an historical context.

Payne, M. (2000). *Narrative therapy: An introduction for counselors.* Thousand Oaks, CA: Sage.

This is a popular introduction to narrative therapy due to clear explanations, useful case transcripts, as well as a practical clinical focus.

Piercy, F. P., Sprenkle, D. H., & Wetchler, J. L., & Associates (1996). *Family therapy sourcebook* (2nd ed.). New York: Guilford Press.

This wide-ranging overview of family therapy approaches is popular among practitioners, students, and professors alike for its clarity and depth of coverage.

Silverstein, L. B., & Goodrich, T. J. (2003). *Feminist family therapy: Empowerment in social context.* Washington, DC: American Psychological Association.

This book focuses on feminist issues in family therapy and places feminist family therapy within its historical context from the perspective of practicing therapists.

Walsh, W. M., & McGraw, J. A. (2002). *Essentials of family therapy: A structured summary of nine approaches.* Denver, CO: Love Publishing.

This is a concise overview of popular systemic approaches to family therapy using a consistent format throughout. The format allows readers to rapidly identify similarities and differences among the models covered.

# 8

# Assessment, Diagnoses, and Treatment Planning

Jo Ellen Patterson
Todd M. Edwards
Stefanie L. Carnes
*University of San Diego*

## TRUTH OR FICTION?

___ 1. *The first contact with a client, though usually made through the telephone, is very important in the therapeutic process.*

___ 2. *A therapist should avoid providing structure in the initial session with a family.*

___ 3. *In the first therapy session, it is not helpful to learn about the solutions the client has already tried.*

___ 4. *As the first session comes to a conclusion, it is helpful for the therapist to offer some comments on the presenting problem.*

___ 5. *Family therapists should have the skills to make a DSM diagnosis.*

___ 6. *A therapist should never ask a client directly about suicidal ideation.*

___ 7. *The circumplex model of family assessment examines family cohesion, family flexibility, and communication.*

___ 8. *When using the circumplex model, therapists should take into consideration a family's life cycle stage and cultural background.*

___ 9. *When working with a couple, it is usually best for the therapist to join with one person more strongly than the other.*

___ 10. *When working with a couple, it is essential for the therapist to develop goals that are agreed upon by the therapist and both members of the couple.*

___ 11. *Family therapists should avoid contact with other professionals involved in the care of their clients.*

___ 12. *When administering a psychometric instrument, the therapist should pay attention to the level of reactivity in a client's responses.*

___ 13. *A treatment plan is usually developed by the end of the second session.*

___ 14. *Treatment plans should never include the therapist's theoretical underpinnings.*

___ 15. *Once a treatment plan is made, it should not be changed.*

In this chapter we will review the essential family therapy skills in **assessment, diagnoses**, and **treatment planning**. The previous two chapters have provided a thorough overview of the major models in marital and family therapy. Our goal is to provide a multi-systemic family therapy approach to assessment and treatment planning in order to locate a fit between theory and the unique treatment needs of each client system.

We will begin with a discussion of the first contact with a family and then review the major stages in an initial session. Next, we will provide an overview of the necessary areas for assessment, including the individual, couple, family, and larger systems. A major challenge for any family therapist is bridging the gaps among the presenting problem, his or her preferred theory or theories, and treatment planning. A blueprint to overcome this challenge is offered along with strategies to plan interventions. Throughout this chapter, it is important to remember that a good assessment and treatment plan are developed by a theoretically sound therapist who uses his or her conceptual model to develop ethical interventions.

## BEGINNING THERAPY

The first contact, which usually takes place on the telephone, has received little attention in the family therapy literature, which is unfortunate due to its importance. Therapy begins during this contact, as you start building a therapeutic relationship and a structure for therapy. The goal of the initial phone conversation is to make an initial contact, gather some preliminary information, and arrange the first session (Weber & Levine, 1995).

After learning about who referred the person, get a brief description of the problem to determine if you can offer assistance. Prospective clients can, at times, be quite expansive in their problem description. Unless someone is in crisis, you need to help the person be as focused as possible while at the same time communicating respect and sincerity. This will help save time and diminish the possibility of bias in favor of one person. If you determine that you will not have the expertise to help a particular client, give the person the names and phone numbers of people and places that can help. If you can help, discuss a structure for the first session.

The structure you establish for the initial session can have a significant effect on the course of therapy. One of the key questions is, "Who will attend the first session?" Napier and Whitaker (1978) believed it essential for all family members to be present from the beginning of therapy and refused to start therapy until all were present. Such an expectation offers the family an orientation to systems thinking (Weber & Levine, 1995). However, few family therapists follow this rigid stance (Berg & Rosenblum, 1977) and instead make the decision about who will attend on a case-by-case basis (Nichols & Everett, 1986). When a client is requesting couples therapy but expresses a desire to attend the first session alone, we highlight the difficulty in switching from individual to couples therapy and encourage both partners to attend the first meeting. Additional information that needs to be discussed during this phone call includes the date, time, and location of the first appointment, check-in process, and fees.

1. A client contacts you and begins discussing a problem in an area in which you have very little expertise. The best course of action is to:
   a. give them names and numbers of people who can help.
   b. tell them you're the wrong person for the job and they should look elsewhere.
   c. invite them in for a session and go for it—you can learn along the way.
   d. let them talk to you on the phone for awhile and get it out of their system.

2. When a client requests couples therapy but would like to attend the first session alone, you should:
   a. meet them for coffee instead of having a "formal" session.
   b. tell them they're clearly not ready for couples therapy and to call you back when they are.
   c. explain the difficulty of switching from individual to couples therapy and encourage them both to attend.
   d. give them a detailed explanation of the concept of triangulation and let them decide what to do.

## What Is the Most Important Task in the Initial Session?

The initial session is often the most important session of the therapy process. It may be the *only* session of the therapy process if you don't accomplish your goals, especially one goal—**joining**. From the first telephone contact, through the first interview and beyond, joining is your most critical task. Minuchin and Fishman (1981) defined joining as "the glue that holds the therapeutic system together" (p. 32). Additional ways of capturing the term joining include building the transference, establishing rapport, building trust, or creating a therapeutic bond. But the bottom line is that if your client does not a) like you at least somewhat, b) have some confidence that you can help him or her, and c) feel slightly more hopeful about the problem leaving the session than he or she felt at the beginning, the therapy is probably over.

Research suggests that the client's view of the therapeutic relationship is one of the most significant factors in therapy outcome (Grunebaum, 1988). In addition to creating safety in the therapy room, a good therapeutic relationship also allows you to take significant risks later in the therapy by challenging clients' stuck patterns. Clients share their most precious secrets with you because of the relationship they have with you. A close therapeutic relationship encourages clients to push themselves to take risks outside of the session and avoid making foolish choices. This therapeutic bond will help energize you even though you are seeing your sixth client of the day and know that it is going to be a difficult and challenging hour.

Skills that inexperienced therapists usually do very well such as listening, expressing empathy and concern, asking questions to better understand, and offering hope are all part of the joining process. For many young therapists, these skills seem natural and easy to express. So they devalue them and move on to asking challenging assessment questions, interpreting their pain, or giving advice about what the clients should do to improve. In their rush, they risk losing the clients. More importantly they might miss one of our favorite parts of being a therapist—getting to know our unique clients and coming to understand their unique problems.

3. The most important thing to work on during the first session is:
   a. obtaining a thorough assessment.
   b. establishing a therapeutic relationship.
   c. developing a detailed treatment plan.
   d. offering some good advice so they don't have to come back.

## How Should I Structure the Initial Session?

Below, we review the five stages of the first session. Each stage is given a suggested allotment of time for a 60-minute session, which is offered as a suggestion not as an inflexible rule. Our suggested format for managing the first session follows similar formats offered by Weber, McKeever, and McDaniel (1985), Weber and Levine (1995) and Nichols and Everett (1986). Having a structured format and maintaining the structure during the first session will help the family see you as a leader who can manage multiple people and multiple issues.

*Stage 1: The Greeting (10 minutes).* The first stage in any first session is the initial greeting, which allows you to introduce yourself, greet each family member, and lower any anxiety the client might be feeling as he walks in your office. This process is critical in laying the groundwork for the joining process described above. Questions such as "Did you have any difficulty finding the office?" initiate social conversation that allows clients to see both your humanness and professionalism. After this contact, it is important to request basic demographic information for each person present (e.g., name, age, relationship to the family). You also will want to orient them to your office, such as seating, the location of the bathroom, and room temperature. After the initial greeting, clients will benefit from an orientation to the format of the session, particularly if you will be videotaping or allowing for observation.

A second critical administrative task that needs to be addressed early is reviewing confidentiality. Clients need to be informed about the confidential nature of therapy and the possible scenarios in which confidentiality will be broken (e.g., child abuse, elder abuse, duty to warn). Clinicians typically have an informed consent form available for clients to review before the session, but it is imperative to review this information at the beginning of therapy. If you will be having individual sessions with family members, particularly children, you will need to define your rules of confidentiality in these specific situations at this time or prior to the individual sessions.

This is also a good time to inquire about previous counseling experience and orient them to the length of the session (e.g., 60 minutes, 90 minutes). Clients who have been socialized to counseling in the past will have a general understanding about the roles of a client and therapist, whereas someone new to counseling may need a more detailed orientation.

*Stage 2: Defining the Problem (25 minutes).* Before jumping into a problem description, you will need to convey to the family that each person will have an opportunity to be heard while the other family members listen. This is obviously important for joining purposes, but it's most important for assessment purposes. You want to give yourself the opportunity to see the problem from different perspectives and each person will provide some information that other family members will not. This may also be the first time family members have heard someone speak about the problem, which provides new information to the family. Another benefit of hearing multiple perspectives is that there may be disagreement about the problem itself. For example, members of a couple sometimes define the problem in different ways. Following the overview of session structure, you can ask a simple question like "What brings you to counseling/therapy" or "How can I help you?" to focus the session (Greenan & Tunnell, 2003).

After hearing each person, it is important to summarize what you heard and respectfully transition to the next person. A problem that can arise during this process is one family member monopolizing the conversation. It is absolutely critical that you provide enough structure to interrupt this process in order to provide space for other family members. You don't want to anger the person who talks excessively, but if you fail to interrupt this behavior the other family members will lose faith in your ability to lead the session.

Once a problem has been elicited, the next step is to get a detailed description of the problem. Oftentimes, problems are introduced in vague terms, such as, "Tommy is lazy," or, "Bonnie doesn't care about me." Unpacking terms or phrases like "lazy" or "doesn't care" makes the problem more vivid. Asking for examples of the problem is one method to learn more about the problem. You also want to listen for what stressors may be making the problem worse and how serious the client thinks the problem is.

During these detailed descriptions, you must also pay attention to the family's interactional patterns, both in the story description and their interactions in the office. One core technique (Seaburn, Landau-Stanton, & Horwitz, 1995) to access these interactions is to ask the family to engage in an enactment (Minuchin, 1974), in which the family members reenact an example of the problem. This will provide important process information that you will want to revisit and highlight in the therapy.

At some point, it is helpful to move away from the presenting problem and map the effects of the problem on a family's life (White & Epston, 1990). For example, you could ask the following: "How is this problem affecting your relationship with your spouse/partner?" and "How is this problem affecting your picture of yourself as a spouse?" Such questions give you a broader view of the family and the relationship complexity that accompanies presenting problems.

4. When clients use vague language to describe a problem ("Tim is rebellious"), the therapist should:
   a. ask the clients to give examples of rebelliousness to further understand the problem.
   b. begin discussing treatment options for rebelliousness.
   c. normalize rebelliousness.
   d. challenge the reality of rebelliousness.

5. What should you do when one family member dominates the conversation?
   a. Let him talk until he's ready to stop, he probably has the most valuable information.
   b. Let him talk, it's not your place to interrupt.
   c. Interrupt so you can talk instead.
   d. Interrupt to make space for other family members.

*Stage 3: Identifying Attempted Solutions (10 minutes).* Ask what solutions have already been tried and find out if any of those solutions have worked. Families may have created and implemented solutions that they describe as unsuccessful. However, it is possible the solution was a good one, but it was implemented in the wrong manner or it was abandoned too early. For example, a parent might have tried a new method of handling temper tantrums, but claims that the child's behavior got worse, which resulted in a return to an old method. The new method may have eventually worked if implementation had continued.

Knowledge about attempted solutions also helps the therapist learn what *not* to suggest, at least initially, in terms of treatment options. For example, a client may have been offended by a previous therapist or other expert telling them to take an antidepressant, get psychological testing, confront a family member or consider hospitalization for the problem. To suggest one of these attempted solutions is a sure-fire way to lose credibility with this family in the first few sessions. In addition to identifying solutions in the initial session, it can sometimes be helpful to ask a family to make a list of attempted solutions for homework between the first and second sessions.

A final element in this stage of the interview is looking for times when the problem was absent or diminished. These times have been referred to as "exceptions to the problem" (O'Hanlon &

Weiner-Davis, 1989) or "unique outcomes" (White & Epston, 1990). Collecting this data can assist you and the family in understanding more about the problem and why it was absent in situations where it was expected to be present.

> 6. Learning about a client's previously attempted solutions helps you:
>    a. identify solutions that have worked in the past.
>    b. identify solutions that may have worked if they hadn't been abandoned so quickly.
>    c. learn what to not suggest as an initial treatment method.
>    d. all of the above.

*Stage 4: Defining Goals (10 minutes).*   Once the problem description and attempted solutions have been adequately explored, you will want to turn to the family's goals for therapy—what does each person want to see changed? Family members will often say what they want to eliminate ("I want dad to stop nagging me") and have a harder time articulating what they want ("I want dad to tell me I'm doing a good job"). Encourage your clients to describe desired changes in positive language (the presence of something) rather than in negative language (the absence of something).

Another important aspect of setting goals is to help the family access some strengths they have that will help them achieve these goals. You can simply ask, "What qualities in your family give you a sense of hope that these goals can be achieved?" Or, ask the family to tell you about a time when they overcame a different challenge and what they learned about themselves that might be useful today. These are just a couple of ways to access strengths.

As the session is nearing completion, this is a good time to offer the family some of your thoughts on the problem and their family. As you have been listening to the family, you have been forming hypotheses. In a nonjargon fashion, it is now time to present some of your thoughts to give the family some indication that you were listening and understanding their problem. Give them some information that they did not have when they walked in your office. This information does not need to be prophetic, but it does need to be thematic, meaning you need to identify the key themes from the client's presentation. It is also helpful to get some feedback from the family members about what you have said.

> 7. Which of the following is an important aspect of goal setting?
>    a. describing goals in positive language
>    b. accessing some family strengths
>    c. instilling a sense of hope
>    d. all of the above

*Stage 5: Developing a Contract (10 minutes).*   As you conclude the session, ask the family members about their experience of the session and what they would like to do next. In an effort to give the family members responsibility for therapy initiative, we want them to tell us if and when they would like to meet again. If the family states an interest in continuing but defers to our judgment regarding the time frame, we will push to see them weekly initially and gradually space the sessions out. If the family wants to think about it or declines treatment with us, we graciously remind them that we are available in the future if needed and offer them the names and contact information of other therapists should they decide to seek services elsewhere.

If an agreement is made to continue, we establish a commitment for the therapy structure that includes scheduling, confidentiality, fees, and cancellations. We also ask the family to sign releases of information to coordinate care with other professionals and retrieve additional information about the family. In many cases, you will want to consult with these professionals at the beginning and throughout the course of therapy. These professionals could include previous or current therapists, family physicians, psychiatrists, school counselors or teachers, lawyers, and probation officers. Collaboration with these professionals is essential to ensuring that your treatment plan will be consistent with the work of others (McDaniel, Hepworth, & Doherty, 1992).

## THE MULTI-SYSTEM ASSESSMENT

As a family therapist, it is likely that you are going to get many different opinions about what to assess and why. You may be asked to assess an individual client, a couple, or a family. You may also be asked to assess for a *DSM* diagnosis, an initial impression about whether the client needs referrals for psychotropic medication, or whether the client needs a referral to a physician, other social services, or testing. In addition, you may be asked to decide if there are legal concerns or payment (insurance) questions. A lot is expected, and you have to decide what you are competent to assess, what referrals you might suggest, and if there are any potential crisis situations such as suicide risk.

In addition, your client may not agree with you about the focus of your assessment and may seek something entirely different. If you don't pay attention to your clients' wishes, they may not return. You also have to consider your clinic's assessment protocol, the payer's assessment guidelines, and the client's resources. Unfortunately, we have seen many situations in which inexperienced therapists are asked to do assessments that are significantly beyond their experience levels or they are required to make an assessment of serious mental illness in a 30-minute session. We have also seen situations where student therapists are encouraged to fit clients' problems into a specific category or situation because that is how the therapy is funded. We urge you to be conservative and circumspect in your assessment process and watch for these subtle ethical dilemmas. Underlying most of these dilemmas are serious economic constraints, not unethical clinics.

8. Which of the following must you consider as you assess a client?
   a. whether or not a referral is necessary
   b. insurance requirements
   c. the client's wishes
   d. all of the above

## How Do I Assess Individuals?

In our experience, assessing individuals is easier than assessing couples and/or families. The therapist's focus remains on one person—regardless of whether the therapist is considering the person's relationships, genetic history, or work struggles. More complicated assessment occurs when you have to assess individuals within a couple or family that is seeing you for therapy. For example, one of us was seeing a couple for therapy and listening to the wife's description of the problem: "He is disorganized, never on time, unable to finish a project, constantly changing jobs, impulsive, and moody." While the couple sought help for their marriage, the therapist began to think about the criterion for attention deficit disorder.

## How Should I Incorporate the DSM Into My Assessment?

Family therapists have only minimal training in assessment skills to make a *DSM* diagnosis. In addition to not having training, they may not have interest in focusing on psychopathology or mental disorders. Systems theory suggests that problems reside in the family system, not in an individual. Thus, conducting an individual diagnosis may be at odds with a family therapist's training.

Nevertheless, we believe that family therapists must have skills to conduct individual diagnoses. This is important because family therapists often end up working in settings where they are required to make an official diagnosis of their clients. In some cases, payment for services depends on making a *DSM* diagnosis. Other mental health professionals use *DSM* terminology to talk about shared clients. A final reason to know how to conduct a *DSM* diagnostic session is because psychotropic medication referrals depend on *DSM* diagnosis.

While a therapist may never become proficient in the subtleties of making a *DSM* diagnosis, he or she can still learn the criteria for the most commonly seen problems. These common mental disorders include: depression; anxiety, including phobias, panic attacks, responses to trauma, and obsessive-compulsive disorder; substance abuse; personality disorders; and eating disorders.

In addition to these disorders usually found in adults, family therapists need to know about the disorders most commonly found in children. Disruptive behavior problems, childhood depression and anxiety, learning disorders such as attention deficit disorder, and pervasive developmental disorders such as Asperger's or autism are common problems in children.

Even if you are not an expert on these diagnoses, you can learn enough information about the subjective and objective symptoms of each diagnosis to identify a patient who *might* have one or more of these problems. Then you could refer the patient to an expert in *DSM* diagnosis. In addition, if a client is acting strange and bizarre and her symptoms are completely unfamiliar to you, consider referral to either a general physician or a psychiatrist.

A complete diagnosis looks at additional client factors. The therapist might want to ask about current or past medical problems that could be influencing the client's problems. The therapist might want to ask about when the client last saw a physician and for what reason. Is the client currently taking any medications—prescribed or not? Did any physical event happen to the client that might coincide with the onset of symptoms? For example, the client might have been in a car accident, had a head injury, started a new medication, or became ill.

The therapist might want to do a brief mental status exam (see Table 8.1) to ascertain whether or not there are cognitive problems. Asking about family history of mental health problems can help the therapist consider genetics as an underlying etiology. While a family therapist is seldom an expert in these areas, he or she can at least have screening skills and know when to refer the client to another mental health professional.

A few final issues that the therapist wants to consider are duration, intensity, and functioning. How long has the problem been going on? How much is the problem affecting the client's daily living? Has the client missed work or school because of the problem? Are other family members significantly affected by the problem or having to compensate for the client's deficits?

9. Why is it important to be able to make a DSM diagnosis?
    a. for payment purposes
    b. for medication referrals
    c. it's the only way to conceptualize a problem
    d. both a and b

**TABLE 8.1**

Short Mental Status Questionnaire

1. What is the date today?
2. What day of the week is it?
3. What is the name of this place?
4. What is your telephone number (or address)?
5. How old are you?
6. When were you born?
7. Who is the President of the United States now?
8. Who was the President just before that?
9. What was your mother's maiden name?
10. Subtract 3 from 20 and keep subtracting 3 from each new number you get, all the way down.

For clients with high school education:

0–2 errors = intact mental function
3–4 errors = mild mental impairment
5–7 errors = moderate mental impairment
8–10 errors = severe mental impairment

Allow one more error if the client has only a grade school education. Allow one less error if the client has education beyond high school.

*Note:* From "The Mental Status Examination," by S. C. Dilsaver, 1990, *American Family Physician, 41*, pp. 1489–1497, and "A Short Portable Mental Status Questionnaire for the Assessment of Organic Brain Deficit in Elderly Patients," by E. Pfeiffer, 1975, *Journal of the American Geriatrics Society, 23*, pp. 433–441. Copyright 1990 by American Academy of Family Physicians. Adapted with permission.

10. When assessing an individual, which of the following questions would be most helpful in examining their mental status?
    a. How can I help you today?
    b. Have you ever been in therapy before?
    c. How have you been feeling lately?
    d. What day of the week is it?

## What Else Should I Consider When Assessing Individuals?

Also, the therapist must consider any dangerous or critical situations. Violence, abuse, suicide risk, substance abuse, and duty to warn (another person about the client threatening his or her life) are all examples of potentially dangerous situations. Often, the client won't bring up these issues initially. In fact, he or she may not mention these issues at all. Instead, the therapist has to be listening for hints or warning signs of these situations. For example, the client may appear quite depressed or angry. This would be a cue that the therapist needs to gently ask about thoughts of suicide or violence. A child might appear afraid of his parent, and this could lead one to ask about physical or sexual abuse.

Asking about these difficult issues may not be enough to elicit the truth. The therapist's rapport with the client and the way the therapist asks the question will strongly influence whether the client responds truthfully. For example, the therapist might ask, "Have you ever thought about hurting yourself?" or, "I've had other clients in your situation who thought about killing themselves, have you ever considered the same ideas?" Even if the therapist asks these questions carefully, the client may not tell the truth. Thus, the therapist has to keep these issues always in the back of his or her mind and maintain a curious, open perspective. The therapist might not find out the truth until later in the therapy.

We mentioned earlier that the client's agenda or concerns that they bring to therapy and the therapist's concerns might differ. Listen to the client's concerns. Explore the client's understanding and beliefs about the problems that brought him or her to therapy. By asking these questions, the therapist discovers the client's strengths, motivation for therapy, expectations about the therapy, and the client's resources that can be used to solve the problem.

11. When assessing individuals, you will need to consider:
    a. suicide risk.
    b. substance abuse.
    c. harm to others.
    d. all of the above.

12. A good way to assess for suicidality is to:
    a. normalize suicidal ideation, then ask the client if he or she has thought about it.
    b. ask the client how he or she is feeling today.
    c. wait for the client to mention it.
    d. all of the above.

## How Should I Assess Families?

Because you have already been exposed to various therapeutic theories for working with families, we are not going to use this section to cover each theoretical perspective on assessment. Rather, we want to describe the Circumplex Model of Marital and Family Systems (Olson, Russell, & Sprenkle, 1989), which integrates diverse systemic concepts in family therapy.

The **circumplex model** (Fig. 8.1) emphasizes family **flexibility** and family **cohesion** in understanding a family's structure and interactional process. As the diagram shows, flexibility—the tolerance for change—ranges from *rigid* to *chaotic*. Cohesion, the level of emotional closeness, ranges from *disengaged* to *enmeshed*. *Communication* is a third dimension that captures how families work out issues related to cohesion and flexibility. The model allows you to develop working hypotheses about family functioning. For example, a family may have a low level of cohesion and too much flexibility (chaotically disengaged), which may be related to poor parental leadership, children who demonstrate out of control behavior, and communication that is unclear. Such a description will undoubtedly inform your treatment plan.

The degree of family cohesion and adaptability is intimately related to a family's life cycle stage. The family life cycle describes the typical stages that a multigenerational family system experiences over time. Family cohesion and flexibility change through the life cycle to hopefully accommodate individual development and normal family transitions. For example, you might expect that families with small children will lean toward more enmeshment and rigidity than families with adolescents, which is appropriate considering the efforts of adolescents to develop more autonomy and freedom.

In addition to family life cycle transitions, families also experience unexpected transitions that can create more chaos or rigidity and push a family towards more togetherness or

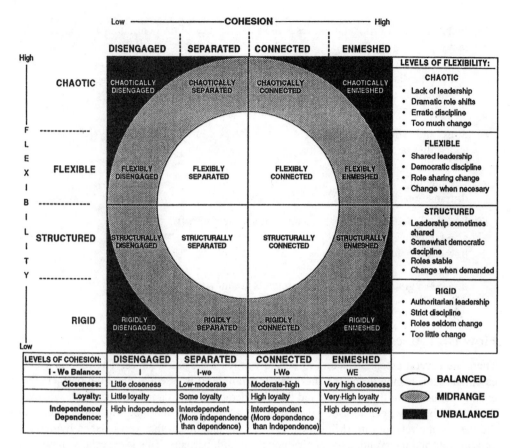

**FIG. 8.1.** Circumplex Model of Family Systems. *Note.* From "Circumplex of Family Systems: Integrating ethnic diversity and other social systems" by D. M. Gorall and D. H. Olson. In *Integrating Family Therapy: Handbook of Family Psychology and Systems Theory* (p. 219), by R. H. Mikesell, D. D. Lusterman, and S. H. McDaniel, 1995, Washington, DC: American Psychological Association. Copyright © 1995 by the American Psychological Association. Reprinted with permission.

separateness. Nichols and Everett (1986) referred to these additional systemic developmental disruptions as **systemic shifts** and **systemic traumas**. Systemic *shifts* refer to subtle changes in the family. For example, a grandparent moving into the family home may disrupt or exacerbate particular patterns. A systemic *trauma* refers to unpredictable life events, such as a death or illness, which shakes the foundation of a family as it attempts to survive in the face of tremendous stress. The ability of a family to work together and accommodate these changes is central to their functioning as a family.

Culture is also an important consideration when evaluating cohesion and flexibility (Gorall & Olson, 1995). According to Olson and Defrain (1997), "If normative family expectations support behavioral extremes on one or both of the [family circumplex] dimensions, the family will function well—as long as its members are satisfied with these expectations" (p. 97). The expression of individuality, for example, will look different for African American and Latino families in comparison to Anglo American families (McGoldrick & Carter, 2001).

13. In the circumplex model, families at the extreme ends of the continuum are considered to be:
    a. functioning at the highest level.
    b. poor candidates for therapy.
    c. vulnerable to problematic behavior.
    d. none of the above.

14. Stress and symptom onset is greatest at which point in the family life cycle?
    a. families with young children
    b. families with adolescents
    c. launching
    d. transitions between stages or life events

15. Which of the following is an example of a systemic shift?
    a. a father being diagnosed with cancer
    b. the birth of a child
    c. marriage
    d. a cousin moving in because his parents are moving out of town

## How Do I Assess Couples?

There are several essential factors to consider when assessing couples. The first and most essential factor is monitoring the **therapeutic triangle**. It is essential that both partners feel equally connected to the therapist, and that the therapist is not taking one partner's side over the other. You may need to use "selective joining" to engage the more distant partner into the therapeutic relationship (Minuchin, 1974). This may mean that you balance homework assignments and interventions to appear equal for both partners. This is especially important during the joining process. As the therapeutic alliance grows with the couple, you may become free to challenge one partner or the other, or use the therapeutic relationship to unbalance the system.

After you have established good rapport with both partners, it is important to assess the relationship history. Hiebert, Gillespie, and Stahmann (1993) recommend the use of a timeline when gathering history about the couple's relationship. While gathering the information you look for themes in the couple's interactions that can be developed into therapeutic goals. Also focus on sequences of interaction and typical behavior patterns common for the couple. In addition to gathering the couple's relationship history, many therapists choose to conduct genograms or use enactments in marital assessment.

In assessing a couple, it is important to evaluate several different aspects of their relationship. The "Seven Cs" (Birchler, Doumas, & Fals-Stewart, 1999) is a useful model for gaining a broader understanding of a couple (Table 8.2). Evaluating these different areas will help you see beyond the presenting problem and have a fuller picture of the couple.

16. What is the most essential factor to consider when assessing couples?
    a. monitoring the therapeutic triangle
    b. providing helpful homework assignments
    c. considering triangles that have been formed in the family
    d. assessing the relationship history

**TABLE 8.2**

The Seven Cs

| | |
|---|---|
| *Commitment* | How committed is the couple to each other? |
| *Caring* | What caring behaviors does the couple display? |
| *Communication* | How effective is their communication? |
| *Conflict Resolution* | How does this couple solve problems, manage anger, and resolve conflict? |
| *Character* | How are the partners doing as individuals? Is there any psychopathology? |
| *Culture* | How is culture affecting their relationship? |
| *Contract* | What expectations does each partner have of the relationship? |

*Note.* Adapted from "The Seven Cs: A Behavioral Systems Framework for Evaluating Marital Distress," by G. R. Birchler, D. M. Doumas, and W. S. Fals-Stewart, 1999, *The Family Journal: Counseling and Therapy for Couples and Families, 7*, pp. 253–264.

17. Why would a therapist need to use "selective joining" in couples therapy?
    a. to engage the more distant partner
    b. to join with the more vocal partner
    c. to form a strong alliance with their preferred partner
    d. a therapist should never use selective joining

18. Which of the following is not one of the "Seven Cs"?
    a. caring
    b. character
    c. compatibility
    d. contract

## What About Assessing Larger Systems?

As a family therapist, you are uniquely positioned to appreciate the interactions within the family and between the family and other systems, such as the school and legal systems. With any family, it is important to learn more about the context in which they live in order to understand how their context affects their lives and to learn how their context can be a resource in therapy. For example, learning about a family's church community may help you understand their values and be considered as a helpful partner in supporting the family through difficult times.

An assessment of larger systems also gives you information about other professionals involved in the care of your clients. Your ability to successfully manage these cross-disciplinary relationships may be as significant to a positive outcome than any single intervention. Eliciting the perspectives of others (physicians, psychiatrists, teachers, probation officers) will inform your assessment and give you direction for treatment planning. Ongoing collaboration with these professionals will ensure that you are working toward a common mission (McDaniel, Campbell, & Seaburn, 1995; Patterson, Peek, Heinrich, Bischoff, & Scherger, 2002; Seaburn, Lorenz, Gunn, Gawinski, & Mauksch, 1996).

19. Which of the following is a contextual factor at work in a family's life?
    a. culture
    b. religious or spiritual beliefs
    c. neighborhood
    d. all of the above

20. The following professionals are important to consider in assessment:
    a. teachers
    b. psychiatrists
    c. other therapists
    d. all of the above

## What Is the Role of Psychometric Instruments?

Using **psychometric assessment** instruments can serve as an important adjunct to clinical interviewing when gathering assessment data. Many excellent assessment tools exist that can serve as quick screening methods for all types of problems facing individuals, couples, families, and children (see Table 8.3). When selecting an instrument, multiple factors should be considered such as ease of administering and scoring, reading comprehension level, length or number of items, costs, availability of the instrument, and level of clinical utility. Measurement issues are also important including the sensitivity, reliability, and validity of the tool. Additionally, you should pay attention to the level of reactivity in the client's responses, such as social desirability and demand characteristics.

There are four basic types of instruments. These include self-report instruments, behavioral measures, physiological measures, and projective tests. Self-report measures, such as surveys are commonly used in clinical practice. For example, the Brief Symptom Inventory is a good tool for assessing suicidality. Behavioral measures involve direct observations by the therapist, such as enactments, which were described earlier. Physiological measures such as galvanic skin response or urinalysis are used less frequently due to the fact that they are expensive and often intimidating to clients. Finally, in projective testing, clients are assessed according to their response to ambiguous stimuli. Examples include the Rorschach inkblot test or a family kinetic drawing.

### TABLE 8.3

A Sample of Clinically Popular Assessment Instruments

| Instrument | Measurement Construct | Method of Measurement | Number of Items | Unit of Analysis |
|---|---|---|---|---|
| Beck Depression Inventory (Beck) | Depression | Self-report | 21 items | Individual |
| Brief Symptom Inventory (Derogatis) | Psychopathology | Self-report | 52 items | Individual |
| Family Kinetic Drawing (Burns) | Family relationships | Projective | Blank paper | Individual child |
| Family Adaptability and Cohesion Evaulation Scale III (Olson, Portner, & Lavee) | Adaptability, Cohesion, & Communication | Self-report | 20 items | Family |
| Dyadic Adjustment Scale (Spanier) | Dyadic Adjustment | Self-report | 32 items | Couple |
| PREPARE (Olson & Schaefer) | Premarital Adjustment | Self-report | 125 items | Couple |

21. Which of the following should be considered when selecting an instrument for assessment?
    a. reading comprehension level
    b. availability
    c. reliability and validity
    d. all of the above

22. One tool useful in screening for suicidality is the:
    a. Beck Suicide Inventory.
    b. Relationship Brief Inventory.
    c. Brief Symptom Inventory.
    d. none of the above.

# TREATMENT PLANNING

Treatment involves integrating all the important information gathered during the assessment process and developing a plan to assist the client with the presenting problems. The therapist determines which family therapy framework he or she will be using to address the client's problems and the appropriate interventions or treatment protocols. Oftentimes this will include balancing the client's wishes, the therapist's preferences, and the payer's guidelines, which can be difficult.

To help you organize your thinking about client's problems and make treatment decisions, we suggest a seven-step process outlined in Table 8.4 (Patterson, Williams, Grauf-Grounds, & Chamow, 1998). During this process the therapist selects a list of problems. This may involve prioritizing issues, which will help focus the treatment. Steps two and three involve assessment of the history of the problem and making a *DSM* diagnosis. Step four entails establishing treatment objectives. The therapist then selects a treatment modality, such as individual, couple, or family work, and selects a framework with corresponding interventions to address the problem. The final stages involve determining the length and frequency of treatment and making outside referrals. While these seven steps provide a broad overview of the treatment process, it is important to examine in greater detail the processes of treatment planning and selecting treatment procedures.

**TABLE 8.4**

Developing an Initial Treatment Plan

---

Step 1: Select a problem list.
Step 2: Examine history of problems and previous/current treatment.
Step 3: Conceptualize the case and make a diagnosis using a DSM-IV multiaxial assessment.
Step 4: Establish long-term treatment goals.
Step 5: Select treatment modality, objectives, and interventions.
Step 6: Determine length and frequency of treatment.
Step 7: Consider referrals to outside resources.

---

*Note:* From *Essential Skills in Family Therapy* (p. 70), by J. Patterson, L. Williams, C. Grauf- Grounds, and L. Chamow, 1998, New York: Guilford Press. Copyright 1998 by Guilford Press. Adapted with permission.

## What Is the Purpose of a Treatment Plan?

Clinicians develop treatment plans to serve as conceptual maps of the progression of treatment. The treatment plan outlines the goals and interventions the therapist intends to use to respond to the client's problems and symptoms. The plan is usually developed within the first three to four sessions. During the assessment process, the therapist pays close attention to recurrent themes, complaints, and problematic interactions or behavior patterns that emerge in therapy. The therapist organizes these issues into a list of goals that are client specific. It is often helpful to include the client in the process of developing goals. This can help instill hope for the client, and sometimes may even be a catalyst in promoting change.

23. One way to instill hope in a client when developing goals is to:
    a. form really difficult goals.
    b. form goals they've already accomplished.
    c. include the client in the process.
    d. not have goals to avoid discouragement.

## How Do I Make a Treatment Plan?

The treatment plan serves to guide the therapist in arranging appropriate timing for their goals and interventions. The most common format for treatment planning includes early phase goals, middle phase goals, and late phase goals. This format helps the clinician be comprehensive and organized in their approach to treatment. Furthermore, the therapist can organize the goals hierarchically, from most important to least important. It can also assist them in avoiding premature or poorly timed interventions. See Table 8.5 for a structured treatment plan outline.

**TABLE 8.5**

Structured Treatment Plan

---

A. Early Phase Goals
  1. Develop the therapeutic alliance
  2. Problem assessment
  3. Crisis assessment (issues of harm, abuse, suicide, homicide, substance use, violence, etc.)
  4. Joint goal setting with the therapist and client
  5. Early referrals (psychiatric evaluation, group therapy)

B. Middle Phase Goals
  1. Presenting problem(s) specifically addressed
  2. Application of theory-specific goals, techniques, and interventions

C. Late Phase Goals
  1. Address long term issues
  2. Solidify gains made during treatment
  3. Strategies for handling future issues, relapse prevention
  4. Referrals
  5. Appropriate termination

---

*Note:* From *Theory-Based Treatment Planning for Marriage and Family Therapists,* by D. R. Gehart and A. R. Tuttle, 2003, Pacific Grove, CA: Brooks/Cole-Thomson Learning.

Treatment plan goals are best articulated using observable or measurable behavioral indicators. The clinician can be even more specific by identifying his or her theoretical underpinnings and proposed interventions to achieve each goal. Gehart and Tuttle (2003) suggest the following format for writing goals:

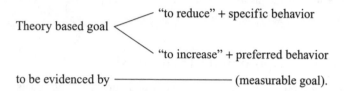

Theory based goal

"to reduce" + specific behavior

"to increase" + preferred behavior

to be evidenced by ——————————— (measurable goal).

Using this format, examples of goals include, "Parent skills training to reduce aggressive conduct to be evidenced by decreased frequency of fighting behavior," or "Strengthen parental subsystem hierarchy to increase parenting skills to be evidenced by decreased triangulation." For an excellent review of incorporating theory into treatment planning see Gehart and Tuttle (2003).

24. One way for a therapist to organize their treatment plan is:
    a. early phase, middle phase, and late phase goals.
    b. most important to least important goals.
    c. most difficult to least difficult goals.
    d. both a and b.

25. Which of the following is an early phase goal?
    a. creating strategies for relapse prevention
    b. application of theory specific goals
    c. specifically addressing the presenting problem
    d. crisis assessment

## What Are the Strengths and Limitations of a Treatment Plan Approach?

There are many benefits to using a structured treatment plan format. Third party payer reimbursement often requires a treatment plan that includes measurable behavioral goals. The plan can assist the managed care company in monitoring treatment progress and keeping therapists accountable. Treatment plans can assist with the continuity of care when multiple providers are active on the same case. Furthermore, the therapist can easily monitor the progress of treatment. A final benefit is that using a treatment plan can provide protection for a clinician from a legal standpoint.

Conversely, a therapist should be mindful of the limitations of treatment planning. Strict adherence to the treatment plan can reduce flexibility and the creative flow of the therapeutic process. A rigid application of the plan may neglect the client's immediate needs, thereby hindering the therapeutic alliance. The therapist's ideal plan may not be congruent with the client's level of motivation or evolving goals. In order to address these limitations, the treatment plan should not be applied rigidly, but should be collaborative, open to revision, and overtly addressed during the therapeutic process.

26. Which of the following is NOT a benefit of using a structured treatment plan format?
    a. The plan can help provide continuity of care when there are multiple providers involved.
    b. Strict adherence to a plan limits flexibility.
    c. It can be used by the insurance company to hold the therapist accountable for progress.
    d. It can provide legal protection for the therapist.

## How Do I Choose Appropriate Treatments?

Once you have conceptualized a case and established your treatment goals, you can decide which treatments would be most helpful. There are many ways to make these decisions and the process of choosing treatments has become more complicated for family therapists today than it was in the past.

In the past, family therapists would traditionally choose a treatment based solely on their theoretical orientation. For example, if I considered myself a "structural family therapist," I would conceptualize the clients' problems in light of this theory and choose the appropriate structural intervention. All clients would be understood and treated from this theoretical perspective.

Today there are multiple influences that help determine the treatment. Recent research has influenced treatment selection. Researchers began to ask, "Which treatment works best for which problem under what conditions?" Then they began doing research to answer this question. The results are a series of treatment protocols that are usually based on *DSM* diagnosis. Professional organizations such as the American Psychiatric Association or the American Psychological Association publish these protocols, and therapists who prefer evidence-based treatments can use them. Additionally, many insurance companies have adopted these protocols, and to obtain reimbursement, it is not uncommon for the therapist to be required to provide a treatment plan that matches these guidelines.

The legal system has also influenced the treatment selection process—mainly through the principles of informed consent. Informed consent refers to the rights that a client seeking therapy has. Basically, the client has the right to know about his or her diagnosis and what treatments exist for his or her problem. The client has the right to help select his or her treatment. To implement this principle, a therapist must know about available treatments, even if the treatments are outside of the therapist's expertise or scope of practice. Then the therapist must "inform" or tell the client about his or her options in as straightforward a manner as possible. This involves discussing what is known about the benefits and risks of any given treatment.

The client can then chose the treatment that he or she wants. There is a benefit to this process. Keeping the client actively engaged in making decisions about his therapy means that the client will stay more motivated than if he is a passive recipient of a treatment dealt out by an omnipotent therapist.

If the therapist cannot provide the treatment, he is ethically obliged to help the client find the professionals that can offer assistance. This may mean referral to a physician for psychotropic medication or to a psychologist for psychological testing. Often, the therapist continues to provide the primary treatment and uses other treatments as adjunctive.

Often, the client, couple, or family comes to the therapist with multiple problems, some of which have treatment protocols and some that have little or no research support. A multi-level intervention is necessary for therapy to be effective. The therapist uses the treatment protocols, the clients' wishes, the multitude of available community resources, knowledge about the clients' resources, and his own good judgment to make treatment decisions. The therapist tries to be holistic in his treatment approach and simultaneously attend to the clients' thoughts and feelings about the treatments.

27. How does informed consent affect the treatment selection process?
    a. The therapist must inform the client about which treatment option has been chosen.
    b. The therapist is more free to try experimental treatments since the client has given consent to treatment.
    c. The therapist must inform the client of treatment options and allow the client to help select the treatment.
    d. The therapist must learn how to be sneaky to obtain consent for the treatment she has chosen.

28. When a client presents with multiple problems, it is important to:
    a. attend to only the worst problem.
    b. consider all of the problems when planning treatment.
    c. refer them to someone who can handle multiple problems.
    d. use the same treatment technique for every problem to provide consistency.

## How Do I Keep Up With Different Treatment Guidelines?

Juggling the clients' wishes, the payer's guidelines, the legal restraints, and one's own good sense can be difficult at times. Often therapists select different treatments at different times, according to short-term and long-term goals. In addition, the therapist is constantly assessing the impact of her treatments, and revising her treatment plan based on the client's responses.

We believe that treatment procedures are changing so rapidly that instead of only teaching our students a specific treatment for a specific problem, we also teach them *how to obtain information* about treatments. We teach them how to do rapid literature searches using new technologies and databases such as the Cochrane Library. However, it is common that students can only find partial data, solutions, and recommendations through the professional literature. These solutions may not match the clients' wishes, resources, or situation. Therefore, clinical judgment remains a critical part of treatment planning.

29. Which of the following does a therapist use in making treatment decisions?
    a. her own good judgment
    b. the clients' wishes
    c. treatment protocols
    d. all of the above

30. Since treatment procedures change rapidly, it's important for therapists to:
    a. keep up to date by researching professional literature.
    b. use only those treatments they learned about in graduate school because the newer ones are less established.
    c. only use clinical judgment and avoid getting caught up in the flavor of the month.
    d. keep up to date by following developments reported in the popular media.

Although assessment and treatment are often discussed as separate activities, the boundaries between them are actually quite diffuse. As the often-quoted saying goes, "Assessment is treatment and treatment is assessment." Assessment and treatment planning are a continual process that will provide your clients with structure, insight, and the activation of their own healing strategies. Your development as a therapist will be partly reflected in the quality and scope of your assessments and treatment planning, which is why it is essential for you to remain actively engaged in the latest research, clinical theory, and legal guidelines. A good assessment and treatment plan will communicate your commitment to the therapy, your competence, and your hope for change.

## ACKNOWLEDGMENT

We would like to thank Marissa Lee for her help with this chapter.

## KEY TERMS

**assessment:** The process of evaluating a client; used to determine a method of treatment or referral.

**circumplex model:** A model used to assess a family's functioning in terms of flexibility, cohesion, and communication.

**cohesion:** The level of unity or closeness in a couple or family.

**diagnosis:** A label used to capture a client's problem. Frequently it is derived through the client meeting specified criteria outlined in the *DSM*.

**flexibility:** The ability and willingness of a person or system to change or adapt.

**joining:** The process of building rapport and accepting a client in order to facilitate the therapeutic process.

**larger system:** The cultural and societal influences on a person.

**psychometric assessment:** The use of psychological tests and inventories to aid in the assessment and diagnosis of a client.

**systemic shift:** A subtle change in the family that is not captured in the traditional family life cycle but may unbalance the family structure and create discomfort.

**systemic trauma:** An unpredictable life event, such as a death or illness, that shakes the foundation of a family as it attempts to survive in the face of tremendous stress.

**therapeutic triangle:** The shape of a therapeutic relationship when a therapist is working with a couple. It is natural, but can be problematic if it becomes unbalanced.

**treatment plan:** A strategy for treatment devised from assessment and diagnosis, used to guide the therapeutic process and evaluate progress.

## DISCUSSION QUESTIONS

1. What are the most important factors to consider in your first contact with a client? How can you use that contact to begin building a therapeutic relationship with the client?
2. What legal, ethical, and therapeutic goals should you focus on in the first interview? What specific techniques might you use to accomplish each goal?
3. What are some advantages of incorporating *DSM* into your assessment?
4. What are some crisis situations you might encounter and how should you assess for them?

5. Describe how you might use the circumplex model in assessing families.
6. Why are each of the "Seven Cs" important in assessing a couple?
7. What are the three parts of a useful treatment plan goal? What does each part contribute to the therapist's treatment planning process?
8. What are the benefits and limitations of using a treatment plan?
9. Choice of treatment can be influenced by the client, the therapist, and by parties other than the client or therapist. What are some of the effects each can have on the choice of treatment?
10. A woman calls you complaining of depressed mood and agrees to bring her family in to meet with you. Describe what the assessment, diagnosis, and treatment process might look like.

## SUGGESTED FURTHER READING

Mikesell, R. H., Lusterman, D. D., & McDaniel, S. H. (1995). *Integrating family therapy: Handbook of family psychology and systems theory*. Washington, DC: American Psychological Association.

This is easily the most comprehensive guide available on family therapy. There are three excellent chapters on assessment.

Morrison, J. (1995). *The first interview: Revised for DSM-IV*. New York: Guilford Press.

A readable, accessible guide to individual assessment. It is particularly helpful for clients presenting with major psychopathology.

Nichols, W. C. (1988). *Marital therapy: An integrative approach*. New York: Guilford Press.

A must read for any therapist preparing to work with couples. Nichols helps readers bridge the gap between theory and practice to prepare them for the challenges associated with couples therapy.

Nichols, W. C., & Everett, C. A. (1986). *Systemic family therapy: An integrative approach*. New York: Guilford Press.

It is unfortunate that a second edition of this book was never written, because it is by far the most theoretically sound family therapy book written to date. It transcends any one model of therapy and teaches the reader how to think and act systemically.

Patterson, J., Williams, L., Grauf-Grounds, C., & Chamow, L. (1998). *Essential skills in family therapy*. New York: Guilford Press.

This book is the perfect companion for the beginning therapist. Experienced therapists can look to the book as a helpful reminder, particularly when preparing for licensing exams.

Weeks, G. R., & Treat, S. R. (2001). *Couples in treatment*. New York: Brunner-Routledge.

Based on the intersystem model of couples therapy, this practical book is an indispensable resource for couples therapists. Whereas most couples therapy books are heavy on theory and light on skills, this book delivers an appropriate blending of theory and skills that will be an immediate help for therapists at any experience level.

## REFERENCES

Berg, B., & Rosenblum, N. (1977). Fathers in family therapy: A survey of family therapists. *Journal of Marriage and Family Counseling, 3*, 85–91.

Birchler, G. R., Doumas, D. M., & Fals-Stewart, W. S. (1999). The seven Cs: A behavioral systems framework for evaluating marital distress. *The Family Journal: Counseling and Therapy for Couples and Families, 7*, 253–264.

Dilsaver, S. C. (1990). The mental status examination. *American Family Physician, 41*, 1489–1497.

Gehart, D. R., & Tuttle, A. R. (2003). *Theory-based treatment planning for marriage and family therapists*. Pacific Grove, CA: Brooks/Cole-Thomson Learning.

Gorall, D. M., & Olson, D. H. (1995). Circumplex model of family systems: Integrating ethnic diversity and other social systems. In R. H. Mikesell, D. D. Lusterman, & S. H. McDaniel (Eds.), *Integrating family therapy: Handbook of family psychology and systems theory* (pp. 163–182). Washington, DC: American Psychological Association.

Greenan, D., & Tunnell, G. (2003). *Couple therapy with gay men*. New York: Guilford Press.

Hiebert, W. J., Gillespie, J. P., & Stahmann, R. F. (1993). *Dynamic assessment in couple therapy*. New York: Lexington Books.

McDaniel, S. H., Campbell, T. L, & Seaburn, D. B. (1995). Principles for collaboration between health and mental health providers in primary care. *Family Systems Medicine, 13*, 283–298.

McDaniel, S. H., Hepworth, J., & Doherty, W. J. (1992). *Medical family therapy: A biopsychosocial approach to families with health problems*. New York: Basic Books.

McGoldrick, M., & Carter, B. (2001). Advances in coaching: Family therapy with one person. *Journal of Marital and Family Therapy, 27*, 281–300.

Minuchin, S. (1974). *Families and family therapy*. Cambridge, MA: Harvard University Press.

Napier, A. Y., & Whitaker, C. (1978). *The family crucible*. New York: Perennial.

Nichols, W. C., & Everett, C. A. (1986). *Systemic family therapy: An integrative approach*. New York: Guilford Press.

O'Hanlon, W. H., & Weiner-Davis, M. (1989). *In search of solutions: A new direction in psychotherapy*. New York: Norton.

Olson, D. H., & DeFrain, J. (1997). *Marriage and the family: Diversity and strengths*. Mountain View, CA: Mayfield Publishing Company.

Olson, D. H., Russell, C. S., & Sprenkle, D. H. (1989). *Circumplex model: Systemic assessment and treatment of families*. New York: Haworth Press.

Patterson, J., Peek, C. J., Heinrich, R. L., Bischoff, R. J., & Scherger, J. (2002). *Mental health professionals in medical settings: A primer*. New York: Norton.

Patterson, J., Williams, L., Grauf-Grounds, C., & Chamow, L. (1998). *Essential skills in family therapy*. New York: Guilford Press.

Pfeiffer, E. (1975). A short portable mental status questionnaire for the assessment of organic brain deficit in elderly patients. *Journal of the American Geriatrics Society, 23*, 433–441.

Seaburn, D., Landau-Stanton, J., & Horwitz, S. (1995). Core techniques in family therapy. In R. H. Mikesell, D. D. Lusterman, & S. H. McDaniel (Eds.), *Integrating family therapy: Handbook of family psychology and systems theory* (pp. 5–26). Washington, DC: American Psychological Association.

Seaburn, D. B., Lorenz, A. D., Gunn, W. B., Gawinski, B. A., & Mauksch, L. B. (1996). *Models of collaboration: A guide for mental health professionals working with health care practitioners*. New York: Basic Books.

Weber, T., & Levine, F. (1995). Engaging the family: An integrative approach. In R. H. Mikesell, D. D. Lusterman, & S. H. McDaniel (Eds.), *Integrating family therapy: Handbook of family psychology and systems theory* (pp. 45–72). Washington, DC: American Psychological Association.

Weber, R., McKeever, J., & McDaniel, S. (1985). A beginner's guide to the problem-oriented first family interview. *Family Process, 24*, 357–364.

White, M., & Epston, D. (1990). *Narrative means to therapeutic ends*. New York: Norton.

# Case Management

Patricia C. Dowds
David G. Byrom
*Family Therapy Institute of Suffolk*

## TRUTH OR FICTION?

___ 1. *About 80% of people benefit from being in any kind of therapy.*
___ 2. *There are common factors to all the different schools of therapy.*
___ 3. *The common factors are more important to patient change than the type of therapy chosen.*
___ 4. *There are over sixty years of research on psychotherapeutic outcome.*
___ 5. *Effectiveness of treatment is not attributable to any particular school.*
___ 6. *The therapeutic relationship is more important to positive outcome than any technique factor.*
___ 7. *Eighty-five percent of change is related to factors other than technique.*
___ 8. *Relationship development skills are crucial to positive outcome.*
___ 9. *Therapy must be collaborative to be effective.*
___ 10. *You can create a "map" of all the community and systemic forces around an individual or family.*
___ 11. *The client must be a partner in goal setting for successful outcome.*
___ 12. *You can determine whether a family needs crisis intervention, short term treatment, or long-term treatment before you begin treatment.*
___ 13. *You can learn therapeutic questioning.*
___ 14. *Patient skills enhancement can be an important part of treatment.*
___ 15. *Termination is a stage of change.*

We looked over our 1,248 books on psychotherapy. The majority of them espouse different treatment orientations with different techniques. We checked the research; there are literally hundreds of orientations (four hundred at last count), and not many of them are in agreement.

So we asked ourselves, "How can we distill thirty useful pages for MFTs who must have received different trainings depending on the orientation of their graduate departments?" When we were new practitioners, we ourselves were often overwhelmed by the great diversity of techniques, models, and opinions voiced as "the way to treat." We expect that either you are similarly overwhelmed, or have chosen one orientation above others so as to create a "workplace."

Despite diversity, disagreement, and major differences in theoretical orientations, therapy works. In this chapter, we share what the research supports, what works for us, and what has been helpful to the students we train and to the clinicians whom we assist with clinical supervision.

We have organized this chapter on case management into two sections: First, we discuss the treatment process using the four common factors that Asay and Lambert (1999) distilled from their reviews of six decades of psychotherapy outcome research. Their work, and the writings of Duncan, Hubble, and Miller (1997a, 1997b, 1999) expounding on the four common factors in the treatment process, have been invaluable in helping therapists see the path through the forest and not wander from tree to tree. This common factors focus gives a constructive addition to any "therapy school." So if you have chosen an orientation, or school, these factors will strengthen your work. If you have not, these factors can be worked with separate from any formal school of psychotherapy.

Second, we present Nancy Boyd-Franklin's (1989) multisystems model as a useful way to organize treatment in any setting. This approach is useful whether treatment takes place in a clinic, school, hospital, home, or private office. It creates a map by which the clinician can conceptualize the family and community systems, and organize outreach and interventions.

## CREATING SUCCESSFUL TREATMENT OUTCOMES—THE COMMON FACTORS

The field of family therapy is as crowded with competing schools as is the overall field of psychotherapy. Starting with Sigmund Freud and his disciples, how to do effective psychotherapy has been a constant debate. There are hundreds of different therapy models, and each claims superior effectiveness. And yet, research has found that these very *different* systems produce very *common* **outcomes**.

There has been a great deal of research on psychotherapy outcomes in the last sixty years. Asay and Lambert (1999) in their review of psychotherapy outcome research found that "What is effective in psychotherapy is attributable to common factors, shared by many schools" (p. 23). They find that there is little doubt that psychotherapy is effective. Treated patients are much better off than those who do not receive treatment. In one meta-analysis, the average treated person was better off than 80% of the untreated individuals (Smith, Glass, & Miller, 1980).

What is not a popular finding is that the effectiveness of treatment is not attributable to any specific school or technique of psychotherapy. Instead, the effectiveness of treatment seems to be attributable to four **common factors**. These factors are: **client factors** and extratherapeutic events, **therapeutic relationship** factors, expectancy and placebo effects, and therapeutic techniques, with therapeutic techniques having the least effect on positive outcome.

Many therapists are very shocked (though some are very relieved and some reply with "of course") to find that outcome is predominantly determined by the client and outside events—not by the techniques or theoretical models. However, therapists can greatly influence these client factors, enabling clients to become productively involved in treatment and utilize treatment for their benefit.

1. The outcomes of psychotherapy treatments have:
   a. received very little attention.
   b. been viewed as art, not science.
   c. been researched for more than years.
   d. depended on the process used.

2. Outcome research has found that:
   a. people get better at the same rate with or without treatment.
   b. About 50% of people in therapy improve.
   c. The average treated person is better off than 80% of untreated individuals.
   d. Therapy does not work.

3. Outcome research has found that:
   a. you must carefully match the individual client to a particular treatment.
   b. only specific treatments work.
   c. there are many patient, therapist, and technique variables to be factored into a successful treatment.
   d. there are four common factors that account for positive outcomes.

The therapeutic relationship is the second most powerful factor. So research returns us to an old position of "Physician, heal thyself first." Expectancy, or hope, is as important as technique in facilitating psychotherapeutic change. And finally, we have technique as one of the lesser factors.

What stands out is that the *relationship* is most basically and powerfully under our influence, as well as how we continue nurturing and working with the ebbs and flows within these therapy relationships throughout our work with our clients. But, we can (and do) play significant roles in facilitating effective outcomes in therapy by understanding and creating ways to nurture clients' strengths and resources and their use of their lines' context and environment, and their expectancies. We play significant roles in facilitating a working relationship to develop treatment goals, to choose appropriate methods of change for each client, and to foster a hopeful therapeutic outcome. We must be comfortable and experienced in the therapeutic techniques we choose, as they are our tools. Because the research shows that 85% of change is related to factors other than technique, this means the beginning therapist, as well as the more experienced clinician, needs to attend to the therapist's life factors such as family of origin, communication skills, and relationship development skills, and must develop the ability to assess treatment and change "readiness."

4. The most important factor *within* a successful therapy is:
   a. the therapists' length of training.
   b. the type of treatment utilized.
   c. the addition of appropriate medications during the course of treatment.
   d. the therapeutic relationship.

5. The most powerful factor that emerges from the sixty years of outcome research is:
   a. outcome is predominantly determined by the client and outside events.
   b. therapists' years of experience.
   c. matching gender of therapist to gender of client.
   d. size of family in treatment.

| Client factors and extratherapeutic events | 40% |
| Therapeutic relationship | 30% |
| Expectancy and placebo effects | 15% |
| Techniques | 15% |

FIG. 9.1. Percentage of Improvement in Psychotherapy Patients as a Function of Therapeutic Factors. *Note.* Adapted from Lambert, M. J., "Implications of Outcome Research for Psychotherapy Integration" in *Handbook of Psychotherapy and Behavior Change* (4th ed.) (p. 97), by J. C. Norcross and M. R. Goldfried (Eds.), 1992, New York: Basic.

We are convinced that the four common factors are the core of all treatment and of all related case management. We are convinced by the research, by our own clinical experience, and by the experiences of our many students. These are the factors that therapists must attend to in order to foster successful therapeutic outcomes. They are ordered for discussion purposes by their relative effect, using the percentages in Figure 9.1, but we argue that the contributing factors are overwhelmingly client-based. Thus, this ordering is for readability purposes only, and does not reflect any judgment of relative importance.

## Being Mindful and Focused on Maximizing the Four Factors

The nearly sixty years of outcome research supports the efficacy of psychotherapy. Therapists must be knowledgeable about the outcome research since our confidence is essential to successful outcomes. In keeping our own hope alive, and in effectively reinforcing the hope of our clients—that their problems are solvable and their suffering can be relieved—we are being therapeutic. This means that being mindful, being continuously conscious of these common factors, and being continuously focused on maximizing the use of all four factors, we can be very, very useful as helpers.

Our hope must be used to keep us listening in optimally open-minded ways to our clients and their contexts, so that the demands and challenges of our work do not lead us to displace our hope and capacity to inspirit others. Doing so could cause us to pathologize, label, or make our very real clients—who are always living, doing, facing, and solving life demands—secondary to our conceptual models and techniques. If we fall into these very human errors, this would be yet another marginalizing of our clients—one of the very contextual/environmental challenges with which they are already struggling.

## Our Clients and Their Contexts

We are convinced by the extensive research, some of which is cited above, that the client is the source of over 70% of the outcome variance in improvement in therapy. Each client's frame of reference is clearly central (the major portion—40%—of outcome success contribution). Because the expectations/placebo effects factors are actually client factors (self-generated healing through the client's own belief and hope), then we must add another 15%, bringing the subtotal to 55%. *And,* clients share at least one half of creating and maintaining the therapeutic relationship. This is another 15%, bringing the estimated total to 70% or more. Review Lambert's (1992) findings as presented in Figure 9.1 and see the clear implications that *the client is the source and agent of at least 70% and the therapist is the source of at most 30%* of what is occurring in the therapeutic relationship and in technique and model use factors.

The extratherapeutic factors include *all* aspects of the client and his or her environment:

- The client's pre-existing strengths, innate capacities for growth, and abilities to find and make use of help and support from other people—all these in combination with chance events occurring extratherapeutically in the client's life.
- The person's abilities, skills, and resources that can be utilized to resolve that client's presenting problem, both within and outside therapy.
- Each client's perceptions and experience of each and all past therapeutic experiences and of the current therapeutic relationship, of their presenting problem and its causes, and of how this current therapy might usefully address the client's goals. This has been has been described in a conceptually useful way as "the client's theory of change" (Duncan, Hubble, and Miller, 1997, p. 23).

Duncan, Hubble, and Miller (1997a, 1997b, 1999)—among the leading proponents of empiricism in informing effective treatment—argue most persuasively that clinicians become mindful of these extratherapeutic factors. We can start with reviewing how we are already validating and nurturing both client strengths and change-producing chance events in the client's environment in our specific clinical work with each client.

As we proceed in this chapter, we describe ways to utilize the rich resources comprising the client's worldview, and, particularly, his or her "theory of change." We believe that valuing the client's view of how change occurs must be continuously drawn upon as we work collaboratively in treatment and that all treatment philosophies and all clinical interventions require that we value in our actual working:

- That the client is the essential and ultimate expert.
- That the collaborative work of therapy can optimally occur only when clinicians are committed to the value that therapy is not something that is *performed* on the client.
- That any therapy is the exchange interpersonally conducted by all participants with the ongoing emphasis being on the quality of the client's participation in the therapy sessions.
- That the clinician has a fundamental responsibility to genuinely respect all of the above, and, to be as creative and persevering as possible to encourage and reinforce the client's participation in the therapy sessions.
- That when we are working as clinicians we have a special privilege. We have the honor to be invited by clients into their worlds, most often into their most intimate lives and during the most vulnerable times in their living.

6. There is extensive research on the source of outcome variance in treatment. Which is the correct finding?
   a. The therapist is responsible for the major part of outcome variance.
   b. The therapist and client are about equal in contribution.
   c. The use of the correct technique accounts for positive outcome.
   d. The client is the source of at least 70% of outcome variance.

7. Extratherapeutic factors include:
   a. family of origin variables.
   b. clients' pre-existing strengths, abilities, and skills.
   c. the client's ability to trust and work with others.
   d. all of the above.

8. If psychotherapy is collaborative:
    a. the client is the essential and ultimate expert on change.
    b. you need a team of therapists.
    c. you need a therapist and a physician.
    d. none of the above.

*A Few Words of Caution.*   In contrast, when we maintain static characterizations of clients—the way diagnoses can be straightjackets for our minds—we are maintaining beliefs in constancy—in permanence—in our clients' presenting problems. Such beliefs on our part, just as on the client's part, tend to mired down and missing the continuous flux, the constant changes that are really in the nature of living and in our environments. These beliefs—this pathologizing the other, the client, and also the clinician at times (countertransference)—have resulted from the medicalization of psychotherapy services. These beliefs in pathology and static diagnoses have developed under the pressure of our culture and with the complicity of our professions. We see this as moving away from the longstanding values of healing and respect. This is further complicated by the current industrialization of health care which turns our clients into commodities and our services into business losses in an attempt to make health insurance profitable. This latter development is also highly antithetical to healing.

The deficit model, which is an outgrowth of the disease model, has been strikingly useful in evolving knowledge and treatments for some physical illnesses. This disease/deficit model has not been at all useful in the very human problems of living. And the labeling is at its most institutionalized worst in the *Diagnostic and Statistical Manual of Mental Disorders* (American Psychiatric Association, 2000) in its claims of mental disorders as conditions within a person. Kenneth Hardy (1999) fittingly called the *DSM* "The Diary of the Socially Maligned." For further reading along this vein we recommend the excellent critique of the *DSM* by K. Tomm of the Dulwich Centre in Australia (1990). The MFT field is the leader in translating problems in living into human/family difficulties—into relational terms—the very essence of how we live. We are grateful for all the voices that give powerful testimony to the realities of being human in the world, of living in a context of many relational experiences and shared influences. We are needed!

9. The extensive medicalization of psychotherapy and of all mental health and substance abuse care, including case management, has been the most major contributor to which of the following?
    a. clinicians forming and maintaining beliefs in the client's problems as permanent and static
    b. pathologizing—using the deficit model institutionalized in the *DSM* series (now *DSM–IV*)
    c. conceptualizing clients and clinical services (and their practitioners) as commodities for the industrialization of health care by insurance and pharmaceutical industries
    d. all of the above

Alarmingly unsupported by scientific fact are the powerfully influential and widespread beliefs and practices that include the *DSM–IV–TR*. For example, how decisions are made about which treatment is appropriate for a particular person is not demonstrated empirically. Nor does this descriptive psychiatry—this classification system—predict outcome of treatment. Similarly unsupported by more than forty-five years of outcome research (which has dramatically improved in its methodologies, designs, and analyses) are, of course, the differential effectiveness of competing therapeutic approaches and the superiority of psychopharmacological over psychological interventions (Hubble, Duncan, & Miller, 1999). Hubble, Duncan, and Miller also report similar outcome confirmation problems with the empirically validated treatments. *Caveat emptor* holds for clients and professionals alike.

10. In assessing which treatment is appropriate for which client, which of the following has been empirically demonstrated to optimize effective outcomes?
   a. a thorough knowledge of *DSM* diagnoses
   b. skillful use of systematized *DSM–IV* diagnosis decision-making methods
   c. relying on what is scientifically conclusive of outcome confirmation by "empirically validated treatments"
   d. maximal use of the "common factors" findings by tailoring these to what we learn from the client

Now, back to what we *can* do, what we know helps, and *what does work* in effective therapy, the collaborative work of the therapist and client.

*Client Empowering.*  Clinicians can help empower the significant (keep the 40% in mind) contribution of extratherapeutic events by:

• Listening for, inviting, and then using the client's own descriptions of these continuous changes to help us choose what to accentuate, what to clarify and expand, and what to reinforce. Attending and conversing with clients give us ways to encourage the further uses of these change events, both when these occur with the client as the agent in some way, as well as when they are seemingly completely outside the client's control and may be capitalized on further by the client's subsequent actions.

• Exploring what is different about better versus worse times in the client's daily living, when presenting problems are minimal or absent, and when the client feels helplessly at the mercy of the problem(s)—the entire spectrum of their experience of their presenting problem(s).

• Creating the necessary foundation within the therapeutic relationship and dialogue for future success in attaining the client's goals by starting from the thesis that the client is the primary agent of change, the most powerful common factor in outcome in psychotherapy (Tallman & Bohart, 1999) and by coming to know the client's own natural, self-healing propensities.

• Getting to know the **client's life contexts**—get to know his or her world outside the influence of the problem. Individuals and families are always so much more than whatever has brought them to therapy.

• Continually attending to client competencies *and* client problems. Madsen (1999) shared a workshop participant's contribution: "Competence is quiet, it is difficult to hear" (p. 26). As Madsen also points out, the evolution of family therapy brings to the present much baggage emphasizing pathology, with the biggest change being in who gets labeled—our thinking needs to move much more to "let's work with the family because they are the most powerful solution" (p. 26).

11. When we work clinically, knowing and being mindful of teachings from the "common factor" enables us to:
   a. have little, or very limited (15% at best), influence in the most potent area of "extratherapeutic events."
   b. continuously use what clients teach us about changes for them—whether these changes seem to occur by chance or by the client as clearly the agent generating change.
   c. listen for, invite, and use clients' perceptions and beliefs about how change occurs in life to help empower them and to cultivate the therapeutic relationship.
   d. "b" and "c" above.

12. Because client factors and extratherapeutic events comprise the most powerful common factor, a reasonable estimate of this client-based outcome variance is _____.
   a. 40%
   b. 55%
   c. 70%
   d. 85%

## Therapeutic Relationship Factors

Not only does Hans Strupp (1995) conclude that "The quality of the interpersonal relationship as context is the *sine qua non* in all forms of psychotherapy" (p. 70), but Orlinsky, Grawe, and Parks (1994) have shown in their extensive review of the process-outcome research that "The quality of the patient's participation in therapy stands out as the most important determinant of outcome.... The therapist's contribution toward helping the patient achieve a favorable outcome is made mainly through empathic, affirmative, collaborative, and self-congruent engagement with the patient. These consistent process-outcome relations, based on literally hundreds of empirical findings, can be considered facts established by more than forty years of research on psychotherapy" (p. 361).

Bachelor and Horvath (1999) argue that *the relationship itself is the treatment*, that having the therapeutic relationship is the treatment. They conclude that the findings across these last four decades show us the following—with excellent implications about the ways therapists can take action:

1. The quality of the therapeutic relationship from the very beginning and throughout its course—with quality defined as mutually determined goals, mutually determined methods, and the client's view of the emotional bond with the therapist—has repeatedly demonstrated much better predictive validity of outcome success than many other variables studied, including the therapist's theoretical orientation experience level, or professional discipline (i.e., psychologist, social worker, professional counselor, psychiatrist).

2. The client's perception of the relationship is a better predictor of outcome than the therapist's assessment of the relationship. The client's assessment of therapist-provided conditions (of accurate empathy, respect, nonpossessive warmth and genuineness) correlates significantly higher with effective outcome than does the therapist's assessment of how well he or she provided those conditions. Clinicians are indebted to the seminal and enduring teachings of Carl Rogers on precisely these therapist-provided "core conditions," and his basic writing on these dimensions deserve reading and rereading (Rogers, 1951, 1957).

3. The ways clients experience empathy are as varied as are the uniqueness of each and every client who interacts with a clinician. "Nurturing" does not seem very important to clients. What does seem relevant to clients is that the therapist has what can be understood as "a cognitive appreciation" of the situations in which clients find themselves, and that the therapist seems to accurately reflect the states of feeling at the time of the incident reported in therapy. This latter defines the "accurate empathy" dimension in number two above.

4. A surprising, and instructive, finding was that no correlation emerged in the literature between the length of the therapeutic relationship and the strength of the therapeutic alliance. So, one most valuable hint from this is that only if we fail early in being relevant to clients and don't match the uniqueness and needs of each client, as described above, then do we need to "build the relationship." More clearly stated, when the unique needs of each client are clarified—when we ask them to help us understand the details of their perceptions of the relationship—then we can strategize together. Together we can see which perceptions diverge and then we can work toward agreement on what is helpful, on what is needed to strengthen the therapeutic alliance from the initial session and throughout the therapy.

13. The therapeutic relationship dimension which best predicts effective outcome is:
    a. accurate matching of client with therapist's theoretical model orientation and therapist rating of the therapeutic's relationship.
    b. the client's view of the emotional bond with the therapist.
    c. the client's assessment of the therapist-provided conditions—accurate empathy, respect, nonpossessive warmth, and genuineness.
    d. both "b" and "c."

14. Accurate empathy offered by a therapist is:
    a. measured by independent judges rating the therapist's ability to validly put him or herself in the patient's life experience and to nurture in ways that were inadequately provided in the patient's family of origin.
    b. the client's perception of the therapist as accurately reflecting their feeling states at the times of the incidents they are reporting in therapy.
    c. what is experienced by the client as a "cognitive appreciation" of their life situations by the therapist.
    d. both "b" and "c."

## Expectancy, Hope, and Placebo in Combination With Technique Factors

These are myriad, and all clearly client-generated (with the therapist's facilitation by what we do together with our clients, as discussed above). When a client engages in a new therapeutic endeavor, that very act, the act of trying something new, encourages hoping, even re-instituting a hoping process in very demoralized people. Clinicians have many ways in which we can, and already do, inspirit and facilitate hoping for and expecting the change that clients desire—as we discussed previously, we work at forming strong alliances from the start, at mutually identifying goals, and at making client strengths integral in the treatment.

The "healing rituals" in which we engage are most critical in that they help clients mobilize and organize their hope and expectancies in ways that contribute to their ability to address methods of change. This is how techniques are powerful—by helping clients have structured and concrete ways (methods) to then use the inspiriting that is under way and draw upon the resources in themselves and in their life contexts to move in change-generating ways.

15. The "placebo effect" factor is:
    a. a misnomer from the medicalization of clinical work and from inaccurate conceptualizing of methodology in outcome research.
    b. the essential role of client expectancies and hope generated by clients from merely engaging in therapeutic endeavors.
    c. the powerful dimensions inherent in therapy "healing rituals" that help clients structure and concretize the change-generating ways available to them from their life contexts, from the therapeutic relationship, and from the therapist's preferred models and techniques.
    d. both b and c.

General suggestions highlighted by Hubble, Duncan, and Miller (1999) are that:

• We "have faith in the efficacy of [the] treatments. . . [to be] the most successful in producing positive placebo effects [client hope and expectancy for desired changes]" (Benson & Epstein, as cited in O'Reagan, 1985, p. 17).

• We should convey to the client our interest in the results of the technique or orientation we are using—typically by asking clients about the usefulness or benefits they found (and did not find) in the particular methods used (e.g., homework assignments). we can routinely ask clients to observe and record any changes. Even directing clients to notice and tell us about what they have noticed potentiates hope and expectancies for change to occur.

• We help clients believe in possibilities—that they can change, that they can begin anew in whatever ways are important to them, that they can become effective agents in directing their lives and attaining desired outcomes.

• We orient treatment toward the future—we can use outcome-focused questions, for example, as de Shazer et al. (1986) described in what they called "focused solution development" (p. 207). Questions that typify this are: "When you become less anxious (or there is less fighting in the family), what will that be like?" "What will be different then?" (Look for just noticeable differences.) "Tell me how the first indication of this will be clear to you (to each of you in the family)?" Possibilities of these questions, and in making the step-by-step process of noticeable change abound.

• All ways to heighten the client's experienced personal agency—the client's felt self-control—must be observed and collaboratively discovered, so that the client's belief in personal control is increased. Listen for and reinforce, with some genuine confirmation, the ways clients talk about having any impact on how their daily living goes. Craft your questions and statements in ways that are clearly based on your belief in the client's impact on what occurs in his or her daily living. One example: "How striking it is that you handled that anxious (conflict) situation in ways to feel safer (not fight)." Or, "How did you decide when that was what was about to happen, and how did you decide to handle it that effective way?" "What more ideas do you have for situations like these?"

## Models and Techniques—What They May Really Offer Us

An indispensable chapter by Sprenkle, Blow, and Dickey (1999) clarifies with applicable details some contributions from marriage and family therapy research to the four common factors. We urge you to read this chapter in particular, of course within the context of all the accompanying chapters which are all similarly helpful in thinking about and practicing effectively as clinicians. In the following sections we use a selected family therapy/family systems model and useful techniques that will flesh out this common factor in more breadth. For now, however, think over the following summary of the essential role of models and techniques.

Throughout the clinical writings and research literature therapists appear to get the most out of specific models and techniques by having ways to practice those *core conditions,* the absolutely essential ingredients that all therapies use and that do truly cut across all orientations as well-demonstrated common factors. Often shared with therapists-in-training is the idea that it is crucial to have a model of therapy, a theory of individual, marital and/or family personality/dynamics/systems which the therapist can hold onto in the demanding interactions of the face-to-face therapy session, especially when the going gets rough. The wisdom in this mentoring advice certainly holds because we need to have our own structure and focus, and we must be able to convey and use structure and focus in our work in sessions and from session to session. Clients, and their therapists, expect change that something different—and successful— will occur. This change can be in exposing oneself to feared situations, in interpersonal risk-taking, raising self-awareness to some useful level, learning to manage anger constructively, attaining sobriety, or any number of hoped-for changes unique to each and every person. We must keep foremost the client's theory of change and the client's readiness for change—and for how much change—over our own preferred and favored techniques.

16. The primary reason that models and techniques are useful for therapists to master and use is:
   a. they enable the therapist to accurately understand clients and their problems and then effectively intervene.
   b. because these are most potent contributors to effective change.
   c. they give therapists ways to continuously practice the "core conditions" of therapy and to have personal structure and focus in challenging face-to-face therapy work.
   d. successful therapy is not possible without adhering to one theoretical orientation.

# A WORKING MODEL TO ORGANIZE THERAPEUTIC INTERVENTIONS

As we have discussed, various factors common to all therapy systems account for the major part of improvement found in clients. The question we now address is, "How will you organize your view of a family system and its connected systems using these treatment factors?"

We find the multisystems model utilized by Boyd-Franklin (1989) and Boyd-Franklin and Bry (2000), to be the most useful across treatment settings (Fig. 9.2). It incorporates structural, behavioral, and problem solving approaches. It focuses the clinician on the full "ecological and systemic context, including the many different institutions, agencies, and systems that have impact on them" (Boyd-Franklin and Bry, 2000, p. 7). Using this model you start by creating a framework that helps you see the networks to which you must establish connections, and which connections you should maintain to organize effective treatment and insure adequate case assessment. Within this model you are free to create traditional psychotherapy treatment plans, which focus on weekly "talking" meetings. This model allows you to expand that process when necessary to include extended family, community, school, and social service systems in

Multisystems

| Level I | Individual |
|---|---|
| Level II | Subsystems |
| Level III | Family household |
| Level IV | Extended family |
| Level V | Nonblood kin and friends |
| Level VI | Church and community resources |
| Level VII | Social service agencies and other outside systems |

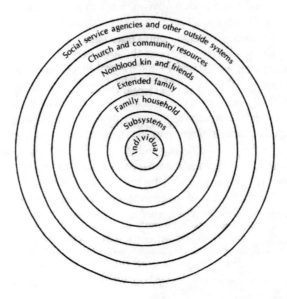

**FIG. 9.2.** The Multisystems Model. *Note.* From *Black Families in Therapy: A Multisystems Approach* (p. 149), by N. Boyd-Franklin, 1989, New York: Guilford press. Copyright 1989 by Nancy Boyd-Franklin. Reprinted with permission.

your treatment plans. This is particularly useful when working in agencies and institutions, but is also important for clinicians in private practice settings.

The multisystems model is a natural extension of the process that began when therapists expanded their vision from inside the individual to the context in which the individual lived—"the family." Now we have expanded from the inside the family to the community and cultural contexts in which the family lives. As therapists once realized that they could not understand the individual outside of the context of his or her family, we now realize that we cannot understand the family outside of the context of the significant community, cultural, or agency influences that they are dependent on, or significantly interact with.

The multisystems model is represented as a series of concentric circles.

The use of this system gives the therapist a concrete map of the significant influences in an individual or family case. This way the therapist can make useful decisions about what systems to reach out to, or at least be knowledgeable about. Another advantage of this approach is that it breaks the pattern of having different therapists and caseworkers for each level. When you have several mental health workers involved with one family, it often contributes to further confusion and disorganization for that family.

Whether the clinician does family treatment in an office, or works in an agency that conducts home-based treatment, the same map applies. It enables a therapist to choose whether it would be helpful to reach out to a caseworker, teacher, or minister—or all three—to help a family mobilize their resources to address problems. It helps ensure that powerful influences in a family's functioning will not be overlooked. It is important to note that this map is useful when working with individuals as well. It also enhances the therapist's ability to look for resources for a client/family.

## Case Example

Karen was an eleven-year-old brought to treatment by her mother. The school had requested treatment due to Karen's high absenteeism. Karen stated she often had stomachaches and had to stay home. If Mom tried to force her to go to school she would have a major temper outburst, often hitting herself and her mother. There was an eighteen-year-old sister and a sixteen-year-old brother at home with Karen, but Mom revealed that Karen's father had left six months previously. There was a divorce and custody battle in progress. When the siblings were brought in at the next session it was clear that they were taking sides in the divorce and fighting with each other. The eldest daughter wanted to stay with Mom. The son wanted to go with Dad. The youngest—Karen—told her father she would go with him, but then became symptomatic. When Dad was brought in he made it clear that he felt the children were better off with him, and told them so. With exploration it was revealed that the court appointed law guardian had interviewed the two youngest children; the eldest had refused to be interviewed. The law guardian was inexperienced and indecisive. The court wanted the custody suit resolved without trial and would take recommendation.

### Interventions

**Level 1. Individual:**   Sessions for Karen

**Level 2. Subsystems:**   Sibling sessions, coparenting sessions

**Level 3. Household:**   Sessions for mother and children

**Level 4. Extended:**   Sessions for father and children

**Level 6. Church and Community Resources:**   Divorce support group for Mom

**Level 7. Outside Systems:**

*School*—Social worker organized a girl's group for Karen's grade and included work on divorce.
*Court*—Supported coparenting sessions, recommended outside evaluation if parents did not resolve custody dispute.

This case shows how an awareness of the multisystemic view leads to the therapist reaching out to facilitate support and other treatments for a family. Not creating false dichotomies among individual, family, and outreach work creates a more cohesive treatment plan. So instead of several therapists, school social workers, court personnel, all of whom may never have time to speak—much less coordinate—treatment, you have one therapist, in touch with all the systems, moving back and forth from individual to family sessions as needed.

17. To organize therapeutic interventions you must focus on:
    a. the primary and extended family.
    b. the identified patient, to alleviate suffering.
    c. social service agencies, to coordinate treatment.
    d. full systemic context, including family, community, schools, and social service agencies.

18. When creating a "map" of a family system and its connected systems:
    a. contact and intervene on all levels.
    b. start at the center and work your way out.
    c. you can choose where it would be helpful to intervene.
    d. assign different therapists to each level.

19. When working from a "multisystemic" view:
    a. have several therapists to share the workload.
    b. use one therapist for work inside the family system, a second for work with agencies outside the family.
    c. always have a separate therapist for the children.
    d. there is one therapist in contact with all important systems.

## Beginning Treatment or How We Set the Measure of Outcome

Treatment begins with the client and the therapist defining a **treatment contract**. The treatment contract is really a process in which the family and the therapist define the problems to be solved, and reach some sort of understanding on the goals of treatment and the method of therapy. This contract can be formal and written, or more an agreement that is clearly understood by all parties. It needs to be formulated in the beginning of treatment before therapeutic interventions begin. While the major goals will probably remain the same, it must be open to discussion as therapy progresses.

This treatment contract is the foundation by which the therapist and the client creates the possibility of change. It is the framework by which they can discuss and evaluate progress in treatment. The formulation of treatment goals needs to be collaborative. As Prochaska (1993) points out in his work on change, the motto for the client is, "When in doubt, don't change" (p. 249). So the therapist needs to not proceed unless the client is a partner in the therapeutic undertaking. This includes the change factors of expectancy and the therapeutic relationship. The client's position is, "Do I believe this journey can happen?" "Do I agree with you on the destination?" "Do I agree on how to travel?" and "Do I think you are a good person for me to make this journey with?" If the answers to these questions are "yes," therapeutic work proceeds very productively.

Therapists facilitate the goal-setting process in families in many different ways. They ask parents to describe how they want their family to be different, they ask each family member to describe how they want things to be different, or in mandated treatment they ask the family what needs to happen to get the referring system to leave the family alone. You need to have each member spell out in detail what would define a good outcome. For families that have little hope, and therefore have difficulty setting goals, you can use a variation of what deShazer (1988) calls miracle questions. This involves asking the client to imagine that a miracle has happened and that their problem is solved. The client must describe to you what would now be different; this difference becomes the treatment goal(s) for this client. There are many variations of miracle questions, including: *magic* questions: "Wave a magic wand and tell me how your son/daughter/spouse, would be different," or, "Look into a crystal ball and describe a good future." A number of therapists (O'Hanlon & Weiner-Davis, 1989) use *presuppositional* questions. Presuppositional questions need to be framed in the client's own language. Some examples of these questions are:

- If therapy is helpful, what will have changed?
- What do you each do differently to get your spouse to stop being angry with you?
- What do you need to see your spouse do differently this week to know they want this marriage?
- What do you need to change to like yourself more?

Another style of goal-setting questions are *scaling* questions. These ask the family to rate the situation and the outcomes to create a hierarchy of goals. Some examples are:

- On a scale of 1 to 10 with 10 being happiness, how important is less arguing to your happiness?
- How would you rate your fighting now? What would be an acceptable level?
- You rated the severity of your fighting as a 7. Is there any other problem you would rate higher?

Hopefully, therapists develop the style of question that personally suits them best. From the answers the clients give to interviewing questions, and the feedback a therapist can provide, the goals of treatment can be set in such a way as to facilitate change and encourage positive outcome.

Once the goals have been agreed on there will need to be some decisions on the length and frequency of treatment. Unfortunately in this age of "managed care," these decisions are often made more by the insurance companies and their case managers than by the client and therapist. Companies set limits on how many sessions they will pay for; they then will often "manage" how many of these sessions will be authorized for payment during a particular course of treatment. While it is of questionable use having people who have never seen the client making treatment decisions, managed care is our most common form of mental health insurance.

20. What is the foundation by which the therapist and the family create the possibility of change:
    a. the treatment setting.
    b. the therapeutic orientation.
    c. the treatment contract.
    d. specific therapeutic interventions.

21. Before the goals of treatment can be formulated, the therapist must:
    a. make a complete diagnosis.
    b. consult with the treatment team, and make a diagnosis.
    c. decide on the type and length of treatment.
    d. have the family collaborate in setting goals.

22. Because the treatment contract defines the goals, methods, and length of treatment:
    a. the therapist needs to be patient and wait for the family to decide what they want.
    b. the appropriate legal forms must be used.
    c. the goals must be matched to appropriate methodology.
    d. the therapist can facilitate this process by the use of careful questioning.

Aside from insurance intrusions, the therapist needs to decide on the treatment length early on. While it can and often will be modified during the course of treatment, it is a mistake to leave it open-ended. The therapist will determine whether the client/family needs crisis intervention, brief therapy, or long-term therapy. Patterson, et al, have an excellent table to determine length of treatment (Table 9.1).

23. Length of treatment is decided:
    a. during the course of treatment by the amount of progress made.
    b. by the insurance company.
    c. the therapist decides the treatment length early.
    d. "when it is over."

## TABLE 9.1

### Length of Therapy Indicators

*Indicators for Crisis Intervention*
1. There is a severe disruption in client or family functioning.
2. Client's response to an event is extremely overwhelmed and highly stressed.
3. An external event has occurred suddenly and caused considerable psychological or emotional instability.
4. Family or client has been traumatized by an external event or a developmental change.
5. Client is in danger of harming self or other.
6. Client's symptoms have intensified to the point of causing incapacitation.

*Indicators for Brief Therapy*
1. Agency or institutional policy dictates a limited number of visits.
2. Client or family's goals are essentially symptom focused.
3. Client or family is receptive to therapy and willing to change.
4. Client or family has additional resources available to support and integrate change.
5. Clear changes in behavior are rapidly observed.
6. Client or family's history is not a primary concern.

*Indicators for Long-Term Therapy*
1. Client's or family's history has significant bearing on presenting problems.
2. Client or family can engage in a longer-term therapeutic relationship.
3. Client's concerns go beyond behavioral issues and involve underlying dynamics or causes.
4. Client's goals for therapy include identifying and sustaining changes during therapy.
5. There is a significant amount of anxiety and concern that warrants longer-term work.

*Note.* From *Essential Skills in Family Therapy,* by J. Patterson, L. Williams, C. Grauf-Grounds, and L. Chamow, 1998, p. 82, New York: Guilford Press. Copyright 1998. Reprinted with permission.

24. An indicator for crisis intervention is:
    a. severe disruption in client or family functioning.
    b. client or family is overwhelmed and highly stressed.
    c. client is in danger of harming self or others.
    d. all of the above.

25. Brief therapy is indicated when:
    a. the family or client has been traumatized by an external event.
    b. clear changes in behavior are rapidly observed.
    c. the family's history has significant bearing on the presenting problems.
    d. none of the above.

26. A therapist should consider long-term treatment over brief treatment when:
    a. the client's symptoms have intensified to the point of causing incapacitation.
    b. the client/family has additional resources available to support change.
    c. the family's concerns go beyond behavioral issues and involve underlying dynamics or causes.
    d. therapy is not working very well.

At this point, the therapist and the family have agreed on how they will work together—they have agreed on what will constitute a good outcome—so now the therapist asks: "How will I help get us to our goal?" While treatment skills and techniques only account for 15% of positive outcome, it is where most of us focus our anxiety. So a discussion of techniques is in order.

## Ongoing Treatment Techniques

The techniques therapists can use to help create change are myriad. For the most part techniques are outgrowths of a particular orientation. Therefore it is difficult to speak of techniques separate from an orientation. Yet every therapist wants to do something helpful, and they want to know what is helpful.

There are sets of **therapeutic skills** that transcend orientations. There are communication and relationship skills that therapists can teach their clients. In this way, they become a part of relationship building, or increasing client competency, and are enhancements to outcome.

27. Treatment techniques:
    a. are the most important part of therapy.
    b. take many years to learn well.
    c. are for the most part outgrowths of a particular orientation.
    d. can be standardized.

### Therapeutic Skills

*Questioning.* One of the primary skills of a psychotherapist is the ability to ask good questions. We discussed earlier the questioning techniques of O'Hanlon and Weiner-Davis (1989), and de Shazer (1988). Tomm (1988) describes the many different sorts of questions a therapist can ask, illustrating how questions are used to get information, assign responsibility, create connections, or challenge a family's perception of reality. He assigns questions to one of four categories:

*Lineal questions:* investigative, content oriented, e.g., Why is your son failing high school?
*Circular questions:* explore relationships, e.g., Who is most upset by his failure?
*Strategic questions:* challenge the family's status quo, e.g., What would happen if both
   parents were upset?
*Reflexive questions*: encourage change, e.g., If your son became successful in school how
   would things be different at home?

Any beginning therapist would be wise to read his work and the work of O'Brian and Bruggen (1985) on circular questioning. Their discussions on using questions to elicit relationship information while challenging a family's status quo are invaluable. What is crucial is that the therapist feels comfortable asking as many questions as they need to understand a family relationship, or to track a problem behavior.

**Task Creation.**   Different orientations will generate tasks either within the therapy session (enactments) or send the family home to try out new behavior (assignments). Either way, the construction of a good task helps the family move from the status quo to new possibilities. Our bias is to have the family begin the work on a new task during the session to provide support and to function as a resource for the family, then send them home to continue working on a new process.

**Joining, Supporting, and Challenging.**   In the course of successful therapy the family must feel that the therapist understands them. The process of careful family-specific questioning along with some empathic comments creates a sense that the therapist "is with them"; this is *joining* or co-creating a working relationship. Some families need support to stabilize them before they can proceed beyond this. Though this is not change producing itself, a family cannot work on change unless there is some stability. Once a family feels out of crisis, the therapeutic relationship will be stronger. This relationship will allow the therapist to respectfully challenge or confront self-defeating or problem behaviors.

28. Therapeutic skills transcend orientations. They include:
    a. questioning
    b. joining, supporting, and challenging.
    c. task creation.
    d. all of the above.

29. One of the primary therapeutic skills is:
    a. questioning.
    b. history taking.
    c. diagnosis.
    d. treatment planning.

**Patient Skills Enhancement.**   Therapists always need to assess, "Does this family/client have the interpersonal skills necessary to create the changes needed?" From there every therapist needs a library of skills training books, groups, or people to facilitate learning. Though every therapist needs to know his or her local parent training groups, couples groups, divorce groups, and substance abuse groups, they need their own resources as well. A therapist needs to know good versus bad conflict techniques, how to encourage assertiveness, how to help parents problem solve together, how to help people express their thoughts and feelings, and so on. So a therapist needs a lifetime of experience when they start! Fortunately there are many great books on fostering skill development.

## Termination

Prochaska (1993) views **termination** as the final stage of the change process, which occurs "when there is zero temptation to engage in the problem behavior, and there is 100 percent confidence that one will not engage in the old behavior regardless of the situation" (p. 253). These high standards would lead to interminably long treatments. Most terminations are done in the spirit of hope, with a door left open for a return if necessary.

If the therapeutic relationship has been a collaborative one, then it follows that termination should be a joint decision. Termination is as important as the initial contract formation stage. Now the challenge is for the family/client to go it alone. Before this happens the therapist and the family need to evaluate what has happened during their work together, what changes have occurred, and what would need to happen to undo all the changes made. A mutual termination is very empowering because both *the family* and *the therapist* have the experience of success.

So a termination also has treatment goals. The family needs to review carefully the changes they have made and the skills they have learned. They need to know what previous behaviors were contributing to their problems. They need to have had the experience of success from their new skills or behaviors. This experience of success will raise the family's sense of being a "successful home," and thereby increase all its members' esteem. Termination is not one session; it is a process of summation and ending of the therapy.

But not all terminations are mutual. Unilateral terminations can be very uncomfortable for both the therapist and the family. A therapist may choose to terminate treatment because they believe that they can no longer be helpful, or because they believe a referral to another facility or specialist is in order. The therapist may decide it is best to transfer a case if it is not possible to agree on the treatment contract, or to establish a good therapeutic relationship; perhaps there are individual differences. When transfer or termination is the therapist's decision, they should give the family notice and be prepared to spend time on this with them. A mismatch of client problem and therapist's skills, or of personality styles between them, should not be experienced by the family as their "failure in therapy."

Some families/clients will chose to terminate without agreement with the therapist. Some will not discuss this, they will just fail to show up for their appointment and disappear. This is generally uncomfortable for the therapist, who may wonder, "Who is to blame." Clients terminate for many reasons, but primarily it is that their priorities on therapy are different than the therapist. They may decide other activities are more important for their time, money, or emotional investment. Or they may experience relief from their difficulties and just stop coming. This sort of termination does not mean a failure on the therapist's part.

30. Termination is the final stage of the change process. It should:
    a. be a joint decision.
    b. have treatment goals.
    c. include a review of changes.
    d. all of the above.

In closing, the research overwhelmingly reminds us of the potency of clients as central play-wrights and actors in their own lives, and therapists as stagehands—as interactive audiences—as people who learn and are "helpers."

## KEY TERMS

**client empowering:** The process of creating within the client an awareness of his or her strengths and capacities to solve their own difficulties.

**client factors:** All aspects of a client—their skills, strengths, capacities, and problems.

**client's life contexts:** His or her world outside the influence of the problem.

**common factors:** Essential ingredients that all therapeutic orientations utilize.

**outcome:** The effects of therapy on the client/family; can be positive or negative.

**patient skills enhancement:** The process of reinforcing existing skills and facilitating new learning within therapy sessions and in the community.

**termination:** A process of summation and ending therapy.

**therapeutic relationship:** The client-assessed interpersonal relationship from first contact onward.

**therapeutic skills:** The entire spectrum of known and learnable contributions which therapists can make for effective outcomes.

**treatment contract:** The collaborative effort of the therapist and the client by which they define the goals and methods of treatment.

## DISCUSSION QUESTIONS

1. Discuss the importance of the therapeutic relationship to positive outcome. What comprises the relationship? How important is it? What can the therapist do to enhance it?
2. What are client factors/extratherapeutic events? Can the therapist influence these? If so, how?
3. Expectancy, or hope, is as important as technique in facilitating change. What would you do to increase hope in a client/family?
4. Discuss some of the ways that we can clinically empower our clients families. What can we do for them, how should we act, and what do we need to have them do?
5. What do models and techniques offer to patients? How much do models and techniques account for therapeutic outcome? How important are they for the therapist?
6. What is the usefulness of using the multisystemic model? How would it organize treatment differently, or change with whom the therapist worked? How would it influence the therapist's understanding of a family?
7. What are the important factors in beginning treatment? What must be decided very early on? Who is involved in these decisions? How can the therapist influence this process?
8. Discuss what indicators (at least four) you would use to decide if a client or family needed crisis intervention.
9. What are some of the therapeutic skills that transcend orientation? Can these be taught? Give examples.
10. Discuss the process of termination. What are the differences between collaborative terminations and unilateral terminations?

## SUGGESTED FURTHER READING

Lerner, H. G. (1997). *The dance of anger: A woman's guide to changing the patterns of intimate relationships.* New York: HarperCollins.

Stone, D., Patton, B., & Heen, S. (1999). *Difficult conversations: How to discuss what matters most.* New York: Viking.

Taffel, R. (2000). *Getting through to difficult kids and parents: Uncommon sense for child professionals.* New York: Guilford Press.

Taffel, R. (2002). *When parents disagree and what you can do about it.* New York: Guilford Press.


## REFERENCES

American Psychiatric Association. (2000). *Diagnostic and statistical manual of mental disorders* (4th ed.). Washington, DC: Author.

Asay, T. P., & Lambert, M. J. (1999). The empirical case for common factors in therapy: Quantitative findings. In M. A. Hubble, B. L. Duncan, & S. D. Miller (Eds.), *The heart and soul of change* (pp. 23–55). Washington, DC: American Psychological Association.

Bachelor, A., & Hovarth, A. (1999). The therapeutic relationship. In M. A. Hubble, B. L. Duncan, & S. D. Miller (Eds.), *The heart and soul of change* (pp. 133–178). Washington, DC: American Psychological Association.

Boyd-Franklin, N. (1989). *Black families in therapy: A multisystems approach.* New York: Guilford Press.

Boyd-Franklin, N., & Bry, B. H. ( 2000). *Reaching out in family therapy: Home-based, school, and community interventions.* New York: Guilford Press.

de Shazer, S., Berg, I., Lipchik, E., Nunnally, E., Molnar, A., & Gingerich, W. (1986). Brief therapy: Focused solution development. *Family Process, 25*(2), 207–222.

de Shazer, S. (1988). *Clues: Investigating solutions in brief therapy.* New York: Norton.

Duncan, B. L., Hubble, M. A., & Miller, S.D. (1997a). *Escape from Babel: Toward a unifying language for psychotherapy practice.* New York: Norton.

Duncan, B. L., Hubble, M. A., & Miller, S. D. (1997b). *Psychotherapy with impossible cases.* New York: Norton.

Hardy, K. (1997). Workshop of Diversity and Family Therapy. Port Jefferson, New York.

Hubble, M. A., Duncan, B. L., & Miller, S. D. (1999). Directing attention to what works. In M. A. Hubble, B. L. Duncan, & S. D. Miller (Eds.), *The heart and soul of change* (pp. 407–447). Washington, DC: American Psychological Association.

Lambert, M. J. (1992). Implications of outcome research for psychotherapy integration. In J. C. Norcross & M. R. Goldfried (Eds.), *Handbook of psychotherapy integration* (4th ed., pp. 94–129). New York: Basic.

Madsen, W. C. (1999). *Collaborative therapy with multi-stressed families: From old problems to new futures.* New York: Guilford Press.

O'Brian, C., & Bruggen, P. (1985). Our personal and professional lives: Learning positive connotation and circular questions. *Family Process, 24,* 311–322.

O'Hanlon, B., & Weiner-Davis, M. (1989). *In search of solutions.* New York: Norton.

O'Reagan, B. (1985). Placebo: The hidden asset in healing. *Investigations: A Research Bulletin, 2*(1), 1–3.

Orlinsky, D. E., Grawe, K., & Parks, B. K. (1994). Process and outcome in psychotherapy-Noch einmal. In A. E. Bergin & S. L. Garfeild (Eds.), *Handbook of psychotherapy and behavior change* (4th ed., pp. 270–378). New York: Wiley.

Patterson, J., Williams, L., Grauf-Grounds, C., & Chamow, L. (1998). *Essential skills in family therapy: From first interview to termination.* New York: Guilford Press.

Prochaska, J. O. (1993). Working in harmony with how people change naturally. *The Weight Control Digest, 3, 249,* 252–255.

Rogers, C. R. (1951). *Client-centered therapy.* Boston: Houghton Mifflin.

Rogers, C. R. (1957). The necessary and sufficient conditions of therapeutic personality change. *Journal of Consulting Psychology, 21,* 95–103.

Smith, M. L., Glass, G. V., & Miller, T. I. (1980). *The benefits of psychotherapy.* Baltimore: Johns Hopkins University Press.

Sprenkle, D. H., Blow, A. J., & Dickey, M. H. (1999). Common factors and other nontechnique variables in marriage and family therapy. In M. A. Hubble, B. L. Duncan, & S. D. Miller (Eds.), *The heart and soul of change* (pp. 329–359). Washington, DC: American Psychological Association.

Strupp, H. H. (1995). The psychotherapist's skills revisted. *Clinical Psychology, 2*, 70–74.

Tallman, K., & Bohart, A. C. (1999). The client as a common factor: Clients as self-healers. In M. A. Hubble, B. L. Duncan, & S. D. Miller (Eds.), *The heart and soul of change* (pp. 91–131). Washington, DC: American Psychological Association.

Tomm, K. (1988). Interventive interviewing: Part III. Intending to ask lineal, circular, strategic or reflexive questions. *Family Process, 27*(1), 1–15.

Tomm, K. (1990). A critique of the DSM. *Dulwich Centre Newsletter, 3,* 5–8.

# 10

# Managing Behavioral Emergencies

Phillip M. Kleespies
Barbara L. Niles
Catherine J. Kutter
Allison N. Ponce
*VA Boston Healthcare System*

## TRUTH OR FICTION?

___ 1. *When a member of a family or couple reports thoughts about harm to self or others, one of the major tasks for the therapist is to determine if the individual's condition is a behavioral emergency as opposed to a behavioral crisis.*

___ 2. *If clinicians have been well trained, they can be expected to predict suicide or violence to others.*

___ 3. *Proximal risk factors can act as precipitants for life-threatening behavior, but are seldom sufficient to explain it.*

___ 4. *If a perfect predictive test for behavioral emergencies were invented, it could easily be validated by using suicide or homicide as an outcome measure.*

___ 5. *Many instances of suicide or violence can be explained by the acute risk factors involved.*

___ 6. *Poor parent-child communication has been associated with adolescent suicidal behavior.*

___ 7. *If a patient or client is depressed but also feels anxious, he or she will be too apprehensive to actually commit suicide.*

___ 8. *Having children under eighteen in the home is considered protective against suicide for depressed patients.*

___ 9. *Male perpetrators of violence against their partners are, generally speaking, no more aggressive outside of their domestic relationship than anyone else.*

___ 10. *Having been victimized in an adult relationship seems related to becoming involved in future violent relationships.*

___ 11. *With domestically violent men, alcohol abuse makes little difference in the likelihood that they will become violent again.*

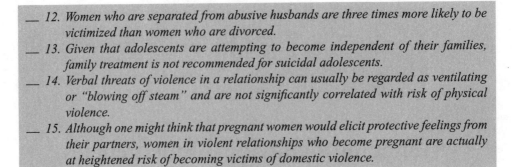

_____ 12. Women who are separated from abusive husbands are three times more likely to be
victimized than women who are divorced.
_____ 13. Given that adolescents are attempting to become independent of their families,
family treatment is not recommended for suicidal adolescents.
_____ 14. Verbal threats of violence in a relationship can usually be regarded as ventilating
or "blowing off steam" and are not significantly correlated with risk of physical
violence.
_____ 15. Although one might think that pregnant women would elicit protective feelings from
their partners, women in violent relationships who become pregnant are actually
at heightened risk of becoming victims of domestic violence.

You have been seeing a couple in therapy for the past five weeks. The woman works for a small company and has recently been advanced to a beginning level managerial position. Her husband is a construction worker who feels left behind by his wife's success. He calls you and says that he has seen his wife having dinner with a man who is a higher level manager at her work. He believes that they are having an affair and he plans to confront her about it this evening. He states that, if there is evidence to support his suspicions, he has had thoughts of killing his wife and then himself. Thus far, he has only had thoughts, and he denies that he has made any definite plans or preparations. How might you respond to such a tense situation?

One of the major tasks for a therapist who is thrust into such an apparently urgent clinical situation is to determine if it is what we refer to as a **behavioral emergency** or whether it might be better termed a **behavioral crisis**. It is important to understand the distinction between these concepts because it drives our thinking, our decision making, and our interventions (Kleespies, Deleppo, Gallagher, & Niles, 1999). A *behavioral emergency* occurs when an individual reaches a state of mind in which there is imminent risk that he or she will do something (or fail to do something) that will result in serious harm or death to self or others. There are at least four types of behavioral emergencies: (1) high risk suicidal states, (2) potentially violent states, (3) situations in which there is grave risk to a relatively defenseless victim (e.g., a child or elder who lives in an abusive home), and (4) situations in which there is high risk to an individual by virtue of his or her very impaired judgment.

A *behavioral crisis,* on the other hand, is a serious disruption of a person's baseline level of functioning such that his or her coping mechanisms are inadequate to restore equilibrium. A crisis is often brought on by an emotionally significant event in which there may be a turning point for better or worse. If the individual cannot resolve the problem that is causing the crisis, typically, a state of anxiety develops. The individual, however, is not necessarily at risk of engaging in life-threatening behavior. A crisis, of course, can contribute to or precipitate a behavioral emergency, but it should not be regarded as sufficient to explain it. There are usually many additional distal and proximal factors that lead down a pathway to life-threatening behavior.

1. A *behavioral emergency* is distinguished from a *behavioral crisis* in that a behavioral emergency involves:
   a. the complete loss of ability to cope.
   b. overwhelming anxiety.
   c. imminent risk of serious harm or death.
   d. the use of very poor judgment.

2. If an individual is unable to resolve a behavioral crisis, he or she typically:
   a. starts to abuse alcohol.
   b. experiences a state of anxiety.
   c. attempts suicide.
   d. dismisses the problem or conflict.

The purpose of this chapter is to review the evaluation and management of behavioral emergencies as they may occur within a couples/family treatment context. Thus, a family member may become suicidal or potentially violent (as noted in the example at the beginning of this section), while another might be the potential victim. How is the family or couples therapist to assess the risk and intervene appropriately in an effort to provide safety? Will the family be a support to its member or members who are at risk, or might family involvement, at this particular time, only aggravate an already tenuous situation? These and many other questions and issues can confront the therapist when working with families or couples in which there is significant conflict and pathology.

## LIMITATIONS ON PRACTICE AND RESEARCH

At the outset, it is important to note that it is not possible, with the methods currently available to us, to predict such statistically rare events as suicide or homicide. For the interested reader, Kleespies and Dettmer (2000) have presented the arguments about the difficulty of predicting such a low base rate event as suicide, and the same arguments apply regarding the prediction of homicide. Thus, the field of risk assessment has shifted its focus from prediction to the more realistic goal of attempting to improve our ability to estimate levels or probabilities of risk.

Likewise, there are definite limitations on research into such life-threatening behaviors as suicide and homicide. Generally speaking, actively suicidal patients or patients who appear to be at imminent risk of violence are excluded from research studies. There is simply no known ethical way to involve such individuals in sound empirical research when the measurement outcome is death or serious injury.

Having said these things, we initially present a heuristic framework for estimating risk in emergency situations. We then use this framework in presenting the available empirical evidence for evaluating and managing suicide risk and risk of domestic violence and victimization.[1] Finally, we provide recommendations for managing situations in which there appears to be imminent risk of life-threatening behavior.

3. It is not possible to predict suicide or homicide because:
   a. there are too many false negatives.
   b. clinicians don't receive the proper training.
   c. clinicians fail to use standardized tests.
   d. the base rate is too low for accurate detection.

---

[1] Child abuse and elder abuse clearly constitute behavioral emergencies in families. Space constraints, however, do not allow us to discuss them in this chapter. The interested reader is directed to other chapters in this volume for presentations on child abuse.

4. It is difficult to conduct research on imminent risk factors for suicide or violence because:
   a. there is no way to collect a sample of patients who have suicidal or violent ideation.
   b. there are few researchers who will work with patients who have suicidal or violent ideation.
   c. it would be unethical to include patients in a study when imminent suicide or violence could be the outcome.
   d. there is no possible research design for such studies.

## A FRAMEWORK FOR ESTIMATING RISK OF LIFE-THREATENING BEHAVIORS

Although they were thinking primarily of estimating risk of suicidal behavior, Rudd and colleagues (Rudd & Joiner, 1998; Rudd, Joiner, & Rajab, 2001) have presented a framework that we propose can be extended to organizing risk factors and estimating risk of life-threatening behaviors more generally. Rudd and associates suggested that the clinician think in terms of predisposing or **distal risk factors**, acute or **proximal risk factors**, and **protective factors**. Extended to life-threatening behavior more broadly, distal risk factors form the groundwork in which suicidal or violent behavior takes root. They make for the necessary threshold that renders the patient vulnerable when proximal risk factors occur. Proximal risk factors, on the other hand, are closer in time to the life-threatening behavior itself, and tend to act as precipitants. They are not, however, in most circumstances sufficient to explain the occurrence of life-threatening behavior. Rather, in combination with a significant set of distal factors, they can lead to the conditions needed for life-threatening behavior to occur. Protective factors are conditions or characteristics (such as good social support or value-based inhibitions) which, if present, may decrease risk of life-threatening behavior, but, if absent, may increase it.

Rudd and Joiner (1998) suggested that the degree of risk for suicide can be estimated by weighing these three types of factors. They presented a gradation of suicide risk ranging from minimal to extreme that we propose may also be a fruitful way of estimating risk for violence or victimization. A person at minimal risk for life-threatening behavior might have no known distal risk factors or proximal risk factors and multiple protective factors, while someone at moderate risk might have some distal factors, some proximal risk factors, and some protective factors that are beginning to weaken. Those in the severe to extreme range, who may have multiple distal and proximal risk factors and lack protective factors, are more likely to be at imminent risk.

5. A framework (cited in this chapter) that may be useful in estimating the risk of life-threatening behavior includes:
   a. psychological testing, medication, and family support.
   b. the use of the clinician's intuition about the degree of risk.
   c. the patient or client's ability to contract for safety.
   d. evaluating and weighing distal risk factors, proximal risk factors, and protective factors.

# EVALUATING ACUTE RISK OF SUICIDE IN THE FAMILY

## Distal Risk Factors for Suicide

*Adults: Psychopathology.* Serious mental illness has emerged as one of the strongest predictors of suicide. Recent literature reviews have summarized findings that over 90% of adults and adolescents who commit suicide suffered from a major psychiatric disorder (Kleespies & Dettmer, 2000; Miller & Glinski, 2000). Further investigation has found that only certain psychiatric diagnoses are associated with a significantly elevated risk of suicide. The above-mentioned reviews identified mood disorders (primarily depression), alcohol abuse, and schizophrenia as the diagnoses most strongly associated with a heightened risk of suicide in adults. An estimated 80% to 85% of adults who complete suicide suffer from at least one of these three diagnoses (Kleespies & Dettmer, 2000). Other diagnoses that have been empirically associated with an increased risk of suicide include posttraumatic stress disorder, bipolar II disorder, and borderline personality disorder.

6. The three psychiatric diagnoses that have the highest risk of suicide for adults are:
   a. schizophrenia, alcohol abuse, and depression.
   b. panic disorder, PTSD, and alcohol abuse.
   c. depression, borderline personality disorder, and heroin abuse.
   d. depression, cocaine abuse, and anxiety disorder.

*Adolescents: Psychopathology and Family Characteristics.* In adolescents, psychopathology and certain family characteristics have emerged as strong predictors of suicidal behavior. Adolescent suicide attempts have been associated with major depression, substance use disorders, and conduct disorders as well as with psychological characteristics such as impulsivity and poor affect regulation (Lewinsohn, Rohde, & Seeley, 1996). In addition, investigators have identified poor parent-child communication and negative family interactions as risk factors for adolescent suicidal behavior (e.g., King, Segal, Naylor, & Evans, 1993).

7. Adolescents with conduct disorders are:
   a. at elevated risk for suicide attempts.
   b. at no elevated risk to harm themselves.
   c. likely to destroy property but unlikely to be a risk to self or others.
   d. at risk of accidental injury but not of intentional self-harm.

*Family History of Suicidal Behavior.* A family history of suicidal behavior has emerged as a significant predictor of suicide attempts (Brent, Bridge, Johnson, & Connolly, 1996). The families of suicidal individuals often exhibit impaired communication and problem-solving skills (McLean & Taylor, 1994), and suicidal behavior might, in some cases, be a learned strategy for communicating with family members or coping with difficult situations. In addition to transmitting a direct risk for suicidal behavior, elevated risk of suicide in family members might, in some cases, be due to the genetic or environmental transmission of characteristics associated with suicidal behavior, such as depression or impulsivity (Brent, 2001).

8. A major predisposing or distal risk factor for suicidal behavior is:
   a. a history of medical illness.
   b. global insomnia.
   c. a family history of alcoholism.
   d. a family history of suicide

## Proximal Risk Factors for Suicide

*Acute Risk Factors for Adults With High Risk Diagnoses.*   Suicide risk profiles vary across different diagnoses (Clark & Fawcett, 1992), and Kleespies and Dettmer (2000) have recently outlined acute risk factors for adults with each of these high-risk diagnoses. In a large prospective study, Fawcett et al. (1987) identified acute risk factors for suicide among individuals with depression, including symptoms of severe anhedonia, global insomnia, severe anxiety, and current alcohol abuse. Among individuals with schizophrenia, prospective studies have found suicide risk associated with hopelessness, depression, obsessive-compulsive features, paranoid ideation, and subjective distress (Cohen, Test, and Brown, 1990; Peuskens et al., 1997). Risk is greatest for male schizophrenic patients under the age of 40, and when these patients are not acutely psychotic but have a heightened awareness of the debilitating aspects of their illness and suffer with depression. The findings of retrospective studies examining risk factors for suicide among individuals with substance use disorders have suggested that comorbid depression and recent loss of a significant relationship are acute risk factors for suicide in this population (see e.g., Murphy, 1992). In addition, suicide among individuals with alcoholism is generally more likely in mid-life and after a prolonged history of alcohol abuse and dependence.

9. Prospective studies have indicated that patients with schizophrenia are at increased acute risk of suicide when they are:
   a. having a psychotic episode.
   b. depressed but not in a psychotic state.
   c. over 50 years of age.
   d. experiencing increased anxiety.

10. Alcoholic patients who commit suicide typically do so:
    a. in their 20s or 30s while attempting to become sober.
    b. in mid-life after years of drinking.
    c. despite having good family relationships.
    d. when they develop cirrhosis of the liver.

*Acute Risk Factors for Adolescents.*   As with adults, only a minority of adolescents with high-risk psychiatric diagnoses attempt or complete suicide, and an acute crisis can usually be identified in the lives of those who do exhibit suicidal behavior. Precipitants include family problems (e.g., physical abuse, disciplinary crisis, parental unemployment, argument with parent), problems in social relationships (e.g., breakup of romantic relationship, argument with friend), the loss of a relative or friend (e.g., through moving or death), the suicide attempt of a friend or relative, legal or disciplinary problems, substance abuse, and serious medical conditions (Lewinsohn et al., 1996; Wagner, 1997).

## Protective Factors for Suicide

Some individuals who appear at a heightened risk for suicide based on a review of risk factors such as those identified above, manage to cope successfully without developing suicidal ideation or behaviors. Observations of such resilience have stimulated interest in identifying protective factors (i.e., characteristics of the individual or the environment that may buffer the impact of stressors). When present, these characteristics increase resilience and decrease the risk of suicidal behavior; when they are absent, the risk is increased. Protective factors are thus important considerations in the assessment of suicide risk. Although the research on protective factors has been limited relative to the investigation of risk factors, several of these protective factors have received empirical support.

*Family Relationships.* Family relationships appear to offer significant protection against suicidal ideation and behavior. In studies of adolescents, family connectedness and cohesion have been identified as the strongest protective factors, significantly lowering the risk of suicidal ideation and behavior (Resnick et al., 1997; Rubenstein, Heeren, Housman, Rubin, & Stechler, 1989). In adults, strong supportive family relationships, being married, and having children under the age of 18 years living at home have also been found to reduce suicide risk (Lester, 1987; Fawcett et al., 1987).

*Social Support Network Outside of the Family.* Supportive relationships outside of the family also seem to confer protection against suicide risk. Friendships have been found protective in adolescents as well as in adults. While supportive relationships with a few close friends have been found protective in adults, acceptance and integration into a social group has been found more protective for adolescents (Rubenstein et al., 1989). In addition, adolescents' sense of connectedness to school has been identified as protective against suicide (Resnick et al., 1997).

*Reasons for Living and Other Protective Factors.* Linehan, Goodstein, Nielsen, and Chiles (1983) identified a set of beliefs that differentiate suicidal from nonsuicidal individuals and developed a scale to assess these reasons for living (e.g., responsibility toward family and children, moral objections to suicide, fears of social disapproval and of the pain involved in suicide). The results of subsequent studies have offered support for the assertion that reasons for living such as those identified above serve as protective factors against suicidal behavior in adolescents and in adults (e.g., Gutierrez et al., 2002; Jobes & Mann, 1999). Other studies have identified additional protective factors including hopefulness and spiritual well-being, a purpose for living, and employment (e.g., Stack, 2000).

11. Empirical studies have found that one of the strongest protective factors against suicide in adolescents is:
    a. family connectedness.
    b. seeing the impact of a peer's suicide on family and friends.
    c. having a great deal of personal freedom.
    d. having employment during after-school hours.

## MANAGING SUICIDE RISK

Strategies for managing suicide risk may be adjusted according to the level of risk involved. While hospitalization is often required for individuals judged to be at imminent risk for suicide, mild to moderate suicidal ideation is usually managed effectively on an outpatient basis, and this section will focus on the outpatient management of suicide risk. Rudd and colleagues outlined suggestions for treating individuals determined to be at mild to moderate risk for suicide and developed an empirically supported treatment program for intervening with individuals exhibiting suicidal behavior (Rudd et al., 2001). These authors suggested that the intensity of outpatient treatment should vary in accordance with risk indicators. For patients at mild risk, they suggested that recurrent evaluation and monitoring of suicidal potential is usually sufficient. For patients at moderate risk, their recommendations include 24-hour emergency availability, an increase in frequency of contact (telephone and/or outpatient visits), frequent assessment of suicide risk and evaluation of the need for hospitalization, and professional consultation as needed. They furthermore suggested that the treatment of mild to moderate suicide risk should include a problem-solving component and target identified skills deficits (e.g., emotion regulation, distress tolerance, impulsivity, interpersonal assertiveness) in addition to other salient issues.

12. If a patient reports active suicidal ideation, the most appropriate immediate response would be to:
   a. ask the patient not to discuss it in the family session.
   b. request a medication evaluation.
   c. evaluate the estimated level of risk and respond accordingly.
   d. hospitalize the patient.

Because family problems have been implicated in both the onset and recurrence of suicidality, Spirito (1997) suggested that family therapy is often the treatment of choice for suicidal behavior. Although a great deal has been written about treating suicidal individuals in individual and group therapy, those interventions that involve family members of suicidal individuals are most relevant to this chapter and will be the focus of the discussion of managing suicide risk.

Family members may play important roles in the treatment process. Contact with the family can reduce social isolation and increase self-esteem, family members may be able to provide important information that the patient is unable or unwilling to provide, and family members may be enlisted to recognize and respond to signs of suicide risk (Kleespies & Dettmer, 2000; McLean & Taylor, 1994). Numerous approaches have been developed to treat suicidal individuals and their families using treatment models based on crisis intervention, family systems, psychodynamic, behavioral, and cognitive-behavioral principles (see Spirito, 1997 for a review). Most of the approaches that have empirical support for their effectiveness have focused on suicidal adolescents and their families.

Rotheram-Borus and colleagues (Rotheram-Borus, Piacentini, Miller, Graae, & Castro-Blanco, 1994) developed a brief cognitive-behavioral outpatient family therapy program for adolescent suicide attempters and their families. Known as Successful Negotiation/Acting Positively (SNAP), this program was designed to address issues of impaired communication and problem-solving skills in these families. Treatment goals include creating a more positive family environment, teaching problem-solving skills, and building coping and conflict negotiation skills. This treatment has been found effective in reducing suicidal behavior in female adolescents who had previously attempted suicide (Piacentini, Rotheram-Borus, & Cantwell, 1995).

Building on this treatment, in a sample of female adolescents who presented for emergency medical care after attempting suicide, Rotheram-Borus et al. (1996) randomly assigned participants to the SNAP treatment program either alone or in combination with a specialized emergency room (ER) intervention designed to increase treatment compliance. The ER program consisted of three components: (1) training ER staff to work with adolescent suicide attempters and their families, (2) showing a videotape to attempters and their families in the ER to provide families with a better understanding of adolescent suicidality and the course of outpatient therapy, and (3) conducting a brief family treatment session in the ER. The combined intervention was associated with improved treatment compliance, improved family functioning, lower levels of both adolescent and maternal depression, and less adolescent suicidal ideation. These findings suggest that training the ER staff to work with suicidal patients and providing patients and families with psychoeducation are, in and of themselves, useful interventions in decreasing suicidal ideation, even before outpatient treatment is initiated.

Miller and colleagues have developed and validated another approach to intervention with suicidal adolescents, a modification of Linehan et al.'s (1991) Dialectical Behavior Therapy program (Rathus & Miller, 2002). In Dialectical Behavior Therapy for Adolescents (DBT-A), adolescents and their parents participated in skills-training groups, with the goal of improving the family environment and teaching parents skills that they ultimately may use to coach their teens. Parents or other family members are also included in individual therapy sessions when family issues seemed paramount. Initial outcome data have found DBT-A more effective than standard treatment in reducing psychiatric hospitalization, increasing treatment completion rates, and reducing suicide attempts and intent to die (Rathus & Miller, 2002).

Brent (2001) summarized the findings across studies and argued that treatment programs characterized by aggressive outreach, psychoeducation, and skills training to improve the family's communication, problem-solving, and emotion regulation are associated with the greatest reductions in subsequent suicidal behavior. Brent also suggested that most treatment approaches have been insufficient to bring about significant long-term change, and he advocated a long-term treatment approach for this often chronic and recurrent condition.

13. For suicidal adolescents, there is empirical evidence for the effectiveness of which of the following treatments?
   a. confrontation and insight oriented therapy.
   b. humanistic and supportive treatment.
   c. supportive group psychotherapy.
   d. cognitive-behavioral treatment and the development of coping skills.

# EVALUATING RISK OF DOMESTIC VIOLENCE AND VICTIMIZATION

## Distal Risk Factors for Abusers/Perpetrators

*Childhood History.* There is consistent evidence that men who are abusive towards their female partners were exposed to more violence in their childhoods than nonabusive men (Hotaling & Sugarman, 1990). In a large scale study, Hanson, Cadsy, Harris, and LaLonde (1997) found that abusive men are more likely to have witnessed their parents hitting each other and to have been physically abused as children. In addition, this study showed that overall violence in the family during childhood (i.e., hitting among children, between parents, and between parents and children) was higher for men who abused than for nonabusive men.

*Previous Aggression.*    The maxim that *previous behavior is the best predictor of future behavior* holds true in the case of violence against a spouse or significant other (Riggs, Caulfield, & Street, 2000). Longitudinal studies have shown that if a person has previously committed violence against his or her partner, it is a major risk factor for future violence in the relationship (Leonard & Senchak, 1996). Verbal abuse, such as threats of physical violence and demeaning insults, is also positively related to physical violence in a relationship (Sugarman, Aldarondo, & Boney-McCoy, 1996). In addition, several studies have illustrated that male perpetrators of violence against their partners are more aggressive in general, not just in the context of their domestic relationships (Barnett, Fagan, & Booker, 1991). Some research (e.g., Hamberger, Lohr, Bonge, & Tolin, 1996), however, suggests that there may be subgroups of maritally violent men, that is, some who are aggressive outside the home and others who do not engage in violence in other contexts.

14. When applied to domestic violence, the maxim that *previous behavior is the best predictor of future behavior*:
    a. means that we have a way to predict domestic violence with great accuracy.
    b. does not apply to the prediction of domestic violence.
    c. means that those who have not engaged in domestic violence in the past will definitely not do so in the future.
    d. means that there is a heightened risk of future domestic violence among those who have engaged in it in the past.

Although they have been much less commonly studied, females who perpetrate violence against their male partners are an important risk group to consider. In most cases, violence by women toward men in relationships coincides with violence by men toward women (Feld and Straus, 1989). Although women are less likely to seriously injure their male partners, violence by women can be an important marker of violence in a relationship. Riggs et al. (2000) have suggested that wives' aggression towards their husbands places them at increased risk for future victimization by their husbands.

15. The perpetration of violence by females against their male partners is:
    a. so infrequent that it is not regarded as a risk factor.
    b. typically disregarded by their male partners.
    c. likely to result in behavior change on the part of the male partner.
    d. likely to coincide with violence of their male partners toward them .

*Personal Characteristics Associated With Risk for Domestic Violence.*    In terms of demographic factors, younger age and lower socioeconomic status have been linked to domestic violence. Unemployment and minority status are also related to increased risk for domestic violence, but this may be due to their association with lower socioeconomic status (Riggs et al., 2000). Psychological characteristics associated with increased risk for perpetration of domestic violence include high levels of anger and hostility and lower levels of assertive behavior (Eckhardt, Barbour, & Stuart, 1997). In terms of psychopathology, the diagnoses of depression, posttraumatic stress disorder (PTSD), borderline personality disorder, and substance abuse have been shown to be associated with men's perpetration of marital violence (Riggs et al., 2000).

Three basic subtypes of batterers have been identified by a variety of researchers: the family-only batterer, the dysphoric/borderline batterer, and the generally violent/antisocial batterer (Hanson, et al., 1997; Holtzworth-Munroe & Stuart, 1994). The family-only batterers are the most similar to well-adjusted men and have fewer adjustment problems, that is, their violence is less severe than the other two subtypes. The dysphoric/borderline batterers are more insecure and dependent in their intimate relationships, have high levels of subjective distress, and moderately severe criminal histories. The most severe type of batterer is the violent/antisocial batterer. These men have extensive criminal histories, are likely to be violent both inside and outside the home, and have highly abusive backgrounds and unstable adult lives.

16. A psychological characteristic that has been associated with the perpetration of domestic violence is:
    a. a low level of assertive behavior.
    b. an inability to cope with sad affect.
    c. a high level of assertive behavior.
    d. a pessimistic outlook on life.

*Relationship Characteristics Associated With Risk for Domestic Violence.* Relationship satisfaction is generally lower for men who are physically violent with their partners than for men in relationships where there is no violence (Riggs et al., 2000). Although there are notable exceptions and many couples in violent relationships—perhaps as many as half—report relationship satisfaction (Bauserman & Arias, 1992; Riggs et al., 2000), research shows that couples reporting relationship distress are at substantially higher risk for violence. The rates of relationship violence in treatment-seeking couples are three to four times higher than general population rates (Vivian & Malone, 1997). Riggs and colleagues (2000) note that clinicians working with distressed couples should therefore assess marital violence on a routine basis.

17. Relationship satisfaction is:
    a. rarely reported by couples in violent relationships.
    b. reported by nearly half of the couples in violent relationships.
    c. reported by a majority of couples in violent relationships.
    d. not conceivable in a violent relationship.

## Distal Risk Factors for Victims/Survivors

*History of Witnessing Parental Violence and Childhood Victimization.* Victimization in domestic relationships has been linked in numerous investigations to experiences with violence in the family of origin. This includes witnessing violence between one's parents (O'Keefe, 1998) and childhood victimization (Ornduff, Kelsey, & O'Leary, 2001). Although there appears to be strong support for the association between witnessing family violence and victimization in childhood and adult relationships, there is considerable debate as to whether either consistently predicts involvement in violent relationships (e.g., Hotaling & Sugarman, 1990). Despite the controversy, the frequency with which an association has been reported suggests that these experiences be taken, advisedly, as risk factors and be used by the clinician as information about the possibility of risk to the client or patient.

18. There is some evidence that perpetrators of domestic violence and victims of domestic violence often have the following experience in common:
    a. a history of having been violent.
    b. a history of substance abuse.
    c. a history of having been exposed to violence as a child.
    d. a history of enuresis as a child.

*History of Victimization in Adult Relationships.* As Quigley and Leonard (2000) have discussed, violence early in marriage appears to be predictive of subsequent marital violence. Prior violence by the same partner is also related to increased risk of minor and severe physical injuries sustained by abused women (Thompson, Saltzman, & Johnson, 2001). The psychological sequelae of relationship violence may include depression, anxiety, and obsessive compulsive disorder (Axelrod, Myers, Durvasula, Wyatt, & Cheng, 1999; Cascardi & O'Leary, 1992; Gleason, 1993). There are also strong suggestions that having a history of being victimized in an adult relationship is related to revictimization in violent relationships (Kemp, Rawlings, & Green, 1991).

19. Violence early in a marriage:
    a. is not usually repeated.
    b. tends to decrease if the perpetrator is remorseful.
    c. is likely to indicate risk of future violence in the relationship.
    d. is more likely to result in a violent reaction from the victim.

## Proximal Risk Factors for Domestic Violence in Couples

Riggs et al. (2000) have detailed a number of possible risk factors for specific incidents of domestic violence in their review of correlates of perpetration and victimization of such violence.

*Pregnancy.* Pregnancy appears to be a time when women may be at increased risk of victimization. Goodman, Koss, and Russo (1993) reported that the incidence of partner violence is 35% higher in pregnant women as opposed to nonpregnant women, and, among women with an abuse history, the risk of abuse during pregnancy triples. In a stratified prospective cohort analysis, McFarlane, Parker, and Soeken (1995) found that 16% of pregnant women in urban prenatal clinics had been abused during the pregnancy. A literature review by Bohn (1990) revealed an incident of abuse during pregnancy in approximately half of all battered women. Although Riggs et al. (2000) have suggested that there are no data that definitively mark pregnancy as a time of risk for women, there appears to be reason to be alert to pregnancy as a possible risk factor for victimization.

20. When battered women become pregnant:
    a. they are at elevated risk of being abused.
    b. they are more likely to be protected by their male partners.
    c. they are more likely to defend themselves against abusive male partners.
    d. they are more likely to become suicidal.

*Alcohol Use.* Evidence is mounting to show that alcohol consumption is often a critical factor in specific incidents of domestic violence. Thus, Fals-Stewart (2003) found that male-to-female aggression was eight to eleven times more likely to occur on days when men drank than on days of no alcohol consumption in a sample of domestically violent men seeking treatment for either domestic violence or for alcoholism. Furthermore, this research showed that violence was more likely during male partners' drinking or shortly after drinking episodes, as opposed to long after the drinking ceased. Researchers continue to speculate about the mechanisms by which alcohol use contributes to violent behavior—whether by increasing proximal conflict, disinhibiting the perpetrator, or eroding the long-term relationship satisfaction (Fals-Stewart, 2003; Riggs et al., 2000). O' Farrell, Fals-Stewart, Murphy, and Murphy (2003) found that partner violence decreased substantially after alcoholism treatment (from 56% to 25%) and that those patients who remained abstinent were only half as likely (15%) to engage in domestic violence as those who resumed some alcohol use (32%).

21. On days when men who have a history of domestic violence abuse alcohol:
    a. the likelihood of male-to-female aggression is increased greatly.
    b. there is less risk to their partners because the greater risk is when they are sober.
    c. they are more likely to direct their violent tendencies outside the home.
    d. the likelihood of male-to-female aggression has been found to be unchanged.

Cunradi, Caetano, and Schafer (2002) found that in the general population, alcohol related problems for men and women were associated with the severity of intimate partner violence. These data are especially relevant since they were collected from a nonclinical, nonhelp-seeking population. Not only is the batterer's substance abuse a strong risk factor for his or her partner becoming the object of violence but it is also related to the extent of physical injuries that are sustained (Thompson, Saltzman, & Johnson, 2001). Sharps, Campbell, Campbell, Gary, and Webster (2001) reported that perpetrator problem drinking was associated with an eight-fold increase in partner abuse and if the perpetrator was actively drinking, the risk of femicide or attempted femicide was doubled.

22. Following treatment for alcoholism, there is evidence that, for those who remain abstinent, the incidence of partner violence is:
    a. entirely eliminated.
    b. decreased but not substantially.
    c. decreased substantially but not entirely.
    d. unchanged.

Couples should be identified as being at risk of violence if the potential abuser is actively using alcohol, especially if the drinking involves a pattern of bingeing and is reaching problematic levels. Male partners who have a history of violence may be substantially more dangerous when they have been drinking; thus advising female partners to avoid conflict while such men are intoxicated would be prudent and may reduce the risk of violence (Fals-Stewart, 2003).

*Termination of a Relationship.*   The termination of a relationship, especially a violent relationship, may be a situation during which a woman is at increased risk of victimization at the hands of her former partner. It has been well documented that women who are estranged from their partners are at increased risk of abuse and even murder (Wilson, Daly, Wright, 1993). Ellis and Wight (1997) also found a positive association between conjugal violence and estrangement. In a 1998 report, the U.S. Department of Justice stated that women who are separated from their husbands have a rate of victimization that is three times higher than divorced women, and the rate is 25% higher for separated women relative to married women (United States Department of Justice, 1998). Given this information, it is especially important for evaluating clinicians to be aware of the status of the client's relationship and to assist the client in assessing his or her personal risk.

23. Women who have obtained a divorce:
    a. are at greater risk of violence from their former partners than women who have only separated.
    b. are at much less risk of violence from their former partners than women who have only separated.
    c. are at no greater or lesser risk of violence from their former partners than women who have separated.
    d. no longer need to be concerned about possible violence from their former partners.

*Perceived Danger.* Riggs et al. (2000) drew on the results of Weisz, Tolman, and Saunders (2000) to conclude that a woman's belief that her husband may become violent should be treated as a strong risk factor for future violence. A woman's previous experiences of violence perpetrated by her partner are likely to have given her a sense of when she is in danger. Weisz and colleagues found that survivors' predictions of future violence were strongly associated with subsequent violence.

24. There are some findings that women who have experienced partner violence have:
    a. become hypersensitive and tend to overreact to potential threat from male partners.
    b. become unable to perceive threat from their male partners.
    c. no better ability to detect risk of partner violence than anyone else.
    d. a good sense of when they are in danger from their abusive partners.

## Protective Factors for Domestic Violence

It is important to realize that the term *protective factor* does not necessarily refer to something that a potential victim might engage in for the purposes of being safe. Rather, protective factors are simply correlates which, if present, may make victimization or violence a less likely occurrence. When clinicians must come to a decision about the level of risk in a particular situation, it can be useful to include those factors that might be associated with decreased risk in the equation.

The empirical study of protective factors for victimization and violence has not been well developed. One study (Rickert, Wiemann, Kissoon, Berenson, and Kolb, 2002) found that physical violence among women seen in a publicly funded family planning clinic was less likely if they had a higher education level, were older at first intercourse and at first childbirth, and used contraceptives at their last intercourse. Among a sample of Mexican-American women, Lown and Vega (2001) found that good social support was associated with less risk of physical abuse.

25. A factor that has been found to be "protective" when assessing for risk of victimization in violent relationships is:
    a. the presence of children under age 12 in the home.
    b. older age at first childbirth.
    c. the threat of obtaining a restraining order.
    d. maintaining a position of passive resistance.

The research on perpetrators of marital violence has been almost exclusively focused on identifying risk factors. In the course of identifying such risk factors, some studies have noted factors that are, in essence, the opposite of the risk factors and would therefore be likely to reduce risk level. Thus, in their large-scale study including a community sample, Hanson et al. (1997) reported that nonabusive men were less likely than abusive men to have experienced violence during childhood, to have antisocial personality features, to be experiencing subjective distress and marital maladjustment, to have attitudes tolerant of spouse assault, and to engage in impulsive behaviors.

## MANAGING HIGH RISK SITUATIONS AND ACUTE INCIDENTS OF DOMESTIC VIOLENCE

Assessing for risk of domestic violence is a matter to be approached with care and empathy. Among the feelings a battered individual may experience when disclosing his or her victimization or concern about future abuse are fear and shame. It is essential for the interviewer to listen calmly and validate the victim's experience. The common elements of methods for assessing potential relationship violence include asking questions about violence and providing an environment in which the client can feel safe to divulge information about abuse. It is very possible that the abused individual has received negative messages about him or herself from the abusive partner. The victim may have been told that he or she deserves to be hurt or cannot make it on his or her own. The interviewer's job is to listen to the story without judging and to help formulate a plan of action if necessary.

Before it is possible to implement a formal intervention with a potential victim of domestic violence, it is necessary to assess and evaluate the risk factors, the estimated level of potential for harm, and the potential victim's safety resources. Any one of the risk factors discussed above might be a warning sign of potential violence; however, as with any assessment, each of the factors must be taken into consideration with other information provided by the client that might increase or decrease the level of risk. It is especially important to encourage the client to analyze his or her partner's potential for violence and his or her own assessment of personal risk.

It is also essential to plan for safety with the potential victim. Dutton (2001) has referred to safety planning as a skill-building process as opposed to an outcome. She described it as a way of thinking that allows the victim to reflect on his or her situation and make plans to diminish the possibility of harm. Safety planning focuses on developing strategies for specific situations (e.g., when the abusive partner is in the home), or for specific points in time (e.g., following a court proceeding). Clinicians can help create safety plans by doing things such as encouraging the client to plan an escape route from his or her residence or keep important documents and belongings in an accessible place should he or she need to leave home on short notice. If the potential victim is a parent whose children live at home, it is also necessary to plan for the childrens' safety. Additionally, it is recommended that the clinician be familiar with community resources such as shelters and women's support centers that the client may access if seeking help.

26. In dealing with situations in which there is a high risk of victimization, it is essential that the partner at risk:
    a. avoid provoking her partner by taking out a restraining order.
    b. develop strategies to keep herself safe when critical events occur.
    c. try to discuss the partner's anger without being too confrontational.
    d. attempt to be tolerant and understanding.

## KEY TERMS

**behavioral crisis:** a serious disruption of a person's baseline level of functioning such that his or her coping mechanisms are inadequate to restore equilibrium.

**behavioral emergency:** a condition in which an individual is at imminent risk of doing something (or failing to do something) that will result in serious harm or death to self or others.

**distal risk factor:** a risk factor that increases risk for later vulnerability to the outcome of interest. It can be viewed as part of the foundation that makes the outcome in question a possibility.

**protective factor:** a variable that correlates significantly with the inhibition of the outcome of interest (e.g., domestic violence, suicide, etc.); or a variable that makes it less likely that the individual will engage in, or experience, such a negative event.

**proximal risk factor:** a risk factor that is more closely associated in time (i.e., within 6–12 months) with the outcome of interest. The combination of distal and proximal risk factors can lead to the necessary and sufficient conditions for the outcome to occur.

**risk factor:** a variable that correlates significantly with the outcome of interest (e.g., domestic violence, suicide, etc.), and was measured prior to the time of the occurrence of the outcome. Risk factors may be categorized as **distal** or **proximal**.

## DISCUSSION QUESTIONS

1. If you had a family in therapy and a male adolescent member of the family reported that he felt suicidal, what considerations would you go through in evaluating and managing the risk involved?
2. Discuss whether it is possible to predict and prevent all instances of patient suicide and patient violence to others, and why you hold your opinion.
3. Discuss why it is so difficult to conduct prospective studies of the imminent risk of suicide and violence.
4. In regard to estimating the risk of a behavioral emergency (e.g., the risk of suicide or violence), discuss how distal risk factors, proximal risk factors, and protective factors might be used in the process.
5. Based on the evidence presented in this chapter, discuss what past and present family problems or issues might suggest greater or lesser risk of suicide.
6. Discuss the treatment interventions that have been found to have empirical support for treating suicidal adolescents.
7. Based on the evidence presented in this chapter, discuss what distal risk factors might suggest greater risk of domestic violence.
8. Based on the evidence presented in this chapter, discuss some of the major proximal factors that might contribute to partner violence.
9. Discuss how you might handle a therapy situation in which the wife of a young couple reports that her husband physically abused her last night.
10. If the estranged husband of a woman patient has begun to stalk her, how would you advise her in terms of maintaining her safety?

## SUGGESTED FURTHER READING

Kleespies, P. (Ed.). (1998). *Emergencies in Mental Health Practice: Evaluation and Management.* New York: Guilford Press.

This book is organized as a curriculum for instruction on evaluating and managing the behavioral emergencies that mental health clinicians most often encounter. It defines the area of emergency practice, outlines the emergency interview, gives specific, evidence-based information about evaluating for short-term risk of suicide and violence, assists with risk management strategies, and highlights the need for the clinician to be able to deal with the impact that work with emergency cases can have on him or her.

Kleespies, P. (Ed.). (2000). Special Section: An Empirical Approach to Behavioral Emergencies.
Part I: Suicidal Behavior and Self-Injury. *Journal of Clinical Psychology, 56* (9), 1103–1205.
Part II: Violence to Others and Interpersonal Victimization. *Journal of Clinical Psychology, 56* (10), 1237–1369.

This two part Special Section expands upon the above-noted book (Kleespies, 1998) and includes articles on youth suicidal behavior, suicide in the medically and terminally ill, violence risk among youth, risk for domestic violence, and evaluation and intervention with victims of rape.

Rudd, M. D., Joiner, T., & Rajab, M. H. (2001). *Treating Suicidal Behavior: An Effective, Time-Limited Approach.* New York: Guilford Press.

The authors of this book present a framework for evaluating risk and protective factors, estimating the risk of suicide, and intervening in a manner consistent with the level of risk. The book outlines an empirically supported, cognitive-behavioral treatment approach to suicidality.

# REFERENCES[2]

Axelrod, J., Myers, H. F., Durvasula, R. S., Wyatt, G. E., & Cheng, M. (1999). The impact of relationship violence, HIV, and ethnicity on adjustment in women. *Cultural Diversity and Ethnic Minority Psychology, 5,* 1173–1182.

Barnett, O.W., Fagan, R., & Booker, J. (1991). Hostility and stress as mediators of aggression in violent men. *Journal of Family Violence, 6,* 217–241.

Bauserman, S. K., & Arias, I. (1992). Relationships among marital investment, marital satisfaction, and marital commitment in domestically victimized and nonvictimized wives. *Violence and Victims, 7,* 287–296.

Bohn, D. K. (1990). Domestic violence and pregnancy: Implications for practice. *Journal of Nurse Midwifery, 35,* 86–98.

Brent, D. A. (2001). Assessment and treatment of the youthful suicidal patient. *Annals of the New York Academy of Sciences, 932,* 106–131.

Brent, D. A., Bridge, J., Johnson, B. A., & Connolly, J. (1996). Suicidal behavior runs in families: A controlled family study of adolescent suicide victims. *Archives of General Psychiatry, 41,* 888–891.

Cascardi, M., & O'Leary, K. D. (1992). Depressive symptomatology, self-esteem, and self-blame in battered women. *Journal of Family Violence, 7,* 249–259.

Clark, D., & Fawcett, J. (1992). Review of empirical risk factors for evaluation of the suicidal patient. In B. Bongar (Ed.), *Suicide: Guidelines for assessment, management, and treatment* (pp. 16–48). New York: Oxford University Press.

Cohen, L., Test, M., & Brown, R. (1990). Suicide and schizophrenia: Data from a prospective community study. *American Journal of Psychiatry, 147,* 602–607.

Cunradi, C. B., Caetano, R., & Schafer, J. (2002). Alcohol-related problems, drug use, and male intimate partner violence severity among U. S. couples. *Alcoholism: Clinical and Experimental Research, 26,* 493–500.

Dutton, M. A. (2001). Understanding risks to women of intimate partner violence. *National Center for Post-Traumatic Stress Disorder Clinical Quarterly, 10,* 11, 14–16.

Eckhardt, C., Barbour, K. A., & Stuart, G. L. (1997). Anger and hostility in maritally violent men: Conceptual distinctions, measurement issues, and literature review. *Clinical Psychology Review, 17,* 333–358.

Ellis, D., & Wight, L. (1997). Estrangement, interventions, and male violence toward female partners. *Violence and Victims, 12,* 51–67.

Fals-Stewart, W. (2003). The occurrence of partner physical aggression on days of alcohol consumption: A longitudinal diary study. *Journal of Consulting & Clinical Psychology, 71,* 41–52.

Fawcett, J., Scheftner, W., Clark, D., Hedeker, D., Gibbons, R., & Coryell, W. (1987). Clinical predictors of suicide in patients with major affective disorder. *American Journal of Psychiatry, 144,* 1189–1194.

---

[2] A more extensive reference list for this chapter is available from the first author (P.M.K.). The interested reader can request the list by sending an e-mail message to: Phillip.Kleespies@med.va.gov

Feld, S., & Straus, M. (1989). Escalation and desistance of wife assault in marriage. *Criminology, 27*, 141–161.

Gleason, W. J. (1993). Mental disorders in battered women: An empirical study. *Violence and Victims, 8*, 53–68.

Goodman, L. A., Koss, M. P., & Russo, N. F. (1993). Violence against women: Physical and mental health effects. Part I: Research findings. *Applied and Preventive Psychology, 2*, 79–89.

Gutierrez, P., Osman, A., Barrios, F., Kopper, B., Baker, M., & Haraburda, C. (2002). Development of the Reasons for Living Inventory for young adults. *Journal of Clinical Psychology, 58*, 339–357.

Hamberger, L. K., Lohr, J. M., Bonge, D., & Tolin, D. F. (1996). A large sample empirical typology of male spouse abusers and its relationship to dimensions of abuse. *Violence and Victims, 11*, 277–292.

Hanson, R. K., Cadsy, O., Harris, A., & LaLonde, C. (1997). Correlates of battering among 997 men: Family history, adjustment and attitudinal differences. *Violence and Victims, 12*, 191–208.

Holtzworth-Munroe, A. & Stuart, G. L. (1994). Typologies of male batterers: Three subtypes and the differences among them. *Psychological Bulletin, 116*, 476–497

Hotaling, G. T., & Sugarman, D. B. (1990). A risk marker analysis of assaulted wives. *Journal of Family Violence, 5*, 1–13.

Jobes, D. A., & Mann, R. E. (1999). Reasons for living versus reasons for dying: Examining the internal debate of suicide. *Suicide and Life-Threatening Behavior, 29*, 97–104.

Kemp, A., Rawlings, E. I., & Green, B. L. (1991). Post-traumatic stress disorder (PTSD) in battered women: A shelter sample. *Journal of Traumatic Stress, 4*, 137–148.

King, C. A., Segal., H., Naylor, M., & Evans, T. (1993). Family functioning and suicidal behavior in adolescent inpatients with mood disorders. *Journal of the American Academy of Child and Adolescent Psychiatry, 32*, 1198–1206.

Kleespies, P. M., & Dettmer, E. L. (2000). An evidence-based approach to evaluating and managing suicidal emergencies. *Journal of Clinical Psychology, 56*, 1109–1130.

Kleespies, P., Deleppo, J., Gallagher, P., & Niles, B. (1999). Managing suicidal emergencies: Recommendations for the practitioner. *Professional Psychology: Research and Practice, 30*, 454–463.

Leonard, K. E., & Senchak, M. (1996). Prospective prediction of husband marital aggression within newlywed couples. *Journal of Abnormal Psychology, 105*, 369–380.

Lester, D. (1987). Benefits of marriage for reducing risk of violent death from suicide and homicide for White and non-White persons: Generalizing Gove's findings. *Psychological Reports, 61*, 198.

Lewinsohn, P. M., Rohde, P., & Seeley, J. R. (1996). Adolescent suicidal ideation and attempts: Prevalence, risk factors, and clinical impressions. *Clinical Psychology Science and Practice, 3*, 25–46.

Linehan, M. M., Armstrong, H. E., Suarez, A., Allmari, D., & Heard, H. L. (1991). Cognitive-behavioral treatment of chronically parasuicidal borderline patients. *Archives of General Psychiatry, 48*, 1060–1064.

Linehan, M. M., Goodstein, J. L., Nielsen, S. L., & Chiles, J. A. (1983). Reasons for staying alive when you are thinking of killing yourself: The Reasons for Living Inventory. *Journal of Consulting and Clinical Psychology, 51*, 276–286.

Lown, E. A., & Vega, W. A. (2001). Prevalence and predictors of physical partner abuse among Mexican American women. *American Journal of Public Health, 91*, 441–445.

McFarlane, J., Parker, B., & Soeken, K. (1995). Abuse during pregnancy: Frequency, severity, perpetrator, and risk factors of homicide. *Public Health Nursing, 12*, 284–289.

McLean, P. D., & Taylor, S. (1994). Family therapy for suicidal people. *Death Studies, 18*, 409–426.

Miller, A. L., & Glinski, J. (2000). Youth suicidal behavior: Assessment and intervention. *Journal of Clinical Psychology, 56*, 1131–1152.

Murphy, G. (1992). *Suicide in alcoholism.* New York: Oxford University Press.

O' Farrell, T. J., Fals-Stewart, W., Murphy, M., & Murphy, C. M. (2003). Partner violence before and after individually based alcoholism treatment for male alcoholic patients. *Journal of Consulting and Clinical Psychology, 71*, 92–102.

O'Keefe, M. (1998). Factors mediating the link between witnessing interparental violence and dating violence. *Journal of Family Violence, 13*, 39–57.

Ornduff, S. R., Kelsey, R. M., & O'Leary, K. D. (2001). Childhood physical abuse, personality, and adult relationship violence: A model of vulnerability to victimization. *American Journal of Orthopsychiatry, 71*, 322–331.

Peuskens, J., DeHert, M., Cosyns, P., Pieters, G., Theys, P., & Vermote, R. (1997). Suicide in young schizophrenic patients during and after inpatient treatment. *International Journal of Mental Health, 25*, 39–44.

Piacentini, J. C., Rotheram-Borus, M. J., & Cantwell, C. (1995). Brief cognitive-behavioral family therapy for suicidal adolescents. In L. VandeCreek, et al. (Eds.), *Innovations in clinical practice: A sourcebook, Vol. 14* (151–168). Sarasota, FL: Professional Resource Press/Professional Resource Exchange, Inc.

Quigley, B. M., & Leonard, K. E. (2000). Alcohol and the continuation of early marital aggression. *Alcoholism: Clinical and Experimental Research, 24*, 1003–1010.

Rathus, J., & Miller, A. (2002). Dialectical behavior therapy adapted for suicidal adolescents. *Suicide & Life-Threatening Behavior, 32*, 146–157.

Resnick, M. D., Bearman, P. S., Blum, R. W., Bauman, K. E., Harris, K. M., Jones, J. et al. (1997). Protecting adolescents from harm: Findings from the National Longitudinal Study on Adolescent Health. *Journal of the American Medical Association, 278*, 823–832.

Rickert, V. I., Wiemann, C. M., Kissoon, S. D., Berenson, A. B., & Kolb, E. (2002). The relationship among demographics, reproductive characteristics, and intimate partner violence. *American Journal of Obstetrics and Gynecology, 187*, 1002–1007.

Riggs, D. S., Caulfield, M. B., & Street, A. E. (2000). Risk for domestic violence: Factors associated with perpetration and victimization. *Journal of Clinical Psychology, 56*, 1289–1316.

Rotheram-Borus, M. J., Piacentini, J. C., Miller, S., Graae, F., & Castro-Blanco, D. (1994). Brief cognitive-behavioral treatment for adolescent suicide attempters and their families. *Journal of the American Academy of Child and Adolescent Psychiatry, 33*, 508–517.

Rotheram-Borus, M. J., Piacentini, J. C., van Rossem, R., Graae, F., Cantwell, C., Castro-Bianco, D., et al. (1996). Enhancing treatment adherence with a specialized emergency room program for adolescent suicide attempters. *Journal of the American Academy of Child and Adolescent Psychiatry, 35*, 654–663.

Rubenstein, J. L., Heeren, T., Housman, D., Rubin, C., & Stechler, G. (1989). Suicidal behavior in "normal" adolescents: Risk and protective factors. *American Journal of Orthopsychiatry, 59*, 59–71.

Rudd, M. D., & Joiner, T. (1998). The assessment, management, and treatment of suicidality: Toward clinically informed and balanced standards of care. *Clinical Psychology: Science and Practice, 5*, 135–150.

Rudd, M. D., Joiner, T., & Rajab, M. H. (2001). *Treating suicidal behavior: An effective, time-limited approach.* New York: The Guilford Press.

Sharps, P. W., Campbell, J., Campbell, D., Gary, F., & Webster, D. (2001). The role of alcohol use in intimate partner femicide. *American Journal on Addictions, 10*, 122–135.

Spirito, A. (1997). Family therapy techniques with adolescent suicide attempters. *Crisis, 18*, 106–109.

Stack, S. (2000). Suicide: A 15-year review of the sociological literature. Part I: Cultural and economic factors. *Suicide and Life-Threatening Behavior, 30*, 145–162.

Sugarman, D. B., Aldarondo, E., & Boney-McCoy, S. (1996). Risk marker analysis of husband-to-wife violence: A continuum of aggression. *Journal of Applied Social Psychology, 26*, 313–337.

Thompson, M. P., Saltzman, L. E., & Johnson, H. (2001). Risk factors for physical injury among women assaulted by current or former spouses. *Violence Against Women, 7*, 886–899.

U.S. Department of Justice (1998). Violence by intimates: Analysis of data on crimes by current or former spouses, boyfriends, or girlfriends. Washington, DC: Bureau of Justice Statistics.

Vivian, D., & Malone, J. (1997). Relationship factors and depressive symptomatology associated with mild and severe husband-to-wife physical aggression. *Violence and Victims, 12*, 3–18.

Wagner, B. M. (1997). Family risk factors for child and adolescent suicidal behavior. *Psychological Bulletin, 121*, 246–298.

Weisz, A. N., Tolman, R. M., & Saunders, D. G. (2000). Assessing the risk of severe domestic violence: The importance of survivors' predictions. *Journal of Interpersonal Violence, 15*, 75–90.

Wilson, M., Daly, M., & Wright, C. (1993). Uxoricide in Canada: Demographic risk patterns. *Canadian Journal of Criminology, 35*, 263–291.

# COMMON CLIENT PROBLEMS

PART

# III

# DISTRESSED COUPLES

# 11

# Conflict and Disenchantment

Edward F. Kouneski
David H. Olson
*University of Minnesota*

## TRUTH OR FICTION?

\_\_\_ 1. *Using multiple methods, empirical research has classified couples into five types: some are happy, others are distressed.*

\_\_\_ 2. *When a couple is described as stable, it means that both partners have a sense of psychological well being.*

\_\_\_ 3. *Even happy couples have many disagreements and conflicts.*

\_\_\_ 4. *Couples who are disenchanted, or devitalized, rarely attempt to resolve conflict.*

\_\_\_ 5. *Husbands are more realistic than wives are when describing problems in the relationship.*

\_\_\_ 6. *Conflicted couples report more partner abuse than devitalized couples.*

\_\_\_ 7. *Any relationship problem can be solved if couples try their best to cooperate.*

\_\_\_ 8. *If a relationship problem cannot be solved, it is wise to ignore it.*

\_\_\_ 9. *Distressed couples move from conflict to disenchantment in predictable ways.*

\_\_\_ 10. *Complaining about a partner's behavior is not the same as blaming them for a problem in the relationship.*

\_\_\_ 11. *Contempt corrodes a relationship faster than defensiveness.*

\_\_\_ 12. *While actively listening to a partner describe a problem, it is important to suggest ways to solve it.*

\_\_\_ 13. *To help resolve conflict, couples can brainstorm ten or more possible solutions, discuss each, and select one solution to try right away.*

\_\_\_ 14. *A positive action during conflict is to pause the discussion whenever negative behavior is displayed.*

\_\_\_ 15. *Positive behavior during conflict interaction does not include laughing at yourself.*

Unwittingly, couples in distress are on a path that leads from conflict to disenchantment. Each day lived with unresolved issues, negativity, and tension takes them a step closer. Once there, affection for each other and hope in the relationship are lost. The journey takes a toll on each person's health and their children's well being. Marital distress contributes to depression and other psychiatric disorders, compromises immune system functioning, increases vulnerability to disease and illness, and has damaging effects on children's social and emotional development (Gottman, 1998).

These couples can turn back from disenchantment, but it becomes more difficult the longer they wait. How they interpret and approach conflict determines the course of their relationship more than what they argue about or how many disagreements they have. Even happy couples have disagreements, and some have many, but they approach conflict as an opportunity to show that the relationship matters. For happy couples, conflict serves a useful purpose. It punctuates important issues and lets each person stake a claim to the relationship, in effect saying "I'm in this for good, so let's work this out." By giving conflict a positive meaning, couples see more clearly that what they choose to say or do during a conflict matters.

Distress can be prevented if couples recognize early signs of trouble, such as disagreeing on *how to resolve* a problem, not sharing their true concerns and feelings, bickering over many trivial issues, or arguing just to get their own points across (Olson & DeFrain, 2003). If the warnings are ignored, as conflicts go unresolved, couples may soon find themselves blaming each other instead of taking responsibility for their problems—and growing increasingly bitter, resentful, and hostile. As conflicts intensify, valid complaints get erased by criticism, insults, and personal attacks, and these are met by a continual vigilance to defend and protect one's self. Eventually, couples see no choice but to turn away from each other, facing distance and loneliness (Gottman, 1999).

As a family therapist, you will find that these are challenging cases. Too often, couples seek help when the relationship seems beyond repair. To give you a more complete understanding of **couples in distress**, this chapter describes findings and implications from research on couple types conducted with the **ENRICH Inventory** (Kouneski & Olson, 2004; Olson & Fowers, 1993) and by Gottman (1993). It also incorporates insights from Gottman's (1998, 1999) research on marital processes.

ENRICH (the acronym for enriching relationship issues, communication, and happiness) is a relational assessment instrument backed by extensive research. Its norms were calculated with data from more than 250,000 culturally and ethnically diverse couples. The inventory is used by therapists to profile couples on multiple characteristics of their relationship, focusing on strengths and issues (Olson & Olson, 1999). One of its unique features is an empirically derived couple **typology**.

The **ENRICH couple typology** identifies three types of *happy, stable* couples and two types of *distressed, unstable* couples. This distinction is supported by findings from longitudinal research, which revealed that couples classified as distressed at the start were most likely to be separated or divorced three years later (Fowers, Montel, & Olson, 1996).

Research with ENRICH relies on **self-report** data gathered from large, national samples of couples who completed the inventory in couples therapy or at marriage enrichment workshops. Gottman's research relies on **observational** procedures to code the interactions of couples as they complete assigned tasks in a laboratory setting. Gottman's typology classifies couples based on communication styles used during conflict interactions. In addition, his research identifies marital processes that make a relationship healthy or dysfunctional.

These two approaches are vastly different yet they share a common goal—to understand why some marriages succeed and others fail. From different perspectives—insider (self-report) and outsider (observation)—they provide unique, complementary findings. Both represent significant developments in the study of marriage preceded by a long history of typological research.

Typological research has advanced much since Terman (1938, cited in Gottman, 1998) made a pioneering effort. Initially, couple typologies were intuitively derived from in-depth, personal interviews with couples and could not be replicated. Later, empirical methods were introduced and over time became more sophisticated. Yet no typology had wide appeal. Researchers saw that typologies had great potential but were uncertain that potential could ever be realized. This perspective changed when Fitzpatrick (1984) introduced an innovative, rigorous method for classifying couples by their styles of communication. She demonstrated how to capture the complexity of intimate relationships and influenced many other researchers, including Gottman. The new efforts, with ENRICH and by Gottman, have brought couple typologies even closer to their full potential by firmly linking research to practice.

From the profiles of couples presented in this chapter, family therapists can glean insights for developing intervention strategies and actions. Knowing a couple's type, and its associated characteristics, can inform a therapist's initial hypotheses to be tested and reformulated during the course of therapy. By tailoring treatment goals to specific types of couples, with a sound assessment tool, therapists can increase the chances for successful outcomes (Beach & Bauserman, 1990).

1. Disenchanted couples are_____.
   a. disillusioned
   b. relieved
   c. flexible
   d. neutral

2. The most useful typologies are based on _____.
   a. a sound assessment tool
   b. a multidimensional framework
   c. an empirically tested method
   d. all of the above

3. Typologies do NOT promise_____.
   a. insights for treatment planning
   b. realistic profiles of couple types
   c. successful outcomes in therapy
   d. none of the above

## COUPLE CHARACTERISTICS

The ENRICH typology (Fig. 11.1) was derived using cluster analysis with dyadic scores on ten core scales from the ENRICH Inventory. The scales represent domains that were identified after an extensive review of the literature on marital distress. All were proven reliable for research and clinical use (Olson, 1996). The dyadic (**positive couple agreement**) scores reflect couple consensus on what is working well in the marriage.

### Core Profile

Figure 11.1 illustrates the core profile of each couple type. The scales represent either *skills* (Communication, Conflict Resolution), *intimacy* (Family and Friends, Sexual Relationship,

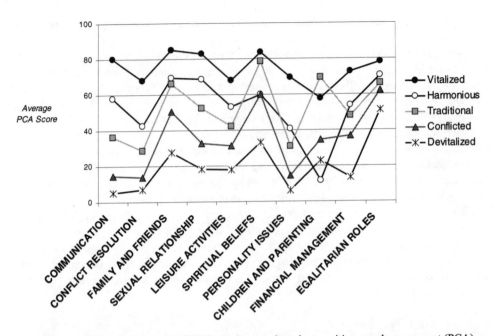

**FIG. 11.1.** Core profile of the ENRICH couple types based on positive couple agreement (PCA) scores—the percentage of items that couples rated as a positive quality in their relationship. (*Source.* Kouneski, 2002.)

Leisure Activities, Spiritual Beliefs), or *stressors* (Personality Issues, Children and Parenting, Financial Management, Egalitarian Roles). Each scale had a large effect in discriminating the types (Kouneski, 2002). The most powerful discriminators, in order, were the two skills, communication and conflict resolution, and a stressor, personality issues. The next most powerful discriminators were three forms of intimacy (social, sexual, and recreational) and another stressor, children and parenting.

4. Which ENRICH scale most effectively discriminates the five couple types? (See Fig. 1.)
   a. communication
   b. egalitarian roles
   c. leisure activities
   d. sexual relationship

5. The core profile of ENRICH couple types does NOT examine_____.
   a. stressors
   b. skills
   c. intimacy
   d. behaviors

## Expanded Profile

To expand its clinical relevance, the ENRICH Inventory was modified, adding items and scales that assess *couple dynamics*, *relationship behaviors*, and *psychological well-being*

**TABLE 11.1**

Expanded Profile of the ENRICH Couple Types

| | Proportions of Couples by Type | | | | |
|---|---|---|---|---|---|
| | *Vitalized* | *Harmonious* | *Traditional* | *Conflicted* | *Devitalized* |
| *Dynamics* | | | | | |
| Couple Closeness | | | | | |
| Both high | 98.4 | 92.7 | 75.6 | 34.8 | 8.2 |
| Both low | .1 | .4 | 1.3 | 13.4 | 38.8 |
| Couple Flexibility | | | | | |
| Both high | 87.8 | 66.7 | 43.9 | 14.9 | 2.1 |
| Both low | — | — | .9 | 11.7 | 34.5 |
| *Behaviors* | | | | | |
| Assertiveness | | | | | |
| Both high | 95.4 | 74.1 | 51.8 | 13.7 | 4.0 |
| Both low | .2 | .3 | 1.9 | 15.0 | 33.1 |
| Avoidance | | | | | |
| Both high | .2 | 1.1 | 4.3 | 17.5 | 36.2 |
| Both low | 85.9 | 58.2 | 28.9 | 9.3 | 2.1 |
| Partner Dominance | | | | | |
| Both high | .2 | 2.8 | 7.3 | 35.3 | 64.1 |
| Both low | 77.1 | 31.6 | 13.0 | 1.6 | .1 |
| *Well Being* | | | | | |
| Self-Confidence | | | | | |
| Both high | 78.5 | 57.5 | 41.1 | 22.6 | 11.2 |
| Both low | .7 | 2.2 | 5.0 | 17.2 | 29.5 |
| Happiness in Life | | | | | |
| Both | 88.7 | 76.1 | 65.9 | 34.2 | 15.8 |
| Neither | 2.1 | 4.3 | 8.0 | 23.7 | 40.7 |
| One only | 9.3 | 19.6 | 26.1 | 42.1 | 43.5 |

*Note:* Categorical labels of "both high" and "both low" indicate whether both partners had high or low individual percentile rank scores (based on national norms). Not displayed is the proportion of couples with moderate or mixed scores.

(Olson & Olson, 1999). Subsequently, analyses were conducted to see if the ENRICH typology could predict additional characteristics of the types (Kouneski, 2002; Kouneski & Olson, 2004).

Table 11.1 displays an expanded profile of each couple type. Couple dynamics were measured by two scales, *Closeness* and *Flexibility*. These scales match two constructs, cohesion and adaptability, from the **circumplex model of marital and family systems** (Olson, 2000). Relationship behaviors were measured by three scales, *Assertiveness*, *Avoidance*, and *Partner Dominance*. Psychological well being was measured by the *Self-Confidence* scale, composed of items on self-esteem and mastery, and a single item, *Happiness in Life*. All of these measures were significantly important predictors of couple type, as were two categorical variables (not displayed), the presence of children and the incidence of partner abuse; these are discussed later as special cases for intervention.

6. In the expanded profile (see Table 2), Vitalized and Harmonious couples are most alike in _____.
   a. closeness and flexibility
   b. closeness and happiness
   c. assertiveness and self-confidence
   d. self-confidence and happiness

## ENRICH COUPLE TYPES

### Happy, Stable Couples

#### Vitalized Type

**Vitalized couples** are the happiest type, with the most relationship strengths and the lowest risk of divorce. They are the most skilled in communication and conflict resolution and have the highest levels of intimacy (social, sexual, recreational, and spiritual). They are the most successful in preventing stressors from interfering with their relationship.

Vitalized couples are the most emotionally connected of the types and the most flexible in adapting to change or stress. They are highly assertive and rarely engage in avoidant or controlling behaviors. These couples are the most likely to understand and respond to each other's needs in the relationship. They have mutually high levels of self-confidence, and they share a sense of happiness and enjoyment in life.

#### Harmonious Type

**Harmonious couples** are happy, with many relationship strengths and a low risk of divorce. They are somewhat skilled in communication and conflict resolution. They have moderate to high levels of intimacy. Notably, they are satisfied with their sexual relationship and their social connections. They handle some stressors better than others. Financial management and personality issues are potential problem areas. (Unlike other couple types, many Harmonious couples do not yet have children; this explains their low level of agreement on parenting.)

Harmonious couples are as close but not as flexible as Vitalized couples. They are somewhat assertive. Typically, they do not avoid conflict. Occasionally, they engage in controlling behaviors. Both partners tend to be self-confident, reporting that they enjoy their lives.

#### Traditional Type

**Traditional couples** are somewhat happy, with more external than internal assets and a low risk of divorce. They are low in agreement on communication and conflict resolution skills (internal assets), but they are highly compatible in spiritual beliefs and parenting practices. They value being part of a religious community and maintaining close connections to family and friends (external assets). They are not very satisfied with their sexual relationship and leisure activities. They have two potential sources of stress: personality issues and financial management.

Traditional couples are nearly as close but not as flexible as Harmonious couples. They tend to be avoidant and controlling at times. There is evidence of some unhappiness and low self-confidence in these marriages.

## Distressed, Unstable Couples

### Conflicted Type

**Conflicted couples** are unhappy, with few strengths and a high risk of divorce. Besides lacking skills in communication and conflict resolution, they experience low levels of intimacy. Spiritual intimacy is not as low as other forms of intimacy. Of the stressors, personality issues rank as the most problematic, followed by incompatible parenting beliefs and practices (see Figure 11.1).

Conflicted couples are disconnected emotionally, and they see the marriage as inflexible and unchanging. They have difficulty asserting what they want or need in the relationship. One partner tends to be more avoidant or more domineering and controlling than the other. Their sense of well-being is fragile. In many of these marriages, one or both of the partners lacks self-confidence and the capacity to feel happy and enjoy life.

### Devitalized Type

**Devitalized couples** are the unhappiest, least satisfied type, with the highest risk of divorce. They avoid communication and conflict resolution. They have the lowest levels of intimacy and the least capacity to deal with stressors of all the types. Personality issues, financial management, and children and parenting are all major sources of stress.

These couples function as disengaged and rigid. They are much less assertive than other types. Both partners view each other as domineering, and one or both partners strictly avoid bringing up issues. In fact, *twice* as many Devitalized as Conflicted couples reported mutually high levels of avoidance and partner dominance; and many more Devitalized couples reported feeling unworthy, incompetent, and unhappy in their lives (see Table 11.1).

7. Traditional couples are MOST compatible (see Fig. 1) in _____.
   a. communication and sexual relationship
   b. family and friends and financial management
   c. children and parenting and spiritual beliefs
   d. spiritual beliefs and egalitarian roles

8. Conflicted couples are LEAST compatible (see Fig. 1) in _____.
   a. sexual relationship, leisure activities, and egalitarian roles
   b. family and friends, spiritual beliefs, and children and parenting
   c. conflict resolution, personality issues, and financial management
   d. communication, conflict resolution, and personality issues

## Gender Differences

Unlike happy couples, distressed couples have discrepant perceptions of their relationship (Kouneski & Olson, 2004). In Conflicted and Devitalized marriages, wives perceived the marriage as more rigid and less egalitarian than did their husbands, and they reported more problems with communication, personality issues, and children and parenting. Husbands reported more satisfaction than their wives, who were not as idealistic as their husbands. The discrepancies were greater for Devitalized than Conflicted couples.

## Satisfaction and Stability

Longitudinal research on couple types (Fowers, Montel, & Olson, 1996) found that Traditional couples were not as satisfied in their marriages as Harmonious couples but Traditional were more stable (i.e., less likely to divorce) than Harmonious. Next to Vitalized, Traditional was the second most *stable* type and Harmonious the second most *satisfied* type. This finding suggests viewing satisfaction and stability as distinct concepts. It also invites more investigation into which couple characteristics are uniquely associated with relationship satisfaction and marital stability.

There are some clues in the core profile (see Figure 11.1) that suggest: a) *satisfaction* may be most influenced by shared positive perceptions of communication, conflict resolution, and personality differences (Harmonious is next to Vitalized in these areas); b) *stability* may be uniquely associated with shared spirituality and compatible parenting (Traditional matches or exceeds Vitalized in these areas); and both satisfaction and stability may be influenced by social support from family and friends (Harmonious matches Traditional in this area). These findings and hypotheses suggest an intervention strategy for Conflicted couples, as discussed below.

## Implications for Intervention

### Strategies

Conflicted couples know that their marriage is shaky and they need to move it to more solid ground. A recommended strategy is to build existing strengths and remove a current stressor. The outcome to expect is a change to a more stable type. It is reasonable for Conflicted couples to move one level up, to bring their strengths to a level that matches the Traditional type.

Conflicted couples' greatest strengths are in two areas, *Family and Friends* and *Spiritual Beliefs* (i.e., they have more positive agreement on these scales than others). Their highest stressor is *Children and Parenting*. Notably, Traditional couples, who are solidly stable, have strong positive agreement in each of these areas (see Figure 11.1).

This recommendation emphasizes the need to focus on strengths and stressors that influence stability. As hypothesized, this means making progress in parenting conflicts, spiritual connectedness, and social support. It does not preclude opening moves toward satisfaction (e.g., suggesting communication and conflict resolution exercises or a long term strategy for personality conflicts). Be advised, however, that some couples will resist efforts to increase satisfaction unless they experience a sense of belonging and stability in the marriage, as explained below.

Of all the types, Devitalized couples seem the most discouraged and unmotivated to develop skills in the relationship. Devitalized couples have fewer clear starting points for problem solving than Conflicted couples, who can identify their issues more readily. Unless Devitalized couples can construct a common view of their issues, let alone their strengths, progress in therapy seems unlikely.

Devitalized couples, in effect, have sacrificed their well being to the marriage, and so have many Conflicted couples. The therapist's challenge is to help these couples generate feelings of self-worth and competence. A recent study revealed that persons with low self-esteem tend to adopt negative views of their partner (and the relationship), and their views reflect how they see themselves (Murray & Holmes, 2000). They lack trust and a sense of belonging in the relationship. They fear rejection and avoid becoming closer or more attached to a partner. A therapist's suggestion to increase closeness or intimacy only provokes anxiety.

Instead of aiming to increase couple closeness, the goal of therapy can be to increase flexibility, to help these marriages become less chaotic and rigid. Flexibility is the ability to change and adapt in response to stress. Alleviating stress can make a difference, helping distressed couples to gain more confidence in the relationship, and in themselves. The couples can be encouraged to discuss parenting beliefs and practices, personality conflicts, financial goals, and roles and responsibilities.

A complementary action is to have couples identify stressors in other areas of life (e.g., work satisfaction, career plans, educational aspirations, personal interests and talents) and begin consulting with each other on these problems and opportunities. By going through this process, couples can show support for each other and, indirectly, become more emotionally connected. They will reach a crossing point for healthy functioning when they can maintain a consistent pattern of supportiveness.

## Caveats

No typology fits everyone perfectly. Despite statistical patterns that can be discerned, there will be exceptions, such as cases that fall near the boundary of two types. Within each type, couples may agree on the same percentage of items but differ how they responded to individual items in the ENRICH Inventory. Therefore, it is important to keep each couple's uniqueness in sight.

Some caution should be exercised in communicating a couple's type, because negative labels may be perceived as pathologizing (i.e., fixed and permanent). Some distressed couples have very few positive perceptions of their relationship, and on receiving the label *Conflicted* or *Devitalized*, they may feel disempowered.

9. Conflicted couples can increase marital stability initially by focusing on _____.
   a. conflict resolution and family and friends
   b. egalitarian roles and sexual relationship
   c. children and parenting and spiritual beliefs
   d. financial management and leisure activities

10. Devitalized couples in therapy do NOT quickly learn to _____.
    a. regulate conflict
    b. increase closeness
    c. cope with a stressor
    d. resolve a problem

11. Typologies are useful for _____.
    a. assigning an individual diagnosis
    b. discovering a couple's unique qualities
    c. predicting a couple's outcome
    d. generating ideas for treatment

12. Labeling couples as Devitalized could be _____.
    a. disconcerting
    b. disempowering
    c. enabling
    d. motivating

## Special Cases

### Couples With Children

It is not unusual for any couple to experience relationship changes during the childrearing years. Closeness and intimacy decline after childbirth; and marriage satisfaction dips during adolescence, coinciding with parent–child communication issues (Olson and DeFrain, 2003). Some couples rebound quickly, but not distressed couples. Of all the types, Conflicted and Devitalized couples have the most stress and conflict that revolves around parenting practices. Yet often this is not their reason for seeking therapy.

*Presenting Issue: Child Behavior.* In many cases, a child behavioral problem is the presenting issue. At first, distressed couples may not be ready or willing to consider how conflict or distance in their relationship contributes to the problem. Couple intervention can begin on first contact, when one of the parents calls to schedule an appointment, by requiring that both parents attend the intake session. Therapists are advised to devote part of the session, or a separate session, to meet with the couple, apart from the child; and inquire about how they are doing as a couple and individually. Surprisingly, couples may feel a sense of relief as they put aside child concerns, momentarily, to focus on their own health and well being.

*Presenting Issue: Couple Distress.* When distressed couples first report parenting strains, some therapists may routinely suggest that they make their own relationship a priority (e.g., hiring a babysitter and going out on dates). In many cases, this is useful. The goal is to get emotionally connected in order to stay united in parenting. This is an unlikely fit, however, for couples who do *not* regard themselves, or each other, highly (Murray & Holmes, 2000).

An alternative approach is to resolve parenting issues and let emotional connectedness evolve. A discussion on parenting beliefs can start by asking couples to reflect on how they were raised and parented, to decide which practices (e.g., discipline, supervision and monitoring, involvement, encouragement) they will carry forward or leave behind. After the discussion, couples may find their views not as far apart as they thought.

No matter how close they come to agreement on parenting, couples need to revisit this topic often. As a child grows and develops, parenting practices need to shift, to stay focused on the child's needs. If parents do not connect to discuss these developments, conflict can resurface. It may also spill over to the child with harmful consequences (Olson & DeFrain, 2003).

Finally, another avenue for intervention targets the couple's sense of competence as parents. Attending a parenting education class is an opportunity to develop competency, with a hidden benefit: Some skills learned in the context of parenting are transferable to the relationship.

### Abuse by Partner

Progress in either skill building or problem solving will be difficult, if not impossible, if partner abuse has been identified. When this is identified, it should become the immediate focus of therapy (Gottman, 1999). Therapists are advised to work within their areas of competency and, if necessary, refer the couple to someone with the requisite skills and experience. (See chapter 14 for diagnosing and treating intimate partner violence.)

In a recent study of the ENRICH couple types, Asai and Olson (2000) found a high incidence of abuse among distressed, unstable couples. Most (72%) Devitalized couples and about half (48%) of Conflicted couples were abusive. (Between 5% and 21% of happy, stable couples reported some form of abuse—physical, verbal, or emotional.) Finding Conflicted couples near evenly split (52% were nonabusive), they concluded: Conflict does not always escalate to violence, and some distressed couples can discuss difficult issues without engaging in abusive behaviors.

13. If partner abuse is reported, therapists without competency in this area can help couples:
    a. find a therapist who specializes in partner violence.
    b. explore a history of abuse in their families of origin.
    c. focus on relationship strengths instead of the abuse.
    d. build communication skills to discuss the abuse.

14. Which couples experience childrearing as extremely stressful?
    a. harmonious and traditional
    b. conflicted and devitalized
    c. devitalized and harmonious
    d. conflicted and traditional

## MARITAL PROCESSES

### Conflict Interaction

#### Happy, Stable Couples

Gottman (1993) observed communication styles that couples used during conflict interactions, and he identified three types of happy, stable couples. *Volatile* **couples** are highly affectionate and emotionally expressive. They argue passionately and have intense disagreements, yet they are happy. *Validating* **couples** value companionship and have a strong sense of togetherness. They handle conflict constructively with a moderate level of emotional expressiveness. *Conflict Avoiding* **couples** are committed and share traditional values. They have a low level of emotional expressiveness and prefer to accept rather than resolve disagreements.

Couples mismatched in communication style (e.g., validating and conflict avoiding) will have stressful interactions, and to varying degrees, engage in the classic pursuer–distancer, or demand–withdrawal, pattern (i.e., one partner's need to discuss an issue is greater than the other's).

Of Gottman's types, volatile couples are the most intriguing, because it seems contradictory that volatility does not create distress. Gottman's scientific explanation is that Volatile couples freely express positive sentiment, and these moments far exceed any negative moments (1999). He found that happy couples maintain at least five positive interactions (e.g., acceptance, affection, interest, joy) for every negative interaction. The 5:1 ratio is a threshold, and couples begin to feel distress when they go below it. In fact, highly distressed couples do not have more positive than negative interactions, rather, they have fewer (a .8:1 ratio).

#### Hostile, Unstable Couples

Gottman also identified two types of distressed, unstable couples, **Hostile–Engaged** and **Hostile–Detached**, which resemble the Conflicted and Devitalized types, respectively. These couples have difficulty regulating conflict. Their interactions are marked by intense, negative

**TABLE 11.2**

A Cascade from Conflict to Disenchantment

| *Sequence of Events* |
| --- |

1. One partner views the other's negative behavior as intense and unprovoked. This perception contributes to feeling overwhelmed and flooded with emotions.
2. A strong urge is felt to do whatever possible to escape. The classic *fight-or-flight* response is engaged.
3. Believing that more unprovoked attacks are certain and it is necessary to stay on guard leads to a state of hypervigilance.
4. In this state, negative attributions are common, such as assigning hostile intent to a partner's actions even when they are neutral, not negative.
5. Defensiveness increases, leading to withdrawal.
6. Commitment to the relationship is questioned, and separation begins to be viewed as a viable solution.
7. Perceiving that problems in the relationship are severe, pervasive, and permanent leads to the decision to handle them alone.
8. Action is taken to construct parallel lives. This brings feelings of isolation and loneliness.

*Note:* Adapted from Gottman, 1999.

behavior and affect. *Hostile–Engaged* couples are highly defensive and overtly hostile. *Hostile–Detached* couples are uninvolved and covertly hostile.

In either case, psychological well being suffers. There were differences in self-confidence and happiness between Conflicted and Devitalized couples (see Table 11.1). Devitalized couples were more inclined to report that they feel unworthy, incompetent, and unhappy in their lives; and this experience was common to both partners. To the extent that Conflicted couples are overtly hostile and Devitalized couples are covertly hostile, it appears that the covert form is the most harmful.

15. Conflicted couples MOST resemble Gottmans' _____ type.
    a. volatile
    b. conflict avoiding
    c. hostile–engaged
    d. hostile–detached

## Distance–Isolation Cascade

Table 11.2 shows a continuous series of events that lead from conflict to disenchantment, based on Gottman's (1999) theory of a ***distance–isolation cascade***. At the top of the cascade, one partner views the other's negative behavior as unprovoked and intense; he or she then feels overwhelmed and flooded with emotion. At the bottom of the cascade, couples feel isolated and lonely and see no solution other than to separate or divorce.

### Corrosive Behavior

The cascade is prompted by negative behaviors such as criticism, contempt, defensiveness, and stonewalling, which Gottman (1998) referred to as the *Four Horsemen of the Apocalypse* (Table 11.3). Some behaviors are more corrosive than others. Relationship satisfaction is

**TABLE 11.3**

Negative and Corrosive Behaviors

*"Four Horsemen of the Apocalypse"*

1. *Criticism*. Denigrating a partner's character or personality by assigning blame to them for problems in the relationship.
2. *Contempt*. Expressing extreme hostility and intending to do harm to a partner by insulting or emotionally abusing them.
3. *Defensiveness*. Continually whining and making excuses, denying responsibility for any part played in contributing to a problem.
4. *Stonewalling*. Emotionally shutting down, withdrawing, and avoiding interaction with a partner, notably when conflict is intense.

*Note:* Adapted from Gottman, 1999.

most affected by wives' criticism, husbands' stonewalling, and both husbands' and wives' defensiveness or contempt.

## Conflict Escalation

As negative behaviors accumulate and are not balanced by positive moments, couple conflict escalates to a more destructive level marked by the exchange of negative affect. Gottman's (1999) term is ***negative affect reciprocity***: When a partner expresses hostility, the other does too. At this level, **negative attributions** and perceptions take hold; for example, couples perceive negativity as inherent to the relationship, or they attribute it to a partner's character flaw. (In contrast, happy couples perceive each other's negativity as situational and attribute it to being overtired or stressed.) An attempt to repair the interaction only provokes more negativity. Apologies are not made after these arguments. Couples stay disconnected.

## Physiological Effects

Conflict interactions of high intensity are complicated by physiological effects, such as a rise in blood pressure and stress hormones. Physiological **reactivity** creates a heightened state of arousal, which impedes a person's ability to process information (Gottman, 1999). According to Gottman (1998), men experience strong effects, which may explain why they tend to avoid conflict.

16. A sign of defensiveness is _____.
    a. emotionally shutting down
    b. denying responsibility
    c. expressing hostility
    d. all of the above

17. Which negative behaviors are most damaging?
    a. husbands' stonewalling, wives' criticism, either partner's defensiveness or contempt
    b. husbands' stonewalling, wives' defensiveness, either partner's criticism or contempt
    c. husbands' criticism and stonewalling, wives' defensiveness and contempt
    d. husbands' contempt, wives' criticism, either partner's defensiveness or stonewalling

## Suggestions for Intervention

Gottman (1998) discussed what to expect in the first session with distressed couples. In summary, they may express extreme dissatisfaction, display no signs of affection, reveal dissimilar goals and values, call conflict pointless, and show low self confidence.

### Immediate Goal

Gottman (1999) believes that couples need to immediately experience how to create a dialogue on longstanding issues. He seeks dramatic change in the first session and schedules it to last three hours. He advises couples that there are perpetual problems, such as personality conflicts, and it is best *not* to ignore them. Dealing with a perpetual problem is much like learning to adjust with a permanent physical illness or disability. It cannot be cured but it can be managed by discussing and adopting coping strategies. Gottman emphasizes that couples return to this discussion regularly, to discuss how the strategies are working and make other adjustments as needed.

### Treatment Focus

For future sessions, there is some flexibility in choosing an intervention. Gottman (1999) advises behavior, perceptions, and physiology all have reciprocal effects; therefore, a change in one area will bring about change in the other areas. A therapist may choose to intervene on negative behaviors that corrode the relationship by increasing the balance of positive-to-negative interactions; or challenge the couple's negative perceptions and attributions, which escalate conflict; or focus on physiological reactivity, teaching couples to initiate soothing and calming techniques for each other and themselves.

### Action Plan

Couples therapy often focuses on building communication skills. This is a good place to start, but it is not a final outcome. For couples in distress, skill building alone may have only temporary effects; for lasting effects, it must be complemented by pattern change. Learning to use communication skills is an intermediary step toward altering dysfunctional patterns of behavior and the marital processes that enable them.

For example, Gottman (1999) found a consistent pattern. Distressed wives tended to initiate conflict and their husbands tried to avoid it. Also, wives started these discussions harshly, and their husbands were not influenced by their opinions. Communication skills can help alter this pattern. Wives can learn how to raise issues gently and kindly, and husbands can learn how to become meaningfully involved in the discussion (e.g., by showing interest, listening closely).

Based on Gottman's (1999) insights, there are two highly important goals for distressed couples to achieve.

1. *Be less tolerant of negative behavior*. Distressed couples become sensitized to negativity, and respond to it only if it escalates. They need to recognize this behavior sooner, before it intensifies (i.e., lower their threshold for negativity). It is also important to reach an understanding that the behavior must be dislodged quickly.
2. *Increase positive affect in conflict and everyday interactions*. To imbue positivity into their relationship, couples need to become curious about each other's point of view, and show active interest and acceptance. They need to find humor in their interactions, and be open to expressing joy.

To use a sports metaphor, couples can tackle the problem from high (increasing positivity) and low (reducing negativity). Distress will fade as they experience more positive than negative moments in the relationship and consistently exceed the magic ratio (5:1).

18. In the first therapy session, distressed couples will:
    a. express extreme dissatisfaction.
    b. show few or no signs of affection.
    c. describe different goals and values.
    d. all of the above.

19. What can couples do about a perpetual problem?
    a. dismiss it as unsolvable
    b. continue to try to solve it
    c. discuss how to cope with it
    d. ignore it until it worsens

## TOOLS FOR PRACTICE

ENRICH is a component of the **PREPARE/ENRICH program** for marriage and couples education. It is useful for both prevention and clinical intervention. ENRICH is aligned with strength based approaches to couples therapy that emphasize behavioral change to build skills and competencies in an intimate relationship. Its philosophy is to empower couples to effect change. It encourages couples to openly discuss issues and strengths in the relationship, to practice assertiveness and active listening skills, and to transform conflict interaction into a positive experience.

20. The ENRICH program offers:
    a. a philosophy of empowerment.
    b. practical tools for skill building.
    c. insights for therapeutic intervention.
    d. all of the above.

21. Objectives of the ENRICH program do NOT include:
    a. encouraging open discussion of issues.
    b. resolving all of the problems identified.
    c. increasing strengths in the relationship.
    d. teaching couples to actively listen.

### Relational Assessment

The ENRICH Inventory is an essential part of the program. This 165-item questionnaire is administered separately to both partners. Individual responses are compared to determine how close they are in agreement. Sample items are shown in Table 11.4. The couple's score on an item is coded in one of three ways. These distinctions are useful for treatment planning. *Positive agreement items* represent strengths in the relationship that serve as resources to call upon in resolving issues. *Negative agreement items* suggest that a couple has the same view of a

**TABLE 11.4**

Comprehensive Relational Assessment: Based on the ENRICH Inventory

| Scales | Sample Items |
| --- | --- |
| *Core Profile* | |
| Communication | "My partner is a very good listener." |
| Conflict Resolution | "At times, I feel some of our differences never get resolved." |
| Family and Friends | "I really enjoy spending time with my partner's family." |
| Sexual Relationship | "I am satisfied with our openness in discussing sexual topics." |
| Leisure Activities | "My partner has too many activities or hobbies." |
| Spiritual Beliefs | "Sharing spiritual values helps our relationship remain strong." |
| Personality Issues | "My partner sometimes makes comments that put me down." |
| Children and Parenting | "We agree on how to discipline our children." |
| Financial Management | "We have trouble managing money." |
| Egalitarian Roles | "I do more than my share of the household tasks." |
| *Expanded Profile* | |
| Closeness | "We consult each other on all important decisions." |
| Flexibility | "We are creative in handling our differences." |
| Assertiveness | "I can express my true feelings to my partner." |
| Avoidance | "I go out of my way to avoid conflict with my partner." |
| Partner Dominance | "Sometimes I am concerned about my partner's temper." |
| Self-Confidence | "I can do just about anything I decide to do." |

*Note:* All scales contain ten items, except the last four, which contain eight items.

problem; these can be starting points for problem solving. *Disagreement items* reveal divergent perspectives and sometimes reflect uncertainty or a reluctance to reveal one's true concerns.

22. The term "positive couple agreement" refers to _____.
    a. a dyadic score
    b. similar perceptions
    c. couple consensus
    d. all of the above

23. The term "negative agreement" refers to problems on which couples have _____.
    a. the same perspective
    b. intense disagreement
    c. found a solution
    d. not reached consensus

24. "I can express my true feelings to my partner" is an example of _____.
    a. assertiveness
    b. conflict resolution
    c. emotional intimacy
    d. self-confidence

25. "We consult each other on all important decisions" is an example of _____.
    a. assertiveness
    b. couple closeness
    c. egalitarian roles
    d. partner dominance

**TABLE 11.5**

Constructive Conflict Resolution

*A 10-Step Procedure for Couples*

1. Set a time and place for discussion.
2. Clearly define the problem or issue of disagreement.
3. Have each person acknowledge their own part in contributing to the problem.
4. List past attempts that were not successful to resolve it.
5. Brainstorm at least ten ideas for possible solutions.
6. Discuss and evaluate each of the possible solutions.
7. Agree on one solution to try.
8. Have each person identify how they will work toward this solution.
9. Schedule a follow-up meeting to discuss progress.
10. Reward each other for collaborating to reach the solution.

*Source.* Olson and Olson, 2000.

## Communication Skills

The *Wish List* exercise is one of several used in the ENRICH program (Olson & Olson, 1999). It encourages couples to be assertive and use active listening skills. Each partner makes three requests—one at a time, taking turns—for something they would like their partner to change or do more often. The speakers are encouraged to use "I" statements to describe how they experience a problem behavior. The listeners are encouraged to paraphrase the content of the request and reflect the partner's feelings and concerns. In this exercise, it is not necessary to reach an agreement. Active listening takes effort. It is not a natural form of communication (Gottman, 1998); however, it is useful. It prepares couples to accept influence from each other, because couples intentionally listen to understand each other's perspective.

## Conflict Resolution

### Procedure

The ENRICH *Ten Steps for Resolving Couple Conflict* are displayed in Table 11.5. This procedure was developed after reviewing current research and theory on conflict resolution (Olson & Olson, 1999). This procedure encourages individual reflection, self-disclosure, and personal commitment. Couples first solve a disagreement with the therapist present. Their assignment is to select another problem to discuss at home and report on their progress at the next session. Couples are informed that the goal is for both partners to be satisfied with the outcome. This requires a willingness to discuss issues openly, explore alternatives, and make decisions together.

26. Using the 10-step conflict resolution procedure, for an identified problem couples do NOT discuss:
    a. behavior that contributes to it.
    b. past attempts to solve it.
    c. how to sabotage the agreed solution.
    d. how to achieve the agreed solution.

**TABLE 11.6**

Positive Conflict Interaction

*Guidelines for Couples*

1. Bring an open mind, truly intent on understanding your partner's perspective.
2. Let yourself feel affection for your partner and genuinely express it.
3. Notice times when you can compliment your partner, and carry through.
4. Show active interest with body language (e.g., leaning in, looking each other in the eye).
5. Stay focused on the issue in the present, without bringing up issues from the past.
6. To be assertive, state what you need or want, simply and directly.
7. Retell your message, if uncertain that it was heard.
8. To actively listen, reflect back, or paraphrase, what you heard.
9. Ask clarifying questions, if necessary, to fully understand your partner's concerns.
10. Resist attacking, blaming, or withdrawing.
11. Devise a list of rules for fair fighting and agree to cry "foul" when they are violated.
12. Whenever necessary, call a brief "time-out" and return to the discussion.
13. Take responsibility for your own feelings and behavior.
14. Avoid threats and ultimatums.
15. Use humor appropriately to relieve tension, and be able to laugh at yourself.

*Note:* Adapted from Olson and DeFrain, 2003.

## Guidelines

Guidelines on how to argue constructively are useful for distressed couples, because their conflicts are marked by negativity and they do not easily reach agreements. For constructive conflict interaction, many strategies have been recommended (see Olson & DeFrain, 2003), such as those listed in Table 11.6. Gottman (1999) advises that couples make and accept repair attempts (e.g., apologizing, making amends) as often as needed during the discussion. He also emphasizes the need for couples to dislodge disruptive, negative behaviors before they are reciprocated (e.g., cry "foul"); and if couples miss these opportunities, therapists must intervene.

27. Tips for couples to argue constructively do NOT include:
    a. actively listening to a partner's concerns.
    b. using body language to communicate nonverbally.
    c. crying "foul" to interrupt a partner's hostile behavior.
    d. avoiding humor if the argument intensifies.

28. Behavior that disrupts problem solving does NOT include:
    a. complaining about hurt feelings.
    b. keeping silent when criticized.
    c. bringing up past issues.
    d. blaming your partner.

29. To communicate active interest *nonverbally* without provoking hostility:
    a. make eye contact, recline back.
    b. glance away, recline back.
    c. make eye contact, lean forward.
    d. glance away, lean forward.

30. An idea can be turned into a solution if a partner avoids:
    a. persuading the other to accept it.
    b. judging it by first impressions.
    c. suggesting too many ideas.
    d. all of the above.

---

In this chapter, we have closely examined the characteristics of happy and distressed couples by describing the healthy and dysfunctional processes in these marriages to show the path from conflict to disenchantment. We have emphasized using an empirically sound relational assessment tool and the value of using a typological framework in clinical practice to inform intervention. A typology must be intuitively appealing, so that you can see it fitting naturally into your own theoretical framework. It must also make an authentic impression on couples, reflecting the reality they are experiencing in their relationship.

Science often illuminates the wisdom in proverbs. Leo Tolstoy (1992) opened his novel *Anna Karenina* with, "All happy families resemble one another, each unhappy family is unhappy in its own way." Of the ENRICH couple types, Vitalized couples embody the ideal family. Positive interactions and relationship strengths fill their marriages. Harmonious and Traditional couples have strengths too but these need to be solidified and expanded in order to sustain a happy, stable marriage. Absorbed by miseries, Conflicted and Devitalized couples do not appreciate or value their relationships, but change is possible if they begin again to care for each other's well being. With research insights on what makes marriages succeed or fail, family therapists can help couples create a vision of marital happiness toward which the partners can aspire.

## KEY TERMS

**circumplex model of marital and family systems:** Supported by theory and research, describes couple dynamics in two essential areas: closeness (cohesion) and flexibility (adaptability). Couple communication skills facilitate change, for example, to increase closeness.

**closeness:** An indicator of couple functioning based on the Circumplex Model. Close couples are emotionally connected and rely on each other for support.

**conflict avoiding couples:** Highly committed couples that prefer to accept rather than resolve disagreements; a happy, stable type identified by Gottman.

**conflicted couples:** A dissatisfied, unstable ENRICH type with some compatibility on spirituality, family connections, and friendships. They have many personality issues, unresolved conflicts, and communication problems (similar to Hostile–Engaged).

**couples in distress:** Extremely unhappy, dissatisfied with their relationship, and unstable,— likely to divorce. Two types are Conflicted and Devitalized.

**devitalized couples:** The most dissatisfied and unstable ENRICH type with no clearly identifiable strengths. In a state of disenchantment: disillusioned and disengaged (similar to Hostile–Detached).

**distance–isolation cascade:** A sequence of events that leads from conflict to disenchantment, prompted by intense conflict over an extended period of time.

**ENRICH Inventory:** A multidimensional, self-report questionnaire used for relational assessment and treatment planning. Identifies issues at various levels, for example, individual, couple, and contextual.

**ENRICH couple typology:** An empirically derived typology of couples based on cluster analysis with positive couple agreement scores on ten scales from the ENRICH Inventory.

**flexibility:** An indicator of couple functioning based on the circumplex model. Flexible couples share leadership and make decisions together.

**Four Horseman of the Apocalypse:** Refers to four negative behaviors that corrode a couple's relationship—criticism, contempt, defensiveness, and stonewalling.

**harmonious couples:** A highly satisfied, somewhat stable ENRICH type with moderate communication skills, an enjoyable sexual relationship, and close connections to friends and family.

**hostile–detached:** Covertly hostile couples, disengaged from conflict; a distressed, unstable type identified by Gottman.

**hostile–engaged:** Overtly hostile couples, continually engaged in conflict; a distressed, unstable type identified by Gottman.

**negative affect reciprocity:** An exchange of negative affect, for example, when one person expresses hostility, the other responds in kind. Signals conflict has escalated to a new, high level.

**negative attributions:** Negative perceptions and interpretations of a partner's behavior, for example, assigning hostile intent to neutral behavior.

**observation:** A research method typically applied in a laboratory setting that relies on coding the behavior of couples interacting on an assigned task.

**positive couple agreement (PCA):** A dyadic score that represents the percentage of items partners rate similarly as a positive aspect of the relationship.

**PREPARE/ENRICH Program:** A preventive approach to couples therapy, widely used for marriage and couples education. Encourages couples to openly discuss issues and build relationship strengths.

**reactivity:** A physiological response induced after intense, longstanding conflict. Causes heightened states of arousal that impede information processing abilities.

**self-report:** A research method that relies on questionnaires to identify individual beliefs, attitudes, perceptions, and behaviors.

**traditional couples:** A somewhat satisfied, highly stable ENRICH type, with highly compatible views on spirituality, parenting, and family connectedness (similar to Conflict Avoiding type).

**typology:** A system of classification placing couples into distinct groups, or types.

**validating couples:** Closely connected couples that value companionship and are effective at problem solving with moderate displays of emotion; a happy, stable type identified by Gottman.

**vitalized couples:** The most satisfied, stable ENRICH type with excellent communication and conflict resolution skills and very few personality conflicts.

**volatile couples:** Highly affectionate, emotionally expressive couples that argue passionately; a happy, stable type identified by Gottman.

## DISCUSSION QUESTIONS

1. Summarize the characteristics of happy and distressed types of couples.
2. Describe how Conflicted and Devitalized couples differ from each other.
3. Describe an intervention strategy for couples unmotivated to build conflict resolution skills.

4. Discuss intervention strategies for distressed couples who are raising children.
5. Relying on their profile, explain why Devitalized couples are the most abusive type.
6. Explain why Volatile couples are happy—not hostile—even though they have intense conflict.
7. Discuss two observational findings that cannot be revealed by a couple's self-report.
8. Describe what happens during the cascade from conflict to disenchantment.
9. Outline an approach to help couples constructively engage in conflict.
10. Discuss the strengths and limitations of using couple typologies in therapy.

## SUGGESTED FURTHER READING

Berger, R., & Hannah, M. T. (Eds.) (2000). *Preventive approaches in couples therapy*. Philadelphia: Brunner/Mazel.

An informational resource on marriage and couples education programs. Identifies prevention principles and practices relevant to clinical intervention.

Doherty, W. J. (2001). *Take back your marriage: Sticking together in a world that pulls us apart*. New York: Guilford Press.

A practical guide helping married couples handle common stressors and everyday concerns they face in contemporary society.

Gottman, J. M. (1999). *The marriage clinic: A scientifically based marital therapy*. New York: W.W. Norton.

A resource to understand the dynamics of couple interaction and effective ways to intervene. Contains checklists and questionnaires for relational assessment.

Olson, D. H., & Olson, A. K. (2000). *Empowering couples: Building on your strengths*. Minneapolis: Life Innovations, Inc.

A workbook for couples to build a happy, stable relationship. Contains couple exercises and assignments useful in therapy and provides a framework for conducting couple workshops.

## REFERENCES

Asai, S. G., & Olson, D. H. (2000). *Spouse abuse and marital system: Based on ENRICH*. Retrieved May 11, 2003, from Life Innovations, Inc. Web site: http://www.lifeinnovations.com/pdf/abuse.pdf

Beach, S. R. H., & Bauserman, S. A. K. (1990). Enhancing the effectiveness of marital therapy. In F. D. Fincham & T. N. Bradbury (Eds.), *The psychology of marriage* (pp. 402–419). New York: Guilford Press.

Fitzpatrick, M. A. (1984). A typological approach to marital interaction: Recent theory and research. *Advances in Experimental Social Psychology, 18*, 1–47.

Fowers, B. J., Montel, K. H., & Olson, D. H. (1996). Predicting marital success for premarital types based on PREPARE. *Journal of Marital and Family Therapy, 22*, 103–119.

Gottman, J. M. (1993). The roles of conflict engagement, escalation, and avoidance in marital interaction: A longitudinal view of five types of couples. *Journal of Consulting and Clinical Psychology, 61*, 6–15.

Gottman, J. M. (1998). Psychology and the study of marital processes. *Annual Review of Psychology, 49*, 169–197.

Gottman, J. M. (1999). *The marriage clinic: A scientifically based marital therapy*. W. W. Norton: New York.

Kouneski, E. F. (2002). *Five types of marriage based on ENRICH: Linking intrapersonal and interpersonal characteristics*. Unpublished doctoral dissertation, University of Minnesota, Twin Cities.

Kouneski, E. F., & Olson, D. H. (2004). A practical look at intimacy through the lens of the ENRICH couple typology. In D. J. Mashek & A. Aron (Eds.), *Handbook of closeness and intimacy* (pp. 117–133). Mahwah, NJ: Erlbaum.

Murray, S. L., & Holmes, J. G. (2000). Seeing the self through a partner's eyes: Why self-doubts turn into relationship insecurities. In A. Tesser, R. B. Felson, & J. M. Suls (Eds.), *Psychological perspectives on self and identity* (pp. 173–198). Washington, DC: American Psychological Association.

Olson, D. H. (2000). Circumplex Model of Marital and Family Systems. *Journal of Family Therapy, 22,* 144–167.

Olson, D. H. (1996). *PREPARE/ENRICH counselor's manual: Version 2000*. Minneapolis, MN: Life Innovations, Inc.

Olson, D. H., & DeFrain, J. (2003). *Marriages and families: Intimacy, diversity, and strengths* (4th ed.). New York: McGraw-Hill.

Olson, D. H., & Fowers, B. J. (1993). Five types of marriage: An empirical typology based on ENRICH. *The Family Journal: Counseling and Therapy for Couples and Families, 1*, 196–207.

Olson, D. H., & Olson, A. K. (1999). PREPARE/ENRICH program: Version 2000. In R. Berger & M. T. Hannah (Eds.), *Preventive approaches in couples therapy* (pp. 196–216). Philadelphia: Brunner/Mazel.

Tolstoy, L. (1992). *Anna Karenina* (L. S. Maude & A. Maude, Trans.). New York: Knopf.

# 12

# Separation, Divorce, and Remarriage

Craig A. Everett
*Arizona Institute for Family Therapy*

Steve E. Livingston
*Florida Department of Education*

Lee Duke Bowen
*Mercer University School of Medicine*

## TRUTH OR FICTION?

___ 1. *The divorce rate for second marriages is higher than for first marriages.*

___ 2. *Divorce is a systemic process that has distinct and predictable stages for most couples and families.*

___ 3. *The pre-divorce phase is a time of reorganization for couples and families.*

___ 4. *The spouse being left in a divorce usually feels a sense of relief.*

___ 5. *Children experiencing divorce commonly struggle with feeling guilty or responsible for their parents' divorce.*

___ 6. *Retaining control in the decision-making process is a primary advantage of using divorce mediation.*

___ 7. *Utilizing the adversarial divorce process increases cooperative co-parenting after the divorce.*

___ 8. *Divorce education programs consist of information and skill-building programs.*

___ 9. *Sustained reliance on the use of fantasy to solve marital dissatisfaction is helpful.*

___ 10. *Physical separation is the least dramatic part of the divorce process.*

___ 11. *Pseudo-reconciliation is an effective therapeutic technique.*

___ 12. *Some separated couples consider reconciliation in their marriage in reaction to entering the legal process of divorce.*

___ 13. *The entrance of a remarried partner can create an imbalance in the system.*

___ 14. *Parents are responsible for the well-being of children throughout the divorce process.*

___ 15. *Partners who experience increased ambivalence never experience feelings of anger toward one's partner.*

Divorce is a social phenomenon that touches a significant proportion of American families each year. It has been estimated that up to 75% of individuals and families seeking services from marriage and family therapists are dealing with issues related in some way to relationship and family dissolution. Therefore as a family therapist you must have a sound systemic theoretical and clinical foundation in the areas of separation, divorce, and remarriage to successfully treat families experiencing divorce. The goals of this chapter are as follows:

1. To explain the divorce process from a systemic perspective,
2. To present clinical intervention strategies for use with divorcing families,
3. To present concepts and terms related to the divorce process, and
4. To assist in your preparation for licensure as a marriage and family therapist.

1. Which of the following is *not* cited as a reason for divorce replacing death as the most common ending for marriage?
   a. increased life span
   b. changes in the legal system
   c. changing roles for men
   d. changing biopsychosocial roles for women

## THE POTENTIAL FOR DIVORCE—THE DEMOGRAPHICS

The potential for divorce in the United States continues to be high. Historically and across all cultures, those who entered marriage expected that the marriage would last a lifetime. The American culture has supported marriage and it has been estimated that about 90% of the adult population will marry at least once in their lifetime. However, during the twentieth century, divorce has replaced death as the most common reason for the end of marriages. The population's increased lifespan, changing biopsychosocial roles for women, changes in social values, and changes in the legal system have been cited as responsible for the shift to divorce as the endpoint of most marriages (Pinsof, 2002).

The rate of divorce increased dramatically in the last half of the twentieth century, peaking in 1985 at 55% of U.S. marriages (Cherlin, 1992). Recent demographics indicate that divorce rates have leveled off since the 1980s, maintaining a rate of approximately 50% of first marriages. The divorce rate for second marriages is higher with an average of approximately 60% ending in divorce.

A variety of other developmental and demographic variables also affect the divorce rates (NCHS, 1998). For example, the highest divorce rates occur in marriages within the first seven years and as children reach adulthood and leave the nuclear home. Other variables related to family dynamics and divorce include the following:

- The younger the age at the time of first marriage, the greater the rate of divorce.
- The shorter the length of courtship, the higher the rate of divorce.
- The rate for Caucasians in the United States is approximately 50%.
- The rate for African Americans in the United States is higher at 60%.
- The rate is lower for individuals who reported a religious affiliation.
- Additional variables that increase the divorce rate include a family's history of divorce, substance abuse, mental illness, financial stress, individual immaturity, and developmental life crises.

# THE DIVORCE PROCESS I—THE STAGES

Marriage and family therapists view divorce as a systemic process that has distinct and predictable stages. Early sociological and clinical works tended to focus solely on independent causes of divorce and its consequences for *individuals*. These works often failed to take into account the systemic nature of divorce or its identification as a particular phase in a *family's* life cycle. The literature has gradually shifted to focus on the broader systemic nature of divorce and understanding it as a crisis within the larger process of the family's development. Divorce precipitates a **transitional life crisis** that influences all levels of the family's system (i.e., its **subsystems** and family-of-origin system). The crisis affects not only the individual members (i.e., parents and children), their social support systems, and intergenerational members, but also relationship patterns, the definition of subsystems, and **external** and **internal** boundaries.

2. All of the following are systemic components that are important to the assessment of divorcing couples and the development of systemic treatment plans *except*:
   a. family rules.
   b. family boundaries.
   c. attorney selection.
   d. intergenerational influences.

For the clinician, evaluating the interactive process of the family and using a thorough systemic assessment is critical for assisting families and individuals in surviving and adjusting to this difficult life crisis. The clinician must be able to assess the family's life experiences systemically across a continuum from pre-divorcing interactions to post-divorcing adjustments. Systemic components important to this assessment and the development of treatment strategies include (Nichols, 1996; Nichols & Everett, 1986):

- **Family roles**
- **Family rules**
- The **system's hierarchy**
- Family **boundaries-open, closed,** and **diffuse**
- Systemic and intergenerational **alliances** and **coalitions**
- Intergenerational influences
- External family support systems

## The Stages of the Divorce Process

The clinical literature has identified at least three major **stages of the divorce process** (see Everett & Volgy, 1991; Kaslow, 1981; Kaslow & Schwartz, 1987; Sprenkle & Gonzalez-Doupe, 1996):

*Stage 1*—Pre-Divorce Issues
*Stage 2*—The Decision to Divorce
*Stage 3*—Post-Divorce Restructuring and Remarriage

In the following sections we will describe the components of each stage, their clinical aspects, and potential clinical interventions.

3. An increasing sense of marital dissatisfaction is most often a precursor to which of the following?
   a. the separation process
   b. the remarriage process
   c. the celebration process
   d. the recommitment process

## Stage 1—Pre-Divorce Issues: Emotional Decoupling

This is a time in the relationship during which a spouse, or the couple jointly, begins to experience a variety of emotions that reflect a growing dissatisfaction or unhappiness with the marriage. These emotions may range from doubt and frustration to anger and depression, and may lead to a variety of distancing behaviors that are associated with a decline in marital intimacy and an increase in marital dissatisfaction (Kressel, 1985). This increasing sense of marital dissatisfaction is often a precursor to separation. It may also evolve due to a broad range of stressors. The accumulation of these stressors is called *clustering* (Guerin, Fay, Burden, & Kautto, 1987).

A spouse's growing dissatisfaction with the marriage and resultant distancing in the relationship is referred to systemically as a process of **emotional decoupling** (Everett & Volgy, 1991). Gradually this decoupling leads to a spouse's disengagement from expected family and couple roles, and a withdrawal of loyalties to the family system. Specific steps in this pre-divorce stage are described by Everett & Volgy (1991).

4. Feelings of ambivalence usually involve all but one of the following:
   a. doubt
   b. anxiety
   c. certainty
   d. fear

5. The more one engages in the fantasy solution to problems in one's marriage:
   a. the more one loves one's partner.
   b. the more one distances from one's partner.
   c. the less likely that outside issues will negatively impact the relationship.
   d. the less likely one will choose to distance from one's partner.

**Heightened Ambivalence.**    *Ambivalence* is an alternation of feelings of love and hate experienced toward a spouse. These alternations of emotions lead to a lack of consistent feelings toward the spouse and serve to increase feelings of doubt about the partner or doubt about the continuation of the relationship (Nichols & Everett, 1986). As these emotions accumulate, one member of the couple may indulge in fantasies of escaping the relationship to one's family of origin or beginning a relationship with an "old flame." Such fantasies usually result in temporary relief; but the more one invests in such fantasy solutions (Guerin et al., 1987), the more one distances emotionally from the spouse. The confusing part of the ambivalence for clinicians is that these negative feelings toward the spouse may occur with oscillations of positive feelings.

At this stage, the children may begin to sense an increase of tension between their parents. They may pull away from one or both parents in an attempt to defend themselves from tension and anxiety or they may respond with increased clinging behavior in an attempt to seek reassurances that all is well.

6. The distancer in the marital relationship:
   a. becomes the pursuer.
   b. tries to get the pursuer to stop pursuing.
   c. is the partner who experiences the ambivalence.
   d. is the hurt member of the relationship.

7. As the unhappy spouse continues to distance from one's partner such distancing behaviors are likely to become:
   a. more progressive in nature.
   b. more regressive in nature.
   c. less problematic for the partner who does not want the marriage to end.
   d. less drastic in nature.

8. Pursuing behaviors include all of the following *except*:
   a. waiting for one's partner to call.
   b. calling the partner several times a day.
   c. seeking to spend more and more time with the partner.
   d. planning increased family activities which includes the partner.

*Distancing.* Ambivalence leads to distancing behaviors on the part of the disenchanted spouse. This spouse may begin to spend increased time in independent activities and less time in joint activities with the family. This distancing is progressive and the disenchanted spouse may withdraw from expressions of affection and may also fail to respond to gestures of affection or intimacy from the partner. The partner who is feeling "rejected" may begin to pursue the "distancing" partner with telephone calls, flowers, or dates.

Children whose parents are experiencing this phase will often side with the confused or "rejected" parent and distance themselves emotionally from the "distancing" parent. This early side taking on the part of children can create dysfunctional loyalties that can potentially have seriously negative consequences in later custody disputes and personal adjustment.

9. The process of separation usually begins:
   a. when one member of the couple moves out.
   b. when all financial matters are settled.
   c. when one member escapes into fantasy of life without the partner.
   d. when the divorce is settled.

*Pre-Separation Fantasies and Actions.* This period occurs when the disenchanted spouse begins to think seriously about leaving the increasingly dissatisfying marriage. For the disenchanted partner this fantasy may involve images of becoming involved with another partner. Other fantasies may range from returning to one's family of origin to the death of the partner. The indulgence in such "fantasy solutions" (Guerin et al., 1987) creates further emotional distance in the marriage leading to more disengagement from the partner and often the beginning of the separation process.

10. One of the most dramatic events in the process of separation and divorce is:
    a. when partners self-disclose to each other.
    b. when one partner empties the joint checking account.
    c. when one partner no longer refers to his spouse as mother.
    d. when one partner physically moves from the couple's home.

***Physical Separation.*** The decision by one spouse to physically leave the family's home is perhaps the most dramatic event in the entire process of separation and divorce. Family members can no longer deny the gravity of the situation. Many "rejected" spouses whose partners leave the home report feeling "overwhelmed and helpless" and others report an inability to concentrate on their continuing parenting roles with their children.

For children, physical separation represents the first overt action that their parents may be considering a divorce. A child's potential responses to the separation will depend upon a variety of variables including: age, gender, developmental level, stability, roles in the family, degrees and severity of conflict, and intergenerational and social support. Children experiencing this stage may appear terrified, sad, depressed, and anxious.

***Pseudo-Reconciliation.*** Many spouses experience high levels of anxiety or loss following a physical separation. They may suddenly find themselves isolated and alone. If such feelings and emotions become intense enough the spouses may move back in together precipitously to soothe feelings of loneliness and fear. Such a move tends to expose children to a renewal of false hope and causes the parents to temporarily minimize or deny problems and issues that led them to the point of separation. Rarely does this pseudo-reconciliation last. Eventually the original unresolved issues and surface again.

***Pre-Divorce Fantasies.*** If the couple fails at reconciliation and again experiences disillusionment, each partner may begin to imagine separate lives and may begin to talk more openly regarding plans to divorce.

For children, the chaos and uncertainty that stem from separation, pseudo-reconciliation, and separation again can provoke expressions of intense anger and acting out behaviors directed toward both spouses or toward other children at school. Children may also demonstrate a variety of symptoms ranging from academic and behavioral problems to somatic complaints and increased distancing from the home.

11. Which of the following is *not* a stage in the pre-divorce phase of the divorce process?
    a. blended family formation
    b. heightened ambivalence
    c. distancing
    d. pseudo-reconcilitation

## Stage 2—The Decision To Divorce: Structural Decoupling

The decision to divorce initiates a new phase of the decoupling process. Divorce requires couples to negotiate a variety of difficult decisions that include emotional, legal, financial, social, and parental issues. This marks the end of the former nuclear structure and the beginning of the reorganization of the divorced family's structure (Storm & Sprenkle, 1982). This has been referred to systemically as ***structural decoupling*** (Everett & Volgy, 1991). Couples reaching this stage of the divorce continuum are more likely to finalize the legal divorce. Specific steps in this stage are as follows (Everett & Volgy, 1991).

12. With regard to making the decision to divorce:
    a. both spouses usually desire the divorce at the same time.
    b. both spouses usually want to be the one that moves out.
    c. one spouse usually does not care.
    d. spouses rarely make a decision to divorce similtaneously.

13. The conflict experienced by spouses in their decision to divorce may impact the children how?
    a. They are glad the focus is not on them.
    b. They will seek to spend less time at home.
    c. They are vulnerable to psychotic episodes.
    d. They may feel that they have caused their parents' problems.

*Decision to Divorce.* The decision to divorce is usually reached by one spouse and the potential for reconciliation at this point is greatly diminished. The couple's cohesive and collusive bonds that kept them hesitant to let go begin to unravel (Dicks, 1967) and more anger and rage may be expressed.

Children are most at risk during this phase for long-term emotional problems. Parents may become so embroiled in their anger and bitterness with one another that the needs and pain of the children are overlooked or ignored. The children may even feel that they are responsible for the problems and break-up of their parents' marriage.

14. Children tend to interpret ambivalence of either spouse in the process of separation and/or divorce as:
    a. potential for reconciliation.
    b. potential for getting a new home.
    c. potential for having an increase in resources.
    d. potential for never seeing one parent again.

*Recurring Ambivalence.* Ambivalence may reoccur during this stage as couples begin to experience the complexity of the legal process and their own anxiety from their physical separation. It may fuel children's hopes of a reunified family and they may reexperience increased levels of anxiety. Special efforts may need to be directed toward the children as they are caught in this prolonged process.

*Potential Disputes.* Legal matters associated with decoupling and involving the settlement of such issues as financial agreements, property settlements, child custody and access, and child support have potential for negative interactions.. There are two potential methods available to spouses for reaching a divorce settlement: *mediation* and the *adversarial legal process*. We discuss these at length in a separate section.

15. Post-divorce restructuring includes all of the following *except:*
    a. remarriage.
    b. post-divorce co-parenting.
    c. blended family formation.
    d. heightened ambivalence.

## Stage 3—Post-Divorce Restructuring and Remarriage: Structural Recoupling

This final stage in the divorce process begins with the completion of the legal divorce and the family beginning to adjust to the settlement, both custodial and financial, that will define their ongoing post-divorce system and interaction. This stage has been referred to systemically as *structural recoupling* (Everett & Volgy, 1991).

Family members must begin to adjust to new family roles and a new structure. The former spouses and children must begin to cope emotionally with two parental households and develop new social networks (Kaslow & Schwartz, 1987). Parents must deal with the emotional adjustment of "letting go" of their former intimate relationship. Steps in this stage are as follows (Everett & Volgy, 1991).

**Post-Divorce Co-Parenting.**   This is a critical task in which both parents must learn to work together in communicating and decision-making to successfully co-parent their children. To facilitate this, parents must find a comfortable format and structure by which they "recouple" and learn to work together as parents. Everett (Everett & Volgy, 1991) often tells parents at this stage: "Now you must learn how to still be parents when you are no longer lovers or companions."

The success of this stage requires the spouses to let go of past anger and hurt feelings, and create an atmosphere where they can manage basic logistics for the children, that is, day-to-day decisions, transportation, help with homework, and so forth. We know that children's adjustments to the divorce are greatly enhanced when parents create a clear and working post-divorce parenting structure.

16. What percentage of divorced individuals eventually remarry?
    a. 80%–90%
    b. 70%–80%
    c. 60%–70%
    d. 50%–60%

17. When the first of the divorced spouses remarries, there may occur:
    a. few if any feelings of the previous marriage.
    b. a destabilization of the post-divorce family structure.
    c. intense euphoria on the part of all.
    d. few if any gifts.

**Remarriage.**   The data indicate that eventually eight out of nine individuals who have divorced will remarry. When the first of the divorced parents remarries, the balance of the post-divorce recoupling may be in jeopardy and emotional reactivity may arise. The fantasy of reconciliation is eliminated and fears of being replaced by a "new" parent occur. The potential for high conflict is present and may take the form of "brainwashing" to turn the children against their other parent (see a discussion of *Parental Alienation Syndrome,* Gardner, 2001).

This may trigger a child's anger toward the parent who is remarrying, or toward his or her new partner. One may feel the remarrying parent is disloyal and begin to side with the more lonely or sad parent. Residual fantasies of reconciliation by the child are also eliminated.

**Blended Family Formation.**   Following remarriage, the post-divorce family must define new spousal and parent-child subsystems, loyalty issues for children and the remarried parent, internal and external boundaries, interactional patterns, and lines of authority and discipline.

Children often struggle with learning to adapt to new roles with their remarried parent and stepparent, along with retaining their identity with their other parent. Children of all ages are susceptible to becoming caught in the middle of alliances and coalitions that form around the inclusion of a stepparent.

***The Second Remarriage.*** The remarriage of the second former spouse does not typically create the same systemic crisis as above. However, it often represents the final "letting go" of all but a residual hope held by the children that their parents might reconcile. Systemically, this second remarriage helps to structurally rebalance the post-divorce system.

***Dual-Family Functioning.*** The remarriage of the second spouse and the restabilization of both family systems provides a structurally balanced system that has been called the ***binuclear family*** (Ahrons, 1979; Ahrons & Rogers, 1987). This expanded system now contains two sets of spousal and parent–child subsystems, and four intergenerational systems, all sharing the ongoing parenting responsibilities for the children. The task of structural recoupling continues with new opportunities to embrace a stable and cooperative co-parenting system.

## THE DIVORCE PROCESS II—MEDIATION VS. LITIGATION

When a spouse reaches a decision to divorce she or he must decide how to proceed with the legal issues. These issues typically include a settlement of financial matters and personal property as well as parental issues involving the custody, access, and financial support of the children. There are two methods for reaching a final settlement: the **mediated divorce** and the **adversarial divorce**. These choices are critical in defining a family's experience of the divorce process.

## The Mediated Divorce

### *What Is Mediation?*

*Mediation* is a process of settling disputes by parties voluntarily, outside the court system, with the aid of a trained third party. Divorce mediation is the process of couples voluntarily reaching agreement on issues related to property, finances, and children with the aid of a third party trained in negotiation and dispute resolution skills.

18. The benefits of a mediated divorce include all of the following *except*:
    a. enhances communication.
    b. improves individual financial gain.
    c. addresses the needs of all parties.
    d. provides a model for future conflict resolution.

### *What Are the Advantages of a Mediated Divorce Agreement?*

Mediation was first made available to divorcing couples in the 1970s (Haynes, 1981; Kressel, 1985). It allowed couples to retain control over their decision making and shape a settlement that fit their needs and those of their children. The success of parents in completing a mediated settlement also avoided the anger and animosity that often occurs during an adversarial process. It has been observed that this process also teaches negotiation skills that can promote future communication and decision making as co-parents. While not all disputes can be settled through mediation, the benefits are clear for parents who utilize it.

Folberg and Taylor (1984) summarized several benefits of divorce mediation as follows:

- Enhances communication
- Maximizes the exploration of alternatives
- Addresses the needs of all parties
- Reaches an agreement perceived by the parties as fair
- Provides a model for future conflict resolution

## Who Are Divorce Mediators?

Divorce mediators come from two distinct fields: mental health and law. Certification as a mediator is available through a number of organizations that provide their members with specialized training. While a professional who offers services as a divorce mediator should have training in family systems, family development life cycles, and child development, as well as be aware of the legal issues in divorce, many professionals are self-trained or untrained in these areas. Some clinicians develop collaborative mediation teams with family law attorneys.

## What Are the Stages of Divorce Mediation?

Divorce mediation is a multistage process that allows couples to reach their own divorce agreement in the areas of property, finances, and children. While mediators may differ in their own styles, there is a consistency to the general stages of the mediation process. Most mediation begins with a stage of interaction that facilitates relationship and trust building.

> 19. In divorce mediation, it is most helpful to deal with which issue first?
>     a. finances
>     b. children
>     c. property
>     d. taxes

The literature indicates that it is beneficial to begin divorce mediation by addressing the issues involving children first. Parents may be more effective in overcoming their anger and resentment regarding the divorce when their children's well-being is addressed. This sequence promotes more effective resolution of financial concerns later in the mediation process. The early sessions provide a time to educate parents about parenting and structural choices including issues such as custodial alternatives access plans, holidays, vacations, and so forth. The impact of these options on their children is also discussed.

As early as the second session, an outline of the preliminary agreement may be drafted and distributed to each party for review. This is updated after each session. Financial issues relating to the children including child support, health care and dental insurance, taxes, and life insurance are incorporated. The division of finances and property are usually the final issues to be mediated since they tend to facilitate more reactivity from couples. While many states have tried to separate the decisions regarding children and the family's finances, the mediator is aware that negotiation regarding finances may be used as leverage in the areas of child custody and access. Once agreement is reached, the final document is written as a "memorandum of understanding," signed by all parties, and often attached to the final divorce order.

## The Adversarial Divorce

In some divorces, issues may be present that are too complicated to settle in mediation, or the spousal animosity may be too great to allow them to mediate in good faith. The alternative is the use of the adversarial process and the legal/judicial system to settle the divorce. Here each spouse retains their own attorney who becomes their advocate, and who seeks to gain the best possible settlement for their client. The respective attorneys may negotiate what they believe their clients should settle for, but when this is not possible the disputed case goes to a hearing with a judge. Here each spouse's side is presented, often with a great deal of personally damaging details, and with a final decision offered by the court.

20. Which of the following patterns of parental behavior is harmful to children?
   a. One or both parents tries to get the children to side with them.
   b. One or both parents tries to maintain a nonblaming stance toward the partner.
   c. One or both parents focus on the needs of the children.
   d. One or both parents are disappointed with each other.

21. All of the following are disadvantages of an adversarial divorce *except*:
   a. loss of control over the divorce process.
   b. increased animosity.
   c. negativity makes co-parenting more difficult later.
   d. the opportunity for cooperative negotiations.

### What Are the Disadvantages of the Adversarial Divorce Process?

The adversarial divorce process, and often the role of attorneys, tends to support spouses' animosity and the expression of hurtful and angry feelings (Kressel, 1985). Often erroneous charges are made against a former partner in such areas as physical or sexual abuse to gain an advantage in court. Increased conflict at this stage makes effective co-parenting more difficult, even after the court process is completed (Kaslow & Schwartz, 1987). The spouses often lose sight of the best interests of their children, often trying to get the children to side with them against the other parent (**triangulation**). Many couples who pursue the adversarial process are never satisfied with the outcomes and tend to go back to court with considerable frequency for modifications, or simply to harass the former partner.

### What Is the Role of the Therapist in Adversarial Divorce?

The role of a therapist in an adversarial divorce is limited. Most couples engaging in this process do not seek couple or family therapy during this period of their divorce. We believe that family therapy interventions would be helpful at this time but the lack of spousal cooperation diminishes participation and effectiveness. Some attorneys and court related programs refer highly conflicted families for clinical work.

Some clinicians may be involved in these adversarial proceedings by performing custody evaluations for the courts. These are very specific evaluations that require considerable experience by the therapists and familiarity with their ethical roles within the legal process. We should note that the American Association for Marriage and Family Therapy (AAMFT) considers it unethical for marriage and family therapists to assume a dual role of therapist to the family, children, or couple *and* to provide custody evaluations to the court for these client families (2002). It can also be deemed unethical for a therapist who has worked clinically with a parent or children to make recommendations regarding custodial issues.

Overall, the reader can see that the choice by a divorcing couple to pursue a mediated settlement versus that of an adversarial divorce can have lasting effects on their future interaction and ability to co-parent.

## THE DIVORCE PROCESS III—CLINICAL ISSUES FOR INDIVIDUALS, COUPLES, AND CHILDREN

### Issues for Individual Divorcing Spouses

The effect of divorce on individual partners varies according to their prior roles and experiences in the marriage and their position in the divorce process. These individuals may experience a variety of emotions ranging from high levels of stress and disequilibrium to loss and grief to hurt and animosity. In most cases, one partner has typically made the decision to "leave" the marriage and the other partner must struggle with feelings of "being left." It is important for the clinician to recognize this decoupling process and understand the unique clinical needs of the couple at this time (Crosby, 1989; Everett & Volgy, 1989; James, 1989; Nichols, 1989).

22. All of the following are typical of the spouse "leaving" *except*:
    a. feelings of relief, guilt, doubt, and anxiety.
    b. feeling further along in the emotional separation and grief process than the spouse being left.
    c. dealing with the shock of the suddenness of the divorce decision.
    d. a desire to proceed quickly with the divorce to "get it over with."

### *The Partner Leaving*

The partner choosing to leave the relationship may experience a variety of feelings including relief, guilt, doubt, anger, and anxiety. This spouse may have been questioning and distancing (decoupling) in the relationship for some years and is thus further along in the emotional separation and grief process than their partner. This "leaving" partner is more likely to experience the recurring ambivalence described earlier as a result of guilt associated with initiating the divorce. Upon entering into the legal phase of the divorce, this spouse may want to proceed through the legal process quickly in order to "get it over with" and, in order to relieve their sense of guilt or anxiety, may agree prematurely to an inequitable settlement. If this spouse has an ongoing extramarital relationship, she or he may also approach ending the marriage with some urgency.

23. The primary clinical task of the spouse "being left" is to:
    a. get revenge.
    b. deal with the process of ending the relationship and "letting go."
    c. try to hold on as long as possible.
    d. work in therapy to be the kind of person their spouse would take back.

## The Partner Being Left

This partner typically experiences fear, anger, rage, anxiety, depression, and abandonment in relation to the divorce being thrust upon them. This partner may be more likely to experience the acute grief that accompanies a new loss. The decision by their partner often comes as a surprise. The sudden sense of loss can easily turn to anger, rage, and vindictiveness. This partner will need to focus on dealing with the ending of the relationship and "letting go." Of course this process as a satisfactory adjustment can take some years to achieve.

## Issues for the Divorcing Couple

The decision to divorce intensifies the decoupling process for the relationship. The clinician needs to recognize that the primary emotional and structural features for a couple in this stage are a loss of trust, loyalty, and protection. The collusive bond that formerly provided a sense of protection has diminished, leaving a sense of aloneness. This has been described as a period of mourning exhibited by feelings of anger, guilt, a sense of failure, and diminished self-worth (Kressel, 1985). Both spouses may experience a heightened sense of vulnerability that can lead to the expression of anger and rage. As the couple begins to face the legal aspects of the divorce process and work with attorneys, recurring ambivalence may surface, initiating a period of reappraisal of the relationship. However, this ambivalence typically subsides and most couples proceed to divorce.

## Clinical Interventions for Divorcing Couples and Individual Spouses

The following are a variety of clinical issues on which therapists can focus their work:

- Beginning the process of emotionally decoupling for the spouses
- Developing skills in communication and negotiation for future co-parenting
- Helping couples minimize their impulses to punish each other in seeking revenge for their hurt and anger
- Planning for the divorce by providing information about the legal process
- Dealing with intense personal feelings such anger, sadness, and abandonment
- Learning effective ways to deal with children during this time of disorganization
- Helping couples identify their ambivalence and understand its underlying causes as couples revaluate their relationship
- Explore intergenerational issues related to ambivalence
- Making referrals to attorneys and divorce mediators

## Issues in the Divorce Process for Children

Children experience a wide range of emotions in response to the divorce of their parents and these are related to their ages and developmental stages. Common reactions reported in children experiencing divorce include anger, fear, sadness, depression, guilt, rejection, regression, school problems, and physical complaints. They may feel powerless in relation to the divorce and may attempt to stop it by using guilt, anger, illness, or threats. Most children's concerns about divorce revolve around issues of security, safety, protection, and continuity (See Everett & Volgy, 1991; Kaslow & Schwartz, 1987; Nichols, 1984).

24. The counseling process for children experiencing divorce should focus on all the following *except*:
    a. expressing feelings.
    b. developing coping strategies.
    c. negotiating custody arrangements.
    d. dealing with guilt.

25. All of the following are clinical interventions used by marriage and family therapists for divorcing couples *except*:
    a. dealing with intense feeling such as anger, sadness, and abandonment.
    b. non-systemic individual therapy, excluding other family members.
    c. learning effective ways to deal with children during times of disorganization.
    d. beginning the process of emotional decoupling for spouses.

26. Clinical methods for helping children who are experiencing divorce express emotions include all the following *except*:
    a. talking.
    b. artwork.
    c. analysis.
    d. play therapy.

## Clinical Interventions for Children and Their Divorcing Parents

Working with children in therapy during the divorce process can be critical to their emotional adjustment and survival. Many children going through this process will display symptoms of withdrawal and clinical depression, or begin acting out at school, with peers, or at home. The following is a summary of areas of clinical interventions with children and their parents:

- Expressing emotions by talking, artwork, and play therapy
- Providing reassurance that they are not going to be abandoned or lose either parent (if this is true)
- Reestablishing trust with their parents
- Understanding that the divorce is not their fault, reducing feelings of guilt
- Improving communication with their parents and other family members
- Developing confidence and positive feelings of self worth
- Dealing with feelings of loneliness
- Developing trust that they will be survive the divorce
- Helping them learn that they do not need to rescue or be responsible for either of their parents' own personal adjustment to the divorce
- Identifying additional supportive resources with grandparents or other family-of-origin members

27. Clinical interventions important for working with post-divorce parents include all of the following *except*:
    a. learning effective conflict resolution skills.
    b. understanding the needs of children experiencing divorce.
    c. learning skills for keeping children out of the middle of disputes.
    d. trying to reunite parents and revive their marriage.

Here are some clinical interventions to focus upon when working specifically with the post-divorce parents:

- Improving communication skills
- Learning effective conflict resolution skills
- Learning skills for keeping children out of the middle of disputes
- Cooperative co-parenting that focuses on the best interest of children and the restructured family
- Developing flexibility
- Understanding the needs of their children as they experience the divorce
- Controlling destructive reactivity in relation to the divorce

## CLINICAL AND EDUCATIONAL RESOURCES FOR THE DIVORCING FAMILIES

### Divorce Therapy

Divorce therapy is recognized as a systemic intervention focused on helping couples and families negotiate the stages of the divorce process. We define divorce as a part of the family life cycle—it cannot be treated independently from the whole family system. Some marital and family therapists specialize in working with divorcing families in general while others may specialize in working with the post-divorce adjustment of the spouses or the post-divorce adjustment of the children. However, most specialists in the field tend to view this work, that is, divorce therapy, as primarily a component of systemic family therapy and not as a distinct specialty (Kaslow, 1981; Nichols, 1996; Nichols & Everett, 1986).

### Divorce Education Programs

Divorce education programs have increased dramatically in the United States over the past 15 years. Their goal is to help various components (i.e., single parents, remarried parents, stepparents, and children) of the divorced family with their respective post-divorce adjustments. Current estimates have indicated that nearly one-half of counties in the United States currently provide divorcing parents with educational programs that focus on maintaining healthy family relationships and assisting their children through the divorce process (Geasler & Blaisure, 1999). It has been estimated that such programs sponsored by county court systems throughout the country have tripled over the past ten years (Arbuthnot, 2002).

Many states have legislation that requires parental participation, where there are minor children, in divorce education programs before a divorce can be finalized. Such programs may be offered by court sponsored programs or community service agencies. Many other support groups for divorcing spouses and parents are offered in communities by such programs as *Divorce Recovery* and *Parents Without Partners*.

28. Divorce education programs focus on all the following issues *except*:
    a. effective co-parenting.
    b. family of origin/intergenerational issues.
    c. individual post-divorce adjustment issues.
    d. specific issues and needs for children of divorce.

29. Common reactions in children experiencing divorce include all the following *except*:
    a. guilt.
    b. fear.
    c. stability.
    d. sadness.

## What Are the Components of Divorce Education Programs?

Divorce education programs are designed to assist both parents and children with the difficult adjustment to divorce. These programs have been developed to educate parents about individual post-divorce adjustment, effective co-parenting, and specific issues (such as children's feelings of guilt, sadness, and fear) and needs for children of divorce (Kirby, 1998). Some divorce education courses tend to focus on providing information to parents while others may focus on skill building in parenting roles. Most programs are short term, lasting from one meeting to several weeks.

---

Divorce is a complex phenomenon that affects all aspects of the intergenerational family system. It has become so common in our culture that we now define it as a potential component in the family's developmental life cycle. The role of the marital and family therapist can be crucial in helping divorcing and post-divorce families negotiate this experience and emerge in a relatively healthy manner. In this chapter, we have identified the basic aspects of the divorce process. We believe that the identification of these stages of divorce, their effects on family members, and the potential areas of therapeutic interventions can become an important resource for both the therapist and the family alike.

## KEY TERMS

**advesarial divorce:** The process whereby divorcing spouses enter litigation represented by attorneys to settle matters of child custody, property settlements, etc.

**alliances:** A bond formed between two members of a family system for mutual support.

**boundaries:** Invisible lines around family systems or subsystems that define both who is within the system and who is without and the manner by which feedback passes into and out of the system.

**external boundaries:** An invisible line/marker that differentiates the nuclear system from its intergenerational system and environment.

**internal boundaries:** An invisible line/marker that differentiates each of the internal subsystems, that is, spousal, parent–child, and sibling.

**open boundaries:** Delineations that allow a flexible exchange of feedback.

**closed boundaries:** Delineations that deflect feedback and either keep it isolated within the system or prevent it from entering the system.

**diffuse boundaries:** Delineations that fail to control or limit feedback; external feedback becomes intrusive.

**binuclear family:** A termed coined by Connie Ahrons to reflect the dual systems in a post-divorce step- or blended family.

**coalitions:** A bond formed by two or more family members typically directed negatively against another member, such as in scapegoating a child.

**divorce process:** The emotional and structural changes and adjustments that a divorcing family experiences during the divorce.

**emotional decoupling:** A systemic term coined by Everett and Volgy to describe the process by which divorcing spouses must learn to let go of their prior attachments and relationship. It also describes the children's experiences of letting go of the familiarity of their former intact family system.

**family roles:** Functions that define expectable behaviors in the family, for example, parent, caretaker, mediator, and so forth.

**family rules:** Standards that define expectations or rules within the family and that characterize an emotional climate or mandate specific behaviors, for example, "children should be seen and not heard."

**mediated divorce:** The process whereby divorcing spouses work with a mediator or therapist in a cooperative manner to plan their divorce settlement, which can include decisions regarding child custody and access and the division of personal property, assets, and debts.

**structural decoupling:** A systemic term coined by Everett and Volgy to describe the structural changes that must occur in the family system at the time of separation and divorce, for example, living in single-parent households.

**structural recoupling:** A systemic term coined by Everett and Volgy to describe the process that occurs between divorcing parents who must learn to reconnect in emotional and practical ways in order to share parenting roles and access with their children.

**subsystems:** A family system is composed of three internal systems: spousal, parent–child, and sibling. An intergenerational subsystem is often identified to include family-of-origin members. Each subsystem has properties similar to the overall family system.

**stages of divorce:** A sequence or pattern outlining the experiences of spouses and children who are going through the divorce process.

**systemic hierarchy:** The relative power assigned to members of a family within an intergenerational system that can include children and grandparents.

**transitional life crisis:** A turning point (brought on, in this case, by separation and divorce) for the family system resulting in a transitional period before the system can re-stabilize.

**triangulation:** A Bowenian concept that defines the process in families whereby two members, often in conflict, pull a third member into their interaction, often a child, in order to diffuse their dispute.

## DISCUSSION QUESTIONS

1. Divorce has replaced death as the most common ending for marriages. Increased lifespan, changing women's roles, changes in social values, and changes in the legal system have been listed as major contributing factors in this shift. What other variables might help explain this increase in divorce and what are potential clinical implications for therapy with families?

2. Discuss the range of emotions experience by spouses during the emotional decoupling stage. How do these affect marital intimacy?

3. How does ambivalence impact each member of the couple in the separation/divorce process? How does it impact children?

4. How does pursuing and distancing impact the marital relationship? What function does it serve?

5. How does the use of fantasy solution by one partner negatively impact the relationship?
6. Discuss the concept of pseudo-reconciliation and its relevance to separating and divorcing couples.
7. The point at which a couple reaches a decision to divorce is considered to be one of the most critical and potentially damaging times for children in the family. What dynamics occur with the couple that impact children negatively?
8. Divorce mediation has been used successfully to help couples settle the difficult issues associated with divorce. What are the benefits of a mediated divorce and in what situations may mediation be less effective?
9. AAMFT's current ethical standards discourage the dual relationship of a therapist providing therapy to divorcing families and also performing court-ordered custody evaluations for those same families. Why is it wise to separate these two clinical roles?
10. How do divorce education programs differ from traditional therapy and what are the primary benefits of divorce education programs to divorcing families?

## SUGGESTED FURTHER READING

Crosby, J. F. (Ed.). (1989). *When one wants out and the other doesn't: Doing therapy with polarized couples*. New York: Brunner/Mazel.

A thoroughly clinical and comprehensive edited work that identifies the struggles of divorcing families.

Everett, C. A., & Volgy Everett, S. (1991). Treating divorce in family therapy practice. In A. S. Gurman & D. P. Kniskern (Eds.), *Handbook of family therapy: Vol. II* (pp. 508–524). New York: Brunner/Mazel.

Identifies practical issues for the clinician working with divorcing families from an integrative family systems perspective.

Everett, C. A., & Volgy Everett, S. (1995). *Healthy Divorce—Fourteen stages of separation, divorce and remarriage*. New York: John Wiley.

A book written for divorcing families that defines fourteen stages they will experience as they proceed through the divorce process with help given on protecting the children and learning to become co-parents.

Folberg, J., & Taylor, A. (1984). *Mediation: A comprehensive guide to resolving conflict without litigation*. San Francisco: Jossey-Bass.

A thoughtful explanation and review of the issues and methods involved in mediation with divorcing families.

Kaslow, F., & Schwartz, L. (Eds.). (1987). *The dynamics of divorce: A life cycle perspective*. New York: Brunner/Mazel.

A helpful edited work that discusses many issues regarding divorce from a developmental perspective.

Nichols, W. C. (1996). *Treating people in families: an integrative framework*. New York: Guilford Press.

While not focused solely on divorce, a good overview for clinicians in understanding the basic issues in treating families and the conflict that can lead to divorce.

## REFERENCES

Ahrons, C. (1979). The binuclear family: Two households, one family. *Alternative Lifestyles, 2,* 499–515.
Ahrons, C., & Rogers, R. (1987). *Divorced families: A multidisciplinary developmental view*. New York: Norton.
American Association for Marriage and Family Therapy. (2002). *The American Association for Marriage and Family Therapy Code of Ethics*. Washington, DC: Author.
Arbuthnot, J. (2002). A call unheeded: Courts' perceived obstacles to establishing divorce education programs. *Family Court Review, 40*(3), 371–382.
Cherlin, A. J. (1992). *Marriage, divorce and remarriage*. Cambridge: Harvard University Press.

Crosby, J. F. (Ed.). (1989). *When one wants out and the other doesn't: Doing therapy with polarized couples.* New York: Brunner/Mazel.

Dicks, H. V. (1967). *Marital tensions.* New York: Basic Books.

Everett, C. A., & Volgy, S. (1989). The assessment and treatment of polarizing couples. In J. F. Crosby (Ed.), *When one wants out and the other doesn't* (pp. 67–92). New York: Brunner/Mazel.

Everett, C. A., & Volgy, S. (1991). Treating divorce in family therapy practice. In A. S. Gurman & D. P. Kniskern (Eds.), *Handbook of family therapy: Vol. II* (pp. 508–524). New York: Brunner/Mazel.

Folberg, J., & Taylor, A. (1984). *Mediation: A comprehensive guide to resolving conflict without litigation.* San Francisco: Jossey-Bass.

Gardner, R. A. (2001). *Therapeutic interventions for children with parental alienation syndrome.* Cresskill, NJ: Creative Therapeutics.

Geasler, M. J., & Blaisure, K. R. (1999). 1998 Nationwide survey of court-connected divorce education programs. *Family and Conciliation Courts Review, 37*(1), 36–63.

Guerin, P., Jr., Fay, L., Burden, S., & Kautto, J. (1987). *The evaluation and treatment of marital conflict: a four-stage approach.* New York: Basic Books.

Haynes, J. M. (1981). *Divorce mediation: A practical guide for therapists and counselors.* New York: Springer.

James, B. E. (1989). Marital therapy with polarized couples. In J. F. Crosby (Ed.), *When one wants out and the other doesn't* (pp.191–207). New York: Brunner/Mazel.

Kaslow, F. (1981). Divorce and divorce therapy. In A. S. Gurman & D. P. Kniskern (Eds.), *Handbook of family therapy: Vol. I.* (pp. 662–696). New York: Brunner/Mazel.

Kaslow, F., & Schwartz, L. (Eds.). (1987). *The dynamics of divorce: A life cycle perspective.* New York: Brunner/Mazel.

Kirby, J. (1998). Court-related parenting education divorce interventions. *Human Development and Family Life Bulletin, 4*(2), 21–30.

Kressel, K. (1985). *The process of divorce: How professionals and couples negotiate settlements.* New York: Basic Books.

National Center for Health Statistics. (1998). *Cohabitation, Marriage, Divorce, and Remarriage in the United States* (DHHS Publication No. PHS 2002-1998). Washington, DC: U.S. Government Printing Office.

Nichols, W. C. (1984). Therapeutic needs of children in family systems reorganization. *Journal of Divorce, 7*(4), 23–44.

Nichols, W. C. (1989). Polarized couples: Behind the façade. In J. F. Crosby (Ed.), *When one wants out and the other doesn't* (pp.1–21). New York: Brunner/Mazel.

Nichols, W. C. (1996). *Treating people in families: an integrative framework.* New York: Guilford Press.

Nichols, W. C., & Everett, C. A. (1986). *Systemic family therapy: An integrative approach.* New York: Guilford Press.

Pinsof, W. (2002). The death of "till death do us part": The transformation of pair-bonding in the 20th century. *Family Process, 41*(2), 135–157.

Sprenkle, D. H., & Gonzalez-Doupe, P. (1996). Divorce therapy. In F. P. Piercy, D. H. Sprenkle, J. L. Wetchler, and Associates (Eds.), *Family therapy sourcebook* (2nd ed. pp. 181–219). New York: Guilford Press.

Storm, C. L., & Sprenkle D. H. (1982). Individual treatment in divorce therapy: A critique of an assumption. *Journal of Divorce, 5,* 87–97.

# 13

# Sexual Problems

## Joan D. Atwood
*Hofstra University*

___ *14. Most successful sex therapies include a cognitive-behavioral component.*
___ *15. Renal problems can be a contributing factor to erectile dysfunction.*


# THE HISTORY OF SEX THERAPY

The demand for treatment for sexual problems has increased in the past three decades. This is in large part due to increased public knowledge that effective treatments are available and to the growing recognition that these problems are comparable to other behavioral difficulties and therefore often respond to behavioral treatment (Hawton, 1985). There is also increased awareness within the fields of marriage and family therapy, social work, and clinical psychology that sex therapy should be a primary part of the training.

Presently, it is important for you to be familiar with the widely accepted theoretical orientations currently used to treat sexual problems. They are the psychoanalytic, the cognitive–behavioral, including the newer sex therapies, and the systemic. It is important for you to also consider how "normal" sexuality or at least the physiological aspects of the human sexual response are defined.

1. Traditionally, there are three theoretical orientations used to treat sexual problems. They are:
   a. the psychoanalytic, the cognitive-behavioral, and the systemic.
   b. the psychoanalytic, the cognitive-behavioral, and the adlerian.
   c. the psychoanalytic, the cognitive-behavioral, and the object relations model.
   d. the psychoanalytic, the cognitive-behavioral, and the Masters and Johnson model.


## The Psychoanalytic Perspective

Prior to 1970, the treatment of sexual problems was based on anecdotal observations and was considered the domain of psychiatry. The typical therapies for sexual problems that evolved from this tradition are dyadic. The focus is not on only the sexual symptom, but also on a more complete understanding of the person's mental life. The first implication of the psychoanalytic view of sexual dysfunction is that the dysfunction itself is not the problem. It is only a symptom of a deeper, underlying pathology. The second implication is that sexual problems are symptomatic of an underlying, deeper personality conflict that requires intense psychiatric therapeutic intervention and resolution. For example, a psychoanalytic interpretation of premature ejaculation would be that the man with this problem has intense, unconscious feelings of hatred toward women. Such a man supposedly has orgasms rapidly because it satisfies his sadistic impulses, and ensures that his partner will receive little or no pleasure from the act. Vaginismus in women, severe muscular contractions which prevent the penis from entering the vaginas, from this view is seen as one way a woman may deal with her penis envy—which is thought to occur in all girls during the phallic stage of development. Their problem is an expression of their unconscious desire to castrate their partner.

2. Which perspective focuses not on the sexual symptom, but rather on achieving a more complete understanding of the person's mental life?
   a. systems theory
   b. the new sex theory

> c. the Masters and Johnson model
> d. the psychoanalytic perspective

The therapeutic goal is not just to relieve the symptom, but to resolve its infrastructure—the underlying conflict. Insight, understanding, mastery, and psychological growth are highly valued therapeutic goals. Symptom removal used by the other therapeutic approaches are considered "transference cures" or "suggestion," likely to be followed by symptom substitution. This psychodynamic or psychoanalytically based treatment approach requires a lengthy treatment often with questionable outcomes. After the evaluation phase, a married patient with a sexual problem is usually seen alone as interpersonal problems within the marital relationship tend to be viewed as the acting out of the patient's internal conflicts.

## The Masters and Johnson Model

With the Masters and Johnson (1970) publication of *Human Sexual Inadequacy,* a new approach emerged, one that appeared to be an effective treatment approach of much shorter therapeutic duration. This new approach, representative of the cognitive–behavioral approach, challenged psychoanalytic attitudes and suggested a radically different therapeutic approach. In this view, sexual dysfunctions are perceived as learned disorders rather than symptoms of underlying personality disorders. The dysfunctional man or the woman with an orgasmic disorder is viewed as a person who was exposed to an environment that taught him or her to be anxious in a particular situation. In addition, while the psychoanalytic view would see the man's sexual problem, his interpersonal relationships, and his attitudes toward his parents as understandable in terms of one single underlying conflict, the cognitive–behavioral view would suggest that each aspect of the man's functioning might be caused by separate variables. The rapid acceptance of this new form of therapy by both the lay and professional public testified to the inadequacy of psychoanalytic tradition to deal with the widespread presence of sexual problems.

> 3. Which model of sexuality views sexual dysfunctions as learned disorders rather than symptoms of underlying personality disorders?
>    a. psychoanalytic perspective
>    b. the new sex therapy
>    c. systems theory
>    d. Masters and Johnson model

In addition, at that time, there were very little data on human sexuality practices utilizing good methodology with generalizeable samples. There was even less exploration into effective treatment approaches. Masters and Johnson's (1966, 1970) data represented the first study examining sexual functioning and dysfunctioning. Their work suggested a number of interesting possibilities for dealing with dysfunctions. Both partners were included in the treatment. The concerns of each partner were considered without placing blame for the dysfunction. The symptoms belonged to the marital pair, not to the symptom bearer. They believed that the psychological mechanisms of dysfunction were largely related to current rather than past influences, for example, performance anxiety, spectatoring, anger at the dysfunctional spouse. A new emphasis was placed on social forces, such as cultural expectations that prevent the normal development of female or male sexual expression, or religious orthodoxy, rather than on past intrapsychic causes. They believed that male and female co-therapy teams were uniquely suited to fostering communication and mutual understanding between spouses. They felt the therapy team was also more effective in identifying and dealing with the high frequency of serious interpersonal problems. Correction of misinformation and imparting of knowledge were facilitated by co-therapists.

Their model did not go without criticism, primarily from Zilbergeld and Evans (1980) and their publication of *The Inadequacy of Masters and Johnson*. Zilbergeld and Evans challenged Masters and Johnson's outcome statistics, as well as their research methodology. They felt that Masters and Johnson worked primarily with highly motivated and educated middle class couples, many of whom were health professionals in their community. Second, they felt that the Masters and Johnson model did not really measure success rates; instead it measured vaguely defined failure rates. However, the Masters and Johnson treatment model still forms the basis of most sex therapy programs today.

4. Who of the following challenged Masters and Johnson's outcome statistics and their research methodology as well?
   a. De Silva
   b. Hawton
   c. Helen Singer Kaplan
   d. Zilbergeld and Evans

## The New Sex Therapy

*The New Sex Therapy* written by Helen Singer Kaplan (1979) involved a synthesis of the theory and procedures of psychodynamic theory with the more behavioral perspectives. The symptoms are considered the disorder. For the most part, the relationship, not the individuals, is seen as the problem and involves the couple. If one of the partners cannot tolerate the anxiety or change, then this treatment based on behavioral principles will not work. The goal here is more limited than traditional psychodynamic therapies as the focus is on alleviating symptom distress rather than personality overhaul.

5. Which approach involved a synthesis of the theory and procedures of psychodynamic theory with the more behavioral perspectives?
   a. systems theory
   b. Helen Singer Kaplan's
   c. the Masters and Johnson model
   d. the psychoanalytic perspective

## Systems Theory

There has been little effort to elaborate the conceptual connections between the family theories and theories of sexual behavior. Systems theorists generally see sexuality as a symptom or a metaphor of more essential couple issues such as poor communication, hostility and competitiveness, or sex role problems. Even in those cases where the sexual dysfunction is not related to relationship problems, the couple's emotional relationship is often damaged by the sexual problems. Feelings of guilt, inadequacy, and frustration usually accompany sexual dysfunction.

6. Which perspective generally sees sexuality as a symptom or a metaphor in order that the
   couple might avoid dealing with the more essential couple issues?
   a. systems theory
   b. the new sex therapy
   c. the Masters and Johnson model
   d. the psychoanalytic perspective

The major approaches to sex therapy can be separated into two camps. On the one hand, using the Masters and Johnson and the newer sex therapies' model, the sexual issue presented is the problem to be worked on. On the other hand, using the psychoanalytic and the more systemically based therapies, sexual dysfunction is seen as a manifestation of some underlying unconscious conflict or as a metaphor or a symptom of a problemed relationship. These two major divisions represent the division between the fields of sex therapy and couples therapy. However, it does not make sense to train people to practice marriage and family therapy without giving them adequate training in human sexuality. And it is not fruitful to train people to practice sex therapy without giving them the context in which to apply it.

## MULTICULTURAL INFLUENCES

Keep in mind that the above approaches assume that sex is a primary way of exchanging pleasure, that it is a natural activity, that both partners are equally involved, that people should be educated about sexuality, and that communication is a necessary factor in sexual relationships. However, culture also has a great influence on sexual attitudes, sexual scripts, and behavior. In equalitarian relationships, the major goals are sexual pleasure and psychological disclosure and intimacy. But, for example, in Hispanic cultures, men are permitted to engage in sexually pleasureable activities but the norm for women is "purity." In these cultures, women are required to be sexually pure and virtuous. Sex is seen as an obligation to satisfy the husband's needs. For the men, sexuality is an expression of their manliness.

All of us have ideas about sexuality infused with our own value system based on the sociocultural milieu. Therapists carry with them their own sexual scripts and the therapy itself is grounded in the cultural environment. It is crucial for the therapist to keep in mind that clients have their own ideas about the meaning of their sexuality, what role gender plays, and what a good sexual relationship is for them. They also have ideas about what constitutes sexual dysfunctions, what causes them, what the role of a good therapist is and what the goals of therapy should be. In sum, the therapist needs to be respectful of what the clients bring to therapy in terms of their own definitions and meanings.

## THE HUMAN SEXUAL RESPONSE CYCLE

One of Masters and Johnson's (1966) major contributions was the first description of the physiological responses that occur during the human sexual response cycle. To gain a better understanding of sexual dysfunctions, it is important to first grasp sexual functioning.

Individuals generally progress sequentially through the four phases of the human sexual response cycle.

7. The two general responses to sexual stimulation are.
   a. plateau and orgasm
   b. vasocongestion and myotonia
   c. arousal and ejaculation
   d. none of the above

1. *The Excitement Phase* is characterized by increased penile and vaginal vasocongestion.
2. *The Plateau Phase* occurs when there is maximal enlargement and congestion of pelvic organs. In women, the orgasmic platform occurs as the uterus elevates. In men, secretions from Cowper's gland occur. This liquid secretion contains semen and may cause impregnation even though it is prior to ejaculation. Immediately prior to ejaculation, there is a period called *ejaculatory inevitability* when the he is no longer able to voluntarily inhibit ejaculation.

8. There are four phases of the human sexual response cycle according to Masters and Johnson. Which of the following is *not* one of their phases?
   a. plateau phase
   b. resolution phase
   c. the desire phase
   d. the excitement phase

3. *Orgasm* consists of involuntary contractions occurring at 0.8-second intervals in both the penis and vagina. The frequency of contractions is related to the subjective report of intensity of orgasm (Atwood & Gagnon, 1987). Respondents reported more subjectively intense orgasms the more contractions they had.

9. Which of Masters and Johnson's four phases involve involuntary contractions?
   a. orgasm
   b. excitement phase
   c. plateau phase
   d. desire phase

4. *The Resolution Phase* consists of a return to a resting state. For men, there is a **refractory period** whereby the excitement phase cannot recur. This refractory phase increases with age. For women, no such phase is evident suggesting a physiological basis for multiple orgasms.

10. In which phase of Masters and Johnson's model does maximum engorgement and congestion of the pelvic organs occur?
    a. plateau phase
    b. resolution phase
    c. desire phase
    d. the excitement phase

For a complete description of the changes that occur during these phases, see Masters and Johnson's *Human Sexual Response* (1966).

There are two generalized responses to sexual stimulation: vasocongestion and myotonia. *Vasocongestion* refers to increased blood flow to the penile and vaginal area and *myotonia* refers to increased muscle tension. These generalized responses occur in both men and women.

In addition, both genders experience tachycardia whereby heart rate increases from about 70 beats per minute to about 180 beats per minute. Both men and women experience a *sex flush* during sexual stimulation and orgasm. This refers to a blushing of the face, neck, chest, and arms. Please keep in mind that while there is much overlap, there is also variation between individuals and between genders in the human sexual response. Women tend to be more varied in their response than males. Some proceed to orgasm similar to the male response; others proceed to the plateau phase and move into the resolution phase without orgasm; and some are multi-orgasmic. Also, women tend to spend more time in the excitement phase and their resolution phase is not as long as the man's. The vaginal and penile *plethysmographs* are devices used in the laboratory to measure vasocongestion (Geer & Quartararo, 1976). Basically, a plethysmograph is a photo light sensor. It indirectly measures blood volume density. If there is an increased amount of blood in the penile or vaginal area, less light is reflected. If there is a decreased amount of blood, more light is reflected.

## Kaplan's Triphasic Model

Helen Singer Kaplan (1974, 1979) proposed a tri-phasic model of human sexuality consisting of a *desire phase*, an *excitement phase* and a *resolution phase*. She also believed that the sexual dysfunctions could fall into one of these categories and that these categories are separate and distinct, that is, one phase can function well even if the individual is having problems with the other. Adding the desire phase to the human sexual response cycle was an important contribution because in many cases sexual desire is not always present. This phase expanded the Masters and Johnson's model and has been incorporated into Kaplan's basic paradigm. Zilbergeld and Evans (1980) believed that both Masters and Johnson's and Kaplan's models ignored the cognitive and subjective aspects of the sexual response. Their four components of the sexual response cycle are as follows:

1. *Interest or desire* defined as how frequently a person wants to engage in sexual activity
2. *Arousal* defined as how excited one gets during sexual activity
3. *Physiological readiness* (erection or vaginal lubrication, orgasm)
4. *Satisfaction* (one's evaluation of how one feels during intercourse and/or orgasm). Thus they were interested in the cognitive elements of people's sexual experiences.

11. Who of the following theorists put forth a tri-phasic model of human sexuality?
    a. Freud
    b. Masters and Johnson
    c. Helen Singer Kaplan
    d. None of the above

## SEXUAL PROBLEMS

*Sexual dysfunctions* or *problems* are impairments or disturbances in sexual desire, arousal, or orgasm. It is important for you to consider the social aspect of sexuality—what is considered dysfunctional may vary from person to person, from couple to couple, and society to society.

In addition, there are many couples who would consider their sexuality normal and therefore would not become a part of a clinical population; and yet, some of them may report their sexual behavior as less than satisfactory. Frank, Andersen, and Rubinstein (1978) reported that 80% of their happily married couples reported that their sexual relations were happy and satisfactory even though 40% of the men reported erectile or ejaculatory problems and over 60% of the women reported problems with arousal or orgasm.

Several factors appear to be associated with sexual dysfunctions: sexual ignorance (Bancroft, 1989), a person's attitude about sex and sexual activity (Spence, 1991; Zilbergeld & Evans, 1980), anxiety level (Bancroft, 1989), fear of performance (Masters & Johnson, 1970), and the quality of the couple's relationship (Woody, 1992).

12. Which of the following are considered to be factors associated with sexual dysfunction?
    a. sexual ignorance
    b. attitudes about sex
    c. anxiety level
    d. all of the above

Fears of performance are a significant factor in sexual difficulties. *Spectatoring* (Masters & Johnson, 1970) refers to the tendency of the person to watch (and possibly judge) him or herself during sexual activity rather than enjoy the sexual activity. This may lead to inhibited sexual action and enjoyment or true failure.

Some sexual problems are caused by or associated with physical factors. The relevance of such factors as prolonged alcoholism, diabetes, aging, neurological damage, drugs, and so on to sexual activity is well established (Bancroft, 1989; Kolodny, Masters, & Johnson, 1979).

## CLASSIFICATION OF SEXUAL PROBLEMS

Many useful classifications of sexual dysfunctions exist (see American Psychiatric Association, 1987; Bancroft, 1989; De Silva, 1992, 1994; Hawton, 1985; Kaplan, 1974; Masters & Johnson, 1970). See Table 13.1 for a simple classification.

Sexual problems may be considered *primary* (total, present in all circumstances) or *secondary* (situational, present in some circumstances only), depending upon whether the individual has ever been asymptomatic. A man with primary impotence has never had the ability to maintain a successful erection and ejaculation. The anorgasmic female has never had an

**TABLE 13.1**

Sexual Dysfunctions

| Males | Females |
|---|---|
| Low sexual interest | Low sexual interest |
| Erectile dysfunction | Lack of response |
| Premature ejaculation | Anorgasmia |
| Retarded ejaculation | Vaginismus |
| Dyspareunia | Dyspareunia |
| Sexual aversion | Sexual aversion |

orgasm. Secondary problems occur when the individual was sexually functional and then because of situational factors develops the dysfunction, such as when premature ejaculation happens in sexual intercourse but not during masturbation.

13. Which of the following characterize an individual *who was* sexually functional and then because of situational factors develops a dysfunction, such as when premature ejaculation occurs in sexual intercourse but not during masturbation?
    a. primary
    b. secondary
    c. reactive
    d. chronic

The two major male areas of dysfunction include disorders of potency and ejaculation.

14. The two major male areas of dysfunction include disorders of.
    a. potency and arousal
    b. potency and ejaculation
    c. arousal and ejaculation
    d. dyspareunia and ejaculation

## Impotence or Erectile Dysfunction

*Impotence* or *erectile dysfunction* is defined as the inability to achieve or maintain an erection. Primary impotence tends to be rare and according to Masters and Johnson (1970) occurs in 1% of men under age 35. Secondary erectile dysfunction is said to occur if erection is insufficient to result in sexual intercourse. This occurs approximately 25% of the time. The basic premise of the therapy for this disorder is that anxiety disrupts erectile response. Thus, the object of therapy is to diminish the anxiety sufficiently *but not totally*.

15. Which of the following is defined as the inability to achieve or maintain an erection?
    a. sexual aversion or sexual phobia
    b. retarded ejaculation
    c. erectile dysfunction or impotence
    d. dyspareunia

The current psychological treatment for erectile dysfunction is the use of sensate focus or touching supplemented with cognitive techniques used to promote relaxation, positive self-statements, sexual fantasy, and the restoration of self-confidence. For men with lifelong erectile problems, individual psychodynamic treatment has been suggested along with the sex therapy. In general, men with erectile dysfunction pay more attention to how much of an erection they have and less attention to their feelings of arousal.

16. Which of the following has been suggested for men with lifelong erectile problems?
    a. couples therapy
    b. individual psychodynamic treatment
    c. sensate focus exercises
    d. positive self-statements

The treatment of erectile dysfunction has become increasingly medical in the past ten to fifteen years. Drugs, devices, and surgery dominate the field. Recently there has been a report of successful treatment using an adrenergic antagonist drug. Also Sildenafil (Viagra), a Type-V phosphodiesterase inhibitor, has been demonstrated to be an effective medication for the treatment of erectile dysfunction via arteriolar smooth muscle relaxation in the corpus cavernosum, which increases blood flow to promote penile tumescence. When this drug is successful as a treatment for erectile dysfunction, it is important to explore with the couple the changes that have occurred in the marital relationship as a result. For example, unrealistic expectations, inadequate information regarding sexuality, and marital difficulties could be problems associated with poor outcomes. In some cases, marriages may even dissolve following successful sexual results due to medical or psychotherapeutic intervention. It is possible that the marriages were stable around the sexual dysfunction and when the dysfunction was removed, instability ensued.

17. Which of the following is true?
    a. Current psychological treatment for erectile dysfunction has changed very little.
    b. Men with erectile dysfunction pay more attention to how much of an erection they have and less attention to their feelings of arousal.
    c. The treatment of erectile dysfunction has become increasingly more medical in the past 10 to 15 years.
    d. All of the above

While most urologists believe that the vast majority of erectile problems have an organic basis (LoPiccolo, 1992), there are several problems with this view. For example, it is often quoted that 50% to 90% of erectile problems have an organic basis. But this definition is usually made without examination of age. If one looks at men under the age of 50 with erectile dysfunction, the percentage drops drastically. The other problem is inattention to normal changes in the erectile response that occur with age. Kolodny et al. (1979) found that healthy men over age 50 who report good sexual function have tumescence tests that look as abnormal as men reporting erectile dysfunction.

18. It is often quoted that _____ of erectile problems have an organic basis.
    a. 50%–90%
    b. 60%–90%
    c. 70%–80%
    d. 60%–80%

It is important to note that even when urologists see a man with a purely psychological basis to their sexual problem, they often prescribe medical non-surgical treatment such as intracavernous injection therapy or vacuum erection devices. Their rationale for doing this is that their patients will not go to a mental health professional or there are no sex therapists in their community or that sex therapy is too expensive and there is no insurance coverage. There is some evidence that a combination of sex therapy with injection therapy might be helpful in helping a man alleviate his anxiety, which would help him later achieve firmer erections without the medication (Kaplan, 1987). But, these studies tend to downplay an important side effect of injection therapy—the incidence of *fibrosis* (scarring of the soft tissue of the penis). Severe cases of fibrosis that occur in about a third of men using injection therapy can cause pain and curvature of the penis with erection. Support for men with erectile dysfunction can be obtained from Impotence Anonymous (a national organization located at 119 South Rush Street, Maryville, TN 37801). This organization offers therapy for men and their partners.

## Premature Ejaculation

Kolodny, Masters, and Johnson (1979) believed that *premature ejaculation* affects 15% to 20% of all men. A common definition is: given a normal, healthy, functioning female, premature ejaculation is the inability to delay ejaculation long enough to bring the partner to orgasm.

19. Kolodny, Masters, and Johnson believed that premature ejaculation affects _____ of men.
    a. 15%–20%
    b. 25%–30%
    c. 35%–40%
    d. 45%–50%

The treatment of premature ejaculation assumes it is possible to exert conscious control over ejaculation and the man can learn to prolong erection even when sexually aroused. The main components of this treatment program involve couple communication and the increasing ability of the male to perceive impending orgasm.

The "squeeze" technique, a common approach used for this disorder, involves the couple engaging in foreplay until the male achieves erection. He lets his partner know when he is approaching the feeling of orgasmic inevitability. The partner then can use the *squeeze technique*, which is just gently squeezing below the glans of the penis, or stopping intercourse before ejaculation. The exercise can be repeated several times. This tends to take away the impending feeling of the inevitability of orgasm. Next, intercourse is suggested with the female in superior position so that the squeeze technique may be more easily applied and intercourse can be interrupted. In addition, several self-help techniques have been proposed. For example, the use of a condom seems to help lower the sensitivity of the penis because the glans is not stimulated directly. Some men drink an alcoholic beverage to decrease the rapidity of their response; others masturbate before intercourse knowing that the second orgasm will take longer. Kaplan (1974) suggests using the stop-start technique first developed by Semans (1956).

## Retarded Ejaculation or Ejaculatory Incompetence

*Ejaculatory incompetence* is the inability of an erect penis to ejaculate. Masters and Johnson (1970) say that it occurs in less than 5% of men, usually those who are younger and sexually inexperienced. If a man has never ejaculated within the vagina, he is said to have *primary* ejaculatory incompetence. If he has been able to ejaculate in the vagina previously but currently cannot, then he has *secondary* ejaculatory incompetence. These men may be able to ejaculate via masturbation or oral sex.

20. If a man has never ejaculated within the vagina, he is said to have which type of ejaculatory incompetence?
    a. primary
    b. secondary
    c. reactive
    d. chronic

One unintended side effect that could occur with this disorder is that the man is able to maintain sexual intercourse for long periods of time without ejaculating. This may be considered positive by both him and his partner. On the other hand, in some cases he may begin to question his partner's sexual abilities. Or the woman may feel that her partner is not physically attracted to her.

Sensate focus exercises are used to treat retarded ejaculation. *Sensate focus* is basically "touching." Partners touch each other first in nonerogenous zone areas focusing on the plea- surable sensations. This enables the man to focus on his sexual and sensual feelings. In a stepwise fashion, men learn to ejaculate via masturbation alone, then by masturbating with his partner present, and then having his partner masturbate him to the point of ejaculatory inevitability and eventually inserting the penis in the vagina to actually ejaculate.

## Low Sexual Interest

Based on her observations that the lack of motivation to have sex was a crucial factor in unsuccessful sex therapy cases, Kaplan (1979) labeled *low sexual desire* as a dysfunction. In the case of the man, there is no erection and no urge to engage in sexual behavior. In the case of the woman, she experiences a lack of sexual arousal. Physically, she does not lubricate vaginally and there is no change in the vaginal size to accommodate the penis. The causes of low sexual interest may include organic as well as psychogenic factors. Approximately 10% to 20% of men with low sexual interest have pituitary tumors that cause too much production of the hormone prolactin. This hormone reduces the amount of testosterone and can lead to low sexual interest or erectile dysfunction. Sexual unresponsiveness can also be caused by psychogenic factors such as shame, poor self-esteem, a bad relationship, guilt, embarrassment about sexual activity or one's body, or a history of sexual abuse. Before any treatment can begin, etiological factors must be identified.

21. Based on her observations that the lack of motivation to have sex was a crucial factor in unsuccessful sex therapy cases, Kaplan (1979) is responsible for the labeling of which of the following as a sexual dysfunction?
    a. low sexual desire
    b. sexual aversion
    c. erectile dysfunction
    d. dyspareunia

The goal here is to create a nondemanding, relaxed, and sensuous environment in which mutually sexually gratifying activity can take place. For the woman, the sensate focus exercise is critical to assist her in relaxing and in some cases to help her learn about her own sexuality. Female superior position is often helpful because it increases female sensitivity. But a review of the current treatment programs for sexual desire disorder reveals that current approaches are more eclectic than the original Master and Johnson's behavioral techniques (see Leiblum & Rosen, 1988).

## Anorgasmia or Orgasmic Dysfunction

Not all women experience orgasm. This is known as *anorgasmia* or *orgasmic dysfunction*. Orgasmic dysfunction occurs in a woman who is sexually responsive but who does not reach orgasm when aroused. Many women report that they enjoy sexual intercourse even though they do not achieve orgasm.

22. Which of the following occurs in a woman who is sexually responsive but who does not reach orgasm when aroused?
    a. sexual aversion
    b. dyspareunia
    c. vaginismus
    d. anorgasmia

Kaplan (1974) reports that approximately 8% of women are anorgasmic by any means for unknown reasons. Approximately 10% of women are coitally anorgasmic (Kinsey, Pomeroy, Martin, & Gebhard, 1953). Only 30% to 40% of women report that they regularly experience orgasm through sexual intercourse without having the clitoris manually stimulated at the same time (Hite, 1976). Only about 5% of the cases of orgasmic dysfunction are the result of organic factors (Kolodny et al., 1979). The organic causes involved are usually diabetes, alcoholism, hormone deficiencies, or pelvic infections. The other 95% are the result of psychogenic causes such as guilt, shame, and guilt associated with sexual activity. These states of mind tend to interfere with a woman's ability to relax.

In general, the basic task of the therapist is to facilitate the woman to let go of an over-controlled response. This involves maximizing clitoral stimulation, while at the same time diminishing those forces that inhibit orgasm. The major objective is for the woman to have an orgasm. Masturbation is encouraged. Vibrators may be used. She is encouraged to fantasize and to try thrusting movements. She is encouraged to use Kegel exercises (starting and stopping the flow of urine) to strengthen the muscles used in orgasm. Once the woman has achieved an orgasm, she may work with her partner. First, he will manually stimulate her. Next the *bridge technique* can be used. Here he continues to stimulate her clitoris during intercourse. Female superior position is used because this maximizes female stimulation and allows her freedom of movement. The therapist should incorporate systemic and psychodynamic marital therapy into the sex therapy sessions. The outcome studies report that there is more success with women who have never had an orgasm than with women who enter therapy because they want to increase their ability to have orgasms with their partners (DeAmicis, Goldenberg, LoPiccolo, Friedman, & Davies, 1985; Hawton & Catalin, 1990).

## Vaginismus

*Vaginismus* is defined as the involuntary spastic contraction of the outer one-third of the vagina. Vaginismus may cause severe pain (dyspareunia) causing the woman to avoid sexual activity. Kolodny, Masters, and Johnson (1979) estimate that 2% to 3% of all postadolescent women have vaginismus. Generally, they do not have a problem with sexual arousal. The causes of vaginismus are usually psychogenic and related to shame, fear, and embarrassment. Dyspareunia can sometimes lead to vaginismus. Masters and Johnson (1970) found that vaginismus is associated with erectile dysfunction in a woman's partner, strong religious teachings against sexuality, homosexual feelings, a history of sexual assault, and negative or hostile feelings for one's partner.

23. Which of the following occurs in females and is defined as the involuntary spastic contraction of the outer one-third of the vagina?
    a. sexual aversion
    b. dyspareunia
    c. vaginismus
    d. anorgasmia

The successful treatment of vaginismus most often utilizes behavioral techniques focused on modifying a conditioned response. Often vaginal dilators progressing in size are used, combined with Kegel exercises to teach control of circumvaginal muscles, cognitive restructuring to alleviate guilt about sexuality or to resolve past sexual trauma, and attention to systemic marital issues or intrapsychic problems. The dilators are generally used in the doctor's office with or without the partner present. The woman must learn to allow the presence of the dilator without the conditioned fear response. The goal is to decrease the woman's fear and anxiety sufficiently so that penetration can occur. Encouragement and support from the partner is crucial (Lazarus, 1989; Leiblum, Pervin, & Cambell, 1989).

## Dyspareunia

*Dyspareunia* is painful intercourse and it may occur in men as well as women. In men, dyspareunia may be caused by infection in the penis, foreskin, testes, urethra, or the prostate, as well as allergic reactions to spermicidal creams or foams. Some men complain of sensitivity to the string of the IUD if their partner has an intrauterine device. They experience dyspareunia as pain in the penis, testes, or glans area. In women, dyspareunia may be caused by pelvic inflamatory disease, endometriosis, tumors, rigid hymen, yeast infections, creams, or many other reasons.

While many women experience pain at some points during sexual intercourse, dyspareunia is chronic. The pain could manifest as a burning sensation or cramping. It could occur externally in the vaginal area or internally in the pelvic area. Masters and Johnson estimate that approximately 1% to 2% experience dyspareunia on a regular basis.

24. _____ is painful intercourse occurring in men as well as women.
    a. sexual aversion
    b. dyspareunia
    c. vaginismus
    d. anorgasmia

## Sexual Aversion

Some people have an irrational fear—a phobia—of sexual activity. There are little data concerning the prevalence of the disorder or success of any type of treatment program. Individuals with this disorder respond to sexual activity in a phobic way. When they are approached for sexual behavior, they may experience nausea, stress reaction, increased heart rate, muscle tension, or diarrhea. Sexual aversion is usually caused by severe negative attitudes toward sexuality expressed by the individual's parents during childhood (LoPiccolo, 1992). Also related is consistent pressuring by a partner or gender confusion in men (Kolodny et al., 1979). Many clients with sexual aversion disorder have a history of childhood molestation or adult sexual trauma.

Most clinicians would agree that treatment of sexual aversion should include some sort of systematic desensitization to the aversive sexual behavior, along with an introduction and focus on the ability to experience sexual pleasure. Treatment techniques also include suggestions for avoiding flashbacks in sexual situations and the necessity of recovering memories in psychotherapy. Kaplan's (1987) model of sexual phobias broadened the concept of aversion to sex. She suggested pharmacological treatment as an important adjunct to sex therapy. Her view, however, still needs to be empirically tested.

## DIAGNOSIS AND ASSESSMENT

Couple therapists dealing with sexual issues address the following four areas of assessment:

1. Identifying organic causes
2. Identifying psychological issues
3. Examining interpersonal factors
4. Assessing systemic issues

### Organic Factors

Organic factors may be the direct cause, the primary cause, or a contributing factor in sexual functioning. Even in sexually dysfunctional clients who are seemingly organically intact, there are usually some biophysiological processes implicated in the sexual dysfunction. (For a more detailed description of these factors, the reader is referred to Kolodny et al., 1979.) For this reason, the therapist should have a basic knowledge of the potential organic factors that can cause sexual symptoms.

There are also physical causes of sexual dysfunctions. Some of the more relevant ones are: biochemical/physiological disorders, tumors, anatomic or mechanical interference such as endometriosis or prostatitis, postsurgery with neurological or vascular, some neurological disorders. In males, vascular disorders may cause erectile problems by interfering with vascular flow to the penis, endocrine disorders can depress sexual drive by decreasing androgen levels, and genetic or congenital disorders such as **Klinefelter's syndrome** may also result in impotence, as can undescended testes. Drugs and medication may have a direct or indirect effect on sexual functioning. When a person is physically ill or impaired, they generally are not in the mood for sexual activity. Assessment and diagnosis should include some of these relevant questions:

1. Is there a physical disease or disability? (e.g., renal failure, circulatory problems, diabetes).
2. Does the partner of the person who is presenting the sexual dysfunction have a disease? The person may be responding to the partner's postcardiac vulnerability, cancer, prostatectomy, or mastectomy.
3. Is the client taking any drugs that could affect sexual function? (e.g., hypertensive medicine, alcohol, methadone).
4. Has the person had any surgery such as prostate gland removal or vulvectomy?
5. Is there an escalation in the aging process that is impairing sexual functioning?

### Psychological Issues

Briefly, psychological issues refer to the complex and unique elements in each individual that can shape sexual attitudes and behavior (e.g., adequate or inadequate sex information and education). The psychological sequences that mediate most dysfunctions are an unwillingness to make love, an inability to relax, and an inability to concentrate on sensation. A major assessment issue here is to identify the inhibitions that block sexual desire. The most common inhibitions are anxiety, guilt, and reaction to sexual trauma. Once they are identified they need to be conveyed to the couple in a nonblaming, nonjudgmental manner.

Generally speaking, psychological issues involved in sexual dysfunction are early sexual attitudes and experiences such as early rape or incest, lack of information about sexuality, situational factors such as unemployment, communication problems, or intrapsychic issues such as performance anxiety or depression.

Some other information relevant to assessing psychological factors is exploring the person's sexual history including a psychosexual/developmental overview/exploration of the client's childhood personal history and religious upbringing and obtaining information on their current sexual behavior as well as their attitudinal and cognitive factors.

## Interpersonal Issues

Interpersonal issues can affect sexual functioning through ineffective sexual communication (e.g., not openly discussing sexual needs).

It is also important for therapists to carefully evaluate the couple's general relationship at the beginning of therapy. Some sexual dysfunction is usually exhibited by couples in marital distress. Focusing on marital problems helps to facilitate more rapid changes in both marital and sexual functioning.

## Systemic Issues

Although the couple's relationship should be carefully evaluated at the beginning of therapy and some sexual dysfunction is usually exhibited by couples in marital distress, these dysfunctions, however, could play various important roles in the maintenance of the marital system, for example, they may divert the couple from other family interactions (Atwood, 1993; Crowe & Ridley, 1990). They may help the couple to maintain emotional distance. They may provide the couple with outlets for power positions or hostility, and so forth. They may sustain role specific behavior. In these cases, treating the sexual dysfunction in a sex therapeutic modality alone is likely to meet with failure in that the sexual dysfunction must be sustained in order to maintain the stability of the marriage. This type of conceptualization enables the therapist to assess and understand the place of influences within the marriage in the etiology and maintenance of the sexual dysfunction, the relative strength of relationship enhancing forces that could potentially facilitate and support the process of sex therapy, and the relative strength of relationship diminishing forces that would potentially inhibit and perhaps even undermine the process of sex therapy. Therefore, a comprehensive and multi-dimensional approach to the treatment of sexual dysfunctions must include a thorough evaluation of the marital relationship. Focusing on marital problems helps to facilitate more rapid changes in both marital and sexual functioning.

25. Which sex therapy approach includes an evaluation of the marital relationship?
    a. Masters and Johnson
    b. psychoanalytic
    c. systemic
    d. a and c only

## TREATMENT CONSIDERATIONS

The general program most widely used in sex therapy is the conjoint therapy of Masters and Johnson (1970) modified in its detail by Bancroft (1989; see also Gilliam, 1987; Spence, 1991; Wincze & Carey, 1991). Some basic assumptions of this approach are as follows:

1. *The problem is believed to be a joint problem.* It is never really the problem of one person if that person is in a relationship. This does not necessarily imply causality or fault, but rather, that when in a relationship, what one person does has an impact on the other.

2. *Sex is seen as a natural function.* Sexual behavior is enormously affected by social learning, family definitions and values, individual personality dynamics and biology; but it is also considered a natural function. The reflexes of sexual behavior are present from birth. Erections happen; vaginal lubrication happens. These reflexes are not taught; they occur automatically.

3. *The couple is educated in sexual knowledge.* Couples are given information about anatomy, physiology, different coital positions, and so forth. Here it is important to work hand in hand with medical personnel to distribute accurate information regarding any organically based etiology of the sexual dysfunction.

4. *Some of the anxiety is reduced.* The couple is told not to engage in intercourse at this time. This removes the immediate pressure to perform and thus tends to reduce anxiety. Relaxation skill training may be used.

5. *The couple is taught to develop sexual communication skills.* Generally sexual difficulties are concomitant with communication difficulties. It is helpful to include both partners when assisting the couple with more constructive communication techniques.

26. Which of the following concepts characterizes the Masters and Johnson therapy approach?
    a. the problem is believed to be a joint problem
    b. sex is seen as a natural function
    c. the couple is educated in sexual knowledge
    d. all of the above

## The Basic Concepts

*A Biopsychosocial Approach.*   The Masters and Johnson model recognizes the importance of the underlying physiological and anatomical bases of human sexual behavior. In addition, it takes into account the clients' mental health status and physical functioning, as well as providing a basis for answering client's questions related to sexual anatomy and physiology.

*Dual-Sex Therapy Teams.*   Masters and Johnson believed that a dual-sex therapy team of a male and a female therapist is important because only a female can understand female sexuality and only a male can understand male sexuality.

27. Which of the following model of sex therapy utilizes a dual-sex therapy team?
    a. Masters and Johnson
    b. psychoanalytic
    c. systemic
    d. object relations

*A Rapid Treatment Approach.*   The Masters and Johnson treatment program consists of an intensive daily treatment format that occurs over two weeks.

*History Taking and Initial Assessments.*   History taking occurs the first day with each therapist interviewing the same sex partner. This session typically lasts from 1 to 2 hours. In this session, a detailed social history is taken as well as a detailed sexual history. After a break, the partners are interviewed by the therapist of the opposite sex. Next, there is a thorough medical examination.

*Beginning Treatment.*   The basic therapy program of Masters and Johnson involves two weeks away from home and work devoted completely to therapy. While this approach has good success rates, it is impractical and too expensive for most couples. But there are some common aspects of most sex therapy programs:

1. Usually there is a period of coital abstinence to reduce performance anxiety and facilitate communication.
2. There is a focus on giving and receiving pleasure rather than on orgasm per se.
3. Sensate focus exercises involving tactile stimulation are used. These exercises are the cornerstone of any sex therapy program. They begin with an emphasis on nonverbal and then on verbal communication.
4. The couple is encouraged to find a mutually agreed-upon time and place to focus on their sexual interaction without distractions. They are encouraged to spend time together engaging in communication and nongenital touching.
5. They are asked to verbalize to their partner how the touching feels and what aspects they like. They are asked to fondle and touch each other for the specific purposes of giving and receiving pleasure. Again, the emphasis is not on sexual intercourse, nor is it on orgasm.
6. Handriding techniques are used to assist the couple in showing each other what feels pleasurable. Here the partners take turns placing a hand on his or her partner's hand and gently moving the partner's hand over the body showing what is pleasurable. For example, the wife will guide the husband's hand across her body showing him what is pleasurable to her.

28. Common aspects of most sex therapy programs involve which of the following?
    a. a period of coital abstinence
    b. focus on giving and receiving pleasure
    c. sensate focus exercises
    d. all of the above

29. Handriding refers to:
    a. writing one's feelings about sexuality on the bedroom wall.
    b. verbalizing to one's partner what he or she likes sexually.
    c. partners taking turns placing his or her hand on the hand of his or her partner and gently moving the partner's hand over the body showing what is pleasurable.
    d. physical exercises using the hands that help identify nonerogenous zones.

As therapy progresses, the therapist encourages additional exercises. Genital stimulation is suggested, and the couple is encouraged to discuss how they feel. The exercises progress in a nondemanding manner eventually to sexual intercourse. Couples are asked to explore alternative positions and discuss which ones are preferable. Rest periods are suggested as sexual tension mounts in order to prolong sexual pleasure.

There is a sequencing of sexual activities and techniques that facilitate success. Specific techniques are suggested that will meet the specific needs of the couple—for example, the squeeze technique for premature ejaculation.

## WHEN TO REFER

Under any circumstances, it is important for the marriage and family therapist to have a basic understanding of sexual dysfunction etiology. The therapist who does not have specific training in sexual therapy should refer when the following conditions are present:

1. Clinical depression underlying the sexual complaint.
2. Significant past psychiatric history.
3. Problems complicated by homosexual conflict or gender confusion, overt or latent.
4. Patients who present with marked personality or characterological disorders.
5. Primary sexual dysfunction.

30. Which of the following situations indicate when a therapist should refer?
    a. clinical depression
    b. significant past psychiatric disorder
    c. gender confusion
    d. all of the above

## CASE EXAMPLE

*Linda and Mark came for therapy. They said they argued about anything and everything. Married 3 years, they were twenty-two and twenty-five respectively and had just bought a house. They were financially stable and each had their own careers. During the session it was discovered that Mark prematurely ejaculated the majority of times they had sex. This was frustrating to both of them and unusual because prior to their buying the house, this was not a problem.*

Several types of therapy could be relevant in this situation. Using Masters and Johnson's approach, a cognitive-behavioral focus could be implemented. In this case, the couple would be encouraged to not have sexual intercourse initially. This way, most of the anxiety around performance would be removed. Next, they would be told to practice sensate focus techniques, first using nonerogenous zone touching and proceeding to erogenous zone touching. Then, once they were successful at this process, they would use the woman-on-top position and apply the squeeze technique when Mark reported the inevitability of orgasm. Linda would decide when penetration would occur and sexual intercourse would follow.

Another approach more social constructionist in nature (see Atwood, 1993) could be utilized instead. Here the couple's meaning systems would be explored. First, the therapist would question how the couple saw their marriage. What did it mean to them to be married? In this case, it was learned that both Linda and Mark saw marriage as a commitment to each other and to a particular lifestyle. They had planned while they were engaged to proceed into the marriage and then to buy a house and then to have a baby. As it turned out, when questioned about having a child, both reported they were afraid. Buying the house signaled to both of them that the next step in their definition of "married" would be to have a child. While not unusual, Linda and Mark were relatively young and knew from their older friends that having a child meant they would have to curtail a lot of activities they loved doing. It is not a far jump to realize this was at the base of Mark's premature ejaculation. Using this approach, the focus of attention was the couple's meaning systems. Their belief about the meaning of marriage was explored along with an expansion of the idea that marriage must progress along certain lines.

---

Long term follow-up studies of couples who have received sex therapy show considerable variation in outcomes among different types of sexual problems (DeAmicis et al., 1985; Hawton & Catalin, 1990). In terms of male problems, sex therapy appears to produce satisfactory results in both the short and long term for erectile dysfunctions, but less sustained results for premature ejaculation. Men with low sexual desire appear to have a very poor prognosis. With regard to female problems, the result of sex therapy for vaginismus are excellent and sustained, whereas the results of treatment of desire disorders are often disappointing, especially in the long term.

Prognostic significance in sex therapy is the quality of the couples' general relationship; pre-treatment motivation, especially of the male partner; the degree of attraction between partners; and early progress in terms of carrying out homework assignments.

Of relevance to the psychological treatment of sexual dysfunctions is the explosion that has occurred in physical treatments, especially the use of intracavernosal injections and vacuum devises for men with erectile dysfunctions. Though these undoubtedly represent important advances in treatment, especially for men with organic disorders, it is worrying that some clinicians are readily using them to treat apparent psychogenic cases. In the future, there should be more collaboration between those therapists experienced in psychologically based treatment approaches and those such as urologists who largely provide only physical treatment.

The most pressing need in the field is for the development of an understanding of low sexual desire. It appears that there is no physiological factor present in healthy premenopausal women that could be responsible for the disorder. Marital therapy might help couples experiencing this and other difficulties. In addition, the fields of couples therapy and sexual therapy need to have more of an overlap in training programs.

## KEY TERMS

**impotence:** The inability of a man to achieve or sustain an erection during sexual activity.

**Klinefelter's syndrome:** A general abnormality in males in which the sex-determining chromosomes are XXY rather than the normal XY.

**orgasm:** The moment of climax or peak experience during sexual activity.

**plateau phase:** The second phase of the Masters and Johnson description of the human sexual response cycle, describing a high degree of sexual arousal occuring prior to the threshold levels required to trigger orgasm.

**premature ejaculation:** Ejaculation that occurs either prior to, just before, or just after intromission of the penis into the vagina.

**refractory period:** A temporary state following orgasm and ejaculation in the man, in which there appears to be a specific resistance to additional sexual stimulation.

**resolution phase:** Term used by Masters and Johnson to refer to their fourth stage in the human sexual response cycle when the body returns to a sexually unexcited state.

**sex flush:** A description of the skin changes resulting from vasocongestion, often associated with increased sexual arousal.

**sexual dysfunction:** A failure in sexual response.
**vaginismus:** Spasms by the vaginal musculature which prevent entry of the penis.
**vasocongestion:** Congestion of the veins in the genital area resulting in swelling.

## DISCUSSION QUESTIONS

1. Discuss fully the history of sex therapy. What social forces do you think allowed for the progression?
2. Although sexual problems are listed in the *DSM–IV* (*Diagnostic and Statistical Manual*), can you envision a view whereby sexual problems are not considered to be psychological disorders? Give your reasons why or why not.
3. Using the material given in the chapter, discuss a systemic interpretation of three (3) of the sexual disorders.
4. Using Masters and Johnson's model for human sexual functioning, discuss fully the four stages of the human sexual reponse cycle.
5. Discuss why you do or do not believe multicultural influences would affect or influence sexual functioning.
6. In your opinion, how did Helen Singer Kaplan influence the field of sex therapy?
7. List the male and female sexual dysfunctions. Present a discussion on contributory factors that lead to sexual problems.
8. What are some organic or physical disorders that would affect sexual functioning?
9. Why is it important to take a sex history when doing sex therapy? What factors would influence a person's attitudes and values about sexuality and how would this affect his or her sexual functioning?
10. Discuss Masters and Johnson's treatment model in detail, including a discussion of their basic treatment considerations.

## SUGGESTED FURTHER READING

### For Therapists:

Kaplan, H. S. (1995). *Sexual desire disorder: Dysfunctional regulation of sexual motivation.* New York: Brunner-Routledge.

Based on work with 6,000 clients, Kaplan takes an integrated biopsychosocial approach, examining the neurophysiological underpinnings of sexual behaviors as well as the psychodynamic factors and environmental determinants. She also looks at psychiatric disorders that can lead to loss of sexual desire and at organic causes, such as medical conditions, drugs, and aging.

Leiblum, S. R., & Rosen, R. C. (2000). *Principles and practice of sex therapy* (3rd ed.). New York: Guilford Press.

A general sex therapy book that contains a great wealth of information on such topics as sexual dysfunctions and the paraphilias.

### For Couples:

Kuriansky, J. (2001). *The complete idiot's guide to tantric sex.* Alpha Books.

A fun book for couples who want to make a change in their sex lives, it is written in a very clear, detailed, and simple manner and provides tips about how to improve communication, how to make relationships grow, and how to become "one" with each other.

Schnarch, D. (1998). *Passionate marriage: Love, sex and intimacy in emotionally committed relationships*. New York: Henry Holt & Company.

Based on conversations taken directly from Schnarch's (a sex therapist) couples he sees in practice; he believes that the longer a couple has been together, the higher the passion.

## Web sites:

General Information on Sexual Dysfunctions

  http://www.umsl.edu/~s1015655/sexdys.html

Treating Female Dysfunction

  http://www.aafp.org/afp/20000701/127.html

General Information on Sexuality

  http://www.annarborcenter.com/sexuality.html

## REFERENCES

American Psychiatric Association. (1987). *Diagnostic and statistical manual of mental disorders* (3rd ed., rev.). Washington, DC: Author.

Atwood, J. D. (1993). Social constructionist couples therapy. *The Family Journal: Counseling & Therapy for Couples and Families*, 1(2), 116–129.

Atwood, J. D., & Gagnon, J. (1987). Masturbatory behavior in college youth. *Journal of Sex Education and Therapy, 13*(2), 35–42.

Bancroft, J. (1989). *Human sexuality and its problems*. New York: Churchill Livingstone.

Crowe, M., & Ridley, J. (1990). *Therapy with couples: A behavioral systems approach to marital and sexual problems*. Oxford, England: Blackwell.

DeAmicis, L., Goldenberg, D. C., LoPiccolo, J., Friedman, J., & Davies, L. (1985). Clinical follow-up of couples treated for sexual dysfunction. *Archives of Sexual Behavior, 14*, 467–489.

De Silva, P. (1992). Sexual and marital therapy in clinical psychology training. *Bulletin of the British Association of Sexual and Marital Therapists, 8*, 16–18.

De Silva, P. (1994). Psychological treatment of sexual problems. *International Review of Psychiatry, 6*, 163–173.

Frank, E., Anderson, C., & Rubinstein, D. (1978). The frequency of sexual dysfunction in couples. *New England Journal of Medicine, 299*, 111–115.

Geer, J. H., & Quartararo, J. D. (1976). Vaginal blood volume responses during masturbation. *Archives of Sexual Behavior, 5*(5), 403–413.

Gilliam, P. (1987). *Sex therapy manual*. Oxford, England: Blackwell.

Hawton, K. (1985). *Sex therapy: A practical guide*. Oxford, England: Oxford Medical Publications.

Hawton, K., & Catalin, J. (1990). Sex therapy for vaginismus: Characteristics of couples, treatment outcome. *Sexual and Marital Therapy, 5*, 39–48.

Hite, S. (1976). *The Hite report*. New York: Macmillan.

Kaplan, H. S. (1974). *The new sex therapy*. New York: Brunner/Mazel.

Kaplan, H. S. (1979). *The disorders of sexual desire*. New York: Brunner/Mazel.

Kaplan, H. S. (1987). *Sexual aversion and sexual phobias and panic disorders*. New York: Brunner/Mazel.

Kinsey, A. C., Pomeroy, W. B., Gebhard, P. H., & Martin, C. E. (1953). *Sexual behavior in the human female*. Philadelphia: Scunders.

Kolodny, R., Masters, W., & Johnson, V. (1979). *A textbook of sexual medicine*. Boston: Little, Brown and Company.

Lazarus, A. A. (1989). Dyspareunia: A multimodal psychotherapeutic perspective. In S. R. Leiblum & R. C. Rosen (Eds.), *Principles and practice of sex therapy: Update for the 1990s* (pp. 89–112). New York: Guilford Press.

Leiblum, S. R., Pervin, L. A., & Cambell, E. H. (1989). The treatment of vaginismus: Success and failure. In S. R. Leiblum & R. C. Rosen (Eds.), *Principles and practice of sex therapy: Update for the 1990s* (pp. 167–192). New York: Guilford Press.

Leiblum, S. R., & Rosen, R. C. (1988). Changing perspectives on sexual desire. In S. R. Leiblum & R. C. Rosen (Eds.), *Sexual desire disorders* (pp. 1–20). New York: Guilford Press.

LoPiccolo, J. (1992). Postmodern sex therapy for erectile failure. In R. C. Rosen & S. R. Leiblum (Eds.), *Erectile disorders: Assessment and treatment* (pp. 171–179). New York: Guilford Press.

Masters, W. H., & Johnson, V. E. (1966). *Human sexual response*. Boston: Little, Brown and Company.

Masters, W. H., & Johnson, V. E. (1970). *Human sexual inadequacy*. Boston: Little, Brown and Company.

Semans, J. H. (1956). Premature ejaculation: A new approach. *Southern Medical Journal, 49*, 353–358.

Spence, S. H. (1991). *Psychosexual therapy: A cognitive-behavioral approach*. London: Chapman and Hall.

Wincze, J. P., & Carey, M. P. (1991). *Sexual dysfunction: A guide for assessment and treatment*. New York: Guilford Press.

Woody, J. D. (1992). *Treating sexual distress: Integrative systems therapy*. Newbury Park: Sage Publications.

Zilbergeld, B., & Evans, M. (1980). The inadequacy of Masters and Johnson. *Psychology Today, 14*(3), 29–43.

# 14

# Intimate Partner Violence

Sandra M. Stith
Karen H. Rosen
*Virginia Tech*

## TRUTH OR FICTION?

___ 1. Partner violence has adverse affects on only those directly involved.

___ 2. Couples therapy may be an appropriate treatment for some couples in which the man is violent toward his partner.

___ 3. Giving your partner the "silent treatment" can be considered emotional abuse.

___ 4. Pushing and shoving are not considered to be acts of physical abuse.

___ 5. All partner violence is considered battering.

___ 6. Clients are usually forthcoming to their therapist about partner violence occurring within their relationship.

___ 7. It is not necessary for you to assess for relationship violence if the client has not identified it as a therapeutic issue.

___ 8. You should ask about the specific details of incidents of partner violence when both partners are in the room.

___ 9. Violent men tend to be a heterogeneous group.

___ 10. Violent men tend have strengths and resources that may be useful to the therapeutic process.

___ 11. Jealousy and poor communication skills are the most frequently cited motivations for hitting one's partner.

___ 12. One way for a victim of abuse to ensure her safety is to leave her abusive partner.

___ 13. All abused women who seek therapy want to leave their abusive partners.

___ 14. A victim who leaves the relationship often experiences a grieving process.

___ 15. Violent individuals should be held accountable for their abusive behavior.

___ 16. Hitting their partner back is a good way for victims to get their partners to stop hitting them.

Family therapists often need to diagnose and treat intimate partner violence. Therefore our chapter is designed to provide you with some of the tools you need to do so effectively. We begin with information about the frequency of intimate partner violence and the devastating impact it can have on all family members. Next, we discuss the types of partner violence. While physical violence, especially severe life-threatening violence, is often what comes to mind when referring to "intimate partner violence," we believe that to be effective in addressing this issue, you need to understand that each form of partner violence can have catastrophic effects on the physical and/or mental health of family members. We also want you to understand why therapists often do not realize that violence is occurring between partners so that you will be prepared to uncover it if it is occurring. We present clear guidelines to assist you in screening for violence in intimate relationships and assessing for severe violence in relationships where violence is occurring.

As a family therapist, you need to be prepared to work with couples in violent relationships, but also with individual clients in violent relationships. Therefore, we discuss offenders and victims and their treatment as well as how conjoint treatment for intimate partner violence can be used appropriately and safely with some couples. Since substance abuse and intimate partner violence often go hand in hand, we include a section on that issue. Next, we offer you some information about countertransference reactions you might experience when working with intimate partner violence and a few tips to help you deal with your reactions. Finally, we encourage you to become actively involved in community coalitions addressing intimate partner violence in your own communities.

While men and women use violence in their relationships at approximately equal rates, this chapter will focus on violence against women for several reasons. First, wives are more likely than husbands to suffer severe physical injuries and serious psychological and emotional consequences. Second, although neither spouse's aggression is acceptable, a woman is apt to use violence as a means of self-defense after experiencing repeated aggression from her husband, while the man is apt to use aggression as a means of controlling his partner (Stets, 1988). Finally, society's encouragement of women to value "relationship at any cost," as well as weak institutional response to domestic violence (Hotaling, Straus, & Lincoln, 1990), often contributes to women deciding to maintain relationships that are at best psychologically damaging and at worst life threatening. Thus, we focus on husband violence.

## HOW OFTEN DOES INTIMATE PARTNER VIOLENCE OCCUR?

Partner violence is a pervasive social problem that has devastating effects on all family members as well as on the larger community. Rates of violence vary based on the sample from which the rates are calculated. The 1995 National Violence Against Women Survey indicated that 22% of women and 7% of men reported being victimized by an intimate partner at some point in their lifetime. Even higher rates are reported from large-scale random sample studies that ask respondents to report on violence in response to *family conflict*. These studies find annual rates as high as 10% to 35% while studies that look specifically at *violent crimes* indicate rates ranging from 0.2% to 1.1% (Straus, 1999). Regardless of the context in which violence rates are calculated, it is clear that partner violence is an all too common occurrence in many American families.

Although this chapter focuses on violence in heterosexual relationships, it is important to remember that partner violence is also a substantial problem in gay and lesbian relationships (Miller, Bobner, & Zarski, 2000). While research on the prevalence of same sex violence is limited, from what we do know, same sex violence seems to be comparable in frequency to heterosexual violence. For example, Island and Letellier (1991) estimate that between 15% and 20% of gay and lesbian couples experience intimate partner violence. However, keep in mind that prevalence rates in same-sex relationships are very difficult to determine and may be underestimated due to general reluctance to report unpleasant private matters and because heterosexism tends to silence gays and lesbians. Thus researchers must rely on the reports of self-selected samples from the gay and lesbian communities.

1. Prevalence rates of intimate partner violence tend to vary widely from one study to another because:
   a. Some researchers tend to exaggerate their findings for political reasons.
   b. Samples and types of questions asked vary from one study to another.
   c. Researchers do not know how to assess for violence.
   d. Violence is no longer a significant problem in the United States.

2. Prevalence rates of violence occurring in gay and lesbian relationships are especially difficult to determine because:
   a. Rates are determined only by reports of self-selected samples from the gay and lesbian community.
   b. Rates are generally based on lesbian samples.
   c. Heterosexism tends to silence gays and lesbians.
   d. All of the above.

# HOW DOES PARTNER VIOLENCE AFFECT FAMILY MEMBERS?

A true accounting of the costs of partner violence is difficult to obtain partly because incidents are thought to be underreported. A consideration of the costs must include medical, mental health, police, legal, and social services to victims and perpetrators; loss of productivity on the job; and negative impacts on children. Indeed, abusive relationships cause significant distress, which decreases individual and family quality of life. Partner violence has significant adverse effects on women's mental and physical health. One study indicated that severely assaulted women had twice as many headaches, four times the rate of depression, nearly six times more suicide attempts, and twice as many days in bed due to illness as women who were not abused (Gelles & Straus, 1990). In addition, it is estimated that 35% of women visit hospital emergency rooms for treatment of injuries caused by partner violence (American Bar Association, 1995).

Partner abuse has been linked to profound and long-lasting negative emotional and behavioral effects on children who witness the abuse (Jaffe & Sudermann, 1995). These children have been found to assault their siblings and their parents, to commit violent crimes outside the family, and to assault their own intimate partners as adults more often than children who have not witnessed violence between their parents (Gelles & Straus, 1990; O'Leary, 1988). Children in families where there is partner abuse are also more likely to be hit by the abuser (Jaffe, Wolfe, & Wilson, 1990).

Intimate partner violence can also have a significant impact on the therapeutic process. One can only imagine the challenges faced by clients who are trying to change within relationships where power and intimidation are already well established. Because abuse is often associated with power and control, you need to address intimate partner violence before any other therapeutic work can proceed.

3. Women who experience abuse from their intimate partner may experience:
   a. suicidal ideations, headaches, and depression.
   b. broken bones.
   c. physical injuries.
   d. all of the above.

4. Children who live in homes where intimate partner violence is occurring have been found to experience all of the following, *except:*
   a. increased likelihood of assaulting their siblings and parents.
   b. increased likelihood of committing violent crimes outside the family.
   c. increased likelihood of being assaulted themselves.
   d. increased likelihood of experiencing serious childhood illnesses.

## FORMS OF ABUSE

For the sake of this chapter the words abuse and violence are being used interchangeably. There are three primary forms of intimate partner violence: physical, emotional, and sexual. Although researchers and clinicians may not always agree on what acts constitute each of these three forms of abuse, we provide basic definitions as a starting point. We view the three forms of abuse as occurring on a continuum from mild to severe based on the offender's behavior. However, we encourage you to keep in mind that any act of violence has the potential to harm the victim and shift the power arrangement in a relationship. Additionally, although we describe them as discrete types of abuse, in reality, a variety of acts from two or all three often co-occur between partners or from one partner to the other in intimate relationships.

### Physical Abuse

**Physical abuse** includes a variety of nonsexual assaultive behaviors. We consider grabbing, pushing, shoving, pinching and biting acts of physical abuse although often clients do not define them as such. Slapping, hitting, and punching are acts of physical abuse that most clients are concerned about. Of course, the most extreme forms of physical abuse such as choking, hitting with an object or assaulting with a deadly weapon (e.g., gun or knife) are acts that have a high potential to cause physical harm to the victim or fear of harm.

### Emotional/Psychological Abuse

**Emotional** or psychological abuse is more difficult to define because it involves acts that have the potential to leave psychological scars that cannot be seen. For the sake of this chapter we are using the terms emotional and psychological abuse interchangeably and defining them broadly. We also note that emotional abuse is usually designed to frighten, control, or disparage a partner. Acts such as yelling, using derogatory terms, put-downs, or name calling systematically damage a partner's sense of self. In an effort to control or manipulate their partner an abuser may threaten to directly harm her or her pet or withhold emotional support such as giving her the "silent treatment." Other forms of emotional abuse include stalking, trying to isolate a partner from family or friends, or withholding economic support as abusers tend to isolate and restrict the partner's independence.

## Sexual Abuse

We broadly define *sexual abuse* as acts that force the partner to have nonconsensual sexual relations. These include forcing one's partner to have sex without a condom, to have oral or anal sex, or to participate in other unwanted sexual acts. By "force" we mean applying undo pressure, threatening violence, threatening to leave the relationship, or using direct physical coercion.

While intimate partner violence may theoretically occur once or rarely between partners in an intimate relationship, it can also become a pattern of assault and coercive behaviors that include all three forms of abuse described above. The term *battering* is often used when these behaviors are severe and repetitive and carry with them elements of fear, oppression, and control.

5. Emotional abuse is difficult to define because it does not produce readily observable scars and is usually designed to:
   a. frighten, control, or disparage a partner.
   b. prepare a partner for physical abuse.
   c. force a partner to have sex.
   d. help the partner leave the relationship.

6. Which of the following are considered physically abusive acts?
   a. grabbing
   b. shoving
   c. slapping
   d. all of the above

## DISGUISED PRESENTATION

Although partner violence is a pervasive problem, family members often hide it from their therapists. O'Leary, Vivian, and Malone (1992) found that only 6% of women seeking counseling indicated on their intake form that marital violence was a significant problem in their relationship. However, when asked to complete a standardized assessment instrument, 53% indicated that their husbands had physically assaulted them. In another study, Stith, Rosen, Barasch, and Wilson (1991), found that while only 12% of 262 families initially reported partner violence as the presenting problem, partner violence was occurring in at least 40% of the families they saw.

Clients have various reasons for not reporting the occurrence of violence in their relationships (Aldarondo & Straus, 1994). Clients may perceive violence as tolerable and therefore not an important issue to bring up in therapy. They may be unaware of the impact violence has on themselves and their relationship. Clients receiving severe forms of violence may be fearful that their partner will become more violent if they tell their therapist about the violence. In addition, clients are often embarrassed and humiliated that violence is occurring in their relationship and may be afraid of their therapist's response to learning about the violence. Every client will be unique in his or her reasons for not reporting or for underreporting violence, but it is your responsibility to use appropriate techniques to assess for partner violence.

Unfortunately, therapists often fail to identify abuse even in the context of clear evidence given by their clients. In a study by Hansen, Harway, and Cervantes (1991), 40% of family therapists failed to recognize severe violence described in vignettes. Unfortunately, these therapists would have left it untreated. Why do therapists often fail to discover that violence is occurring in their clients' relationship? First and foremost, many therapists simply do not ask about abuse. Second, even when they do ask, clinicians may use the terms "violence" or "abuse," terms that most clients do not associate with their relationships. You will increase your chance of detecting violence when you ask clients about specific behaviors such as "grabbing" or "pushing" or using terms such as "getting physical."

7. Which of the following is an explanation for why victims may not tell their therapists they are being abused?
   a. They may be embarrassed about it.
   b. They may be unaware of the impact that the violence has on themselves and their relationship.
   c. They may be fearful that their partner will become more violent if they tell their therapist.
   d. All of the above.

## ASSESSMENT PROCEDURES

The first step in assessing partner violence is to determine if any form of aggression is occurring in the relationship. You should assess every couple seen and include both an oral interview and a written assessment instrument. It is vital that interviews regarding potential interpersonal violence be conducted with each individual separately. When you ask each partner privately about their own and their partner's violence, you are able to compare each person's story and the degree of consensus between stories. You can increase the odds of detecting violence by the language you use. Asking a couple about how conflict is handled in their relationship, what happens when they get angry, or if either partner ever grabs or pushes the other, is more likely to uncover violence if its happening, than asking if the partner is abusive or violent.

Each partner should complete assessment instruments in different rooms so that they can feel safe to report their experiences accurately and so that they will not be endangered by their responses. Many clinicians include a measure of relationship violence in an **intake assessment package**. The most widely used instrument is the Conflict Tactics Scale (CTS) (See Straus, 1979 for actual instrument) which contains 18 items and asks respondents about their own and their partner's behavior. Straus, Hamby, Boney-McCoy, and Sugarman (1996) developed a revised and more comprehensive version of the Conflict Tactics Scale (CTS2) that contains 78 items assessing psychological, physical, and sexual abuse. Both forms of the CTS are appropriate for both offenders and victims.

In addition to using standardized assessment measures, we recommend that you include questions in your intake package, such as, "Does anyone in your family have concerns about the way anger is handled? If so, explain." Or, "Are you ever uncomfortable with the way conflict is handled between adults in your family? If so, explain." If clients indicate some concern about the way anger is handled, you should discuss this issue further in separate sessions.

8. Which is the best way to find out about abuse that is occurring in your client's relationship?
   a. Ask your client, "Is your partner abusing you"?
   b. Ask your client, "Has your partner ever pushed, shoved, or hit you"?
   c. Ask about abusive behavior in a conjoint session.
   d. Do not ask directly about abuse; let the client talk about the abuse when he or she is ready.

9. Screening for partner violence should include all of the following **except**:
   a. On the intake form, ask clients about concerns with the ways anger is handled.
   b. Use a standardized instrument, such as the CTS in the assessment package.
   c. Interview each client separately and ask about the occurrence of specific controlling, emotionally abusive, and physically abusive acts.
   d. Contact family members without the clients' permission to discover unreported partner violence.

## LETHALITY ASSESSMENT

Once violence is identified, you need to assess the degree of danger and potential lethality (Holtzworth-Munroe, Beatty, & Anglin, 1995) by asking about the severity, frequency, and chronicity of the violence; whether it has been escalating; and whether the victim feels safe. The victim's prediction of the risk for severe assault is one of the best predictors of dangerousness (Weisz, Tolman, & Saunders, 2000). However, please note that victims sometimes underestimate the danger they are in.

If violence is occurring, you should also ask whether guns or other weapons are available in the home; if they are, you should require that all weapons be removed from the home during therapy. You should also assess for substance abuse and depression. Substance abuse can increase the risk for severe violence to occur and sabotage treatment. Depression and suicidality (on the part of either partner) can co-occur with partner violence. If the victim decides to end the relationship, the risk for the offender to become suicidal can be especially high.

A lethality assessment should also assess for other forms of abuse including psychological abuse and stalking. Though psychological abuse generally co-occurs with physical abuse, the extent and seriousness of the psychological abuse is an indicator of the victim's safety. Also, stalking can be an indicator of more serious physical abuse or potential for homicide. You will also want to find out if the abusive partner has been violent outside the home. Have there been any arrests or protection orders in the past due to his violent behavior or threats of violence? If restraining or protection orders were in place were they followed? You should also determine each person's history with abuse. Did they witness or experience physical abuse as a child? Do they believe that physical abuse is acceptable? Has there been violence in previous relationships? Knowing about these attitudes and experiences can help you determine appropriate treatment options.

Finally, important protective factors should be assessed. Does each partner have a healthy social support system? Does the offender appear to take responsibility for his actions and to be ready to make changes in his life? These factors interact with the risk factors described above in determining the acceptability of a **conjoint treatment** methodology.

The overall assessment should be undertaken in the context of a working alliance (O'Leary & Murphy, 1999). High dropout rates among this clientele often come from a punitive rather than a supportive approach to assessment and treatment. Both victims and offenders often expect to be blamed. Any good assessment should also assess strengths and resources. The treatment plan that is developed based on your assessment should build on pre-existing strengths and coping strategies.

---

10. If the client reports that abuse is occurring, the therapist should assess the lethality of the violence by asking about:
    a. the severity, frequency, and chronicity of the violence, and whether it has been escalating.
    b. whether the victim has done anything to provoke the offender.
    c. whether the victim has hope that the offender will stop the abuse.
    d. whether the victim loves the offender.

11. What protective factors might lead you to feel more hopeful?
    a. Each partner has a healthy support system and the offender appears to take responsibility for his actions.
    b. The couple is abusing alcohol, but no illegal drugs.
    c. The offender has a high level of depression.
    d. The victim is planning on leaving the offender.

---

## OFFENDERS

As we stated earlier, although both men and women hit their intimate partners, for the sake of this chapter we are focusing on the male offender. Male offenders are a heterogeneous group. They come in all sizes, shapes, socioeconomic and ethnic backgrounds. They may be educated or illiterate, professional or blue-collar workers. Having made this point, we also know that there are a number of risk markers that are associated with perpetrating intimate partner violence, **typologies** of batterers, and characteristics of offenders that could be dealt with in treatment.

## Risk Markers

Much of the risk marker literature focuses on childhood socialization practices suggesting that violence is transmitted from one generation to another by observing or experiencing violence in one's family of origin. Indeed, researchers have found a consistent, yet weak, relationship between family of origin violence and violence perpetrated in adult intimate relationships (Stith et al., 2000). Other socialization influences come from cultural messages about men and women that are transmitted through movies, television, books, fairy-tales, and institutions. These include beliefs that men are entitled to be treated differently than women and they should be powerful and in control while women should be dependent and submissive. Another often-studied risk marker is substance abuse. The use of alcohol and other drugs is consistently related to perpetrating violence and may also predict increased severity and occurrence of homicide (Kyriacou et al., 1999). Other risk markers include demographic characteristics such as age (youth), unemployment, and low income levels.

12. An important risk marker for offenders is:
    a. a belief that men and women should be treated equally.
    b. a belief that people over 30 should not be trusted.
    c. a belief that men should be powerful and in control while women should be dependent and submissive.
    d. a belief that women should not work outside the home.

## Batterer Typologies

Recent research on typologies of batterers have important clinical implications. Jacobson and Gottman (1998) examined only men who had used severe violence and identified two types of batterers, which they label Cobras and Pit Bulls. Cobras tended to have antisocial, criminal-like traits and to be highly aggressive. Pit Bulls tended to be emotionally dependent and insecure as well as impulsive. These researchers are skeptical that batterers can be rehabilitated claiming that batterers are criminals not clients.

On the other hand, Holtzworth-Munroe and Stuart (1994) suggest that three subtypes of batterers exist—family-only, dysphoric/borderline, and generally violent/antisocial—and that tailoring treatment to each subtype of violent men might improve treatment outcome. Family-only batterers are deemed most appropriate for couples treatment and would probably not be considered "batterers" by Gottman because they do not have a pattern of inflicting severe violence against their partners. They are likely to be the least violent of the groups and likely to have problems such as insecure attachment patterns, mild social skills deficits, and low levels of impulsivity. Additionally, family-only batterers tend to have stable marriages and relatively high levels of marital satisfaction.

13. What are the clinical implications of the batterer typology literature?
    a. All batterers should receive the same type of treatment.
    b. Batterers should be treated through the criminal justice system.
    c. Different types of batterers should receive different types of treatment.
    d. It is probably not possible to treat batterers.

## Why Do They Hit?

There are different types of abusive men and a variety of reasons that may explain why they hit. Maintaining or asserting control over his partner is the most often cited motivation for hitting a partner. Batterers sometimes say they feel powerless, and they seem to have a very low tolerance for that feeling or for feeling controlled (Barnett, Miller-Perrin, & Perrin, 1997). Other problems that offenders have which may explain their tendency to hit include poor communication and problem-solving skills, low self-esteem, life stress, depression, and jealousy. Although many violent men claim to be happily married, marital dissatisfaction is often linked to the use of aggression, particularly severe aggression (Boyle & Vivian, 1996).

14. Why do batterers hit?
    a. To maintain or assert control over their partner
    b. Because the victim provokes them
    c. It's their part in the relationship dance
    d. They have been programed to hit because of growing up in a violent home

310 STITH AND ROSEN

## Treatment

Most programs for offenders treat men in psychoeducational groups. Practice guidelines vary but most are based on a conviction about what causes and maintains abuse. Thus, cognitive–behavioral approaches are based on the assumption that abuse-supporting beliefs, lack of behavioral self-control, and poor relationship skills foster abuse. Feminist approaches are based on the assumption that male socialization in the context of societally-sanctioned oppression of women fosters abuse. Attachment-based approaches suggest that abuse arises when childhood attachment injuries are reactivated in contemporary relationships. In practice, most batterers' treatment programs incorporate different theoretical approaches and interventions. Batterers' treatment appears to produce a moderate reduction in recidivism of domestic violence for those who complete the program. However, the dropout rate is usually quite high (Babcock & La Taillade, 2000). Many states have developed minimum standards for batterer treatment programs. Become familiar with those in your state.

15. Which assumptions underlie cognitive–behavioral approaches to treating male batterers?
  a. Male socialization in the context of societally-sanctioned oppression of women fosters abuse.
  b. Abuse-supporting beliefs, lack of behavioral self-control, and poor relationship skills foster abuse
  c. Abuse arises when childhood attachment injuries are reactivated in contemporary relationships
  d. All of the above

## VICTIMS

As is true for offenders, victims come in all sizes and shapes. Indeed, some scholars suggest that any woman could become a victim of abuse because becoming a victim is an insidious process (Rosen, 1996). Although the next section presents some of the risk markers associated with being a victim of abuse, keep in mind that these characteristics do not *cause* abuse.

## Risk Markers

As is the case with offenders, much of the risk marker literature examines whether victims are more likely to have experienced or witnessed violence in their families of origin. Researchers have found weak but consistent support for the intergenerational transmission process related to becoming a victim of abuse (Stith et al., 2000). Women's socialization experiences may lead them to place overriding importance on their relationship and to accept responsibility for its success or failure. They are bombarded by cultural messages about men and women in movies, television, books, fairytales, and institutions much the same as men. Two key risk markers are women's physical violence against their husbands and their substance abuse. Both are not only consistently linked to women being abused but also to the severity of abuse (Gondolf, 1998; Sugarman, Aldarondo, & Boney-McCoy, 1996). Thus, although neither her violence nor abuse of substances causes her to be hit, either may put her in more danger. Some studies also suggest that battered women have higher levels of anger and are more likely to approve of marital violence than are nonbattered women. Additionally, a number of demographic variables are associated with women's abuse, for example, age and lack of social support, education, and employment.

## Why Does She Stay?

Although in some respects this question places the emphasis on the woman's behavior rather than on the offender's, it's a question that bears addressing because a victim's hesitance to leave her abusive partner may bewilder a clinician who has tried to give her good counsel. Economic dependence, relationship commitment, self-blame, lack of social support, and fear are all reasons that need to be addressed. In fact, research shows that leaving an abusive partner may be the most dangerous time for the victim and should therefore not be done without taking safety precautions. Some scholars have used the word *entrapment* to describe the process of becoming a victim that also hampers leaving (Rosen, 1996). Almost without being aware of it, a woman may become entangled in a relationship that is at times destructive but also remains intermittently pleasant and carries with it the hope that things may change.

## Treatment

Most abused women take active measures to stop their abuse including calling the police, fleeing to shelters, or seeking informal or formal advice and support. Keep in mind that when a woman seeks your help she may not identify abuse as a problem and, if she does, she may not want to leave her abusive partner. An abused woman who seeks help may want to know how to survive the abuse or make him stop. She may see the abuse as her fault and will most likely feel ashamed. Thus, you face the dilemma of respecting her wishes without colluding with the violence—condemning the violent behavior without condemning her for staying. We recommend taking a strong position against violence while taking a nonjudgmental position about her decision to stay.

Helping the abused woman keep herself safe and gain perspective, and empowering her to develop appropriate boundaries are three goals we keep in the forefront. You also need to be aware of community resources for victims and ensure that victims have information about hotlines and domestic violence shelters in the community. Her safety is enhanced if she has a concrete, practical safety plan to put in place if she thinks she may be abused. This plan needs to include a clear escape plan. Where would she go? How would she get there? What number would she call for help? For women who are minimizing the danger, you may need to cite research or examples that make the danger more palpable. Her safety may also hinge on her controlling her own violence if she has been hitting back. You can help her gain perspective about the cycle of violence, who owns the responsibility for violence, what relationship dynamics may keep her stuck, and how she might know when its time to make different choices for herself. In addition, it is important for you to identify and highlight her strengths and resiliencies. Without sacrificing her safety, you can also help her identify small ways that she can begin to take back her life, for example, reconnecting with friends or family, keeping her therapy private, and developing new activities.

Women may seek help after leaving an abusive relationship or they may leave while they are in therapy. In addition to the treatment goals cited above, a woman who has left may need help in maintaining her safety and her decision to leave. She will most likely be tempted to return if he contacts her and asks for a reconciliation or when she becomes lonely and misses him. Therefore, establishing a contingency plan and normalizing the grieving process are relevant treatment options. She will also likely need help with practical matters such as housing, childcare, and obtaining employment as well.

16. What is the primary reason victims stay in abusive relationships?
    a. economic dependence
    b. relationship commitment
    c. fear of offender
    d. all of the above

17. The time when a victim leaves an abusive relationship:
    a. is an exciting and rewarding time for the victim.
    b. is a particularly dangerous time for the victim.
    c. is not particularly stressful for the victim.
    d. is the time when the victim is safest.

## CONJOINT TREATMENT OF INTIMATE PARTNER VIOLENCE

The primary goal of any domestic violence treatment is the cessation of all forms of violence in the relationship. Despite the focus on the couple in conjoint treatment, preserving the relationship should not be a primary goal. Participating in couples treatment may allow some partners to reconsider whether their relationship is viable. Treatment can be considered effective if the violence ceases and the relationship improves, or if the couple separates without a violent incident. A second goal of conjoint treatment should be to increase individual self-control and responsibility. Basic to this goal is a both/and position: each individual is *both* responsible for his or her own behavior *and* understanding that individual behavior affects and is affected by the behavior of others. Although the abuser is held accountable for his actions, interrupting repetitive patterns of behavior that maintain escalating conflict cycles is a powerful tool to deal with the problem.

Regular couples therapy approaches are generally not appropriate for addressing domestic violence. Extra safeguards need to be incorporated into the work to manage the risks. Some of these safeguards include:

1. Accept couples where both partners, in separate interviews, express a strong desire to participate in conjoint treatment and have no fear of their partner's response if they get into a heated discussion.
2. Accept couples where the offender has successfully completed a program designed to specifically address his violent behavior before beginning conjoint treatment.
3. Exclude couples where either partner has a current substance abuse problem.
4. Continuously reassess the appropriateness of conjoint treatment in separate interviews of each partner throughout the treatment process.

18. The primary goal of conjoint treatment of partner violence is:
    a. to improve marital relationships.
    b. to decrease the likelihood of couples divorcing.
    c. to end all forms of violence.
    d. to enhance the quality of life for couples.

19. Which of the following is not a safeguard for conjoint treatment of partner violence?
    a. Couples where the victim, in a private interview, expresses fear of her partner, should be excluded from conjoint treatment.
    b. Couples where either partner has ever shoved, pushed, or slapped their partner should be excluded from conjoint treatment.
    c. Couples where either partner has a current substance abuse problem should be excluded from conjoint treatment.
    d. The safety of conjoint therapy should be continuously reassessed throughout the treatment process.

## Systems Theory and Intimate Partner Violence

Based on systems theory, partner violence is viewed in the context of relationship dynamics and patterns. Considerable controversy surrounds the use of a systemic perspective in the treatment of partner abuse. Some professionals suggest that systems theory blurs the boundaries between the batterer and the battered, and implies that the victim is "co-responsible" for the assault, leading to "victim blaming," and suggesting that the victim did something to deserve the abuse (Stith & Rosen, 1990). However, we find systems theory helpful in understanding partner violence because it focuses on *how* individuals are involved in violent relationships rather than placing blame (Anderson & Cramer-Benjamin, 1999). When assessing violence from a systemic perspective, individual actions and the responses of both partners should be viewed within the context of the violent episodes.

This model assumes that the unit of assessment and intervention is the couple rather than one partner in isolation. For example, Wileman and Wileman (1995) found that violence is reduced when both the man assumes responsibility for his violence and the woman decreases her vulnerability and takes an active role in balancing the power differential in the relationship.

The holistic approach that results from systems theory emphasizes the importance of examining characteristics of individuals involved in the violent relationship, as well as the dynamics that occur within the family context. Relationship characteristics appear to mediate the significance and interpretation given to violence both by the aggressor and the victim. Underlying relationship dynamics may impact each partner's decision to remain in the violent relationship despite the violence, or may play a part in maintaining the violence.

20. Systems theory helps to understand partner violence for all of the following reasons **except**:
    a. It focuses on *how* individuals are involved in violent relationships.
    b. It holds individuals responsible for their actions that contribute to abusive relationships.
    c. It assumes that the couple is the unit for assessment and intervention rather than one partner in isolation.
    d. It assumes the victim is as much at fault for the violence as the offender.

## Why Is Conjoint Treatment Appropriate for Some Couples?

There are a variety of other reasons why conjoint treatment is appropriate for some couples if they intend to remain together. Johnson (1995) identified distinctions between different types of violence occurring in ongoing relationships. He believes that "common couple violence" is characterized by a partner's use of violence that erupts during a specific argument. On the other hand, "patriarchal terrorism" reflects violence embedded in a generalized pattern of a partner's desire for control. As in the earlier discussion of different types of batterers, it has become increasingly clear that not all violent relationships require the same type of treatment.

In addition to treating subgroups of batterers differently, there are also reasons to include female partners in the treatment process. First, most research has found that women initiate and carry out physical assaults on their partners as often as do men (Stith & Straus, 1995). Despite the much lower probability of physical injury resulting from attacks by women, assaults by women are serious. If reciprocal violence is taking place in relationships, treating men without treating women is not likely to stop the violence. In fact, cessation of partner violence by one partner is highly dependent on whether the other partner also stops hitting (Feld & Straus, 1989; Gelles & Straus, 1988). In addition, when women use violence in relationships, they are at greater risk of being severely assaulted by their partners (Feld & Straus, 1989; Gondolf, 1998).

It is also important to remember that violence does not necessarily mean the demise of the relationship. In fact, 50% to 80% of battered wives remain with their abusive partners or return to them after leaving a woman's shelter or otherwise separating from them (Ferraro & Johnson, 1983). While men's treatment groups address men's roles in intimate partner violence, they do not address any underlying relationship dynamics that may impact each partner's decision to remain in the violent relationship, or that may play a part in maintaining the violence. As mentioned earlier, marital discord is a strong predictor of physical aggression toward a partner. Failure to address marital problems increases the likelihood that violence will recur. In fact, failing to assess and provide services to both parties in an ongoing relationship may inadvertently disadvantage the female partner who chooses to stay.

21. Why is conjoint treatment appropriate for some couples if they intend to remain together?
   a. All violent individuals are not alike and treatment needs to be tailored to the individual/couple.
   b. If reciprocal violence is taking place in relationships, treating men without treating women is not likely to stop the violence.
   c. Failure to address relationship problems at some point in the treatment of partner violence puts the couple at risk for continued violence.
   d. All of the above.

## Effectiveness of Conjoint Treatment

Conjoint therapy has been used to treat marital violence for some time now. Results from six experimental studies examining the effectiveness of conjoint treatment of partner violence indicate that violent men who are treated with their female partners (either in individual couple therapy or as part of a multi-couple group) reduced their violence (Stith, Rosen, & McCollum, 2002). In fact, a study by Fals-Stewart, Kashdan, O'Farrell, and Birchler (2002) found that couples therapy for substance abuse was more effective in reducing violence than individual therapy. Brannen and Rubin (1996) found that multi-couple therapy was more effective than gender-specific therapy in reducing violence for male abusers with a history of alcohol problems. Perhaps most importantly, there is no evidence from the six experimental studies conducted to date that women are more likely to be endangered in carefully screened, domestic violence–focused conjoint treatment programs than they are in programs that treat men individually.

22. The results from six experimental studies that compared conjoint treatment for partner violence with alternative treatment approaches found:
    a. Conjoint treatment puts victims at risk for further violence.
    b. Violent men who are treated with their female partners reduced their violence.
    c. Violent men who are treated with their partners escalated their violence.
    d. Conjoint treatment increased the likelihood that couples would remain married.

## SUBSTANCE ABUSE AND INTIMATE PARTNER VIOLENCE

Since a significant proportion of violent incidents involve the consumption of alcohol and/or drugs, we think the co-occurrence of alcohol and violence warrants its own section. Battering husbands tend to have higher rates of alcohol problems than comparison groups (Barnett & Fagan, 1993), and men seeking treatment for alcoholism tend to have higher rates of domestic violence than the general population (O'Farrell & Murphy, 1995). Further, victims of domestic violence often have substance abuse problems themselves. According to one study, between 25% and 50% of violent episodes involve the use of alcohol or drugs (Leonard, 2001) by either the husband or the wife.

Although a strong relationship between using violence and abusing substances by either or both spouses exists, there is considerable controversy as to whether alcohol causes domestic violence, that is, whether curtailing substance abuse will curtail violence. A key argument against alcohol having a causal role in domestic violence is that most studies are methodologically unable to show that the abuse of substances preceded the use of violence—a requirement to show causality. However, in one study, the husband's alcohol use did predict subsequent marital violence but only among couples in which the wife also used substances (Quigley & Leonard, 2000). In any case, several studies suggest that alcohol and aggressive conflict styles (e.g., hostility, reactivity) seem to have a synergistic effect on one another (Leonard, 2001).

Although there is no guarantee that successfully addressing the substance abuse problem will end the violence, failing to address the substance abuse problem may indeed undermine any potential positive outcomes of domestic violence treatment. Therefore, domestic violence treatment should include an alcohol and drug assessment. If it's determined that there is a problem, we recommend that batterers receive alcohol/drug treatment in addition to treatment for their aggression. When working with couples, both partners should be assessed for alcohol/drug abuse problems and referred for substance abuse treatment when indicated. You should obtain a commitment to stop abusing substances as well as a commitment to stop hitting. In fact, we recommend that you make couples work contingent on successful completion of substance abuse treatment for those who are actively abusing substances.

23. Which of the following statements is **not** true?
    a. Battering husbands tend to have higher rates of alcohol problems than comparisons.
    b. Victims of domestic violence often have substance abuse problems.
    c. According to one study, between 25% and 50% of violent episodes involve the use of alcohol or drugs by either the husband or the wife.
    d. Alcohol use has been proven to be the cause of partner violence in most cases.

24. As a clinician working with couples in violent relationships, you should:
    a. Focus on the problem of interpersonal violence and leave the assessment and treatment of substance abuse to a substance abuse professional.
    b. Always assess each partner in a violent relationship for substance abuse problems and make successful treatment for substance abuse a prerequisite for conjoint treatment.
    c. Treat every individual in a violent relationship for substance abuse regardless of whether or not they admit to having a problem with substance abuse.
    d. All of the above.

## PERSON OF THE THERAPIST ISSUES

Spouse abuse challenges many of our basic assumptions about people and forces us to examine our personal beliefs about gender, abuse of power, and therapeutic neutrality. Common scenarios that evoke strong **countertransference** reactions include: listening to clients recount severe episodes of abuse and oppression, working with victims who stay with their batterers despite numerous assaults, working with batterers who refuse to take responsibility for their abuse or who blame the victim, and dealing with intense conflict or threatening behavior during a session. We have observed that situations such as these can evoke strong feelings in therapists sometimes leading to feeling overwhelmed, frustrated, stuck, frightened, incompetent, sad, angry, or powerless. Further, these intense emotional reactions typically precipitate predictable behavioral responses such as blaming the client or oneself, overfunctioning, avoiding toxic issues, becoming judgmental, or distancing. Indeed, the treatment of spouse abuse invites polarized thinking, struggles with moral dilemmas, and emotional trials as well as enormous pressure to "get it right" (Goldner, 1998).

Since intense emotional responses may have a negative impact on the therapeutic process, monitoring your own reactions is particularly important when working with intimate partner violence. In addition to paying attention to your reactions, we recommend that you view them as normal and as valuable information. Does your reaction mirror what is happening with one of your clients? We also recommend that you monitor your behavioral responses to your intense feelings. Are you judging the client? Are you working harder than the clients? If you think your behavior might be impeding your clients' progress or harming the client–therapist relationship, we encourage you to seek supervision. A supervisor will help you gain perspective, discover the source of your strong responses and think of ways to use your reactions more effectively.

25. Therapists' emotional reactions toward clients in violent relationships can precipitate the following response:
    a. blaming the client
    b. overfunctioning
    c. distancing
    d. all of the above

26. Which of the following suggestions are **not** recommended to help therapists deal with intense emotional responses to clients in violent relationships?
    a. monitoring your own reactions
    b. viewing your own reactions as normal and as valuable information
    c. trying to ignore or distract yourself from thinking about your reactions
    d. seeking supervision to assist you in processing your reactions

## COORDINATED COMMUNITY RESPONSE

Partner violence, a complex problem, demands a coordinated community response. Family therapists need to play an active role in this response. It may be more comfortable for you, as a family therapist, to work with clients in your own office rather than deal directly with the dissonance between feminist-based community initiatives and a systemic perspective. However, only by becoming active in community initiatives can you do your part to bridge the apparent gap between frameworks. By working with probation officers, court personnel, domestic violence shelter workers, and staff from men's programs, you can begin to understand each other's perspectives and gain mutual respect. You can volunteer to lead men's groups and victim support groups. Family therapists need to go beyond working to end violence in their own offices and become respected partners in their community's efforts to end abuse.

As increasing attention has been placed upon the problem of domestic violence, every state has developed a coalition against domestic violence. These coalitions receive minimal funding from federal, state, and local governments and rely heavily on the donated time of concerned domestic violence activists and other community members. Most states and or counties have developed standards for treatment of batterers. In some states, these are considered recommendations; in others, they are mandates. Despite the fact that most experts agree that we do not know enough about what treatments work best for whom, twenty states have prohibited couples counseling. Family therapists need to be active participants on task forces that revise domestic violence treatment standards. In any case, you need to be aware of your states' standards and if you do treat couples, use a domestic violence–focused couples treatment targeted to appropriate couples.

27. If family therapists are going to gain credibility in the community as appropriate treatment providers for some couples in violent relationships, they need to:
    a. speak out about the flaws of batterer intervention programs.
    b. become active participants in community coalitions designed to address intimate partner violence.
    c. work quietly in their own offices without becoming involved in the controversy about conjoint treatment.
    d. all of the above.

## KEY TERMS

**battering:** An extreme form of physical violence that includes high levels of emotional abuse, including an attempt on the part of the batterer to control and intimidate the partner. Batterers are almost always men. There are couples who periodically have arguments that escalate into pushing and shoving but never reach the point where the men would be classified as batterers.

**conjoint treatment:** Involves treating individual family members in the room together. It is possible to do couples treatment in which both partners are seen separately. In conjoint treatment, at least some part of the session includes both partners in the room at the same time.

**countertransference:** Emotional reaction, usually unconscious and often distorted, on the part of the therapist to a patient or member of a family in treatment.

**emotional abuse:** Includes a variety of behaviors such as verbal threats, intimidating actions including destruction of property or pets, or humiliating or degrading remarks directed toward the partner. Controlling behaviors, including limiting the partner's access to family and friends and to other resources, are also part of emotional abuse. These behaviors are especially destructive when they occur in a relationship that includes physical violence. Emotional abuse can come to serve the same controlling function that physical abuse does. Although not all men who emotionally abuse their partners are batterers, virtually all batterers also abuse their wives emotionally.

**intake assessment package:** A series of psychological instruments that you might ask clients to complete to ensure that you are diagnosing and treating appropriately. Many clinicians include measures of depression, relationship satisfaction, general life satisfaction, and relationship violence in this package. Some clinicians tailor the tools they are asking clients to complete based on their initial assessment and of course the age of family members coming to therapy.

**lethality assessment:** Assesses the likelihood that the client will be harmed or abused in any way that could cause serious injury or result in death.

**physical abuse:** Any act carried out with the intention of causing another person physical pain or injury regardless of whether an injury actually occurs. These acts range from slapping, shoving, or pushing, to beating up, threatening with or using a weapon on a partner. Both men and women commit these acts.

**sexual abuse:** Acts that force the partner to have nonconsensual sexual relations. These include forcing one's partner to have sex without a condom, to have oral or anal sex, or to participate in other unwanted sexual acts.

**typology:** A theoretically or empirically derived delineation of subgroups within a larger group. For example, a batterer typology describes various subgroups of batterers.

## DISCUSSION QUESTIONS

1. You are seeing a family composed of a married couple, teenage son (age 15), and a daughter (age 8). Discuss how each family member may be affected by the ongoing violence occurring between the couple. Include behaviors that may be overtly and covertly present.
2. What are four explanations as to why clients often fail to disclose to therapists abuse occurring in their relationships?
3. You have been assigned a new couple to treat. According to the staff person who took the phone call from the wife, they are coming to therapy because of "ongoing conflict in their relationship." How would you begin to gather information to help you understand if intimate partner violence is occurring in their relationship? If you were to determine that it was occurring, how would you determine the seriousness of the violence?
4. One of the most difficult issues many therapists struggle with is battered women who return to their abuser. You are meeting with a student therapist who is upset that her client is returning to her abusive husband. What can you tell her to help her understand why this occurs?
5. As a therapist, how might you work with a client currently involved in an abusive relationship to develop a safety plan? Include components that should be included in an effective safety plan.
6. Why is conjoint therapy for intimate partner violence controversial?
7. How might conjoint treatment benefit couples who choose to stay together after violence has occurred?
8. What might be some risk factors associated with conjoint treatment for intimate partner violence? Discuss safeguards you would use to minimize such risk factors.

9. How are substance abuse and partner violence related?
10. Therapists often find themselves experiencing negative countertransference reactions when they work with individuals in violent relationships. Identify what your personal reactions may be when working with individuals in a violent relationship and explain what steps you would take to ensure that the therapeutic process remains effective in light of these feelings.

## SUGGESTED FURTHER READING

Barnett, O. W., Miller-Perrin, C. L., & Perrin, R. D. (1997). *Family violence across the lifespan: An introduction.* Thousand Oaks, CA: Sage Publications.

This book provides a comprehensive review of the literature related to all forms of domestic violence. It includes chapters on battered women and batterers, dating violence, the impact of spouse abuse on children, and an overview of marital violence.

Goodman, M. S., & Fallon, B. C. (1995). *Pattern changing for abused women: An educational program.* Thousand Oaks, CA: Sage Publications.

Although billed as an educational program, this book has many excellent, system-friendly tips for empowering battered women.

Hansen, M., & Harway, M. (Eds.). (1993). *Battering and family therapy: A feminist perspective.* Newbury Park, CA: Sage Publications.

This book provides an overview of domestic violence and has chapters on treating batterers, couples, and victims as well as the impact of domestic violence on children. It also covers ethical and legal issues.

## REFERENCES

Aldarondo, E., & Straus, M. A. (1994). Screening for physical violence in couple therapy: Methodological, practical, and ethical considerations. *Family Process, 33*(4), 425–439.

Anderson, S. A., & Cramer-Benjamin, D. B. (1999). The impact of couple violence on parenting and children: An overview and clinical implications. *The American Journal of Family Therapy, 27,* 1–19.

Babcock, J. C., & La Taillade, J. J. (2000). Evaluating interventions for men who batter. In J. P. Vincent & E. N. Jouriles (Eds.), *Domestic violence: Guidelines for research-informed practice* (pp. 37–77). London: Jessica Kingsley Publishers.

Barnett, O. W., Miller-Perrin, C. L., & Perrin, R. D. (1997). Marital violence: An overview. In *Family violence across the lifespan: An introduction* (pp. 183–207). Thousand Oaks: Sage Publications.

Barnett, O. W., & Fagan, W. (1993). Alcohol use in male spouse abusers and their female partners. *Journal of Family Violence, 8,* 1–25.

Boyle, L. H., & Vivian, D. (1996). Generalized versus spouse-specific anger/hostility and men's violence against intimates. *Violence and Victims, 11*(4), 293–317.

Brannen, S. J., & Rubin, A. (1996). Comparing the effectiveness of gender-specific and couples groups in a court-mandated spouse abuse treatment program. *Research on Social Work Practice, 6*(4), 405–424.

Fals-Stewart, W., Kashdan, M., O'Farrell, T. J., & Birchler, G. R. (2002). Behavioral couples therapy for drug-abusing patients: Effects on partner violence. *Journal of Substance Abuse Treatment, 22,* 87–96.

Feld, S. L., & Straus, M. A. (1989). Escalation and desistance of wife assault in marriage. *Criminology, 27,* 141–161.

Ferraro, K. J., & Johnson, J. M. (1983). How women experience battering: The process of victimization. *Social Problems, 30*(3), 325–339.

Gelles, R. J., & Straus, M. A. (1988). *Intimate violence.* New York: Simon & Schuster.

Gelles, R. J., & Straus, M. A. (1990). The medical and psychological costs of family violence. In M. A. Straus and R. J. Gelles (Eds.), *Physical violence in American families* (pp. 425–430). New Brunswick, N.J.: Transaction Publishers.

Gondolf, E. W. (1998). The victims of court ordered batterers. *Violence Against Women, 4,* 659–676.

Goldner, V. (1998). The treatment of violence and victimization in intimate relationships. *Family process, 37*(3), 263–286.

Hansen, M., Harway, M., & Cervantes, N. (1991). Therapists' perceptions of severity in cases of family violence. *Violence and Victims, 6* (3), 225–235.

Holtzworth-Munroe, A., Beatty, S. B., & Anglin, K. (1995). The assessment and treatment of marital violence: An introduction for the marital therapist. In N. S. Jacobson & A. S. Gurman (Eds.), *Clinical handbook of couple therapy.* New York: Guilford Press.

Holtzworth-Munroe, A., & Stuart, G. L. (1994). Typologies of male batterers: Three subtypes and the differences among them. *Psychological Bulletin, 116* (3), 476–497.

Hotaling, G. T., Straus, M. A., & Lincoln, A. J. (1990). Intrafamily violence and crime and violence outside the family. In M. S. Straus & R. J. Gelles (Eds.), *Physical violence in American families* (pp. 431–470). New Brunswick, NJ: Transaction Publishers.

Island, D., & Letellier, P. (1991). *Men who beat the men who love them: Battered gay men and domestic violence.* New York: Harrington Park Press.

Jacobson, N., & Gottman, J. (1998). *When men batter women: New insights into ending abusive relationships.* New York: Simon & Schuster.

Jaffe, P. G., & Sudermann, M. (1995). Child witnesses of woman abuse: Research and community responses. In S. M. Stith and M. A. Straus (Eds.), *Understanding partner violence: Prevalence, causes, consequences and solutions* (pp. 213–222). Minneapolis: National Council on Family Relations.

Jaffe, P. G., Wolfe, D., & Wilson, S. K. (1990). *Children of battered women.* Newbury Park: Sage.

Johnson, M. P. (1995). Patriarchal terrorism and common couple violence: Two forms of violence against women. *Journal of Marriage and the Family, 57*(2), 283–294.

Kyriacou, D. N., Anglin, D., Taliaferro, E., Stone, S., Tubb, T., Linden, J. A., et al. (1999). Risk factors for injury to women from domestic violence. *The New England Journal of Medicine, 341,* 1892–1898.

Leonard, K. E. (2001). Domestic violence and alcohol: What is known and what do we need to know to encourage environmental interventions? *Journal of Substance Use, 6,* 235–247.

Miller, A. J., Bobner, R. F., & Zarski, J. J. (2000). Sexual identity development: A base for work with same-sex couple partner abuse. *Contemporary Family Therapy, 22*(2), 189–200.

O'Farrell, T. J., & Murphy, C. M. (1995). Marital violence before and after alcoholism treatment. *Journal of Consulting and Clinical Psychology, 63,* 256–262.

O'Leary, K. D. (1988). Physical aggression between spouses: A social learning theory perspective. In V. B. Van Hasselt & R. L. Morrison (Eds.), *Handbook of family violence* (pp. 31–55). New York: Plenum Press.

O'Leary, K. D., & Murphy, C. (1999). Clinical issues in the assessment of partner violence. In R. Ammersman (Ed.), *Assessment of family violence* (pp. 46–94). New York: Wiley.

O'Leary, K. D., Vivian, D., & Malone, J. (1992). Assessment of physical aggression against women in marriage: The need for multimodal assessment. *Behavioral Assessment, 14*(1), 5–14.

Quigley, B. M., & Leonard, K. E. (2000). Alcohol and the continuation of early marital aggression. *Alcoholism: Clinical and Experimental Research, 24,* 1003–1010.

Rosen, K. H. (1996). The ties that bind women to violent premarital relationships: Process of seduction and entrapment. In D. D. Cahn & S. A. Lloyd (Eds.), *Family violence from a communication perspective* (pp. 151–176). Thousand Oaks: Sage Publications.

Stets, J. E. (1988). *Domestic violence and control.* New York: Springer-Verlag.

Stith, S. M., & Rosen, K. H. (1990). Family therapy for spouse abuse. In S. M. Stith, M. B. Williams, & K. Rosen (Eds.), *Violence hits home: Comprehensive treatment approaches to domestic violence* (pp. 83–101). New York: Springer Publishing Company.

Stith, S. M., Rosen, K. H., Barasch, S. G., & Wilson, S. M. (1991). Clinical research as a training opportunity: Bridging the gap between theory and practice. *Journal of Marital and Family Therapy, 17*(4), 349–353.

Stith, S. M., Rosen, K. H., & McCollum, E. E. (2002). Domestic violence. In D. H. Sprenkle (Ed.), *Effectiveness research in marriage and family therapy* (pp. 223–254). Alexandria, VA: American Association for Marriage and Family Therapy.

Stith, S. M., Rosen, K. H., Middleton, K. A., Busch, A. L., Lundeberg, K., & Carlton, R. P. (2000). The intergenerational transmission of spouse abuse: A meta-analysis. *Journal of Marriage & the Family, 62,* 640–654.

Stith, S. M., & Straus, M. A. (1995). Introduction. In S. M. Stith & M. A. Straus (Eds.), *Understanding partner violence: Prevalence, causes, consequences, and solutions* (pp. 1–11). Minneapolis: National Council on Family Relations.

Straus, M. A. (1999). The controversy over domestic violence by women: A methodological, theoretical, and sociology of science analysis. In X. B. Arriaga & S. Oskamp (Eds.), *Violence in intimate relationships* (pp. 17–44). Thousand Oaks: Sage Publications.

Straus, M. A., (1979). Measuring intrafamily conflict and violence: The Conflict Tactic Scale (CTS). *Journal of Message and the Family, 41,* 75–88.

Straus, M. A., Hamby, S. L., Boney-McCoy, S., & Sugarman, D. B. (1996). The Revised Conflict Tactics Scales (CTS2): Development and preliminary psychometric data. *Journal of Family Issues, 17,* 283–316.

Sugarman, D. B., Aldarondo, E., & Boney-McCoy, S. (1996). Risk marker analysis of husband-to-wife violence: A continuum of aggression. *Journal of Applied Social Psychology, 26*(4), 313–337.

Weisz, A. N., Tolman, R. M., & Saunders, D. G. (2000). Assessing the risk of severe domestic violence: The importance of survivors' predictions. *Journal of Interpersonal Violence, 15*(1), 75–90.

Wileman, R., & Wileman, B. (1995). Towards balancing power in domestic violence relationships. *Australian & New Zealand Journal of Family Therapy, 16*(4), 165–176.

# CHILD AND ADOLESCENT ISSUES

# 15

# Developmental Disabilities

Robert M. Hodapp
*Vanderbilt University*

Jaclyn N. Sagun
*UCLA Neuropsychiatric Institute*

Elisabeth M. Dykens
*Vanderbilt University*

## TRUTH OR FICTION?

___ 1. *Although many children with disabilities show problems in only one functional domain, problems often co-occur.*

___ 2. *Based on the functional classification of developmental disabilities, a child with a learning disability is classified as having a major sensory impairment.*

___ 3. *Williams syndrome and Prader–Willi syndrome are examples of genetic causes of mental retardation, which result in etiology-related patterns of physical–medical and behavioral characteristics.*

___ 4. *According to the stress-and-coping family model, parents repeatedly experience unexpected stressors related to raising a child with a disability, which parents eventually learn to accept and cope with.*

___ 5. *Research on families concludes that all parents and families of children with disabilities have negative experiences and that they do not fare as well as families of children without disabilities.*

___ 6. *In contrast with "between-group" studies, the "within-group" model of research identifies characteristics within single groups that might lead to different outcomes.*

___ 7. *"Active-based" coping and "emotion-based" coping are types of parental coping styles that help determine how well a parent will fare in raising a child with a disability.*

___ 8. *Regardless of the type of parental coping style and degree of external support families receive, it is the severity of the child's disability that ultimately determines how successful a family will function.*

___ 9. *Compared to most other families, most families of children with disabilities are un-der increased amounts of stress and often face special problems that rarely confront other families.*

___ 10. *Most families of children with disabilities require clinical services, such as individ-ual, family, or couples therapy.*

___ 11. *The balance and type of support families need depend on the individual parents themselves, as well as the age of the child and parent–child experiences.*

___ 12. *In a self-contained classroom setting, students with disabilities are mostly or totally separate from regular classes and a special education teacher typically provides all of the instruction.*

___ 13. *Least restrictive environment (LRE) allows for full-time integration with nondis-abled children, as well as part-time integration with a resource room or specialist.*

___ 14. *A behavior plan is the most integral component in an Individualized Education Plan (IEP) for students with disabilities.*

___ 15. *In addition to school-based services, families of children with disabilities can also receive supportive services provided by many states.*

Although they reside in every town and city in the country, children and adults with develop-mental disabilities are, to most people, an afterthought. Few couples plan on giving birth to a child with disabilities, and fewer still consider the extra challenges (compared to typically developing children) necessary to raise these children. And yet, the family issues associated with children with disabilities go beyond overcoming lack of awareness. Parents and families need to understand the particular disability that their child has, the emotional and practical issues that the child elicits, and the many different supports available. Many professionals have even compared the experience of having and raising a child with disabilities to entering into a new and foreign country.

This chapter gives you necessary information for helping parents and families adapt to this foreign country of developmental disabilities. Starting with a few basics about what develop-mental disabilities are, you will then learn about how families have been conceptualized in disability studies and interventions. We end the chapter by providing information about more practical issues: what help may be needed at which ages, and where and how you can link parents, families, and helping professionals to the appropriate resources.

## DEVELOPMENTAL DISABILITIES: THE BASICS

Although disabilities are rarely considered by most people, many different types of disabilities exist. An exact count is hard to come by, but several thousand different problems cause devel-opmental disabilities in children. Indeed, the chances are high that you will see one or more persons with a developmental disability in your clinical practice. If you do not see persons with disabilities themselves, you may still encounter parents, siblings, or others who are intimately involved with such persons.

How do you get a handle on the many different types of developmental disabilities? Most professionals think of three major categories of disability when they consider developmental disabilities. These include: (a) problems in cognition, language, or academic achievement, (b) sensory problems, and (c) motor problems. As Table 15.1 illustrates, however, even these three broad categories include many different examples. Still, this type of functional categorization helps one to begin to understand the child and his or her problems.

**TABLE 15.1**

Functional Classification of Developmental Disabilities

| Problems in Cognition, Language, or Academic Achievement | Sensory Problems | Motor Problems |
|---|---|---|
| Mental retardation | Deafness | Cerebral palsy |
| Chromosomal disorders | Hearing loss (hard of hearing) | Spina bifida |
| Metabolic disorders | Hearing impairments (e.g., | Epilepsy |
| Traumatic brain injury | external otitis, otitis media) | Spinal cord injuries |
| Learning disabilities (e.g., | Blindness | Muscular dystrophy |
| dyslexia, developmental | Low vision (partially sighted) | Juvenile rheumatoid arthritis |
| aphasia) | Visual impairments (e.g., | Scoliosis |
| Speech disorders | glaucoma, cataracts, | |
| Language disorders | nystagmus, color and night | |
| Specific language impairment | blindness, strabismus) | |
| Pervasive developmental | Deaf-blindness | |
| disorders (e.g., autism, | | |
| Asperger's syndrome, Rett's | | |
| disorder, childhood | | |
| disintegrative disorder, | | |
| pervasive developmental | | |
| disorder not otherwise | | |
| specified) | | |
| Attention deficit hyperactivity | | |
| disorder | | |

1. Functional classification of developmental disabilities include sensory problems, motor problems, and:
    a. cognitive problems.
    b. language problems.
    c. academic achievement problems.
    d. all of the above.

Other issues also deserve mention. First, even though Table 15.1 separates the three different functional categories, children with disabilities often display more than one problem. Approximately half of children with cerebral palsy also show mental retardation, some with visual impairments show hearing problems, and one-third or more with mental retardation show significant emotional or behavioral problems. Although many children show problems in only one functional domain, problems often co-occur.

2. What major area of impairment in functioning is involved in children with cerebral palsy?
    a. sensory problems
    b. motor problems
    c. medical problems
    d. cognitive, language, academic achievement problems

3. Most major disability types can be further categorized according to:
   a. severity of intellectual impairment.
   b. type of associated medical conditions.
   c. degree of impairment.
   d. type of cause.

A second issue concerns how to categorize individuals within a major class. One method considers the person's degree of impairment. Within mental retardation, individuals have historically been categorized as having mild, moderate, severe, or profound mental retardation. Within hearing impairments or visual impairments, the degree of either hearing loss or visual loss comprises the main way to classify people. Within motor impairments, one speaks of both the number and side-of-body of affected limbs (Batshaw, 2002). See Table 15.2.

4. Individuals with mental retardation have historically been classified according to levels of:
   a. intelligence quotient (IQ).
   b. adaptive functioning.
   c. support services needed.
   d. academic achievement.

5. Hearing impairments are classified based on:
   a. type of hearing device used.
   b. type of cause.
   c. degree of intellectual impairment.
   d. degree of hearing loss.

A final issue concerns the cause or etiology of specific problems. In each major disability type, problems may arise from a wide variety of causes. Some involve difficult or exceptional environmental circumstances (e.g., fetal alcohol syndrome, or FAS), others involve genetic abnormalities. Mental retardation alone has over 1,100 different genetic causes, many of which result in etiology-related patterns of physical–medical and behavioral characteristics (Dykens, Hodapp, & Finucane, 2000). Individuals with Prader–Willi syndrome thus show extreme hyperphagia—or excessive eating—such that the main cause of death in this syndrome continues to be complications due to obesity. Although Table 15.3 limits itself to a few types of mental retardation, many causes also exist for deafness–hearing impairments, visual impairments, and motor impairments.

6. All of the following are causes of mental retardation *except:*
   a. genetic abnormalities.
   b. congenital heart defects.
   c. difficult environmental circumstances.
   d. Down syndrome.

7. What is a main feature in Prader–Willi syndrome that often leads to obesity?
   a. seizure disorders.
   b. hypercalcemia.
   c. hyperphagia.
   d. heart problems.

**TABLE 15.2**

Degrees of Impairment

| Mental Retardation | Hearing Impairments | Visual Impairments | Motor Impairments |
|---|---|---|---|
| *Severity based on level of intellectual impairment* | 1. Deaf—profound hearing losses greater than 70 decibels that result in severe oral speech and language delay or that prevent the understanding of spoken language through hearing | 1. Legally blind— visual acuity of 20/200 or less in the better eye even with correction | 1. Acute—a serious state of illness or injury from which someone often recovers with treatment |
| 1. Mild (IQ 55–59 to approximately 70) | | 2. Low vision—visual acuity falling between 20/70 and 20/200 in the better eye with correction | 2. Chronic—a permanent condition |
| 2. Moderate (IQ 40–54) | 2. Hard of hearing— hearing losses in the better ear of 25 to 70 decibels; those who benefit greatly from amplification through hearing aids and who communicate primarily through spoken language | | 3. Episodic—occurring in episodes; a temporary condition that will pass but may recur |
| 3. Severe (IQ 25–39) | | | 4. Progressive—a disease or condition that worsens over time and from which one seldom or never recovers with treatment |
| 4. Profound (IQ < 25) | | | |
| *Severity based on level of support needed* | *Degrees of Hearing Loss:* | | |
| 1. Intermittent | 1. Slight—15 to 25 decibels | | |
| 2. Limited | 2. Mild—25 to 30 decibels | | |
| 3. Extensive | 3. Moderate—30 to 50 decibels | | |
| 4. Pervasive | 4. Severe—50 to 70 decibels | | |
| | 5. Profound—71 decibels and greater | | |

**TABLE 15.3**

Genetic Disorders of Mental Retardation (MR)

| Genetic Syndrome | Physical–Medical Characteristics | Behavioral Characteristics |
|---|---|---|
| Down syndrome | Congenital heart defects, vision and hearing problems, growth problems, hypothyroidism, diabetes, orthopedic problems, dental problems, gastrointestinal malformations, celiac disease, epilepsy, leukemia, skin conditions, delayed gross motor skills, decreased muscle tone, respiratory infections, constipation | Mild to severe MR, significant language delays (receptive generally better than expressive language), poor verbal short-term memory skills, strong visual-memory skills |
| Fragile X syndrome | Ophthalmic disorders, orthopedic abnormalities, ear infections, heart murmur, seizure disorders, enlarged testicles, hyperextensible joints | Moderate to severe MR for males and mild MR for females, hyperactivity, short attention span, perseverative speech, stereotypic behaviors, sensory processing problems, poor eye contact and social skills |
| Williams syndrome | Cardiac problems (e.g., supravalvular aortic stenosis [SVAS], peripheral pulmonary disease, hypertension), hyperextensible joints, decreased muscle tone, hypercalcemia, constipation, abdominal pain, renal problems, vision problems (e.g., strabismus), hyperacusis | Mild to moderate MR; relative strengths in language, auditory short-term memory, and facial recognition; affinity for music, sociable personalities; impairments in visual-spatial functioning, perceptual planning, and fine motor control; high rates of anxiety and fears |
| Prader–Willi syndrome | Hyperphagia, obesity, hypopigmentation, hypotonia, growth hormone deficiency, sleep disturbances, heart and circulation problems, diabetes, joint problems, temperature regulation problems, hypogonadism | Mild to moderate MR, visual processing strengths, relative weakness in visual and short-term memory, fondness for jigsaw puzzles, high rates of obsessions and compulsive behaviors, impulsivity, temper tantrums |
| Smith–Magenis syndrome | Vision problems, sleep problems, decreased sensitivity to pain and temperature, scoliosis, chest abnormalities, congenital heart defects, seizures, hearing impairments, urinary tract anomalies | Mild to moderate MR, sequential processing weaknesses, strengths in achievement, delays in speech acquisition, impulsivity, aggression, hyperactivity, stereotypies, self-injurious behaviors |
| 5 p- (Cri-du-chat) syndrome | Hypotonia, feeding problems, regurgitation, respiratory and ear infections, severe constipation, cardiac abnormalities, voice hypernasality, vision problems, dental malocclusion | Moderate to profound MR, better developed receptive than expressive language, relative slowing in rate of adaptive skill acquisition, strengths in socialization skills, hyperactivity, inattention |

8. Individuals with Williams syndrome show relative strengths in all areas *except:*
   a. language skills.
   b. auditory short-term memory.
   c. visual-spatial functioning.
   d. facial recognition.

9. Which behavioral characteristic is very common among individuals with Fragile X syndrome?
   a. anxiety and fears
   b. hyperactivity
   c. obsessions and compulsions
   d. aggression

# FAMILY ISSUES: THE CHANGING PERSPECTIVE

## Changing Research Methods

In recent years, studies of families of children with disabilities have changed in two important ways. First, the focus has shifted from a negative, pathological perspective to one emphasizing the disability as a stressor, with both positive and negative effects. Second, methods of research have shifted from between-group studies to examining within-group correlates.

### *From Pathology to Stress and Coping*

Although families of children with developmental disabilities have been a focus of study for many years, the modern field of parenting children with disabilities arose in the early 1960s. At that time, two views dominated. In the first, Freud's concept of mourning was used to postulate that mothers experienced a "maternal mourning reaction" to the birth of a child with disabilities. From this view arose several stage theories that, although differing slightly, noted that most parents react to the child with disability's birth with shock, then depression or anger, and finally with acceptance. An alternative view held that such strong emotional reactions were not stage-bound, per se, but could arise at unexpected times, with events or milestones that repeatedly reminded parents that they were not parenting a "typical" child.

10. According to stage theories, which is the correct order of emotional reactions parents experience to the birth of a child with disabilities?
    a. shock → depression/anger → acceptance
    b. depression/anger → denial → acceptance
    c. denial → acceptance → depression/anger
    d. shock → denial → acceptance

Whether one believed in a stage-like progression or recurrent flare-ups, both views considered parenting the child with mental retardation as a negative experience. So too was other family research negative in orientation. Comparing mothers, fathers, couples, siblings, or families as a whole to families of same-aged typically developing children, these studies concluded the following:

- Mothers of children with mental retardation were more often depressed, more preoccupied with their children, and had more difficulty handling anger at their children.
- Fathers experienced neurotic-like "role constriction," and depression and neuroticism in general.
- Couples showed lower levels of marital satisfaction.
- Siblings were thought to suffer from greater amounts of maladaptive behavior—psychopathology due to the "role tensions" involved in having too many adult responsibilities thrust upon them during the childhood years.
- Families were "stuck" in earlier stages of family development and were considered to be "economically immobile." At least some of this economic immobility was thought to be due to costs of health care, special equipment (e.g., wheelchairs), and extra educational or medical interventions.

11. Based on studies comparing families of children with disabilities to families of same-aged typically developing children, all of the following were found to be true for families of children with disabilities *except:*
    a. Mothers were more often depressed.
    b. Siblings suffered more behavior psychopathology.
    c. Couples showed lower levels of marital satisfaction.
    d. Parents lacked appropriate coping skills.

By the early 1980s, this more negative view was changing, and the child with mental retardation was beginning to be conceptualized as a stressor in the family system (Hodapp, 2002). By using the metaphor of a "stressor," the child with mental retardation could bring about either negative or positive effects. That child could bring the family together and help each individual grow and develop, or instead could cause problems for one or more family members or the family system as a whole.

12. In the stress-and-coping view of families of children with disabilities, the "stressor" refers to the:
    a. sibling reactions.
    b. child with mental retardation.
    c. financial demands of the child's disability.
    d. change in parental employment.

As a result of this change in perspective, the past 20 years have seen a more positive perspective toward parents and families of children with disabilities. Granted, many of these families continue to have problems. The issues, however, are whether all families of children with disabilities must necessarily be "disabled families," and whether all families are the same. The emerging consensus is that, like all families, families of children with disabilities do indeed differ one from another. See Table 15.4 for a summary of this movement from pathology to stress-and-coping in family studies.

## *From Group Differences in Pathology to Within-Group Correlates of Coping*

A second, related change involves the ways in which studies are performed. In earlier years, most studies adopted a **"between-groups"** approach. Studies therefore compared families of

**TABLE 15.4**

Family Studies Movement from Pathology to Stress-and-Coping

| | How Families Were Viewed | Research Orientation | Research Findings on Families of Children With Disabilities |
|---|---|---|---|
| Pathology | 1. Stage-bound emotional reactions: shock → depression/anger → acceptance<br>2. Parents repeatedly experienced emotional reactions at unexpected times | Compared families of children with disabilities to families of same-aged typically developing children | Mothers and fathers—depressed<br>Couples—lower levels of marital satisfaction<br>Siblings—more maladaptive behavior<br>Families—economic immobility |
| Stress-and-Coping | Child with MR is "stressor" in the family system; may engender negative or positive effects | Examined different families of children with disabilities | Some parents and families coping well<br>Families differ from one another |

children with disabilities to families of same-aged children without disabilities. Researchers then focused on mothers, fathers, siblings, or family relations to see how parenting the child with disabilities adversely affected their families.

Although between-group studies continue to be important, recent years have seen as well a rise in what have been called **"within-group"** studies. Within-group studies look only at one group, attempting to identify characteristics within that single group that might lead to different outcomes. In studies of families of children with disabilities, researchers began to search for specific protective factors in parents, social support systems, or children themselves that might lead to more adequate parental coping.

13. All of the following are true for within-group studies on families of children with disabilities *except:*
    a. examine only one single group.
    b. identify characteristics that might lead to different outcomes.
    c. search for protective factors in parents that might lead to more adequate coping.
    d. compare depression among parents of children with disabilities to parents of children without disabilities.

14. Which factor(s) determine(s) how well parents of children with disabilities cope?
    a. parent coping styles
    b. degree of external support available
    c. child's social skills
    d. all of the above

For example, there now seems to be some consensus on the role of parental problem-solving styles for successful coping. Simply stated, parents can be divided into two types. The first type adopts a more *active, problem-solving* approach to raising their child with disabilities. These are parents who, though affected by parenting a child with disabilities, attempt to integrate their emotions with active, practical activities that they can perform to help their children. In contrast, parents of the second type have been called *emotion-based* copers. This latter group includes parents who either perseverate on their negative emotions or, conversely, who deny that they have any emotions regarding parenting their child with disabilities. In several studies, parents of children and adults with disabilities who show the more problem-solving based coping styles have been found to be less depressed.

15. Which parental factor has been associated with lower depression among parents of children and adults with disabilities?
   a. emotion-based coping style
   b. active, problem-solving coping style
   c. denial of problems
   d. underestimating problems

In addition to parents' own styles of problem-solving, a second important factor appears to be the degree of external support parents receive from others. Although most of these supports make sense intuitively, they are nonetheless effective. For example:

- Mothers in good versus bad marriages cope better.
- Two-parent families cope better than do one-parent families.
- Families who are of higher socioeconomic status do better.
- The presence of a well-developed support system—either of family or friends—seems helpful to many parents.

16. Each of the following factors contribute to more successful parental coping *except:*
   a. presence of well-developed support system
   b. higher socioeconomic status
   c. one-parent family households
   d. good quality of marriage

Finally, parental coping seems influenced by factors intrinsic to particular children with disabilities. Children who are more dependent on their parents—as well as those showing a lack of social responsiveness, unusual caregiving demands, or aggressiveness—are most problematic for parents. Conversely, children with more sociable, appealing characteristics may lead to better coping from parents and other family members. It may be the case, for example, that many younger children with Down syndrome—who are considered by others to have more sociable, positive personalities—have parents who feel both less stressed and more rewarded by their child compared to parents of children with other disabilities. Thus, characteristics of the parents, the family support system, and children themselves all relate to better or worse family functioning. See Table 15.5 for a summary of factors affecting parental coping.

One thus sees a fairly mixed picture. On one hand, most families are doing fairly well. Most couples do not divorce; most mothers, fathers, and siblings are not depressed. In addition, several different factors—in the parents, in the family's support system, and in the children themselves—predispose parents and families to more successful coping. Yet compared to other families, most families of children with disabilities are under increased amounts of stress. As shown in Table 15.6, these families often face problems related to money, to information, and to being overwhelmed emotionally. In short, parents and families of children with disabilities are not all having problems, nor are they all doing wonderfully. We need to reach a more balanced, reasoned approach that recognizes both the strengths and vulnerabilities of these families.

**TABLE 15.5**

Factors Affecting Parental Coping

| Parental Coping Styles | Family Support System | Child Characteristics |
|---|---|---|
| Active, problem-solving based coping style | Quality of marriage | Level of dependency |
| Emotion-based coping style | Number of parents in household | Social responsiveness |
| | Socioeconomic status | Caregiving demands |
| | Presence of well-developed support system of family and friends | Aggressiveness |

**TABLE 15.6**

Problems Experienced by Some Families of Children with Developmental Disabilities

| Financial Hardships | Lack of Information | Being Overwhelmed Emotionally |
|---|---|---|
| Financing needs of children with severe to profound MR or with multiple disabilities | Parents lacking adequate knowledge about specific problems and outcomes associated with their child's DD | Children with DD are vulnerable to experiencing abuse and neglect (four times more likely than nondisabled age-mates) |
| Medical cost | Child's educational programs not adjusted to meet the child's special needs | Maltreatment often first occurs during preschool or elementary school period |
| Problems with health care coverage | | |
| Costs of babysitting or respite care | Parents are the sole providers of information about child's needs in the school setting | |

17. Families of children with disabilities often experience special problems that rarely confront other families, some of which include financial difficulties, lack of information, and:
   a. being emotionally overwhelmed.
   b. having to deal with their child's behavioral problems.
   c. lack of social support available.
   d. high rates of parental depression.

## Changing Service Perspectives

Service provision to families has also changed in several important ways.

### Movement From Clinical to Supportive Services

In earlier periods, mothers, fathers, siblings, and families overall were thought to have psychiatric or relational problems that required therapy. But recent studies indicate that most families do not require therapy, but, instead, some degree of support. Such support can come in many forms, and can be provided by different people across different settings. Some families need a supportive person—either a professional or a friend—who will simply listen, thereby validating the many conflicting feelings parents and siblings experience as they parent the child with disabilities. Other families need the emotional support provided from sharing experiences with other parents of children with the same disorder. Some families need a short break—a respite—from the full-time care of their child with disabilities. Still others require either information about their child or about raising children with their child's condition, or help in negotiating the various social service systems.

18. Parents of children with disabilities usually require which types of support(s)?
   a. emotional support
   b. informational support
   c. tangible support
   d. some of each type of a through c

Whatever support is needed, however, support is a multi-faceted phenomenon. In general, support has been conceptualized as being of three types: emotional, informational, or tangible (see Table 15.7). All parents require some of each type of support, although the balance of "who needs what, when" probably depends on the individual parents themselves, as well as on how old the child is and what experiences parents and children are having.

19. What type of support is respite care?
   a. emotional support
   b. informational support
   c. tangible support
   d. all of the above

Moving from therapy to support is not simply a change of name. Instead, the philosophy underlying the "support revolution" concerns empowering parents, giving parents emotional resources, and knowledge of their child, of social service systems, and of how to negotiate. The goal is for parents themselves to advocate for their child. Empowering families helps to make parents themselves the experts, as opposed to professionals per se. Later, when children with disabilities become adults, they should gradually be able to advocate for themselves.

20. The "support revolution" aims to:
   a. empower parents to be advocates for their child.
   b. give parents emotional resources.
   c. provide knowledge of social service systems and how to negotiate them.
   d. all of the above.

**TABLE 15.7**

Types of Supports for Families of Children with Developmental Disabilities

| Emotional | Informational | Tangible |
|---|---|---|
| Extended family, friends, neighbors | DD-specific organizations | Social services |
| Parent support groups | Newsgroups | State and agency services |
| Church | World Wide Web sites | Client's rights advocates |
| | | Respite care |

## Movement Toward Increased Help in Dealing With Appropriate Social Services

When parents give birth to a child with disability, they must negotiate the service-delivery system. In every state, parents thus begin dealing with such agencies as the Department of Developmental Disabilities (differently named from state to state), and with that department's various agencies or centers, who actually administer the funds and programs. Later, during the school years, parents work most closely with their child's school district, school administrators, and teachers. After the school years, transition and adult services enter in. These departments and services are generally unknown to most people in the general public.

As these interactions proceed, parents are suddenly faced with a wide array of rights and responsibilities. Consider schools, the main service-provider from the time that the child is aged 3 to 21 years (Hallahan & Kauffman, 2003). Federal laws such as **Public Law 94-142** (Education for All Handicapped Children Act of 1975) and the **Individuals with Disabilities Education Act**, or IDEA (passed in 1990; amended in 1997) now provide as a right a free, appropriate public school education for all children with disabilities. As Table 15.8 shows, parents need to be aware of an entire gamut of hearings, appeals, and procedures.

21. An IEP evaluation multidisciplinary team must always include at least one:
    a. social worker.
    b. psychologist.
    c. occupational therapist.
    d. speech-language pathologist.

22. How often should an IEP be written?
    a. every 2 years
    b. every other year
    c. at least once per year
    d. at least once every 6 months

**TABLE 15.8**

Individualized Education Program (IEP) Process

1. To determine whether their child has a disability, parents or teachers request an initial evaluation. Parental consent required prior to an evaluation.
2. Child evaluated by a multidisciplinary team consisting of a psychologist and some of the following: speech-language pathologist, occupational therapist, physical therapist, and social worker.
3. Multidisciplinary team follows specific guidelines for appropriate evaluation procedures as part of IDEA. Many tools, as well as parental input, used to determine if the child has a disability.
4. IEP developed—involves a written plan that maps out the goals that the child is expected to achieve over the course of the school year. IEP must contain measurable annual goals, which address both academic and nonacademic concerns and be based on the student's current level of educational and behavioral functioning.
5. IEP created by a team consisting of professionals, the child's parents, and the child (when appropriate).
6. A new IEP written at least once per year; modified as often as needed based on assessments of child's progress.
7. Parents are informed of the progress toward achievement of annual goals as often as parents of children without disabilities are.

The culmination of such hearings and procedures then results in the child's actual placement within a specific educational setting. But as Table 15.9 illustrates, such placements can be in many different settings. Philosophically, however, all children should be educated in what is termed the *least restrictive environment* (LRE). LRE allows for full-time integration with nondisabled children, part-time integration with a resource room or specialist, special classes within a public school, and even special classes or special residential schools when necessary to meet the child's educational needs.

23. The name of the educational environment in which the student receives instruction from the special education teacher for only part of the school day, and is integrated most of the school day with the regular teacher is a:
    a. resource class.
    b. self-contained class.
    c. special day school.
    d. residential school.

24. What students are mostly served in special day and residential schools?
    a. students with visual and hearing impairments
    b. students with learning disabilities
    c. students with language problems
    d. students with severe or profound physical/mental/behavioral disabilities

In whatever setting education takes place, teachers, administrators, and parents must agree on the various goals, services, and practices that will be put in place to educate the student with disabilities. Such goals and practices are codified in the child's **Individualized Educational Plan** (IEP), which has been developed out of the series of legal hearings and appeals mentioned above. See Table 15.10 for descriptions of elements that should be formally entered within each child's IEP document.

25. For all students with disabilities, the following elements must be formally entered within each child's IEP document *except:*
    a. present levels of performance.
    b. communication needs.
    c. measurable goals and objectives.
    d. assessment status.

## Movement Toward Life-Span Services

Although we often think of disabilities as pertaining mostly to children, children with disabilities eventually grow up to become adults. Indeed, over the past few decades, the life spans of persons with many different disorders have increased greatly. More and more, persons with disabilities are living into their middle-age and even old-age years, and service-delivery systems have had to adapt.

26. What is the focus of transition services?
    a. training on the use of communication devices
    b. helping junior high students transition to high school
    c. teaching skills needed for independent living and working
    d. providing social skills training

**TABLE 15.9**

Least Restrictive Educational Environments

| Type of Placement | Major Features of Placement | Type of Students Typically Served |
| --- | --- | --- |
| Regular Class Only | Regular teacher meets all needs of student; student totally integrated; student may not be identified or labeled | Student with mild learning disability, emotional/behavioral disorder, or mild MR; student with physical disability |
| Special Educator Consultation | Regular teacher meets all needs of student with only occasional help from special education consultant(s); student totally integrated; student may not be identified or labeled | Student with mild learning disability, emotional/behavioral disorder, or mild MR |
| Itinerant Teacher | Regular teacher provides most or all instruction; special teacher provides intermittent instruction of student and/or consultation with regular teacher; student integrated except for brief instructional sessions | Student with visual impairment or physical disability; student with communication disorder |
| Resource Teacher | Regular teacher provides most instruction; special teacher provides instruction part of school day and advises regular teacher; student integrated most of school day | Student with mild to moderate emotional/behavioral, learning, or communication disorder or hearing impairment |
| Diagnostic–Prescriptive Center | Special teacher in center provides most or all instruction for several days or weeks and develops plan or prescription for regular or special education teacher; following diagnosis and prescription, student may be partially or totally integrated into regular school or class | Student with mild disability who has been receiving no services or inadequate services |
| Hospital or Homebound Instruction | Special teacher provides all instruction in hospital or home until student is able to return to usual school classes (regular or special) from which he or she has been temporarily withdrawn; student separated from regular school for short period | Student with physical disability; student undergoing treatment or medical tests |
| Self-Contained Class | Special teacher provides instruction in special class of students; regular teacher may provide instruction in regular class for part of school day; student mostly separated from regular class | Student with moderate to severe MR or emotional/behavioral disorder |
| Special Day School | Special teacher provides instruction in separate school; also may work with teachers in regular or special classes of regular school; student mostly separated from regular school | Student with severe or profound physical or mental disability |
| Residential School | Same as special day school; special teacher also works with other staff to provide a total therapeutic environment; student mostly in special setting | Student with severe or profound MR or emotional/behavioral disorder |

Adapted from Hallahan & Kauffman, 2003.

**TABLE 15.10**

IEP Components

| For All Students | For Some Students |
|---|---|
| Present levels of performance | Transition—including transfer of parental rights |
| Measurable goals and objectives | to students |
| Assessment status | Behavior plan |
| All needed services fully described (amount, | English as a second language (ESL) needs |
| frequency, etc.) | Braille |
| Progress reporting | Communication needs |
|  | Assistive technology |

Adapted from Bateman, B. D., & Linden, M. A. (1998). Better IEPs: How to develop legally correct and educationally useful programs (3rd ed.). Longmont, CO: Sopris West.

**TABLE 15.11**

Work Settings for Adults with Disabilities

1. *Competitive (unsupported) employment*—on company payroll with benefits; without trainer or support.
2. *Job placement, or transitional support into regular employment*—short-term help from an agency (e.g., state vocational rehabilitation agency), in finding and getting adjusted to a job.
3. *Supported employment*—job placement, training, and continuing support for as long as necessary in an integrated community business. Supported employment can be in the form of an individual placement or a group model of several workers, such as an enclave or mobile work crew. Workers earn minimum wage or better.
4. *Volunteer work*—unpaid work that is preferred or chosen by an individual for reasons other than "daily support" which is usually done for community service organizations. Workers with disabilities cannot volunteer to do work that would pay a wage to employees without disabilities.
5. *Sheltered work*—work done in a sheltered workshop where the majority of the workers are disabled and earn subminimum wages. Sheltered workshops can offer a variety of employment and evaluation services, such as work adjustment training, vocational evaluation, long-term sheltered employment, and work activity programs.
6. *Work activity center-based or nonintegrated day programs*—focus on "prevocational" skills such as motor tasks or self-care skills.
7. *Day activity or adult day care center-based, nonintegrated programs*—usually have a therapeutic or nonvocational emphasis, depending on the funding source.

One of the most widespread adaptations has involved **transition services**. To simplify slightly, transition services focus on skills needed for independent living and working. The goal is that, upon graduation, young adults with disabilities might be able to live either on their own or in a community group home, and to be competitively employed in the community. To live independently, students are taught to shop for clothes or food within a budget, to use the post office, to understand schedules and take public buses or trains, and to visit a doctor or dentist. To be able to be hired by community businesses (i.e., to be "competitively employed"), students are trained in a variety of vocational skills. Such training addresses more general issues as being punctual, courteous, and on task, as well as providing actual practice in working in unskilled or semi-skilled jobs within the community. The range of potential work and residential settings is described in Tables 15.11 (work) and 15.12 (residential).

**TABLE 15.12**

Residential Settings for Adults with Disabilities

1. *Developmental Centers*—state institutions permanently housing many people with severe to profound levels of mental retardation.
2. *Community Residential Facilities*—also called *group homes,* accommodate small groups (3–10 people) in houses under the direction of "house parents." Placement can be permanent or can involve temporary arrangements to prepare individual for independent living.
3. *Supported living*—persons with mental retardation receive supports to live in more natural, noninstitutional settings such as their own home or apartment.

27. The type of work setting in which adults with disabilities are provided with continuous training and support as they work in an integrated community business while earning minimum wage or better is called:
    a. a day activity program.
    b. sheltered work.
    c. supported employment.
    d. volunteer work.

28. Which of the following best describes "supported living" residential settings for adults with disabilities?
    a. large institution where many people are permanently housed
    b. group homes that accommodate small groups of people
    c. hospital ward where individuals have little or no contact with others
    d. apartments or homes where individuals receive supports to live in natural, noninstitutional settings

## PRACTICAL ISSUES

We end this chapter by expanding our discussion of the needs of children and their families over the life span and providing some preliminary resources to get you started in supporting families of children with disabilities.

### Stages of Child's Life and Family Needs

Children and families have different needs at different points during the child's life. Let's discuss the three major periods separately.

29. Which period in a disabled person's life entails the most comprehensive of all services?
    a. infancy
    b. early childhood
    c. school age
    d. adult years

### *Early Childhood Years (0–3)*

In addition to finding out and dealing with the child's condition, parents are faced with the child's need to develop basic cognitive, linguistic, and social skills. In order to assist in these

**TABLE 15.13**

Child–Family Needs During Period of 0–3 Years

|  | *Needs* | *Resources* |
|---|---|---|
| *Child* | Evaluation: physical, motor, cognitive, linguistic, social-emotional; early intervention services | Multidisciplinary evaluation, resulting in Individualized Family Service Plan (IFSP), with child and family receiving either center- or home-based early intervention services for set number of hours per week |
| *Mother* | Emotional support, caregiving behaviors | Support groups by disability, region, and etiology; part of evaluation for early intervention, intervention services, and IFSP |
| *Family* | Support, financial assistance, information | Support groups, depending on problem, state developmental disabilities or insurance payment for some services; hospitals, agencies, groups |

developments, pediatricians, social workers, and other social service personnel generally put parents in touch with their state's Department of Developmental Disabilities. Through this (or a similar) state agency, parents and their children receive early intervention services.

In an attempt to aid children in the years before formal schooling, federal law now mandates early intervention services throughout the United States. In American early intervention services, Part H of Public Law 99-457—the Education of the Handicapped Amendments of 1986—calls for an **Individualized Family Service Plan** (IFSP). This plan involves a "statement of family strengths and needs relating to enhancing the development of the family's handicapped infant or toddler" (Krauss & Hauser-Cram, 1992). The family system is thereby acknowledged as important—even critical—for the provision of services during the preschool years. See Table 15.13.

## School-Age Years (3–21)

The school-age years probably entail the most comprehensive of all services. Under the aegis of local school districts—and of federal laws governing "free, appropriate public education"— many potential services are available. Such services also have the benefit of being free to parents (as are all services provided by the public school system) and of being coordinated through the school. In this sense, schools are "one-stop" service providers.

In addition to school-based services, families can sometimes receive supportive services from their state. Many states, for example, provide **respite care** services for families who need a break from full-time care. Camps, arts organizations, and other local, state, and national groups also provide services either to children themselves or to their families (see Table 15.14).

## Adult Years (21+)

In addition to the work and residential needs described above, we need to emphasize certain differences between school and adult services. A first issue involves navigating the adult-service system. During the school years, many services for the child are handled by the school within the child's IEP—a one-stop shopping, coordinated system of services. In contrast, adult services are usually under the control of the state's department of disabilities, but contracted out to individual service providers. An adult with disabilities may therefore go to one site for vocational services, another for speech-language therapy, yet others for medical, dental, occupational, or physical therapies.

**TABLE 15.14**

Child–Family Needs During Period of 3–21 Years

|  | Needs | Resources |
|---|---|---|
| Child | Evaluation, referral, and Individualized Educational Program (IEP) | School system: involves legal process of evaluation and placement (notification, hearings, appeals if necessary); information on transition to adult services as child nears age 21 (and school services end) |
| Family | Support, financial assistance, information | Local and national groups; state departments in some states; includes respite care, camps, art (e.g., Very Special Arts) or athletic activities (e.g., Special Olympics); scholarships for adolescents with some disabilities (deafness, blindness) |

**TABLE 15.15**

Offspring Needs During Adulthood

|  | Needs | Resources |
|---|---|---|
| Offspring | Residential services, work | Both run by state developmental disability departments (parents and offspring have major say concerning whether residential or work placements are appropriate) |
| Family | Support, information, guardianship issues | Continuation of many of the services provided during the school years; particularly for individuals with severe disabilities, provisions for residential and work status after parents can no longer serve as legal guardians |

A second point concerns the degree to which adult services are mandated by federal law. In contrast to most school-related services—which are covered under federal education law—adult services are not as directly mandated by the federal government. Compared to school services, then, adult services in most states are not as plentiful or as easy to access. Such services are also more susceptible to cutbacks that often occur in state programs during times of economic downturn.

30. All of the following are true of services for adults with disabilities *except:*
   a. they are mandated by the federal government.
   b. they are usually under the control of the state's department of disabilities.
   c. they are susceptible to cutbacks in funding.
   d. they are "person-centered."

Still, as Table 15.15 illustrates, many different services are potentially available to adults with disabilities. In contrast to services during the childhood years, such services are

**TABLE 15.16**

Support and Informational Organizations

---

National Information Center for Children and Youth with Disabilities (NICHY)
P.O. Box 1492
Washington, DC 20013
(800) 695-0285
www.nichcy.org

Association of Retarded Citizens of the US (The ARC)
100 Wayne Avenue, Suite 650
Silver Spring, MD 20910
(301) 565-3842
www.thearc.org

American Association on Mental Retardation (AAMR)
1710 Kalorama Road, NW
Washington DC 20009-2683
(800) 424-3688
www.aamr.org

Council for Exceptional Children (CEC)
1110 North Glebe Road, Suite 300
Arlington, VA 22201-5704
(888) CEC-SPED
www.cec.sped.org

Association of University Centers on Disabilities (AUCD)
8630 Fenton Street, Suite 410
Silver Spring, MD 20910
(301) 588-8252
www.aucd.org

The Association for Persons with Severe Handicaps (TASH)
29 West Susquehanna Avenue, Suite 210
Baltimore, MD 21204
(410) 828-8274
www.tash.org

Clearinghouse of Disability Information (CDI)
Office of Special Education and Rehabilitation Services
Switzer Building, Room 3132
330 C Street, SW
Washington, DC 20202-2524
(202) 334-8241
www.health.gov

Resources for Children with Special Needs, Inc.
116 E. 16th Street, 5th floor
New York, NY 10003
(212) 677-4650
www.resourcesnyc.org

CAPP National Parent Resource Center
Federation for Children with Special Needs
95 Berkeley Street, Suite 104
Boston, Massachusetts 02116
(617) 482-2915 *or* (800) 331-0688

---

(Continue)

**TABLE 15.16**

(Continued)

---

National Parent Network on Disabilities (NPND)
1727 King Street, Suite 305
Alexandria, Virginia 22314
(703) 684-6763
www.npnd.org

Sibling Information Network
1775 Ellington Road
South Windsor, CT 07074
(203) 648-1205

National Organization for Rare Disorders (NORD)
55 Kenosia Avenue
PO Box 1968
Danbury, CT 06813-1968
(203) 744-0100
(800) 999-6673 (voicemail only)
www.rarediseases.org

Association for Children with Down Syndrome
4 Fern Place
Plainview, NY 11779
516-933-4700 x100
www.acds.org

National Down Syndrome Society
666 Broadway
New York, NY 10012
(800) 221-4602
www.ndss.org

National Fragile X Syndrome Foundation
PO Box 190488
San Francisco, California 94119
(800) 688-8765
www.fragilex.org

Prader-Willi Syndrome Association
5700 Midnight Pass Rd.
Sarasota, Florida 34242
(800) 926-4797
www.pwsausa.org

The Williams Syndrome Association
P.O. Box 297
Clawson, MI 48017-0297
(800) 806-1871
www.williams-syndrome.org

---

person-centered as opposed to family-centered. Since these services are now going to adults (as opposed to children) with disabilities, the adults themselves have the final say over what services are necessary and appropriate.

## Resources: Who, What, and How to Attain

In addition to formal educational and residential services, parents and children with disabilities also benefit from the many parent support groups that have become prominent over the past several decades. The largest educational organization is the Council for Exceptional Children, which is committed to the educational needs of children with all types of developmental disabilities. Besides organizations concerned with all children with disabilities, numerous groups also exist for parents of children with different types of disabilities. As Table 15.16 shows, national organizations exist for children with many different disabilities and their families. Within certain disabilities (e.g., mental retardation), organizations exist even for children with different specific causes (e.g., Down syndrome, Prader–Willi syndrome). Most of these groups organize annual national conferences. Parents, researchers, and service providers all attend these conferences, providing interchanges of needs, experiences, and information rarely available in other contexts. If parents, researchers, and service providers are to be linked in a common partnership, more such forums are necessary.

---

We began this chapter with the metaphor of disabilities as a foreign country. And, as in any foreign country, the language, customs, and practices differ. Still, many children with disabilities and their families do cope well, and are able to receive the emotional, informational, and tangible supports that they need. Using this chapter as an initial guidebook, you too are started on your way to becoming more aware of children with disabilities and their families, and to assisting these families as they travel along this new and different terrain.

## KEY TERMS

**active problem-solving coping style:** Form of parental coping where emotions are integrated with active, practical activities to help their children.

**Americans with Disabilities Act (ADA):** Civil rights legislation for persons with disabilities ensuring nondiscrimination in job application procedures, hiring, firing, advancement, compensation, job training, and other terms, conditions, and privileges of employment.

**between-groups studies:** Study design that compares different groups of subjects.

**emotion-based coping style:** Form of parental coping involving either perseveration on negative emotions or the denial of emotion regarding parenting their child with disabilities.

**Individualized Education Plan (IEP):** Formal written document describing children's skills and stating goals for services as well as strategies for achieving those goals; required for a child to receive special education and related services.

**Individualized Family Service Plan (IFSP):** Plan to provide services for young children with disabilities (under 3 years of age) and their families; drawn up by professionals and their parents; similar to an IEP for older children.

**Individuals with Disabilities Education Act (IDEA):** The Individuals with Disabilities Education Act of 1990 and its amendments of 1997 replaced PL 94-142. A federal law stating that to receive funds under the act, every school system in the nation must provide a free, appropriate public education for every child between the ages of 3 and 21, regardless of how seriously he or she may be disabled.

**least restrictive environment (LRE):** Legal term referring to the fact that students with disabilities must be educated in as normal an environment as possible.

**Public Law 94-142 (Education for All Handicapped Children Act of 1975):** First federal law guaranteeing a free, appropriate public education to all children with disabilities between the ages of 3 and 21.

**respite care:** Short term, temporary care provided to people with disabilities so that their families can take a break from the daily routine of caregiving.

**transition services:** Services for teens and young adults with disabilities focusing on developing skills needed for independent living and working.

**within-group studies:** Study design that compares subjects within one single group.

## DISCUSSION QUESTIONS

1. Think of the different types of disabilities you've encountered during your clinical training. Determine the specific areas of functioning that are affected in each and classify them based on the functional categorization of disabilities.
2. You have a client with mental retardation who has an IQ of 45 and a genetic disorder. Which classification system of mental retardation would you use to evaluate the types of treatments your client would benefit from and why?
3. What are some of the positive effects a child with mental retardation could bring to his or her family system and how would you use such factors in working with these types of families?
4. What types of information would you obtain from parents of a child with mental retardation to get an idea of how well the family is adjusting to the demands of having a child with a disability?
5. Look up information on the service-delivery system in your state (e.g. Department of Developmental Disabilities, regional centers, etc.). Identify possible barriers of access to these services that individuals with disabilities and their families may encounter and determine how you could help parents negotiate them.
6. What type of transition services, work environments, and residential settings could an 18-year-old young adult with Down syndrome benefit from?
7. A parent comes to you with their 2½-year-old daughter who is displaying signs of significant developmental delays. Given that this child is in her early childhood years, what type of evaluation or services would you offer them?
8. What are some common school-based services and supportive services available for children with disabilities and their families in your state?
9. What are some adult services that are directly mandated by your state's laws?
10. Find the basic contact information on national organizations and/or support groups for each disability type listed in Table 15.1. Based on this experience, will it be easy or hard for parents to do the same?

## SUGGESTED FURTHER READING

Batshaw, M. (2002). *Children with disabilities* (5th ed.). Baltimore: Paul H. Brookes.

Provides medical, genetic, and developmental features of children with a variety of developmental disabilities. A great resource for medical and nonmedical practitioners.

Dykens, E. M., Hodapp, R. M., & Finucane, B. (2000). *Genetics and mental retardation syndromes: A new look at behavior and treatments.* Baltimore: Paul H. Brookes.

Up-to-date summary of cognitive and adaptive strengths and weaknesses, psychopathologies, and family issues in persons with genetic diagnoses. Offers many treatment and intervention guidelines for families, schools, and professionals.

Hallahan, D. P., & Kauffman, J. M. (2003). *Exceptional learners: An introduction to special education.* Boston: Allyn & Bacon.

Offers an accurate and easy-to-digest snapshot of the field of special education.

Hodapp, R. M. (1998). *Development and disabilities: Intellectual, sensory, and motor impairments.* New York: Cambridge University Press.

Summarizes developmental and family concerns of children with developmental disabilities, including those with sensory and motor impairments, and mental retardation.

# REFERENCES

Batshaw, M. (2002). *Children with disabilities* (5th ed.). Baltimore: Paul H. Brookes.
Dykens, E. M., Hodapp, R. M., & Finucane, B. (2000). *Genetics and mental retardation syndromes: A new look at behavior and treatments.* Baltimore: Paul H. Brookes.
Hallahan, D. P., & Kauffman, J. M. (2003). *Exceptional learners: An introduction to special education.* Boston: Allyn & Bacon.
Hodapp, R. M. (2002). Parenting children with mental retardation. In M. Bornstein (Ed.), *Handbook of parenting: Vol. 1* (2nd ed., pp. 355–381). Hillsdale, NJ: Erlbaum.
Krauss, M. W., & Hauser-Cram, P. (1992). Policy and program development for infants and toddlers with disabilities. In L. Rowitz (Ed.), *Mental retardation in the year 2000* (pp. 184–196). New York: Springer-Verlag.

# 16

# Behavioral and Relationship Problems

Thomas L. Sexton
Alice E. Sydnor
Marcy K. Rowland
*Indiana University*

James F. Alexander
*University of Utah*

## TRUTH OR FICTION?

___ 1. *Evidence suggests that children's emotional and behavioral problems are associated with relational problems.*

___ 2. *Many clinical settings no longer rely on the DSMIV–TR or the ICD-10.*

___ 3. *A clinician should dismiss traditional assessment and focus solely on theoretically based family dynamics.*

___ 4. *A multidimensional approach to assessment is more likely to produce an understanding of the client that contributes to successful treatment choices and family-based intervention.*

___ 5. *Externalizing problems present similarly from child to child.*

___ 6. *The presentation of ODD and CD may vary across developmental stages of the child.*

___ 7. *Children who report a lack of closeness, support, and affection from their parents are more likely to experiment with drugs or alcohol.*

___ 8. *For family therapists, the "client" is the child or adolescent exhibiting the problem behavior.*

___ 9. *Current treatments target clinically meaningful syndromes or situations with a coherent conceptual framework underlying the clinical intervention.*

___ 10. *Only three family therapy approaches met the criteria of a 'best practice' as set forth by the Blueprint project.*

___ 11. *Functional family therapy considers the family relational system as its primary focus.*

___ 12. *MST was derived from social–ecological models of behavior, family systems, and social learning theory.*

___ 13. *Brief structural strategic family therapy was the first family therapy intervention developed to treat childhood depression.*

___ 14. *Early MDFT sessions utilize individual therapy with the adolescent before sessions with the entire family.*

___ 15. *Family-based intervention models are becoming the treatment of choice for many of the common clinical problems experienced by children and adolescents.*

## THE RANGE OF CHILDHOOD AND ADOLESCENT CLINICAL PROBLEMS: CLINICAL SYMPTOMS AND FAMILY RELATIONAL PATTERNS

Both the developmental psychopathology and the treatment literatures note the role of family and other social systems in child and adolescent behavior problems. Some authors describe the role of these systems in terms of *risk factors* in such a way that suggests they contribute to child and adolescent problems. Others discuss the impact of child and youth behavior problems on various social systems (parent(s)/family, school, community), and others note the important roles that parent(s)/family can play in therapeutic change. As a result, there is growing support for the view that many, if not most, of the clinical issues of children and adolescents prevalent in clinical practice that appear to be individual in nature (e.g., substance abuse, anxiety disorders, depression, agoraphobia, conduct disorders) may be more accurately viewed as family based (Kaslow, 1996) and are most successfully treated with family-based interventions (Alexander, Holtzworth-Munroe, & Jameson, 1994; Gurman, Kniskern, & Pinsof, 1986; Sexton, Alexander, & Mease, 2003).

Perhaps the clearest example involves the acting out, externalizing behavior problems of children and adolescents, most often termed *conduct disorders*. These represent one of the most frequent clinical referrals for children and adolescents to psychological treatments (Kazdin, 1997), and are generally seen as difficult to treat. In addition, because of the often **comorbid** nature of such problems as disruptive behavior disorders (drug involvement, conduct problems, delinquency), many treatment systems and therefore many seemingly distinct populations of clients are often involved. Given the multiple participants, the complex relationships, and different perspectives inherent in treating such problems, family-based interventions are particularly well equipped to play an important role in professional mental health services to these populations (Kaslow, 1996). However, even interventions that treat an individual child (e.g., play therapy) or youth (e.g., individual psychotherapy) must understand the powerful processes that influence their client even though these influences are not directly "in the treatment room." Thus the daunting task for child and adolescent therapists and other treatment planners is to identify clearly the clinical problem presented, to assess systematically the important dimensions and systems important to the problems, and to translate the central clinical issue into treatment plans that provide the highest likelihood of successful therapeutic outcomes. This is particularly important for treatment gains to be maintained for the long term.

To accomplish these complex clinical tasks, family and other therapists must have knowledge of the range of childhood and adolescent problems that present in one or more of a variety of situations (home, school, community), the relational and multiaxial assessment systems that will help them understand these presenting symptoms, and the available treatment options from which they might choose in order to successfully intervene.

The goal of this chapter is to provide family therapists and related professionals (e.g., case managers, triage teams) with the necessary information to successfully assess and treat the most common clinical problems of children and adolescents. The first section of the chapter reviews the specific clinical issues from the perspective of both the primary diagnostics system (*DSM–IV*) and a relational, or family-based, understanding. In the final section we review the range of broad and specific currently available treatment intervention models that can successfully be applied to the clinical problem of children and adolescents.

## UNDERSTANDING CHILDHOOD AND ADOLESCENT PROBLEMS

The classification and assessment of child and adolescent emotional problems have received increasing attention recently (Alexander & Pugh, 1996; Hawkins, Catalano, & Miller, 1992). This work has led to a major shift in the conceptualization and assessment of child and adolescent disorders. The exclusively intrapersonal etiological models of emotional and behavioral problems are being replaced by multisystemic **ecosystemic** approaches that view specific behaviors of the child or adolescent as inexorably tied to the broader family relational and social context in which they occur (Robbins et al., 2003). The shift in etiological perspectives is based on the growing empirical evidence suggesting that a vast number of children's emotional and behavioral problems are associated with relational problems in the family, peer, and school systems (Lytton, 1990; Parker & Asher, 1987; Rubin & Mills, 1991).

1. Which of the following best describes a multisystemic ecosystemic approach?
   a. an approach that focuses on the ecosystemic context of child and adolescent clinical problems
   b. an approach that is influenced by core nerological, biological, and learning histories
   c. an approach that complements the interpersonal etiological model of emotional and behavioral problems.
   d. an approach which views individual behaviors of the child or adolescent as inexorably linked to the social context in which it occurs

Despite the growing understanding of a need for a relational focus for understanding the **etiology** of most child and adolescent problems, most clinical settings exclusively rely on the field's most widely used classification systems, which are based upon intrapsychic and individual etiological models of clinical problems that is, the *Diagnostic and Statistical Manual of Mental Disorders* or *DSM–IV–TR* (American Psychiatric Association, 2000) and the *International Classification of Diseases* or *ICD-10* (World Health Organization, 1992). However, it has become increasingly clear that the assessment and understanding of the clinical problems of children and adolescents are related to the dynamics of family interactions. As a result, evaluating and understanding these problems is both qualitatively and quantitatively more complex than typical and traditional clinical assessment (Synder, Cavell, Heffer, & Mangrum, 1995).

Furthermore, it is important for therapists and other professionals such as case managers to understand that traditional models are limited in ways that make it difficult to adequately describe multiple problems experienced from multiple perspectives that exist within a complex relational family system and successfully choose family-based treatments (Alexander, Sexton, & Robbins, 2002; Borduin, Schaeffer, & Heiblum, 1999). At the same time, it is not helpful to dismiss traditional assessment and diagnosis in favor of an exclusive focus on theoretically based family dynamics, any more than the neurologist would dismiss the systems in which a child or youth with various neurologically based information processing deficits exists. In actual practice, it is critical for treatment providers to be able to identify the specific clinical profiles *and* understand the associated family relational process in order to successfully identify appropriate treatment intervention programs. A multidimensional approach is more likely to produce an understanding of the client that contributes to successful treatment choices and successful family-based intervention.

The behaviors often seen as clinical problems experienced by adolescents and children fall along a continuum from those with an internalized focus (mood and anxiety disorders) to those that have an externalized focus (conduct, oppositional defiant, substance abuse). In each case, the specific clinically significant behavior (e.g., drug abuse) is accompanied by a range of family relational patterns that serve as "context" for the "problem." In the following sections we focus on the most common clinical problems experienced by children and adolescents—externalizing behavior problems. Other clinical problems are covered elsewhere in this volume. We first identify the **prevalence** of the disorder, the common clinical features, and the underlying family relational patterns that support these problems. Table 16.1 integrates the diagnostic symptoms and labels (*DSM–IV–TR*) and the common relational patterns associated with the disorder in more detail.

**TABLE 16.1**

Child Symptom Classifications

| Primary Symptom Categories | Classifications | |
|---|---|---|
| | DSM | Family Relational |
| Externalizing Behavior Problems | Conduct Disorder, Oppositional Defiant Disorder | Parental rejection or hostility, low parental monitoring, inconsistent parental discipline, marital discord, high family/sibling conflict, maladaptive parenting strategies |
| Performance/Attention Problems | Attention Deficit/ Hyperactivity Disorder | Inappropriate parental expectations for achievement or behavior, inappropriate levels of family control, high levels of parent–child conflict related to functional problems of ADHD, chaotic homelife, directive and controlling parenting strategies |
| Mood Problems | Depression | Lack of cohesion and support in family, controlling and conflictual parenting, insecure parent–child attachment, child maltreatment, ineffective conflict resolution, impaired communication patterns |
| Anxiety Problems | School Phobia, Separation Anxiety | Overly involved/intrusive parents, enmeshed parent–child relationship, parent overreliance on child |

## EXTERNALIZING BEHAVIOR PROBLEMS: OPPOSITIONAL DEFIANT DISORDER, CONDUCT DISORDER, AND SUBSTANCE ABUSE

Externalizing behavior problems present differently from child to child, but are typically manifested as deficits in social skills, including the formation and maintenance of peer relations, aggressive behavior, bullying, intimidation, underachievement in school, or low frustration tolerance (Alexander & Pugh, 1996; Altepeter & Korger, 1999; Herbert, 1991). Externalizing behaviors fall into three categories: oppositional defiant disorder and conduct disorder, problems with drugs and alcohol, and difficulties of behavior and attention (Costello & Angold, 1996; APA, 2000). The problems are so common that up to one-half of all clinical referrals of children and adolescents are based on reports of such externalizing behaviors (Kadzin, 1987; Robins, 1981). See Tables 16.1 and 16.2 for a complete summary of the symptoms and relational patterns associated with these clinical issues.

**TABLE 16.2**

Adolescent Symptom Classifications

| Primary Symptom Categories | Classifications | |
|---|---|---|
| | DSM | Family Relational |
| Externalizing Behavior Problems | Conduct Disorder, Oppositional Defiant Disorder, Alcohol and Drug Use | Parental rejection or hostility, low parental monitoring, inconsistent parental discipline, marital discord, high family/sibling conflict, maladaptive parenting strategies, parental disinterest and lack of involvement, parental deviance, lack of closeness and support |
| Performance/Attention Problems | Attention Deficit/ Hyperactivity Disorder | Inappropriate parental expectations for achievement or behavior, inappropriate levels of family control, high levels of parent–child conflict related to functional problems of ADHD, chaotic homelife, directive and controlling parenting strategies |
| Mood Problems | Depression and Suicide | Lack of cohesion and support in family, controlling and conflictual parenting, insecure parent–child attachment, child maltreatment, ineffective conflict resolution, impaired communication patterns |
| Anxiety Problems | Obsessive Compulsive Disorder, Social Phobia | Overly involved/intrusive parents, enmeshed parent–child relationship, parent overreliance on child, highly rigid families, emphasis on instrumental morality |
| Eating/Image Problems | Anorexia Nervosa, Bulimia Nervosa | Family emphasis on achievement and perfection, family concern with appearance, parental concern with body image |

2. Which of the following is *not* a category of externalizing behavior problems?
   a. oppositional defiant disorder
   b. problems with drugs and alcohol
   c. childhood depression
   d. difficulties of behavior and attention

3. About how many of clinical referrals of children and adolescents are based on reports of externalizing behavior?
   a. one-third
   b. one-fourth
   c. one-tenth
   d. one-half

## Oppositional Defiant Disorder and Conduct Disorder

According to the *DSM–IV–TR*, oppositional defiant disorder (ODD) is characterized by a pattern of defiant, uncooperative, negativistic, and noncompliant behavior, usually in the home and in interactions with adults or peers that the child knows well. Defiant behaviors are manifested by stubbornness, an inability to negotiate with peers, inflexibility, and an unwillingness to compromise. ODD may develop in a child as young as age 3, and is usually evident by age 8.

Conduct disorder (CD) is characterized by a pattern of consistently violating the basic rights of others or accepted social norms. Children diagnosed with CD may show little empathy for the feelings and concerns of others, may misperceive neutral events or statements as aggressive and respond aggressively, and may try to blame their peers for their own disruptive or destructive behavior. Symptoms of conduct disorder may appear in preschool, but are more likely to emerge from middle childhood to middle adolescence (Alexander & Pugh, 1996). Comorbid disorders are common with both ODD and CD, including attention deficit/hyperactivity disorder, mood disorders, child-onset mania, and developmental disorders (see also Altepeter & Korger, 1999, for a review of ODD and CD).

4. Which of the following best desribes the characteristic pattern of conduct disorder?
   a. defiant, uncooperative, negativistic, and noncompliant behavior.
   b. increased somatic complaints and decreased attention to physical appearance
   c. consistently violating the basic rights of others or accepted social norms
   d. none of the above

The presentation of both ODD and CD may vary across developmental stages of the child, ranging from irritability and nonadaptability in infants, to impulsivity and restlessness in toddlers, with increasingly noncompliant and aggressive behavior in school-aged children (Altepeter & Korger, 1999). In practice, a younger child is more likely to be referred to as oppositional, with symptoms usually evident before age 8 and no later than early adolescence. There are estimates that 2% to 16% of the child and adolescent population is diagnosed with ODD, whereas CD occurs in approximately 5% to 20% of adolescents (APA, 2000). Although ODD is more common in boys than in girls before puberty, gender differences do not maintain in postpubertal children and adolescents. Gender differences remain with CD adolescents however, occurring two to three times more frequently in boys than in girls (Altepeter & Korger). More specifically, rates for boys under 18 years range from 6% to 16%; for girls, rates range from 2% to 9% (APA, 2000).

Adolescents with ODD typically exhibit chronic emotional, behavioral, and social malad-justment, which appears to continue throughout the life span (Loeber, 1991). Although these types of externalizing behaviors present differently from child to child, they generally include losing one's temper, arguing with adults, deliberately annoying others, being vindictive, and appearing angry and resentful (APA, 2000). Other associated features which violate social norms may include stealing, being expelled from school, running away, rape, drug/alcohol use, and sexual promiscuity (Altepeter & Korger, 1999). Problems with low self-esteem, mood lability (Blau, 1996) and depression may also be present, perhaps with suicidal ideation or at-tempts (Altepeter & Korger). As a result of these and other delinquent behaviors, adolescents with ODD often experience rejection from peer groups. Consequently, there may be increased loyalty to delinquent peer groups, who encourage each other into more deliberate acts of delin-quency and isolation from other peers, thus widening the path to delinquency (Altepeter & Korger; Gormly & Brodzinsky, 1993).

Research widely suggests that there are at least two major forms of CD: aggressive early onset and nonaggressive late onset (Loeber, 1991; McGee, Feehan, & Thomas, 1992; Robins, 1966). There is a marked difference between the two forms. Children on the early-onset trajec-tory are likely to be more aggressive, temperamental, and have accompanying attention deficit disorder, hyperactive and impulsive behaviors, and learning difficulties than late-onset adoles-cents. Aggression seems to be a hallmark of this constellation, with the onset of aggressive behaviors usually occurring prior to adolescence (Loeber, 1991). The late-onset pathway to CD consists of patterns that are more concealing, nonaggressive problems; such as delinquency, experimentation with drugs, sex, alcohol, and shoplifting and these behaviors are more likely to desist after adolescence (Lahey, Loeber, Quay, Frick, & Grimm, 1992). A larger percentage of these adolescents are girls compared with the larger proportion of boys in the early-onset trajectory (McGee et al.). Although late-onset adolescents have frequent involvements with the police during adolescence compared with those who show early onset, they are far less aggressive (Lahey et al.).

5. Which of the following describes children with late-onset conduct disorder?
   a. children who are likely to have problems such as concealing, experience with drugs, sex, alcohol, and shoplifting, and other nonaggressive problems
   b. children who are likely to have accompanying anxiety disorders
   c. children who typically have parent–child relational problems, including inappropriate parental expectations and overprotective parenting
   d. none of the above

The diagnostic criteria delineated by the *DSM* fails to capture the complexity of the reci-procity between the child's behavior and his or her environment. The *DSM* classifies the externalizing behaviors of the individual with little consideration of the effects of the nature of the family relations on the child (Borduin et al., 1999). Indeed there is now substantial evi-dence to suggest that the context of the behavior must be considered before making a diagnosis (Alexander & Pugh, 1996). For example, the behavior of the youth may be influenced by the amount of structure in the environment, the unfamiliarity of the environment, or the presence of the caregiver, among other things (Altepeter & Korger, 1999). Borduin et al. suggest that fam-ilies of children and adolescents displaying externalizing behaviors may experience parental rejection or hostility in the family, low parental monitoring of child behavior or inconsistent parental discipline, marital discord, and high family or sibling conflict. Additional relational factors that influence the development of conduct disorders in children and adolescents include maladaptive early relationships with adults, or maladaptive parenting, including abuse, neglect, or multiple foster care placements (Famularo, Kinscherff, & Fenton, 1992).

6. Relational problems associated with ADHD include:
   a. a lack of family cohesiveness.
   b. parental deviance.
   c. inappropriate levels of family control.
   d. a highly structured homelife.

## Alcohol and Drug Use and Abuse

Research widely indicates that the majority of teenagers in the United States have experimented with mood-altering substances by the time they reach twelfth grade (National Institute on Drug Abuse [NIDA], 1992). Indeed, alcohol and drug use has become a major health and social problem in the United States, with 60% of high school seniors having used illicit drugs and approximately three million problem drinkers (Brown, Aarons, & Abrantes, 2001).

7. Approximately how many high school students are considered to be problem drinkers?
   a. one million
   b. two million
   c. three million
   d. 60%

There is increased recognition that substance use and abuse among adolescents is related to relational problems with parental, peer, and school systems (Dembo et al., 1990). Children who report a lack of closeness, support, and affection from their parents are more likely to begin to use drugs and to maintain the abuse of those drugs (Kandel, 1978). Additional family factors linked with adolescent substance abuse include parent–adolescent conflict (Needle, Glynn, & Needle, 1983) and lack of family cohesiveness (Hundleby & Mercer, 1987). Similar research has noted three major areas of relational problems among families of adolescent substance abusers: parental deviance or antisocial behavior, including alcohol abuse; parental disinterest and lack of involvement with their child or adolescent; and lack of closeness and supportive interactions between parents and children (Sadava, 1987). Parents may also impact adolescent substance abuse indirectly through their impact on peer group selection (Brown, Mott, & Stewart, 1992). Thus, the relational patterns within the family and peer group systems seem to be an important factor in the development of substance use and abuse.

8. How does the presenting problem of alcohol and substance abuse inform therapists about family relational patterns?
   a. It signifies a lack of support and cohesions within the family system.
   b. It may be related to parental disinterest with their adolescent.
   c. It signifies parental overinvolvement with their adolescent.
   d. both a and b

## CLINICAL INTERVENTION PROGRAMS FOR CLINICAL PROBLEMS OF CHILDHOOD AND ADOLESCENTS

Family therapy has a wide range of approaches that can be brought to bear on the clinical problems of childhood and adolescence. Most family-based intervention models share the assumption that problem behaviors are inexorably tied to the relational behavior patterns of the family systems in which they exist (Hazelrigg, Cooper, & Borduin, 1987; Sexton & Alexander, 2002). In family-based models the primary focus of attention is on the identifiable, functional characteristics of clients and relationships to classify clinical problems, to identify desirable treatment goals, and to determine research outcomes. For most family therapists the "client" is a relational system within which the individual resides. Thus, family therapy is not simply another therapeutic modality but a fundamentally different way of construing human problems dictating different therapeutic interventions that focus on the interpersonal system of problem behaviors in order to promote systemic change (Sexton & Alexander, 2003).

9. Which of the following is considered to be the "client" in functional family therapy?
   a. the adolescent exhibiting the problem behavior
   b. the parents of the adolescent
   c. the relational system within which the individual resides
   d. the relationship between the parents

Choosing the correct treatment options from the range of theoretical "schools" and the more recent clinical models of practice can be a daunting task. The clinical problems facing family therapists are most often complex profiles comprised of manifest individual behavior problems (manifest symptoms) expressed within a multifaceted relational system (latent symptoms). Current treatment options range from traditional "theory based" interventions to the current clinical models that are based on systematic practice and accountability, with a focus on outcome and specific mechanisms of change (Alexander et al., 2002). In the arena of childhood and adolescence problems, there has been significant research in the last decade that clearly identifies a range of clinical models with particularly good outcomes. In the current era of accountability, these models can serve as a helpful guide to matching treatments with clinical problems that can now be seen as "best practices." These models have become the "treatment of choice" for many of the problems faced by children and adolescents.

In this section, we briefly review the evolution of family therapy approaches from broad theory to specific clinical models. We follow with a brief review of specific treatment approaches for the common problems of childhood and adolescence in order to help family therapists know the current "best practices" in their domain of childhood and adolescent treatment.

## From "Schools" to Specific Clinical Models: The Evolution of Family Therapy

The theoretical frameworks of family therapy have evolved since its beginnings in the late 1940s and early 1950s. The early founding constructs of systems theory, **cybernetics,** boundaries, communication and **information processing, entropy** and negentropy, **equifinality** and **equipotentiality, morphostasis** and **morphogenesis,** openness and closeness, and **positive** and **negative feedback,** were all ways to understand the "relational system" of the family.

These founding concepts became embodied in the early first generation of family therapy theory that included approaches such as structural family therapy (Minuchin, 1974), strategic family therapy, communications approaches, family-of-origin models, and psychodynamic approaches. These first generation theoretical models represented a heterogeneous group of interventions best divided into two types: pragmatic and aesthetic (Alexander et al., 2002). *Pragmatic* models had specific goals, objectives, and outcomes while *aesthetic* models had more general therapeutic intentions and nonspecific goals. (See Nichols & Schwartz, 1995; Sexton, Weeks, & Robbins, 2003, for further discussion of traditional theoretical models of practice.)

10. Which of the following describes pragmatic models of family intervention?
    a. having specific goals, objectives and outcomes
    b. having specific goals, but no specific outcomes
    c. having general therapeutic intentions and nonspecific goals
    d. having specific therapeutic intentions and general goals

11. Which of the following are *not* early founding constructs of family therapy?
    a. Freud's concept of intrapsychic processes
    b. systems theory/cybernetics
    c. communication and information processing
    d. equifinality and equipotentiality

12. Which of the following are considered first generation family therapy theories?
    a. structural family therapy
    b. strategic family therapy
    c. family-of-origin models
    d. All of the above

During the ensuing two decades the early "schools" of family therapy have given way to more specific, systematic, and well-articulated clinical models. The evolution toward integrated clinical models is based on repeated findings that found little evidence supporting the **efficacy** of theoretical approaches and thus made it clear that broad and global therapeutic orientations did not represent the important and distinguishing characteristics that differentiated effective and ineffective interventions (Alexander et al., 1994; Sexton, Alexander, et al., 2003). The current family therapy models are, unlike early theoretical, eclectic, or common factors approaches, based on a theoretical and conceptual basis of problem etiology and therapeutic change, specific well-articulated procedures for change, outcome evidence that demonstrates the success of the intervention, and process studies that demonstrate the mechanisms that lead to change within the intervention (Kazdin, 1997). Current treatments are not broad and general approaches but instead treatment models that target clinically meaningful syndromes or situations with a coherent conceptual framework underlying the clinical intervention, described in sufficient detail to explain the specific interventions and therapist qualities necessary to carry them out (Alexander et al., 1994). As such, it is possible to have high treatment integrity brought about by clinical supervision, treatment manuals, and **adherence** verification throughout the course of therapy. Liddle (1999) notes that while the traditional approaches to family therapy still have an impact on the field, the new family therapy models extend beyond traditional theoretical boundaries, are more comprehensive, and have included the role of ecological factors outside the family in understanding the etiology of problems.

13. Which of the following is the best description of current family therapy models?
    a. based on common factors approaches
    b. based on therapeutic basis of problem etiology and specify well-articulated procedures for change
    c. considered to be eclectic
    d. broad and general approaches that focus on global therapeutic orientations

14. Which of the following are used to produce high treatment integrity?
    a. clinical supervision
    b. treatment manuals
    c. adherence verification
    d. all of the above

The new models of family therapy that have evolved are based on the growing research evidence that suggests that while family therapy is effective for a wide range of clinical problems, all approaches may not be equally efficacious. For example, Kazdin (1997) identified four family-based programs that could be considered promising in regard to essential criteria of an "intervention" program: parent management training, functional family therapy (Alexander & Barton, 1995; Alexander & Sexton, 2002; Sexton & Alexander, 2002, 2003), multisystemic therapy (Henggeler, Pickrel, & Brondino, 1999), and cognitive problem solving skills training (Shure, 1992). In a similar effort, Sexton and Alexander (2002) and Alexander, Sexton, and Robbins (2002) identified a group of well-defined family-based interventions that combine specific treatment protocols (manuals) developed using realistic client populations, in actual clinical settings, within ongoing, systematic programs of research and evaluation. Currently, four clinical interventions meet these FBest criteria: functional family therapy (Alexander & Parsons, 1973), multidimensional family therapy (Liddle, 1992; Liddle & Dakof, 1995), multisystemic therapy (Borduin, Henggeler, Blaske, & Stein, 1990; Henggeler et al., 1991), and structural family therapy (as developed by Szapocznik & Kurtines, 1989). To date, both the promising programs identified by Kazdin (1997) and the FBest intervention programs noted by Sexton & Alexander (2002) are concentrated in the area of adolescent disruptive disorders and the specific accompanying problems of delinquency, drug abuse, and family conflict.

15. Which of the following clinical interventions *does not* meet the "best practice" criteria of a well-defined family-based intervention as defined by the Blueprint project?
    a. functional family therapy
    b. multidimensional family therapy
    c. multisystemic therapy
    d. therapeutic treatment foster care

16. Interventions which meet FBEST criteria include which of the following?
    a. interventions developed using realistic client populations
    b. interventions which utilize manualized treatment protocols
    c. interventions developed in highly controlled university settings
    d. both a and b

The current systematic treatment models for adolescents have also undergone numerous evaluations that have identified useful, evidence-based family therapy intervention programs for use with a range of child and adolescent problems. For example, with the growing social concern for children and adolescents (e.g., conduct disorder, juvenile delinquency, adolescent drug abuse) recent efforts have been devoted to identifying effective approaches to youth violence (Elliott, 1998; U.S. Public Health Service, 2001) and adolescent drug abuse (Model Programs for Substance Abuse and Delinquency Prevention, Center for Substance Abuse Prevention [CSAP], 2000). These efforts are notable in that they combine rigorous methodological standards traditionally associated with efficacy studies with the needs for replicability across diverse clients and in diverse treatment settings more traditionally characteristic of **effectiveness studies.** In the Blueprint project, for example, over 1,000 programs were reviewed and only 11 met the criteria of a "best practice" (Elliot, 1998). The result is an independently determined group of "best practices" for use in the treatment of adolescent and childhood clinical problems which includes three family therapy approaches: functional family therapy, multisystemic therapy, and therapeutic treatment foster care (Chamberlin & Reid, 1998). The Surgeon General's report on youth violence used a methodology similar to that adopted by the center for the Study and Prevention of Violence (CSPV). In their analysis, they identified four "level 1" programs that were effective in the treatment of juvenile violence (U.S. Public Health Service, 2001). These approaches included functional family therapy and multiysystemic therapy, both family therapy interventions.

17. Which of the following best describes the purpose of conducting effectiveness studies?
    a. to determine replicability across diverse clients in diverse treatment settings
    b. to determine efficacy
    c. to scrutinize the model using rigorous methodological standards
    d. none of the above

## Current Clinical Intervention Models in Family Therapy

Current clinical models are increasingly integrative, research-based, and multisystemic. Treatment models for adolescent problems tend to be family therapy models that target the family relational patterns that seem to underly the adolescent externalizing behavioral problems. Treatment models for childhood problems tend to be parent education based models based in social learning theory. These models target parent behavior in managing childhood problems and focus on managing and coping with the specific emotional, cognitive, or behavior problems through social learning–based parent behaviors. The majority of effective interventions for childhood clinical problems are family-assisted interventions rather than direct family therapy interventions.

18. Which of the following best describes treatment models for adolescent problems?
    a. parent education–based models grounded in social learning theory
    b. family-assisted interventions
    c. family therapy models that target the family relational patterns underlying behavior problems
    d. individual counseling for the identified patient

19. Which of the following best describes treatment models for childhood problems?
    a. parent education–based models grounded in social learning theory
    b. family-assisted interventions
    c. family therapy models that target the family relational patterns underlying behavior problems
    d. both a and b

In the following sections we briefly review the most current treatment models of family therapy intervention models for use in treating the broad areas of child and adolescent clinical problems. These models are identified here because they meet the criteria noted above and they have demonstrated effectiveness with the common issues of children and adolescents. Thus, these models, when done well, are most likely to produce successful clinical outcomes.

## Specific Approaches for the Clinical Problems of Childhood

*Parent Management Training.* Parent management training (PMT) is a widely used set of family-based interventions used with a wide variety of childhood clinical problems. PMT is based on social learning principles and is designed to help parents develop skills to alter their child's behavior in the home. (Webster-Stratton, 1994; Chamberlin & Reid, 1998). The primary goal of PMT is to alter negative interchanges between parent and child, thereby promoting prosocial rather than coercive behavior through developing different parenting behavior. Treatment is primarily conducted with parents who are taught to identify and define problem behavior in new ways; develop new prosocial ways of using positive reinforcement, mild punishment, and so forth; and guided practice. Estrada and Pinsof (1995) suggested that PMT is effective for children with attention deficit/hyperactivity disorder (ADHD), anxieties and phobias, autism, and as an adjunct to pharmacological treatment of hyperactive youth. Kazdin (1997) concluded that it was one of the most promising programs for the treatment of conduct-disordered children. There are several features of PMT that seem to contribute to successful clinical outcomes. Shorter treatments (less than 10 sessions) are not as effective as longer treatments (more than 50–60 hours). In-depth knowledge of social learning principles and specific time out procedures reinforced from in the home enhance treatment. More skilled therapists seem to produce more durable and lasting effects. Families characterized by multiple risk factors tend to show fewer gains than families with fewer risk factors.

Most current interventions designed to address problems of attention (e.g., ADHD) are based on a variation of parent management and parent consultation approaches. For example, most current treatment programs are family-based multimodal programs that combine stimulant medication treatment with parent training or specific behavior modification training skills (Estrada & Pinsof, 1995). Much less is known about family treatments for childhood anxiety. The treatments that do exist are family-assisted interventions based on PMT principles that use cognitive–behavioral intervention strategies. Estrada and Pinsof suggested that successful programs involve parents in the treatment of simple phobias, school phobia, and overanxious disorders. PMT programs are the most common family-based intervention strategies for use with Autistic disorders and pervasive developmental disorders. PMT most often involves a combination of educational interventions (lectures, readings), skills training, home visits that include coaching and reinforcement, and follow-up consultations. The most successful treatment seems to be with children who are least cognitively impaired at the outset of treatment, have families that can actively engage in a demanding treatment program, and attend schools that can support the treatment.

20. The primary goal of Parent Management Training (PMT) is to:
    a. teach parents authoritative parenting strategies.
    b. modify interchanges between parent and child to promote prosocial rather than coercive behavior.
    c. teach children to obey their parents.
    d. work with parents on marital discord.

21. Which of the following childhood problems is least researched from a family treatment perspective?
    a. conduct disorder
    b. anxiety disorders
    c. oppositional defiant disorder
    d. substance abuse

## Specific Approaches for the Clinical Problems of Adolescence

A number of family therapy approaches are in use for a wide range of problems experienced by adolescents. All of these models are family therapy–focused, involving the multisystemic relational systems of the family in treatment.

*Functional Family Therapy.* Functional family therapy (FFT) is a multisystemic family therapy intervention that has as its primary focus and therapeutic entry point in the family relational system. FFT focuses on diverse domains of client functioning (emotional, cognitive, and behavioral) and views clinical "problems" as representative of individual, family, and community risk factors that manifest within ineffective but functional family relational processes. FFT assumes that the symptom is both mediated by and embedded in complex relational sequences involving all other family members and that it has come to serve some legitimate relational outcome (closeness, distance, hierarchy). Change is a phasic process in which each of the three phases of intervention (engagement/motivation, behavior change, and generalization) has a set of therapeutic goals, related change mechanisms that help accomplish those goals, and therapist interventions most likely to activate these change mechanisms. The goal is for change to be systematically guided while clinically responsive. As a *treatment* program FFT has been applied successfully to a wide range of problem youth and their families in various contexts (Alexander & Sexton, 2002; Elliott, 1998; Sexton & Alexander, 2002, 2003). As a *prevention* program FFT has demonstrated success at diverting the trajectory of at-risk adolescents away from entering the mental health and justice systems (Alexander, Sexton, & Robbins, 2000). In both contexts, the target populations are generally youth aged 11 to 18, although younger siblings of referred adolescents may also be seen. Thus the youth range from preadolescents who are at risk to older youth with very serious problems such as conduct disorder, drug involvement, risky sexual behaviors, truancy, and the like. The families represent multi-ethnic, multicultural populations living in diverse communities.

22. Which of the following is the correct order of the phases included in Functional Family Therapy?
    a. behavior change, engagement/motivation, generalization
    b. generalization, behavior change, engagement/motivation
    c. engagement/motivation, behavior change, generalization
    d. behavior change, generalization, engagement/motivation

FFT is a short-term intervention averaging roughly 8 to 12 sessions for mild to moderate cases and up to 26 to 30 hours of clinical service for more difficult cases. The results of published studies suggest that FFT is effective in reducing recidivism (between 26% and 73% with status offending, moderate, and seriously delinquent youth) as compared to both no treatment and juvenile court probation services (Alexander et al., 2000). Of most interest is the range of community settings and client ethnicities that have composed these studies (a more complete list can be found in Alexander et al., 2000). These positive outcomes of FFT remain relatively stable even at follow-up times as long as five years (Gordon, Arbuthnot, Gustafson, & McGreen, 1988) and the positive impact also affects siblings of the identified adolescent (Klein, Alexander, & Parsons, 1977).

*Multisystemic Therapy.*   Multisystemic therapy (MST) is a systematic, manual-driven family-based intervention for youth and families facing problems of juvenile delinquency, adolescent conduct disorder, and substance abuse (Henggeler et al., 1999). MST is an approach derived from social-ecological models of behavior and family systems and social learning theories (Henggeler et al.). It highlights the strengths of individuals, families, and social systems affecting the family in order to raise the level of family functioning and curtail adolescent involvement in delinquent or problem behaviors. Targets of change in MST include individual and family level behaviors as well as outside system dynamics and resources including the adolescent's social network. Treatment interventions are provided on an "as needed" basis focusing on whatever it takes to alter individual, family, and systems issues that contribute to the problem behavior. The typical treatment course for MST implementation ranges from 2 to 4 months. An impressive series of outcome studies has evaluated MST in various contexts with adolescents with varying problems (drug abuse, delinquency, conduct problems, etc.).

23. MST is derived from which theories?
    a. social–ecological models of behavior
    b. family systems theory
    c. social learning theory
    d. all of the above

24. Which of the following are targets of change in MST?
    a. individual level behaviors
    b. family-level behaviors and outside system dynamics and resources
    c. individual and family-level behaviors as well as outside system dynamics and resources
    d. adolescent's social network

25. The primary goal of MST is to:
    a. develop a family-focused problem definition.
    b. connect parents with outside resources to raise the level of family functioning.
    c. help parents develop skills to promote prosocial behavior.
    d. help adolescents dealing with developmental challenges.

*Brief Structural Strategic Family Therapy.*   Szapocznik and his colleagues at the University of Miami were the first to publish a systematic study of a family therapy intervention for adolescent drug use (Szapocznik et al., 1988; Szapocznik & Williams, 2000). The approach was an elaboration of the early structural family therapy approaches. Brief structural strategic family therapy (BSSFT) views adolescent drug abuse as an adolescent's lack of success in dealing with developmental challenges, rigid family structures that prevent natural developmental changes (which parents need to be able to renegotiate as the adolescent grows), and intra-family and acculturation conflict that impact relationships negatively and increase substance abuse. The goals of therapy include changing parenting practices (such as leadership, behavior control, nurturance, and guidance), improving the quality of relationship and bonding between parents and the adolescent, and improving conflict resolution skills.

26. Brief structural strategic family therapy (BSSFT) was first designed to treat which problem?
    a. adolescent drug use
    b. adolescent depression
    c. adolescent anxiety disorders
    d. both a and c

BSSFT uses a variety of strategies and techniques to accomplish its goals. Early work is directed at engaging families to participate. Preliminary phone work is used to determine who will be resistant to treatment and engagement. Initial assessments focus on identifying the normal processes of acculturation and then helping families learn to transcend these differences. Initial family sessions focus on blocking or reframing negativity and promoting supportive interactions. Interventions are commonly done through the parents rather than directly through the therapist (and therefore put traditional hierarchies back into place). Reports from a variety of research studies suggest that BSSFT results in changes in abstinence rates from 7% at admission to 80% at termination. These results were maintained up to the 12-month follow-up.

*Multidimensional Family Therapy.* This multisystemic treatment approach for adolescent substance abuse and its related behavior problems (Liddle, 1992, 1999) has its roots in integrative structural and strategic family therapy but is also a specialized model that integrates the current thinking of drug abuse and delinquency with the notions of structural and strategic family therapy. As such, it adopts a multidimensional focus considering individual, family, and community factors in the development and change of drug abuse problems. The goals of multidimensional family therapy (MDFT) are to improve family functioning and parenting practices, as well as improve relationships between adolescent, family, and larger systems. Early sessions of MDFT utilize individual therapy to help adolescents work through developmental changes in a manner that promotes systems change. The primary goal is to block negative communication such as blaming. Later family sessions seek to promote adaptive parenting through supportive rather than authoritarian family relationships. The primary techniques include the the use of strategic, structural, and developmental tasks.

27. Which of the following is the primary goal of multidimensional family therapy (MDFT)?
    a. to improve family functioning
    b. to block negative communication
    c. to improve parenting practices
    d. to improve relationships between adolescents and their families

Clinical trial studies suggest that MDFT is not only successful in reducing adolescent drug use, but may also make significant impact on prosocial behavior and family functioning. Studies of MDFT have been conducted in diverse locations (Philadelphia, Miami, San Francisco), with ethnically diverse and multiproblem adolescents. For example, Liddle and Dakof (1995) reported one of the few studies that yielded changes in school performance. Adolescents receiving MDFT significantly improved their grade point average by 25%. In addition, MDFT seems to reduce parent–adolescent conflict.

It is increasingly clear that the clinical problems experienced by children and adolescents are complex. The Family-based intervention and assessment system (Fbias) proposed here provides a multisystemic way of understanding these clinical problems, thereby enhancing successful intervention by helping the family therapist focus on the specific problematic behaviors within the family relational systems within which those behaviors are embedded. The Fbias model brings the rich **epidemiological** and clinical perspective of the current behaviorally based assessment of the DSM system together with the family relational perspective of family therapy. Such a multisystemic understanding of clinical problems leads to and promotes the integration of many of the current clinical models of successful intervening with the problems of children and adolescents.

28. Which of the following are the primary domains of therapeutic focus according to the Family-based intervention and assessment system (FBias)?
    a. static and stable biological traits
    b. individual behaviors and family relational systems
    c. the ecosystemic system
    d. learning traits

29. The Family-based Intervention and assessment system is:
    a. an assessment model for diagnosing clinical syndromes.
    b. an assessment model for mapping family genograms.
    c. a multidomain model for understanding the problems of adolescents and children.
    d. none of the above.

Family-based intervention models are becoming the treatment of choice for many of the common clinical problems experienced by children and adolescents. The current clinical models have emerged from the founding principles and early theoretical models of family therapy. The current models of practice are systematic approaches to treatment involving theoretical principles and systematic treatment protocols and have research evidence that suggests they provide a high probability of successful outcome when done well.

## KEY TERMS

**adherence:** The degree to which the therapist follows the treatment model specifically as it is written.

**comorbid disorders:** Two or more disorders affecting an individual at the same time.

**cybernetics:** The comparative study of automatic feedback and control processes in mechanical, electronic, and biological systems; especially processes in which negative feedback keeps the system in a particular state or on course toward a particular goal.

**ecosystemic context:** The context in which an individual lives, including systems such as peers, family, school, and the community, working together as a system.

**effectiveness studies:** Research that shows the treatment to produce the desired effect across populations of clients, with different therapists, across treatment settings.

**efficacy:** The power of a treatment to produce the desired effect; experimental studies usually performed in a laboratory setting using a control group to determine whether or not a treatment works.

**entropy:** A measure of the degree of disorder of a closed system; specification of the number of possible outcomes a given event might have: as the number of possible outcomes increases, the amount of information contained in any one outcome decreases.

**epidemiological:** Pertaining to the study of incidence, frequency, and distribution of mental disorders.

**equifinality:** Arriving at the same end result by means of different pathways.

**equipotentiality:** Different individuals in a system are equally involved in performing specific functions and have the capacity to take over functions from other individuals who are no longer performing their function; having equal potential.

**etiology:** The study of the origins and causes of diseases.

**information processing:** Analyzing tasks and breaking them down into a series of steps between the stimulus and the appropriate response to the stimulus. The information acquired at earlier stages is analyzed and made applicable for later use.

**morphogenesis:** The process by which a system adapts and changes its basic structure in order to survive; movement toward randomness is desirable as it increases survival potential.

**morphostasis:** The means by which a system maintains constancy in the face of environmental variety; a system's homeostatic mechanism.

**negative feedback:** An increase in output causes a decrease in input; a means of correcting deviations to maintain a steady state, a homeostatic mechanism.

**positive feedback:** An increase in output causes an increase in input, promoting change in the system.

**prevalence:** the total number of existing cases of a disorder as a proportion of a population at a specific time.

## DISCUSSION QUESTIONS

1. Compare and contrast Brofenbrenner's ecosystemic model to the F-Bias model.
   a. Explain why early multifaceted models, like Brofenbrenner's, are not adequately integrative.
   b. What is the role of an ecosystemic context within the F-Bias model?
   c. What are the primary domains of therapeutic focus within the F-Bias model?
2. Discuss differences and similarities in the pattern of presenting problems among externalizing disorders in children and adolescents.
   a. Explain how the family, peer, and school relational systems support or contribute to such problems.
3. Discuss the evolution of family therapy models.
4. There are two "level 1" family-based approaches that effectively treat juvenile violence. Discuss the following:
   a. theoretical principles upon which each is based
   b. primary goals of each
   c. strategies or techniques used to accomplish these goals
   d. how relational systems are targeted

## REFERENCES

Alexander, J. F., & Barton, C. (1995). Family therapy research. In R. H. Mikesell et al. (Eds.), *Integrating family therapy: Handbook of family psychology and systems theory* (pp. 199–215). Washington, DC: American Psychological Association.

Alexander, J. F., Holtzworth-Munroe, A., & Jameson, P. (1994). The process and outcome of marital and family therapy: Research review and evaluation. In A. E. Bergin & S. L. Garfield (Eds.), *Handbook of psychotherapy and behavior change* (4th ed., pp. 595–630). New York: Wiley.

Alexander, L. F., & Parsons, B. V. (1973). Short term behavioral interventions with delinquent families: Impact on family process and recidivism. *Journal of Abnormal Psychololgy, 81*(3), 219–225.

Alexander, J. F., & Pugh, C. A. (1996). Oppositional behavior and conduct disorders of children and youth. In F. W. Kaslow (Ed.), *Handbook of relational diagnosis and dysfunctional family patterns* (pp. 210–224). New York: Wiley.

Alexander, J. F., & Sexton, T. L. (2002). Functional family therapy: A model for treating high risk, acting out youth. In F. W. Kaslow (Ed.), *Comprehensive handbook of psychotherapy: Integrative/eclectic, vol. 4* (pp. 111–132). New York: Wiley.

Alexander, J. F., Sexton, T. L., & Robbins, M. S. (2000). Family-based interventions with older, at-risk youth: From promise to proof to practice. *Journal of Primary Prevention, 21*(2), 185–205.

Alexander, J. F., Sexton, T. L., & Robbins, M. S. (2002). The developmental status of family therapy in family psychology intervention science. In H. A. Liddle, D. Santisteban, R. Levant, & J. Bray (Eds.), *Family psychology science-based interventions* (pp. 118–163). Washington, DC: American Psychological Association.

Altepeter, T. S., & Korger, J. N. (1999). Disruptive behavior: Oppositional defiant disorder and conduct disorder. In S. Netherton, D. Holmen, & C. Walker (Eds.), *Child and adolescent psychological disorders: A comprehensive textbook* (pp. 118–138). Oxford, England: Oxford University Press.

American Psychiatric Association. (2000). *Diagnostic and statistical manual of mental disorders: DSM–IV–TR* (4th ed., text revision). Washington, DC: Author.

American Psychiatric Association. (1994). *Diagnostic and statistical manual of mental disorders* (4th ed.). Washington, DC: Author.

Blau, B. I. (1996). Oppositional defiant disorder. In G. M. Blau & T. P. Gullotta (Eds.), *Adolescent dysfunctional behavior: Causes, interventions, and prevention* (pp. 61–82). Thousand Oaks, CA: Sage.

Borduin, C. M., Henggeler, S. W., Blaske, D. M., & Stein, R. J. (1990). Multisystemic treatment of adolescent sexual offenders. *International Journal of Offender Therapy & Comparative Criminology, 34*(2), 105–113.

Borduin, C. M., Schaeffer, C. M., & Heiblum, N. (1999). Relational problems: The social context of child and adolescent disorders. In S. Netherton, D. Holmen, & C. Walker (Eds.), *Child and adolescent psychological disorders: A comprehensive textbook* (pp. 498–519). Oxford: Oxford University Press.

Brown, S. A., Aarons, G. A., & Abrantes, A. M. (2001). Adolescent alcohol and drug abuse. In C. E. Walker & M. C. Roberts (Eds.), *Handbook of clinical child psychology* (3rd ed., pp. 757–775). New York: Wiley.

Brown, S. A., Mott, M. A., & Stewart, M. A. (1992). Delinquency and criminal behavior. In C. E. Walker & M. C. Roberts (Eds.), *Handbook of clinical child psychology* (2nd ed., pp. 677–693). New York: Wiley.

Center for Substance Abuse Prevention. (2000). 2000 annual summary: Effective prevention principles and programs. Retrieved March 1, 2004, from www.modelprograms.samhsa.gov/pdfs/NREPP_summary.pdf

Chamberlain, P., & Reid, J. B. (1998). Comparison of two community alternatives to incarceration for chronic offenders. *Consulting and Clinical Psychology, 66*(4), 624–634.

Costello, J. E., & Angold, A. (1996). Toward establishing an empirical basis for the diagnosis of oppositional-defiant disorders. *Journal of the Academy of Child and Adolescent Psychiatry, 35*(95), 1205–1213.

Dembo, R., Williams, L., La Voie, L., Schmeidler, J., Kera, J., Getreu, A., Berry, E., Genhng, L., & Wish, E. D. (1990). Longitudinal study of the relationships among alcohol use, marijuana/hashish use, cocaine use, and emotional/psychological functioning in a cohort of high-risk youths. *The International Journal of the Addictions, 25*, 1341–1382.

Elliott, D. S. (Series Ed.). (1998). *Blueprints for violence prevention.* University of Colorado, Center for the Study and Prevention of Violence. Boulder, CO: Blueprints Publications.

Estrada, A. U., & Pinsof, W. M. (1995). The effectiveness of family therapies for selected behavioral disorders of childhood. *Journal of Marital and Family Therapy, 21*(4), 403–440.

Famularo, R., Kinscherff, R., & Fenton, T. (1992). Psychiatric diagnoses of maltreated children: Preliminary findings. *Journal of the American Academy of Child and Adolescent Psychiatry, 31*, 863–867.

Gordon, D. A., Arbuthnot, J., Gustafson, K., & McGreen, P. (1988). Home-based behavioral systems family therapy with disadvantaged juvenile delinquents. *American Journal of Family Therapy, 16*, 243–255.

Gormly, A. V., & Brodzinsky, D. M. (1993). *Lifespan human development* (5th ed.). New York: Harcourt Brace Jovanovich.

Gurman, A. S., Kniskern, D. P., & Pinsof, W. M. (1986). Research on marital and family therapies. In S. L. Garfield & A. E. Bergin (Eds.), *Handbook of psychotherapy and behavior change* (3rd ed., pp. 565–624). New York: Wiley.

Hawkins, J. D., Catalano, R. F., & Miller, J. Y. (1992). Risk and protective factors for alcohol and other drug problems in adolescence and early adulthood: Implications for substance abuse preventions. *Psychological Bulletin, 112*, 64–105.

Hazelrigg, M. D., Cooper, H. M., & Borduin, C. M. (1987). Evaluating the effectiveness of family therapies: An integrative review and analysis. *Psychological Bulletin, 101*(3), 428–442.

Henggeler, S. W., Borduin, C. M., Melton, G. B., Mann, B. J., Smith, L., Hall, J. A., et al. (1991). Effects of multisystemic therapy on drug use and abuse in serious juvenile offenders: A progress report from two outcome studies. *Family Dynamics of Addiction Quarterly, 1*(3), 40–51.

Henggeler, S. W., Pickrel, S. G., & Brondino, M. J. (1999). Multisystemic treatment of substance abusing and dependent delinquents: Outcomes, treatment fidelity, and transportability. *Mental Health Services Research, 1*(3), 171–184.

Herbert, M. (1991). *Clinical child psychology: Social learning, development and behavior.* New York: Wiley.

Hundleby, J. D., & Mercer, G. W. (1987). Family and friends as social environments and their relationship to young adolescents' use of alcohol, tobacco, and marijuana. *Journal of Marriage and the Family, 49*, 151–164.

Kandel, D. B. (1978). Convergences in prospective longitudinal surveys of drug use in normal populations. In D. B. Kandel (Ed.), *Longitudinal research in drug use: Emotional findings and methodological issues.* Washington, DC: Hemisphere-Wiley.

Kaslow, F. W. (1996). *Handbook of relational diagnosis and dysfunctional family patterns.* New York: Wiley.

Kazdin, A. E. (1987). Treatment of antisocial behavior in children: Current status and future directions. *Psychological Bulletin, 102*, 187–203.

Kazdin, A. E. (1997). Practitioner review: Psychosocial treatments for conduct disorder in children. *Journal of Child Psychology & Psychiatry & Allied Disciplines 38*(2), 161–178.

Klein, N., Alexander, J., & Parsons, B. (1977). Impact of family systems interventions on recidivism and sibling delinquency: A model of primary prevention and program evaluation. *Journal of Consulting and Clinical Psychology, 45*, 469–474.

Lahey, B. B., Loeber, R., Quay, H. C., Frick, P. J., & Grimm, J. (1992). Oppositional defiant and conduct disorders: Issues to be resolved for *DSM–IV. Journal of the American Academy of Child and Adolescent Psychiatry, 31*, 539–546.

Liddle, H. A. (1992). Family psychology: Progress and prospects of a maturing discipline. *Journal of Family Psychology. Special Issue: Diversity in contemporary family psychology, 5*(3-4), 249–263.

Liddle, H. A. (1999). Theory development in a family-based therapy for adolescent drug abuse. *Journal of Clinical Child Psychology, 28*, 521–532.

Liddle, H. A., & Dakof, G. A. (1995). Efficacy of family therapy for drug abuse: Promising but not definitive. *Journal of Marital & Family Therapy. Special Issue: The effectiveness of marital and family therapy, 21*(4), 511–543.

Loeber, R. (1991). Antisocial behavior: More enduring than changeable? *Journal of the American Academy of Child and Adolescent Psychiatry, 30*, 393–397.

Lytton, H. (1990). Child and parent effects in boys' conduct disorder: A reinterpretation. *Developmental Psychology, 26*(5), 683–697.

McGee, R., Feehan, B. B., & Thomas, C. (1992). *DSM–III* disorders from age 11 to age 15 years. *Journal of the American Academy of Child Psychiatry, 31*, 50–59.

Minuchin, S. (1974). *Families & family therapy.* Oxford, England: Harvard University Press.

Needle, R. H., Glynn, T. J., & Needle, M. P. (1983). Drug abuse: Adolescent addictions and the family. In R. Figley & H. I. McCubbin (Eds.), *Stress and the family* (pp. 37–52). New York: Brunner/Mazel.

National Institute on Drug Abuse. (1992). National high school senior drug abuse survey 1975–1991. Monitoring the future survey. *NIDA Capsules* (NIH Publication No. 99-4180). Washigton, DC: U.S. Department of Health and Human Services, Alcohol, Drug Abuse, and Mental Health Administration.

Nichols, M. P., & Schwartz, R. C. (1995). *Family therapy: Concepts and methods.* Needham Heights, MA: Allyn & Bacon.

Parker, J. G., & Asher, S. R. (1987). Peer relations and later personal adjustment: Are low-accepted children at risk? *Psychological Bulletin 102*(3), 357–389.

Robbins, M., Szapocznik, J., Tejeda, M., Samuels, D., Ironson, G., & Antoni, M. (2003). The protective role of the family and social support network in a sample of HIV-positive African American women: Results of a pilot study. *Journal of Black Psychology, 29*(1), 17–37.

Robins, L. N. (1966). *Deviant children grow up: A sociological and psychiatric study of sociopathic personality.* Baltimore: Williams & Wilkins.

Robins, L. N. (1981). Epidemiological approaches to natural history research: Antisocial disorders in children. *Journal of the American Academy of Child Psychiatry, 20*, 513–544.

Rubin, K. H., & Mills, R. S. (1991). Conceptualizing developmental pathways to internalizing disorders in childhood. *Canadian Journal of Behavioural Science. Special Issue: Childhood disorders in the context of the family, 23*(3), 300–317.

Sadava, S. W. (1987). Interactionist theories. In H. T. Blane & K. E. Leonard (Eds.), *Psychological theories of drinking and alcoholism* (pp. 90–130). New York: Guilford Press.

Sexton, T. L., & Alexander, J. F. (2002). FBEST: Family-based empirically supported treatment interventions. *The Counseling Psychologist, 30*(2), 238–261.

Sexton, T. L., & Alexander, J. F. (2003). Functional family therapy: A mature clinical model for working with at-risk adolescents and their families. In T. L. Sexton, G. R. Weeks, & M. S. Robbins (Eds.), *Handbook of family therapy: The science and practice of working with families and couples* (pp. 323–348). New York: Brunner-Routledge.

Sexton, T. S., Alexander, J. F., & Mease, A. L. (2003). Levels of evidence for the models and mechanisms of therapeutic change in couple and family therapy. In M. Lambert (Ed.), *Handbook of Psychotherapy and Behavior Change* (pp. 590–646). New York: Wiley.

Sexton, T. L., Weeks, G. R., & Robbins, M. S. (2003). *Handbook of family therapy: The science and practice of working with families.* New York: Brunner-Routledge.

Shure, M. B. (1992). *I can problem solve: An interpersonal cognitive problem-solving program.* Champaign, IL: Research Press.

Snyder, D. K., Cavell, T. A., Heffer, R. W., & Mangrum, L. F. (1995). Marital and family assessment: A multifaceted, multilevel approach. In R. H. Mikesell & D. Lusterman (Eds.), *Integrating family therapy: Handbook of family psychology and systems theory* (pp. 163–182). Washington, DC: American Psychological Association.

Szapocznik, J., & Kurtines, W. M. (1989). *Breakthroughs in family therapy with drug abusing and problem youth.* New York: Springer.

Szapocznik, J., Perez-Vidae, A., Brickman, A. L., Foote, F. H., Santisteban, O., Hervis, D., & Kurtines, W. M. (1988). Engaging adolescent drug abusers and their families in treatment: A strategic structural systems approach. *Journal of Consulting and Clinical Psychology, 56*, 552–557.

Szapocznik, J., & Williams, R. A. (2000). Brief strategic family therapy: Twenty-five years of interplay among theory, research and practice in adolescent behavior problems and drug abuse. *Clinical Child & Family Psychology Review, 3*(2), 117–135.

U.S. Public Health Service. (2001). *Youth violence: A report of the surgeon general.* Washington, DC: Author.

Webster-Stratton, C. (1994). Advancing videotape parent training: A comparison study. *Journal of Consulting & Clinical Psychology, 62*(3), 583–593.

World Health Organization. (1992). *The ICD-10 classification of mental and behavioral disorders: Clinical descriptions and diagnostic guidelines.* Geneva, Switzerland: Author.

# 17

# Substance Abuse

Aaron Hogue
Sarah Dauber
Leyla Faw

*The National Center on Addiction and Substance Abuse at
Columbia University*

Howard A. Liddle

*University of Miami School of Medicine*

## TRUTH OR FICTION?

___ 1. *Cigarette smoking is more common than drinking among adolescents.*

___ 2. *The younger a person is when he or she starts using substances, the more likely that person is to develop a substance use disorder.*

___ 3. *Having good social skills can help protect an at-risk adolescent from substance use problems.*

___ 4. *Adolescent substance use is most common in urban areas.*

___ 5. *Research has focused more on identifying protective factors than on identifying risk factors.*

___ 6. *Alcohol is a central nervous system depressant.*

___ 7. *Drug use may negatively affect the user's judgment, thereby increasing the risk of car accidents.*

___ 8. *A depressed adolescent who abuses drugs is at lower risk for suicide than a depressed adolescent who does not abuse drugs.*

___ 9. *Adolescent substance abusers tend to have high levels of anxiety.*

___ 10. *In recent years, the rate of juvenile arrests for drug use violations has increased.*

___ 11. *The most effective drug prevention programs are those that target multiple areas of risk.*

___ 12. *Residential treatment programs differ from inpatient programs in that they are less restrictive and structured and are not set in hospitals.*

___ 13. *The 12-step model is the most effective treatment for adolescent drug abusers.*

___ 14. *Family therapy is more effective than alternative treatments in reducing adolescent*
        *drug use and behavior problems.*
___ 15. *In the presence of certain risk factors, adolescent substance use is inevitable.*

## PREVALENCE AND INCIDENCE OF ADOLESCENT SUBSTANCE USE

In the past decade, there has been tremendous progress in our understanding of how adolescent substance use develops, how to prevent its onset and escalation, how to treat clinical level drug use problems, and how to increase public awareness of the problem and access to intervention programs. Yet, despite these documented advances in scientific and applied arenas, adolescent substance use remains a problem of epidemic proportions in the United States. According to a recent national survey, by 12th grade approximately 80% of youth report at least one exposure to alcohol, 63% to cigarettes, 16% to marijuana, and 9% to other illicit drugs (Johnston, O'Malley, & Bachman, 2002). These figures are strikingly high despite documented underreporting among teenagers. As a family therapist, the odds are high that you will encounter an adolescent substance abuser at some point in your career. [Much of the information cited in this section is taken from the most recent Monitoring the Future Study as well as from a series of CASA reports (see section on further reading).]

1. By 12th grade, approximately ____ % of adolescents have been exposed to alcohol.
   a. 50
   b. 30
   c. 80
   d. 10

## Current Figures and Historical Trends

### Tobacco

Cigarette smoking is the most common form of tobacco use among teens, followed by cigar smoking and smokeless tobacco. More than 60% of high school students have smoked cigarettes. Almost a third of high school students are current smokers, and 14% are frequent smokers. These estimates remain high in spite of recent declines in cigarette smoking since the mid-1990s. Fewer adolescents use smokeless tobacco now than during the mid-1990s when the prevalence rate peaked at about 15% of American adolescents. Currently, 4% of 8th graders and 8% of 12th graders report using smokeless tobacco.

### Alcohol

For every adolescent you will see as a clinician, there is a strong chance that he or she has at least experimented with alcohol. Alcohol is the most widely used drug among adolescents in the United States. Approximately one-fourth of alcohol consumption is attributed to children and adolescents under age 21. More than 80% of high school students report experimenting with alcohol, and over 31% report binge drinking at least once a month. Additional findings suggest that drinking starts early. Nearly one-fourth of all 8th graders report being drunk at least once in their life, and this figure increases to two-thirds by the time adolescents reach 12th grade. Furthermore, 13% of adolescents aged 12 to 17 experienced at least one serious problem related to drinking in the past year (SAMHSA, 1999).

## Marijuana

From 16% to almost half (47%) of all high school students report trying marijuana, and more than one-fourth of high school students are current marijuana users (defined as having used marijuana in the past thirty days). Like cigarette smoking, marijuana use peaked in the mid-1990s and has since declined modestly. Despite the decline in overall rates of use, many adolescents initiate marijuana use as early as middle school. Since the 1970s, the age of initiation has steadily decreased. As is the case with other drugs, earlier age of initiation of marijuana use increases the risk for abuse and related problems later in adolescence.

## Other Substances

Adolescent use of illegal substances other than marijuana rose considerably over the 1990s, reaching a peak in 1997. One in ten high school students reports using a form of cocaine by the end of high school, and 4% say they are current users. Results from national surveys illustrated several trends from the mid-1990s to the present: slight decreases in the use of cocaine, crack, LSD, and inhalants; steady rates of use for heroin and other narcotics; and a sharp rise in the use of ecstasy accompanied by a less pronounced increase in anabolic steroid use.

2. The most common form of adolescent tobacco use is:
   a. cigar smoking.
   b. smokeless tobacco.
   c. cigarettes.
   d. none of the above.

3. The most widely used drug among U.S. adolescents is:
   a. tobacco.
   b. alcohol.
   c. marijuana.
   d. ecstasy.

4. Since the mid-1990s, marijuana use among adolescents has:
   a. slightly increased.
   b. slightly decreased.
   c. stayed the same.
   d. sharply decreased.

# Subgroup Characteristics and Trends

## Gender Differences

There is some evidence that adolescent substance use differs for boys versus girls. Gender differences are reported mostly for alcohol use. Drinking is more common among boys than girls in early adolescence and, to a greater extent, in late adolescence, despite equal amounts of use at age 15. Higher use among boys is consistent with findings that boys hold more positive beliefs toward drinking than do girls. From a historical perspective, the gender difference in drinking appears to be decreasing as alcohol use by girls slowly approaches the levels of use by boys. Boys also demonstrate higher rates of illicit drug use and smokeless tobacco use. Boys and girls report approximately equal rates of cigarette smoking.

5. The tendency for boys to drink more than girls is:
   a. most pronounced during early adolescence.
   b. most pronounced during middle adolescence.
   c. most pronounced during late adolescence.
   d. about the same across the span of adolescence.

## Subgroup Trends

Other than marijuana use, which does not tend to differ across ethnic groups, surveys demonstrate lower rates of substance use for African American adolescents than for White and Hispanic adolescents. In particular, use of cigarettes among African American adolescents is dramatically lower than that among youth of other ethnic groups. Rates of substance use among Hispanics tend to fall between the rates for African Americans and Whites, usually closer to the rates for Whites. With regard to other ethnicities, some research including American Indian/Alaska Native adolescents shows much higher rates of cigarette smoking in this group (28%) than that reported by Whites (16%), Hispanics (10%), Asians (8%), and African Americans (6%).

6. Adolescent cigarette use is lowest among:
   a. African-Americans.
   b. Asians.
   c. Caucasians.
   d. Hispanics.

Recent findings have debunked the myth that substance use is more common in the city. Drug, alcohol, and cigarette use are more common among adolescents in rural America than among those in large urban areas. Eighth graders in rural areas are 83% more likely than their urban peers to use crack cocaine, 50% more likely to use cocaine, 34% more likely to smoke marijuana, 29% more likely to drink alcohol, 70% more likely to get drunk, more than twice as likely to smoke cigarettes, and almost five times more likely to use smokeless tobacco. Rates of use are also higher for rural 10th and 12th graders than for their urban counterparts. Findings of more drug use in rural areas may be related to higher rates of decline in use among urban teens. Overall, these subgroup findings show that clinicians should be sensitive to ethnic and geographical considerations.

7. Adolescent drug use in rural areas is:
   a. less common than in urban areas.
   b. about the same as in urban areas.
   c. more common than in urban areas.
   d. unresearched.

# EFFECTS OF ADOLESCENT SUBSTANCE USE ON ADOLESCENT DEVELOPMENT AND BEHAVIOR

## Physiological and Neurochemical Impact

The chronic use of drugs during adolescence significantly impacts neurological functioning and produces serious physiological symptoms and impairment. An understanding of these physiological effects of substance use may be useful when you are assessing and preparing to treat an adolescent substance user. Specific types of drugs interact with neurotransmitters in the brain and produce a variety of effects on the body.

The use of tobacco introduces **nicotine** into the brain, where it activates the cholinergic receptors, leading to the release of acetylcholine. Nicotine also stimulates the release of dopamine, which leads to the sensation of pleasure. The effects of nicotine on the brain include central nervous system arousal, skeletal muscle relaxation, and activation of the sympathetic nervous system, which leads to an increase in heart rate, blood pressure, and coronary blood flow.

8. Which substance leads to the release of acetylcholine and dopamine?
   a. alcohol.
   b. marijuana.
   c. ecstasy.
   d. tobacco.

In contrast to tobacco, alcohol is a central nervous system depressant. Chronic use of alcohol may lead to a loss of coordination, poor judgment, slowed reflexes, distorted vision, memory lapses, and blackouts. The main active ingredient in marijuana is **THC**. Upon entering the brain, THC binds to cannabinoid receptors, which are located in the cerebellum and the hippocampus, the parts of the brain responsible for coordination of movement and memory. Marijuana also activates receptors in the cerebral cortex, which interferes with the receiving of sensory messages, leading the brain to misinterpret nerve impulses from the sense organs. Short-term effects of marijuana include problems with memory, learning, and problem-solving, distorted perception, loss of coordination, and increased heart rate and anxiety. It is also possible that marijuana use causes changes in the brain that make a person more likely to become addicted to other drugs.

9. All of the following are short-term effects of marijuana use *except:*
   a. distorted perception.
   b. anxiety.
   c. loss of appetite.
   d. loss of coordination.

10. The active ingredient in marijuana is:
    a. nicotine.
    b. THC.
    c. dopamine.
    d. serotonin.

Ecstasy is a substance that is currently increasing in popularity among adolescents. Ecstasy may cause confusion, sleep problems, depression, and anxiety. Chronic use of ecstasy may impair cognitive functioning, including learning, memory, verbal reasoning, and attention.

## Health Risks

### Diseases

Adolescents who use substances frequently are at increased risk for a variety of diseases in both the short and long term. Immediate health consequences of frequent use of marijuana and cigarettes include respiratory problems and chest colds. The long-term effects of chronic substance use in adolescence are more varied and more severe. Specifically, smoking tobacco can cause lung cancer, emphysema, heart problems, and peripheral vascular disease. Chewing tobacco may cause gum damage, tooth loss, and mouth cancers. Chronic alcohol use may cause Korsakoff's syndrome, which is characterized by severe memory loss, sensory and motor dysfunction, and dementia. Alcohol use is also associated with cirrhosis of the liver, heart attack, cancer, stomach ulcers, pancreatitis, and gastritis. Smoking marijuana causes many of the same problems as smoking tobacco and some additional problems, including lung infections and cancer.

Drug use may also increase the risk of contracting a sexually transmitted disease (SAMHSA, 2000). Substance use impairs judgment and reduces inhibitions, both of which may lead the user to engage in risky sexual behaviors, including having multiple partners and not using condoms. These risky sexual behaviors increase the adolescent's risk of acquiring HIV or another sexually transmitted disease. Adolescent drug users who share needles to inject heroin or other drugs are also at increased risk of acquiring HIV.

## Accidents and Suicide

Accidents are the leading cause of death among adolescents. Because of their impact on coordination, alertness, concentration, and reaction time, substances such as alcohol and marijuana have been implicated in a large percentage of traffic and other types of accidents. Adolescents who use drugs may also be at increased risk for suicide. Studies have shown that suicidal adolescents tend to use more drugs than nonsuicidal adolescents. Substance use may intensify a preexisting depressive or psychotic disorder in an adolescent, thereby increasing the risk of suicide. Research suggests that a depressed adolescent who abuses substances is at increased risk of making multiple suicide attempts and of making a medically serious attempt.

## Psychiatric and Psychological Symptomatology

Substance use in adolescents often occurs in conjunction with other psychological disorders or symptoms. This is significant for your work as therapists because people with **comorbid** psychiatric diagnoses tend to require more treatment and have poorer outcomes. The most common disorders to co-occur with adolescent substance abuse are the disruptive behavior disorders, including conduct disorder, oppositional defiant disorder, and attention deficit hyperactivity disorder. These disorders tend to precede the onset of substance use. Substance use in adolescents also often co-occurs with mood and anxiety disorders. The most commonly co-occuring mood disorder in substance-abusing adolescents is major depressive disorder, which usually has a later onset than the substance use. Dysthymia tends to precede substance use. The most common comorbid anxiety disorder is posttraumatic stress disorder. Even those substance-abusing adolescents who do not have a formally diagnosed anxiety disorder tend to have higher levels of anxiety than their non-substance–abusing peers.

11. The most common disorders to co-occur with adolescent substance abuse are:
     a. disruptive behavior disorders.
     b. mood disorders.
     c. personality disorders.
     d. anxiety disorders.

## Psychosocial Functioning

In addition to the effects on physical and psychological health described above, substance use also has consequences in terms of an individual's psychosocial functioning, particularly in the areas of school and work, criminal involvement, and the assumption of adult roles. Adolescents who use marijuana frequently perform poorly in school and are less likely to complete high school. Similarly, alcohol use during adolescence is associated with a reduced ability to learn, academic problems, poor grades in school, and increased likelihood of dropping out. The physical and mental effects of substance use may increase the number of school absences and may prevent the student from performing optimally in school on the days he or she does attend. Adolescents who abuse substances are less likely to be college-bound and are also less likely to participate in prosocial youth activities.

12. Adolescents who use substances are less likely than their nonusing peers to:
    a. drop out of school.
    b. contract a sexually transmitted disease.
    c. die in a car accident.
    d. none of the above.

When an adolescent substance abuser presents for treatment, it is likely that he or she has also had some involvement in the criminal justice system, either as a victim or as a perpetrator. Alcohol use is associated with a greater likelihood of being the victim of a violent crime. Adolescents who abuse alcohol are more likely to be involved in physical fights, run away from home, steal, destroy property, and physically attack others (Greenblatt, 2000). These adolescents are also more likely than their peers to be on probation and to be arrested for breaking the law.

13. Adolescents who abuse alcohol are:
    a. as likely as their peers to commit a crime.
    b. more likely than their peers to commit a crime.
    c. less likely as their peers to commit a crime.
    d. there is no connection between alcohol use and criminal behavior.

The negative effects of adolescent substance use are not limited to the time period of adolescence. Longitudinal research, following adolescent substance users into their adult years, shows that their problems persist. Adolescent substance use may interfere with the successful transition to adulthood and the assumption of adult roles, leading to impaired interpersonal relationships and job performance.

14. Long-term effects of severe adolescent substance use may include:
    a. unemployment.
    b. impaired interpersonal relationships.
    c. single parenthood.
    d. all of the above.

# PATHOGENESIS, ETIOLOGY, AND MAJOR RISK AND PROTECTIVE FACTORS

## Symptom Severity and Progression

The *Diagnostic and Statistical Manual of Mental Disorders* (*DSM–IV*; American Psychiatric Association [APA], 2000) conceptualizes the development of adolescent substance use as a continuum of different levels of use, escalating from experimentation at the low end to substance dependence at the high end. Substance use always begins with initiation and experimentation. These behaviors can then progress to regular use, abuse, and dependence in more extreme cases. Typically, both environmental and personal factors influence the initiation of substance use. Following initiation, the chemical properties of a substance can contribute to increased involvement through its biological interactions with the brain. **Substance abuse** is diagnosed when a person places him- or herself in danger or experiences recurrent, significant problems as a consequence of his or her substance use. **Substance dependence** implies a more serious condition in which the individual may experience tolerance, withdrawal, or other symptoms that negatively affect social and physical functioning. As therapists, you will want to determine your client's level of substance use, as this information will guide your treatment plan.

15. Substance dependence, as defined by the *DSM–IV,* is:
   a. less severe than substance abuse.
   b. more severe than substance abuse.
   c. equivalent to substance abuse.
   d. never present in adolescents.

Another major conceptualization of the development of substance use disorders is referred to as the ***gateway hypothesis***. In this model, alcohol and marijuana represent critical points of entry into the use of other illicit substances. The gateway hypothesis suggests that substance use progresses through four stages: (a) beer or wine, (b) cigarettes or hard liquor, (c) marijuana, and finally (d) other illicit substances. Participation in one stage is necessary for participation in the next stage. Some describe a fifth stage of problem drinking that occurs between marijuana use and other illicit drug use. The gateway sequence is found across gender, race, and ethnicity, and it is observed throughout different historical periods.

16. According to the gateway hypothesis, the first stage of drug use is:
   a. marijuana.
   b. cigarettes or hard liquor.
   c. beer or wine.
   d. cocaine.

17. A possible 5th stage in the gateway hypothesis occurs:
   a. between beer/wine and hard liquor.
   b. between hard liquor and marijuana.
   c. between marijuana and other illicit drugs.
   d. after initiation of cocaine and other illicit drugs.

## Clinical and Diagnostic Figures

Researchers have examined the prevalence of substance use disorders (as diagnosed by the *DSM–IV*) in the general adolescent population. One study found that 13.6% of diagnosed adolescents abused alcohol, 5.6% abused marijuana, 2.6% abused cocaine, 1.6% abused stimulants, and 0.7% abused hallucinogens (Anthony, Warner, & Kessler, 1994). Boys and older adolescents were more likely than girls and younger adolescents to meet *DSM–IV* criteria for a substance use disorder at some point in their lives. Little is known about the types of treatment most often provided for adolescents with substance use problems. Although more than 100,000 adolescents are treated in publicly funded substance abuse programs each year, the number of adolescents who are treated in privately funded programs is not known, nor is the number of adolescents in the community who are in need of treatment.

18. Adolescent substance use disorders are most common in which treatment sector?
    a. Mental Health.
    b. Juvenile Justice.
    c. Education.
    d. Child Welfare.

## Multiple Pathways to Adolescent Substance Use

Every teen at risk possesses a unique combination of factors that increase and decrease the risk for substance abuse at any point in his or her life. Table 17.1 presents a summary of risk and protective factors across several domains. As many researchers have phrased it, there are "multiple pathways" to adolescent substance use. This is an important point for you, as a therapist, to keep in mind. The adolescents that you see may have the same substance abuse problems, but may have very different profiles of risk and protective factors, and may therefore require somewhat different therapeutic techniques. While one teenager might face risk by living in a disorganized community, another might have to overcome low self-esteem or a poor relationship with his or her parents. Risk and protective factors work together to determine the level of risk for an adolescent at any given point in her or his life. For example, an adolescent who lives in a disorganized community might receive support and affection from his or her family to help buffer the risk. When preparing to treat an adolescent substance user, it is important for you to assess not only the variables placing an adolescent at risk, but also the strengths of the adolescent and his or her environment.

## Etiology and Risk Factors

A *risk factor* is a variable in a child's life that increases the probability that he or she will develop a substance use problem. Risk factors include personal characteristics, social situations, and environmental contexts, and they can act independently or together. For example, poor parenting (a risk factor in itself) can increase the likelihood of later effects from negative peer influences. The more risk factors that are present in a child's life, the higher the probability of the child developing a substance use disorder. The risk factors that have been identified fall into the three main categories of etiological theory (Petraitis, Flay, & Miller, 1995).

19. Risk factors:
    a. decrease the chance of a substance use problem.
    b. increase the chance of a substance use problem.
    c. always lead to a substance use problem.
    d. always occur in the same combination.

### Cognitive–Affective

Certain cognitive and emotional characteristics can increase an adolescent's risk for substance use. Cognitive risk factors include positive substance use outcome expectancies, low

**TABLE 17.1**

Risk and Protective Factors for Adolescent Substance Abuse

| | Individual | Microsocial | Macrosocial |
|---|---|---|---|
| *Major Risk Factors* | **Cognitive–Affective**<br>• Low self-esteem<br>• Positive drug-use expectations<br>• Exaggerated estimates of normative drug use<br>• Poor coping skills<br>• Low emotional control<br>**Genetics and Personality**<br>• Genes linked to drug abuse<br>• Tendency to seek out and explore new situations<br>• Angry, aggressive, or impulsive personality<br>• Rebelliousness<br>• Difficult temperament | **Family and Peers**<br>• Parental drug use<br>• Permissive parents<br>• Poor relationship with parents<br>• Low parental monitoring<br><br>**Peers**<br>• Friends use drugs<br>• Friends can easily access drugs<br>• Friends think drugs are positive | **Social/Cultural**<br>• Easy access to drugs in the community<br>• Lack of connection among community members<br>• Positive drug advertising<br>• Media glamorization of drugs |
| *Major Protective Factors* | • Good communication skills<br>• Good sense of humor<br>• Ability to empathize<br>• Feeling in control of the future | • Supportive and affectionate parents<br>• Realistic expectations from parents<br>• Authoritative parenting style<br>• Caring and supportive friends<br>• Conventional friends<br>• Friends who achieve in school | • Supportive adult in the school or community<br>• High community bonding and support<br>• Involvement in extracurricular activities<br>• Positive community role model |

self-efficacy (i.e., an adolescent's perceived ability to resist temptations or urges to drink in high-risk situations), and distorted beliefs about how normal it is for teenagers to use substances. In addition, more global cognitive risk factors include deficits in executive cognitive functioning and general problem-solving skills. Emotional risk factors include coping difficulties, high levels of emotional distress, impulse control problems, and emotion regulation difficulties.

## Family and Sociocultural

This category of risk factors encompasses a wide range of risk factors across family, peers, and community. Having a family history of substance abuse puts a child at twice the level of risk for drinking and four times the level of risk for illicit drug use. A child who is exposed to substance abuse behavior by a caretaker is more likely to use substances. Furthermore, the closer the relationship between parent and child, the more likely the child is to imitate the parent's substance use behaviors. Children with parents who use drugs are also more prone to emotional difficulties and problem behaviors other than substance misuse. Parenting and family management practices also influence adolescent substance use. Research has shown that teens who are not consistently monitored by their parents are at increased risk for substance involvement. Having parents who are permissive about alcohol and drug use also places a teen at higher risk for developing a substance use problem. Family processes can also affect risk for adolescent substance use. When conflict between an adolescent and his or her parents is high, the risk for substance use increases. Child abuse (physical or sexual) is also associated with higher rates of drug use.

Peer influences represent another source of great risk. An adolescent's substance use is often similar to that of his or her peers. Peer influences occur through two processes: socialization and selection. *Socialization* is a process in which social networks influence the initiation of drug use by increasing access to drugs or modeling substance use as a way of coping with stress. Research shows that drug use is more common among teens who have talked to their friends about using drugs, teens who have friends with positive attitudes toward drug use, and teens with friends who use drugs. *Selection* refers to the process of adolescents seeking out peers whose attitudes and behaviors match their own. Selection occurs in several different ways. For example, drug users select friends who are drug users, peer groups restrict membership to only those individuals whose drug use behavior matches that of the group, and friendships can dissolve when drug use behaviors become dissimilar. Research suggests that selection is related to cigarette and alcohol use.

Community factors can also increase an adolescent's risk for substance use. For example, a higher concentration of alcohol establishments, especially in poor or urban areas, is associated with increased risk. In neighborhoods where children do not feel connected to the community, and where families do not become friendly neighbors, risk for substance use is also higher. Other environmental influences include the media, the internet, the fashion industry, and popular culture. These industries often convey images that normalize or glamorize substance use. Over half of students in grades 5 through 12 report that advertising encourages them to drink.

## Genetics and Personality

The third major category of risk includes genetic factors and individual personality and temperament. Identical twins (who share all of their genes) are much more likely to both become alcoholics than fraternal twins who share only half their genes. According to adoption studies, adopted children with biological parents who are alcoholics are twice as likely to become alcoholics than adopted children whose biological parents are not alcoholics. Personality characteristics that place a child at risk for substance use are listed in Table 17.1. Finally, having a difficult temperament, recognizable during infancy and childhood, places teenagers at greater risk for tobacco, alcohol, and marijuana use.

> 20. The temperamental disposition associated with increased risk for adolescent substance use is:
>     a. difficult.
>     b. easy.
>     c. slow to warm up.
>     d. none of the above.

## Protective Factors

When an adolescent possesses one or more risk factors, other, positive factors can interact with these risk factors to lower the level of risk. *Protective factors* act by eliminating or buffering negative risk factors in a child's life. Research on protective factors originally stemmed from findings showing that some adolescents at high risk for substance use problems proved resilient; that is, they did not develop a substance use problem despite the presence of many risks in their lives. Although research on protective factors is minimal compared to that on risk factors, several protective factors have been identified. These can be separated into three main categories: (a) individual variables, (b) family and peer variables, and (c) social and cultural variables.

> 21. Resilient adolescents:
>     a. are not at risk.
>     b. always develop a substance use problem.
>     c. overcome risk.
>     d. are always exposed to fewer risks than nonresilient adolescents.

### Individual Variables

Three main dispositional attributes serve to protect adolescents from developing substance use problems. First, good social skills such as empathy, the ability to communicate, and a sense of humor are found in resilient adolescents. Second, children with high self-esteem and a sense of purpose about their futures are better able to withstand peer pressure and are more resilient to substance use. Third, good coping skills protect against adolescent substance use. Coping skills are the mechanisms by which individuals deal with stress that is often linked to negative events in their lives.

### Family and Peer Variables

Family attributes such as parental support and affection also buffer the risk for substance use in adolescents. A supportive family environment includes high but realistic expectations for achievement, parental monitoring of children's behavior, authoritative parenting style (i.e., showing warmth but also exerting behavioral control), open parent–child communication, and high levels of bonding between parents and children. Having a close, supportive relationship with a parent can decrease the risk imposed by having friends who use drugs. Peers can also be protective. The following peer variables have been shown to lower risk: (a) caring and supportive relationships with peers, (b) peer pressure toward positive behaviors, and (c) peer conventionality and academic achievement.

22. A supportive family environment includes:
    a. permissiveness.
    b. authoritarian parenting style.
    c. authoritative parenting style.
    d. lack of open parent–child communication.

## Social and Cultural Variables

Adolescents who feel connected to their community and participate in community and school events are often resilient in the face of risk. Communities that encourage adolescent participation in community events and impose high but realistic expectations for youth protect against risk for substance use. Positive role models and the opportunity to succeed in school as well as the community can also act as protective factors.

# SOCIAL POLICY AND INTERVENTION APPROACHES

## Social Policy and Juvenile Justice

### Costs to Society

The abuse of substances by both adolescents and adults represents a significant burden on society due to the economic costs associated with treatment and prevention, lost productivity, and crime. In 1992, the total economic cost of alcohol and drug abuse was $245.7 billion (National Institute on Drug Abuse [NIDA], 2002). While information on the economic costs of adolescent drug use in particular is scarce, cost estimates are now available for adolescent alcohol use (Pacific Institute for Research and Evaluation, 1999). The total cost of alcohol use by youth is $58,579 billion per year.

### Adolescent Substance Use and Juvenile Justice

Arrest, adjudication, and intervention by the Juvenile Justice System are often consequences of adolescent drug use. Many of the adolescent substance users that you treat will have had some experience with the Juvenile Justice System. The rate of juvenile arrests for drug use violations has increased in recent years. In 2000, there were 203,900 juveniles arrested for drug abuse violations. From 1988 to 1997, the number of drug law violation cases increased 125%. The majority of these violators were male, and about 40% were under the age of 16. Marijuana is the most commonly used drug for both male and female juvenile detainees, followed by cocaine and methamphetamine. In 1994, the average time served in juvenile correctional facilities was 21 months for drug offenders and 17 months for violent offenders. In 1999, about half of all adolescent admissions to drug treatment were referred by the criminal justice system.

23. The most commonly used drug among juvenile detainees is:
    a. marijuana.
    b. cocaine.
    c. alcohol.
    d. tobacco.

## Prevention Approaches

*Prevention programs* include all programs that focus on delaying the onset of drug use, delaying the progression of use from lower to higher frequency or amount of use, or decreasing the frequency or amount of drug use in nonclinical community samples. Prevention programs in childhood and early adolescence generally focus on *gateway drugs* (tobacco, alcohol, and marijuana). There are three levels of prevention programs. *Primary, or universal, prevention programs* target the general population, and are most often implemented by teachers or peers in a school setting. *Secondary, or selective, prevention programs* target youth considered at risk for abusing drugs. *Tertiary, or indicated, prevention programs* target youth who already display several risk factors for drug abuse and may also display one or more associated problem behaviors. This level of prevention is often considered *early intervention.*

24. A drug use prevention program delivered to all high school students in a particular school is an example of a:
    a. early intervention program.
    b. primary prevention program.
    c. secondary prevention program.
    d. none of the above.

## *Characteristics of Effective Programs*

A thorough review of the empirical evidence on drug prevention reveals the following characteristics of effective prevention programs. Effective programs focus on enhancing protective factors and reducing risk factors. These programs may target either a variety of drugs of abuse or a single area of drug abuse. They include training in general life skills, drug resistance skills, social competency, and strengthening personal attitudes and commitments against drug use. Effective programs are age-specific, culturally sensitive, and community-specific, and use developmentally appropriate interactive teaching methods. Effective programs tend to be long-term, focus on multiple areas of risk, and include booster sessions that reinforce the original program goals.

In order to have a complete understanding of drug prevention, it is also important to know what does not work. Prevention programs that use primarily didactic rather than interactive methods and programs that are atheoretical in nature are not effective. Programs that focus on changing knowledge about drugs and the consequences of drug use, and those that focus on affect or self-esteem, are also not generally effective. Finally, testimonials by former users tend not to be effective.

25. All of the following are characteristics of successful prevention programs *except:*
    a. culturally-sensitive.
    b. includes booster sessions.
    c. focuses on enhancing protective factors.
    d. focuses on knowledge about drugs and consequences of drug use.

## *Examples of Empirically Supported Prevention Programs*

The Life Skills Training Program (Botvin, Baker, Filazzola, & Botvin, 1990) is an example of a universally targeted program. It is a three-year classroom curriculum targeted at middle school or junior high school students. The three main content areas covered by the program are drug resistance skills and information, self-management skills, and general social skills. This program produced 59% to 75% reductions in drug use, with significant reductions in drug use remaining six years posttreatment. Long-term program effects are maintained by booster sessions. This program is effective with both White and inner-city minority youth.

The Strengthening Families Program (Kumpfer, Molraard, & Spoth, 1996) is an example of a selective prevention program. It is a multicomponent family-focused program for six- to ten-year-old children of substance abusers. The program includes a parent training component, a children's skills training component, and a family skills training component. Positive outcomes of this program include reduced family conflict; improved family communication and organization; and reduced youth conduct disorders, aggressiveness, and substance abuse with African American, Asian/Pacific Islander, and Hispanic families.

An example of an indicated prevention program is the Reconnecting Youth Program (Eggert, Thompson, Herting, Nicholas, & Dicker, 1994), a school-based program aimed at high school students who show signs of poor school achievement, the potential for dropping out, and problem behaviors. This program is distinguished from the Life Skills Training program in that it incorporates social support and life skills training, in addition to training in substance use refusal skills. Positive effects of this program include reductions in drug use, depression, and aggression and increases in self esteem, social support, and school performance.

## Treatment Approaches

### Levels of Intervention

The three main levels of intervention for adolescent drug abuse are **inpatient treatment, residential treatment**, and **outpatient treatment**. These three levels represent a range of restrictiveness, with inpatient treatment being the most restrictive setting, and outpatient treatment being the least restrictive setting. According to data collected in 1997, 81% of adolescents entering treatment went into outpatient treatment, 18% went into residential treatment, and 1% went into inpatient treatment (Dennis, Babor, Diamond, Donaldson, Godley et al., 2000). As therapists, you may see adolescents in any of these three settings. An understanding of the different types of treatment settings and interventions will also be helpful if you need to refer an adolescent substance user for further treatment. Within each setting, a variety of intervention types may be provided. These types of interventions are discussed below.

Inpatient programs typically provide services within a hospital or other medically controlled environment. An adolescent substance abuser may be referred for inpatient treatment if he or she presents a danger to self or others, requires acute medical attention, or has a significant coexisting psychopathology. Inpatient programs tend to be short-term, with stays ranging from a few days to a month.

Residential programs are less structured and restrictive than inpatient programs and are not set in hospitals. These programs were established based on the theory that removal from the community and a total commitment to treatment is necessary for the substance abuser to change. An adolescent's stay in a residential program may be either short-term, ranging from one to nine months, or long-term, lasting up to two years. Many residential programs function as **therapeutic communities**, in which the community serves as a surrogate family to the patient, and the goal of treatment is for the individual to adopt the behaviors, values, and life choices associated with a drug-free lifestyle. Research suggests that a longer stay in treatment is associated with more positive outcomes, and that adolescents require more time in treatment than adults in order to achieve a successful outcome. Unfortunately, early dropout from treatment is common among adolescents.

The least restrictive treatment setting is the outpatient setting. Adolescents in outpatient treatment live at home or in a nontreatment residential placement, such as a foster home or group home, and participate in treatment while remaining part of the community. Outpatient interventions range from intensive day-long and partial hospitalization to regular or occasional meetings with a therapist.

26. An adolescent substance abuser who has made several suicide attempts will likely be referred to:
    a. inpatient treatment.
    b. outpatient family therapy.
    c. 12-step meetings.
    d. residential treatment.

## Empirically Supported Types of Interventions

Four main types of interventions for adolescent substance abuse are consistently supported by empirical research: Family therapy, cognitive–behavioral therapy, 12-step programs, and motivational interviewing.

*Family therapy* for adolescent drug abuse is based on family systems theory. This model views problems such as drug use as embedded within the interactional patterns of the family. Treatment includes multiple family members and focuses on the patterns of communication among various family subsystems. Studies consistently find that family-based treatments are more effective than alternative treatments in reducing adolescent drug use and co-occurring behavior problems. The effects of family therapy can last as long as six to twelve months posttreatment. Studies also show that adolescents tend to stay longer in family-based treatments than in alternative treatments, which may be a contributor to their success.

27. All of the following are characteristics of family therapy *except:*
    a. includes multiple family members.
    b. focuses on patterns of communication within the family.
    c. focuses on the adolescent's motivation to change.
    d. views drug use as embedded within the interactional patterns of the family.

One noteworthy family-based treatment approach is *multidimensional family therapy* (MDFT; Liddle, 2000). MDFT is a multicomponent, developmental–ecological treatment for adolescent drug abuse that seeks to reduce symptoms and enhance developmental functioning by facilitating change in several behavioral domains. This approach targets individual behavior patterns, within-family interactions, and interactions between the family and relevant social systems. Specifically, MDFT has four interdependent modules that address multiple aspects of adolescent and family functioning: the *adolescent module* addresses developmental issues such as identity formation, peer relations, prosocial involvement, and drug use consequences; the *parent module* enhances parenting skills in the areas of monitoring and limit-setting, rebuilding emotional bonds with the adolescent, and participating in the teen's life outside the family; the *interactional module* facilitates change in family relationship patterns by helping families develop the motivation and skills to revitalize attachments and interact in more adaptive ways; and the *extrafamilial module* seeks to establish collaborative relationships among all social systems in which the adolescent participates (i.e., family, school, peer, recreational, juvenile justice). MDFT has been recognized as an exemplary intervention model by numerous federal agencies and research institutes (e.g., Center for Substance Abuse Treatment [CSAT], 1999;

Drug Strategies, 2003; NIDA, 1999). It has been tested in controlled outcome studies within a variety of treatment and prevention settings (Liddle & Hogue, 2001) and has proven to be cost effective compared to standard treatment options (Dennis et al., 2000).

*Cognitive–behavioral therapy* (CBT) is based on the assumption that substance abuse is a learned behavior. The goal of treatment is to reduce factors that contribute to the drug use, such as maladaptive beliefs, and to enhance factors that protect against drug use, such as coping skills and academic achievement. CBT therapists focus on developing coping skills, resisting peer pressure, stress and anger management, communication, problem-solving, assertiveness training, self-monitoring, and social network development. CBT interventions are usually carried out within the context of individual therapy with the adolescent.

The *12-step model* is probably the most widely used intervention type. Approximately 75% of inpatient and outpatient treatment programs for adolescents base some part of their program on the 12-step model (Lawson, 1992). Adolescents are also commonly referred to a 12-step program after completing treatment. The 12-step model is based on the disease model of addiction, which views drug use as the central problem that must be dealt with prior to dealing with other associated problems. Treatment consists of group meetings in which the group works through the 12 steps. These include admitting the problem, asking for help, turning the problem over to a higher power, dealing with guilt and anger, and committing to continued self-evaluation. The few studies that exist offer preliminary support for the effectiveness of this model. Posttreatment attendance at 12-step meetings leads to positive outcomes for adolescents. Attendance at these meetings leads to enhanced self-efficacy and motivation to remain abstinent, which in turn leads to positive drug use outcomes.

*Motivational interviewing* (MI) focuses on reducing drug use and other problem behaviors by increasing the adolescent's motivation to change. It is a brief (three to five sessions), nonconfrontational, empathetic approach, which emphasizes developing the adolescent's awareness of the problem and increasing the belief that he or she is able to change. MI is effective in reducing alcohol use and alcohol-related problems in college students at both short- and long-term follow-up, and is also effective for adolescent marijuana abusers (Dennis, et al., 2000).

28. An adolescent who has recently completed a residential treatment program is a good candidate for:
    a. outpatient family therapy.
    b. inpatient treatment.
    c. 12-step meetings.
    d. none of the above.

29. Which of the following treatments is based on the disease model of addiction?
    a. cognitive–behavioral therapy
    b. motivational interviewing
    c. family therapy
    d. 12-step model

## KEY TERMS

**comorbid:** The simultaneous occurrence of two or more psychiatric diagnoses (e.g., substance abuse and depression).

**gateway hypothesis:** A model of the development of substance use disorders in which substance use progresses through stages, and alcohol and marijuana represent critical points of entry into the use of other illicit substances.

**inpatient programs:** Treatment programs that provide services within a hospital or other medically controlled environment.

**nicotine:** The active ingredient in cigarettes.

**outpatient programs:** Treatment programs in which the adolescent participates in treatment while living at home and remaining part of the community.

**prevention programs:** Programs that focus on delaying the onset of drug use, delaying the progression of use from lower to higher frequency or amount of use, or decreasing the frequency or amount of drug use in nonclinical community samples.

**primary (universal) prevention programs:** Prevention programs that target the general population to attempt to prevent the onset of substance use.

**protective factor:** A variable that interacts with risk factors to lower the level of risk for substance use problems.

**residential programs:** Treatment programs in which the adolescent resides at a residential center dedicated to drug use treatment.

**risk factor:** A variable in a child's life that increases the probability that he or she will develop a substance use problem.

**secondary (selective) prevention programs:** Prevention programs that target youth considered at risk for abusing drugs, such as children of drug users or poor school achievers.

**substance abuse:** The *DSM–IV* diagnosis applied to adolescents who place themselves in danger or experience recurrent problems as a consequence of substance use.

**substance dependence:** The *DSM–IV* diagnosis applied to adolescents who may experience tolerance, withdrawal, or other severe symptoms that negatively affect social and physical functioning.

**tertiary (indicated) prevention programs:** Prevention programs that target youth who already display several risk factors for drug abuse and who may also display initial stage drug use or associated behavior problems.

**therapeutic community:** A type of residential treatment program in which the community serves as a surrogate family for the adolescent.

**THC:** The active ingredient in marijuana.

## DISCUSSION QUESTIONS

1. Explain the "gateway hypothesis" and provide both supporting and disputing evidence.
2. Explain the difference between risk factors and protective factors. Describe how they interact, providing an example.
3. Discuss some of the important subgroup differences in adolescent substance use (e.g., ethnicity, geography, gender). How might these differences inform or impact your work as a family therapist?
4. Describe the pathogenesis, or development, of adolescent substance abuse according to the *DSM-IV.*
5. Describe what is meant by the term *multiple pathways* in adolescent substance use research. Provide several examples to illustrate.
6. Discuss the short- and long-term consequences of frequent substance use during adolescence.
7. Discuss the relationship between substance use and psychiatric symptoms/disorders in adolescents. What are the implications of this relationship for treatment?
8. Describe the three levels of prevention programs and provide an example of each.

9. Jane is a 17-year-old girl who has been using marijuana regularly since age 13. Jane has previously been diagnosed with depression and has recently admitted to having suicidal thoughts. Discuss how you would begin to formulate an assessment and treatment plan for Jane. Consider both treatment setting and treatment type.

## SUGGESTED FURTHER READING

### For Further Information on Prevalence and Incidence Rates of Adolescent Substance Abuse

#### *On the Internet*

http://monitoringthefuture.org/

This website provides the most recent findings from the Monitoring the Future study.

#### *In Print*

Center on Addiction and Substance Abuse (CASA) at Columbia University. (2002). *Teen tipplers: America's underage drinking epidemic.* New York: Author.

This report provides recent statistics on alcohol use among adolescents.

Center on Addiction and Substance Abuse (CASA) at Columbia University. (2001). *Malignant neglect: Substance abuse and America's schools.* New York: Author.

This report provides statistics on drug use among adolescents as well as information on consequences of adolescent substance use.

Center on Addiction and Substance Abuse (CASA) at Columbia University. (2000). *No place to hide: Substance abuse in mid-size cities and rural America.* New York: Author.

This report provides information on subgroup and geographic trends in rates of adolescent substance use.

### For More Information on Risk and Protective Factors for Adolescent Drug Use

#### *On the Internet*

http://www.samhsa.gov/oas/NHSDA/NAC97/Table_of_Contents.htm

This website provides information on risk and protective factors for alcohol use.

#### *In Print*

Center on Addiction and Substance Abuse (CASA) at Columbia University. (1997). *Substance abuse and the American adolescent.* New York: Author. Available at the following web address: http://www.casacolumbia.org/ publications1456/publications_form.htm

This paper provides information on risk and protective factors for alcohol as well as other substances of abuse.

Tarter, R. E. (2002). Etiology of adolescent substance abuse: A developmental perspective. *American Journal on Addictions, 11,* 171–191.

This article provides information on the etiology of adolescent substance abuse.

## For Further Information on Prevention and Treatment

### On the Internet

http://www.drugabuse.gov/TB/Clinical/ClinicalToolbox.html

This website provides links to information about treatments for adolescent drug abuse, including treatment manuals and articles on effective approaches to treatment.

### In Print

Bukstein, O. G. (1995). *Adolescent substance abuse: Assessment, prevention, and treatment.* New York: Wiley.

This book provides general descriptions of the various types of treatment and prevention approaches for adolescent substance abuse.

Ozechowski, T. J., & Liddle, H. A. (2000). Family-based therapy for adolescent drug abuse: Knowns and unknowns. *Clinical Child and Family Psychology Review, 3(4)*, 269–298.

This article provides an overview of the current state of knowledge regarding the various family-based approaches for treating adolescent drug abuse, as well as areas in which research is lacking.

Wagner, E. F., & Waldron, H. B. (2001). *Innovations in adolescent substance abuse interventions.* Amsterdam: Pergamon.

This book provides an overview of the main types of treatment for adolescent substance abuse that have received empirical support. Descriptions of the treatments as well as outcome research are described.

## REFERENCES

American Psychiatric Association. (2000). *Diagnostic and statistical manual of mental disorders* (4th ed., text revision). Washington, DC: Author.

Anthony, J. C., Warner, L. A., & Kessler, R. (1994). Comparative epidemiology of dependence on tobacco, alcohol, controlled substances, and inhalants: Basic findings from the national comorbidity survey. *Experimental Clinical Psychopharmacology, 2,* 244–268.

Botvin, G. J., Baker, E., Filazzola, A. D., & Botvin, E. M. (1990). A cognitive–behavioral approach to substance abuse prevention: One-year follow-up. *Addictive Behaviors, 15*(1), 47–63.

Center for Substance Abuse Treatment. (1999). *Screening and assessing adolescents for substance use disorders: Treatment improvement protocol (TIP) Series 31.* (DHHS Publication No. SMA 99-3282). Washington, DC: U.S. Dept. of Health and Human Services.

Dennis, M. L., Babor, T. F., Diamond, G., Donaldson, J., Godley, S. H., Titus, J. C., Tims, F., et al. (2000). *The Cannabis Youth Treatment (CYT) Experiment: Preliminary findings.* A report to H. Westley Clark, Director, Center for Substance Abuse Treatment, Substance Abuse and Mental Health Services Administration, Department of Health and Human Services.

Drug Strategies (2003). *Treating teens: A guide to adolescent drug programs.* Washington, DC: Author.

Eggert, L. L., Thompson, E. A., Herting, J. R., Nicholas, L. J., & Dicker, B. G. (1994). Preventing adolescent drug abuse and high school dropout through an intensive school-based social network development program. *American Journal of Health Promotion, 8*(3), 202–215.

Greenblatt, J. C. (2000). *Patterns of alcohol use among adolescents and associations with emotional and behavioral problems.* Substance Abuse and Mental Health Services Administration.

Johnston, L. D., O'Malley, P. M., & Bachman, J. G. (2002). *Monitoring the future national results on adolescent drug use: Overview of key findings, 2001.* (NIH Publication No. 02-5105). Bethesda, MD: National Institute on Drug Abuse.

Kumpfer, K. L., Molraard, V., & Spoth, R. (1996). The "Strengthening Families Program" for the prevention of delinquency and drug use. In R. Peters & R. McMahon (Eds.), *Preventing childhood disorders, substance abuse, and delinquency* (pp. 241–267). Thousand Oaks, CA: Sage Publications.

Lawson, G. W. (1992). Twelve-step programs and the treatment of adolescent substance abuse. In G. W. Lawson & A. W. Lawson (Eds.), *Adolescent substance abuse: Etiology, treatment, and prevention* (pp. 219–229). Gaithersburg, MD: Aspen Publishers.

Liddle, H. A. (2000). *Multidimensional family therapy (MDFT) treatment for adolescent cannabis users*. (Volume 5 of the Cannabis Youth Treatment (CYT) manual series, 244 pp). Rockville, MD: Center for Substance Abuse Treatment, Substance Abuse and Mental Health Services Administration. (www.samhsa.gov/csat/csat.htm).

Liddle, H. A., & Hogue, A. (2001). Multidimensional family therapy for adolescent substance abuse. In E. F. Wagner & H. B. Waldron (Eds.), *Innovations in adolescent substance abuse interventions* (pp. 229–261). Amsterdam, Netherlands: Pergamon/Elsevier Science.

National Institute on Drug Abuse (1999). *Principles of drug addiction treatment: A research-based guide*. Rockville, MD: Author.

National Institute on Drug Abuse (2002). *NIDA InfoFacts: Costs to Society*. http://www.nida.nih.gov/Infofax/costs.html.

Pacific Institute for Research and Evaluation (1999). *Costs of underage drinking*. Prepared for the OJJDP National Leadership Conference.

Petraitis, J., Flay, B. R., & Miller, T. Q. (1995). Reviewing theories of adolescent substance use: Organizing pieces of the puzzle. *Psychological Bulletin, 117,* 67–86.

Substance Abuse and Mental Health Services Administration. (2000). *Tips for teens*. National Clearinghouse for Alcohol and Drug Information.

Substance Abuse and Mental Health Services Administration. (1999). *Summary of findings from the 1998 National Household Survey on Drug Abuse*. Rockville, MD: U.S. Department of Health and Human Services.

# 18

# Child Abuse and Neglect

Carrie C. Capstick

*St. Luke's–Roosevelt Hospital Center*

Peter Fraenkel

*City University of New York*

## TRUTH OR FICTION?

___ *1. Unintentional physical harm inflicted upon a child is considered physical abuse.*

___ *2. Sexual "experimentation" between children is never considered sexual abuse.*

___ *3. Keeping a child out of school for an extended period without reason is neglect.*

___ *4. Keeping a child in close confinement is a form of emotional, not physical abuse.*

___ *5. Physical abuse is the most common form of child maltreatment.*

___ *6. Because of the parent–child conflict that characterizes adolescence, children between the ages of 12 and 15 are at the greatest risk of child maltreatment.*

___ *7. Domestic violence is a risk factor for abuse and neglect.*

___ *8. Physically disabled children are at increased risk of abuse.*

___ *9. Parents who use drugs or alcohol are at no greater risk of abusing or neglecting their children than non-substance–abusing parents.*

___ *10. Abused and neglected children are at greater risk of developing substance abuse problems than are nonmaltreated children.*

___ *11. The majority of sexually abused children develop psychiatric disorders.*

___ *12. The support of a nonoffending parent mitigates the negative effects of child sexual abuse.*

___ *13. "Parenting training" programs are recommended for physically abusive parents.*

___ *14. Cognitive-behavioral treatment for child abuse and neglect aims to heal the "relational trauma" that follows child maltreatment.*

___ *15. Play sessions may help a child who requires a safe, nonthreatening setting to express his or her feelings associated with being abused.*

Many of our ideas about child maltreatment—physical abuse, sexual abuse, emotional abuse, and neglect—have changed over the past four decades since the mental health field began the serious empirical study of child maltreatment following the seminal paper, "The Battered Child Syndrome," in the early 1960s (Kempe, Silverman, Steele, Droegemueller, & Silver, 1962). We used to believe that the visible signs of abuse, the bruises and broken bones, were the ones that mattered most. Now we know that the invisible psychic wounds can be even more damaging and can forever change a child's sense of safety in the world. We used to think the abuse of children by strangers was more likely and harmful than abuse suffered at the hands of a parent. We have since learned that **child abuse** happens most often within families, and that the rupturing of the trust between a child and an abusive family member is at the core of what makes abuse often so developmentally disruptive and emotionally devastating to the child (Sheinberg & Fraenkel, 2001). We used to worry more about the kids who responded to trauma with overt signs of distress. Now we are equally concerned about the child who appears unaffected.

Although we have made progress in developing a more sophisticated understanding of child maltreatment, many questions remain, such as the degree to which abuse and neglect are responsible for adverse outcomes in children versus the influence of other preexisting characteristics of the child or his or her social environment, or of the often disruptive, traumatic impact on the child and family of disclosure and the events that follow. Along with some of the key questions that persist, this chapter summarizes an already extensive literature on the definitions, risk and protective factors, effects, and treatment of child abuse and neglect. In keeping with the focus of this text, this chapter emphasizes a family systems perspective on abuse and neglect.

1. The study of child maltreatment began in the _____ with pediatrician Henry Kempe and colleagues' seminal paper, "The Battered Child Syndrome."
   a. late 1940s
   b. early 1950s
   c. early 1960s
   d. late 1970s

## HOW ARE DIFFERENT FORMS OF CHILD MALTREATMENT DEFINED?

Definitions of *child maltreatment* vary according to the perspective taken, whether it be legal, psychological, epidemiological, or medical (Erickson & Egeland, 1996). In this chapter, we present definitions adopted by child welfare organizations, reflective of the types of maltreatment reported to such agencies. These definitions are largely consistent with definitions used in research on the causes, effects, and treatment of child maltreatment later reviewed in the chapter. Below are the definitions of the four main types of child maltreatment: physical abuse, sexual abuse, emotional abuse, and neglect.

2. An evaluation of a case of suspected child maltreatment would be primarily concerned with:
   a. evidence that proves the parent intentionally hurt his or her child.
   b. whether the child has suffered harm.
   c. evidence that proves the parent did not know what he or she was doing.
   d. all of the above.

## Physical Abuse

Child *physical abuse* is the intentional or unintentional infliction, or the intended (threatened) but unrealized infliction, of physical harm to a child by an adult as a result of, but not limited to, punching, kicking, beating, biting, burning, or shaking (Wolfe, 1999).

> 3. A mother threatens her child that she will physically hurt him if he doesn't stop misbe-
>    having. This is an example of:
>    a. physical abuse only if she ends up hurting her child.
>    b. emotional, not physical, abuse.
>    c. physical abuse, even if she does not act on her threat.
>    d. psychological maltreatment, not physical abuse.

## Sexual Abuse

*Sexual abuse* refers to any sexual activity with a person when consent is not or cannot be given (Finkelhor, 1979). Because a child is not capable of granting consent, any sexual activity between a child and an adult is, therefore, abuse. Child sexual abuse, thus, includes, but is not limited to intercourse, fondling a child's genitals, exposing a child to genitalia (exhibitionism), or commercially exploiting a child through pornography or prostitution.

> 4. Which of the following is *not* considered sexual abuse or sexual assault?
>    a. two children of the same age, nonaggressively touching each other's bodies
>    b. showing a nine-year-old boy pornography when he has asked to see it
>    c. sexual activity between a man in his thirties and a mature, thirteen-year-old girl who
>       has given consent
>    d. sexual activity between a woman in her thirties and a mature, thirteen-year-old boy
>       who has given consent

## Emotional Abuse

*Emotional abuse* is behavior that compromises the psychological health of a child. Although all abuse may exact an emotional toll on children, certain acts center on emotionally abusive intents and consequences. Sedlack and Broadhurst (1996) in the Third National Incidence Study of Child Abuse and Neglect (NIS) classified three types of emotional abuse:

- close confinement
- verbal or emotional assault
- other or unknown abuse

Locking a child in a closet (close confinement), repeatedly denigrating a child with insults (verbal or emotional assault), or intentionally withholding food or assigning excessive responsibilities (other or unknown abuse) are all examples of emotional abuse according to this classification system.

5. All of the following are considered forms of emotional abuse *except*:
   a. giving a child responsibility of caring for his younger siblings after school until his siblings go to sleep.
   b. repeatedly calling a child a "worthless idiot."
   c. depriving a child of emotional nurturance.
   d. depriving the child of regular meals.

## Neglect

Commonly thought of as an act of omission rather than of commission (Dubowitz, Black, Starr, & Zuravin, 1993; Wolock & Horowitz, 1984), *neglect* occurs when children's basic needs are not met (Black, 2000). Although physical and emotional neglect are the two forms of neglect most commonly discussed, Zuravin (1991) has identified as many as fourteen types of neglect, ranging from educational neglect to refusal to provide mental health care.

6. All of the following are considered types of neglect *except*:
   a. keeping a child out of school for an extended period of time.
   b. not providing proper medical care for a child.
   c. not providing adequate food for a child.
   d. locking a child in a closet.

7. The term *child maltreatment* encompasses the following forms of abuse and neglect *except*:
   a. sexual abuse.
   b. emotional neglect.
   c. medical neglect.
   d. custody battles.

## HOW COMMON IS ABUSE AND NEGLECT?

National studies indicate that close to three million children are harmed or endangered by abuse or neglect each year in the United States (Sedlack & Broadhurst, 1996). According to this estimate, 42 out of every 1,000 children are abused or neglected annually, a rate 85% higher than a comparable study found a decade earlier (Sedlack & Broadhurst). Neglect is the most prevalent form of maltreatment, representing 60% to 70% of all reports in two of the most widely cited national studies of abuse and neglect (Sedlack & Broadhurst; U.S. Department of Health and Human Services, National Child Abuse and Neglect Data System [NCANDS], 2002). The second most common form of child maltreatment is physical abuse (19%–22%), followed by sexual abuse (10%–11%) (Sedlack & Broadhurst; U.S. Department of Health and Human Services, 2002).

## AT WHAT AGE ARE CHILDREN AT GREATEST RISK OF MALTREATMENT?

When all forms of maltreatment are considered, children between the ages of 6 and 8 are at greatest risk of endangerment or harm, followed by children between 9 and 14 years of age (Sedlack & Broadhurst, 1996). However, the risk of specific forms of child maltreatment is different for children of different ages. For instance, although school-aged (ages 6–8) children are nearly twice as likely to be endangered or harmed by maltreatment overall than are infants and toddlers, the latter are more at risk of neglect (Sedlack & Broadhurst). As another example, sexual abuse is quite rare (although it does occur) for children younger than age 3 (Sedlack & Broadhurst).

## WHAT ROLE DOES THE VICTIM'S GENDER PLAY IN RATES OF CHILD MALTREATMENT?

In a recent study (U.S. Department of Health and Human Services, 2002), few gender differences were found in the kinds of maltreatment for which children are at highest risk. One of the differences found was that girls are much more likely to experience sexual abuse than boys. Although this differential is explained by a perpetrator profile made up of mostly heterosexual males, reporting trends suggest that the difference is likely exaggerated. The shame associated with being a male victim of sexual abuse leads to underreporting in boys. In their study of the characteristics of disclosure of children believed to have been sexually abused, DeVoe and Faller (1999) found boys to disclose sexual abuse less often than girls. Additionally, boys are less likely to be represented in psychiatric samples, upon which incidence rates are typically based, because they are more likely to enter criminal justice or substance abuse treatment centers (Putnam, 2003).

Although girls are more likely to experience sexual victimization, boys are at slightly greater risk to receive serious injuries when abused (Sedlack & Broadhurst, 1996). Boys are also at greater risk of emotional abuse than girls (Sedlack & Broadhurst). A relationship between age and gender also exists. Girls are at greatest risk of physical abuse during the ages of 12 to 15, whereas boys are at greatest risk between the ages of 4 and 7 (U.S. Department of Health and Human Services, 2002).

8. Over the past decade rates of child maltreatment have:
   a. decreased by 5%.
   b. increased by 10%.
   c. increased by 85%.
   d. not changed.

9. Children ages _____ are most likely to be the victims of child maltreatment.
   a. 2–4
   b. 4–6
   c. 6–8
   d. 12–14

10. Which of the following is the most common form of child maltreatment?
    a. sexual abuse
    b. neglect
    c. physical abuse
    d. emotional abuse

11. Which of the following may explain low rates of sexual abuse in boys?
    a. Boys are less likely to report sexual abuse because of the intense shame associated with their experience of victimization.
    b. Most perpetrators of sexual abuse are heterosexual men.

c. While girls may come to the attention of the mental health system, where a history of sexual abuse is likely to be identified, sexually abused boys may be more likely to enter the criminal justice system as a result of their abuse-related difficulties.

d. all of the above.

12. When girls are between the ages of 12 and 15 they are most at risk of being physically abused, in contrast to boys who are most at risk between _____ years of age.

a. birth and 3

b. 4 and 7

c. 8 and 11

d. 15 and 18, similar to girls

## WHO IS MOST LIKELY TO ABUSE OR NEGLECT CHILDREN?

Unfortunately, statistics show children are most likely to be maltreated by one or both parents. Mothers acting alone represent 40% of all perpetrators of child maltreatment. Both parents acting together represent the second most common category of perpetrators (19%), followed by fathers acting alone (17%; U.S. Department of Health and Human Services). Family relatives (e.g., siblings, grandparents, uncles, and aunts) are perpetrators in only 5% of all cases, followed by substitute caregivers (e.g., child care workers and foster parents; U.S. Department of Health and Human Services).

In summary, one or both parents are involved in approximately 75% of all maltreatment cases. However, a closer look at the specific forms of child maltreatment alters the findings on the perpetrator's relationship to the victim. For example, while mothers acting alone were responsible for 47% of neglect victims, they were the sole perpetrator in only 4% of sexual abuse cases (U.S. Department of Health and Human Services, 2002). In summary, risk assessment and other preventive measures must look closely at patterns of perpetration with respect to specific forms of abuse and neglect, not only at summary statistics or all forms of maltreatment combined.

13. A child is most likely to be abused or neglected by:

a. a stranger.

b. a mother acting alone.

c. a father acting alone.

d. both parents.

## HOW ARE CHILDREN AFFECTED BY MALTREATMENT?

The effects of abuse and neglect range from short-term (for example, short-lived periods of hypervigilance, impaired attention, emotional upset, and disruptive behavior) to long-term sequelae (such as chronic attentional and affect-regulatory difficulties, substance use disorders, and depression). Effects may be pervasive, impacting emotional, psychological, cognitive, and behavioral functioning, or circumscribed to one or more aspects of functioning. Although varying types of maltreatment share similar psychological and physiological consequences, in part because maltreated children often experience multiple forms of abuse and neglect, there are effects particular to specific forms of maltreatment. For example, cognitive and language delays may be prominent in physically abused children, whereas the betrayal of trust central to sexual abuse may lead to a variety of relationship problems (Edgeworth & Carr, 2000). A few of the short- and long-term effects of child maltreatment are as follows:

- affective disturbances (e.g., PTSD, depression)
- behavioral difficulties (e.g., aggression)
- cognitive impairments/academic problems
- relational difficulties
- medical problems/neurobiological alterations

## WHY DOES CHILD ABUSE AND NEGLECT OCCUR?

### Risk Factors

In recent decades researchers have attempted to identify **risk factors** likely to contribute to the occurrence of child maltreatment. Current theories, such as ecological models of maltreatment (Belsky, 1980), stress multiple contributors, including child, parent, family, societal, and other factors correlated with increased rates of child maltreatment. Although we have used the term *risk factor* as it is appears in the literature, it is important to recognize that these are *correlational* findings, not *causal* conclusions, and to recognize the still preliminary status of much of this body of research. Furthermore, when examining aspects of families or social groups associated with abuse, it is important not to conclude that it is the whole family, or social group, that places a child at greater (or lesser) risk. Below are a few of those factors believed to make maltreatment more likely to take place:

*Child Risk Factors:*

- temperament labeled as "difficult" (Black, 2000)
- physically disabled (Wescott & Jones, 1999)

*Parent Risk Factors:*

- deficits in child management skills (Kolko, 1996)
- Inappropriate developmental expectations of child (Kolko)

*Family Risk Factors:*

- domestic violence (Rumm, Cummings, Krauss, Bell, & Rivara, 2000)
- stress (Emery & Laumann-Billings, 1998)

### Protective Factors

With a vast empirical literature documenting the debilitating effects of child maltreatment on the emotional, psychological, behavioral, and social development of the child, it is difficult not to suppose a clear cause and effect relationship between child maltreatment and poor outcome. However, although negative sequelae have been repeatedly documented, maltreatment as the sole or dominant causal agent has not. Chief among the evidence suggesting mediating factors that influence the development of certain outcomes is the finding that not all children suffer negative outcomes following maltreatment. A study carried out by Kendall-Tackett, Williams, and Finkelhor (1993) revealed that up to 40% of sexually abused children did not evidence expected abuse-related problems. If close to half of children do not suffer long-term negative consequences from maltreatment, what factors are responsible for preventing or moderating the effects of child abuse and neglect? Is it the child? Is it the influence of the family or the community? Below are a few of those factors believed to mediate against or moderate the degree to which maladaptive outcomes result from experiences of child abuse and neglect:

- less severe and chronic abuse (Edgeworth & Carr, 2000)
- low familial stress (Edgeworth & Carr)
- supportive environment (e.g., support of family and community; Widom, 2000)
- early intervention (Widom)
- child's involvement in supportive educational programs (Edgeworth & Carr)

14. Which of the following statements are supported by empirical study?
    a. Almost all sexually abused children develop abuse-related problems.
    b. Less than 5% of sexually abused children develop abuse-related problems.
    c. Less than 40% of sexually abused children develop abuse-related problems.
    d. Only sexually abused girls develop abuse-related problems.

15. Emily is a five-year-old girl who was sexually abused by an uncle between the ages of 3 and 4. Which of the following might help to decrease the likelihood that Emily will develop abuse-related problems?
    a. a supportive relationship between Emily and her mother
    b. taking Emily out of school for a short period of time
    c. helping Emily to confront the uncle who abused her
    d. none of the above

16. Edwin is more likely to experience abuse or neglect *if*:
    a. his father is abusive towards his mother.
    b. he is deaf.
    c. his mother thinks he is an extremely difficult child.
    d. all of the above.

17. Jeff is evaluating a family for risk of maltreatment. Which of the following might suggest that the family is at *high risk*?
    a. There is domestic violence in the home.
    b. Due to chronic unemployment there is a high level of stress in the home.
    c. The parents have poor child management skills.
    d. All of the above.

## WHO IS REQUIRED TO REPORT SUSPECTED ABUSE OR NEGLECT?

Although some states require *any* person who suspects child abuse or neglect to report, the majority of states **mandate reporting** only by those professionals working with children. Physicians, mental health professionals, and school personnel are examples of professionals mandated by law to report suspected child maltreatment. Laws typically mandate reporters to make reports "immediately" or "promptly," typically within 48 hours of suspecting child maltreatment.

## When Does a Report Need to Be Made?

Although guidelines vary according to state, a report is typically mandated when you have "reasonable cause to know, suspect, or believe" that a child has been abused or neglected (National Clearinghouse on Child Abuse and Neglect Information, 2002). This means your decision to report is not dependent on actual knowledge of the abuse. For example, if you observe a pattern of bruises on a child client and suspect physical abuse, even after the child has attributed the bruises to falling down, you are required to report your suspicion; you do not need the child, the parent, or a witness to verify that the bruises were the result of physical abuse. Therefore, you are not to play the role of a forensic investigator, but rather act on your suspicions when you encounter information suggestive of child abuse or neglect. This is not to say that you should not make inquiries (such as asking a parent if bruises resulted from corporal punishment) that would assist in determining if a report should be made. Your concern should be to obtain information that will determine *if a report should be made*, not *whether abuse or neglect has occurred*.

With the exception of one state (Minnesota), child abuse or neglect must be reported regardless of when it occurred. For example, if a thirteen-year-old reported an incident of sexual abuse occurring at the age of 4, it must be reported.

---

18. Four-year-old Oliver displays repetitive, developmentally inappropriate sexual themes while playing. When Oliver's therapist asks him if anyone has ever done these things to him, Oliver begins to cry and refuses to answer. The therapist should:
    a. keep asking Oliver questions until he feels comfortable to speak.
    b. make a report if he suspects that Oliver has been sexually abused.
    c. ask the parents if they can offer insight into Oliver's behavior.
    d. none of the above.

19. A twelve-year-old discloses in therapy that she was sexually abused at the age of 5 and that the relative who abused her moved out of state years ago. The therapist should:
    a. not report the abuse because the child is no longer in danger.
    b. report the abuse, regardless of the perpetrator's whereabouts.
    c. only inform the child's parents of the abuse.
    d. none of the above.

---

## What About Violating Client Confidentiality?

Although a therapist and patient are protected by laws of confidentiality, close to half of the States include provisions that certain privileges (such as confidentiality) do not negate the duty to report in cases of child maltreatment. Accordingly, marriage and family therapists, social workers, psychologists, and other mental health professionals are typically mandated by law to report child maltreatment, even if it involves a breach of confidentiality.

One way to lessen the impact of reporting abuse on one's therapeutic relationship with a child or family is to involve the child and family in making the report. In many cases, child welfare will mandate the child and family to therapy; if you are already working with the family and can maintain a collaborative relationship in spite of the need to report, they may be able to maintain trust and a positive alliance with you.

20. A teacher notices that Anne, a nine-year-old girl, arrives at school every day appearing unwashed and in tattered clothing. Anne also usually "forgets" her lunch and is often absent from school. What should her teacher do?
    a. Report her observations to a child protection agency.
    b. Make an appointment to visit Anne's home to assess for signs of neglect.
    c. Tell Anne that she needs to dress appropriately and remember to bring her lunch.
    d. none of the above.

21. Suspected abuse or neglect should typically be reported:
    a. within 48 hours.
    b. within 48 hours only if the child is in imminent danger.
    c. within 7 business days.
    d. when all of the important details have been gathered.

## HOW ARE CHILD ABUSE AND NEGLECT TREATED?

Because many of the effects of child maltreatment are long-term and may accompany a child into adulthood (e.g., depression, anxiety, interpersonal difficulties), treatment of child victims can be seen as preventive of chronic disorders as much as it is a treatment of current difficulties. Additionally, the prevention of further maltreatment is often a critical component of treatment due to the child's continued dependency on the very caretakers who abused or failed to protect them from maltreatment. Beyond a treatment focus on children and their parents, interventions may also extend to the entire family and even broader influences, such as the community and school setting. In this section we review various approaches to treating child maltreatment, starting with those approaches with the broadest scope, inclusive of family and community influences, to those primarily focused on the child or parents.

22. Treatment of child victims differs from that of adult victims because:
    a. Children often remain in the care of their offenders and therefore prevention of further maltreatment is critical.
    b. Others (e.g., parents) are often the focus of treatment of child maltreatment, not the child victims.
    c. It is more concerned with preventing, rather than treating, abuse-related problems.
    d. All of the above.

## Family Therapy

A family systems approach to child maltreatment is based on the premise that abuse and neglect occur within the context of family relationships. The goals of **family therapy** in the treatment of child maltreatment are to restructure relationships and belief systems in the family to alter the interactional patterns that contribute to abuse and neglect (Carr, 2000). The development of positive communication and problem-solving skills help the family avoid hostile and conflict-laden interactions while enhancing support and cohesion. Not only does a family approach attempt to restore healthy boundaries and effect other changes to prevent further maltreatment, but because parents are so often the offenders, a family systems approach addresses the relational trauma that often follows maltreatment, particularly sexual abuse (Sheinberg & Fraenkel, 2001). The betrayal of trust and safety between the child and offending or even nonoffending parent is a core experience for the child victim and one which can be addressed in a family-centered approach (Sheinberg & Fraenkel). Likewise, strengthening the bond between the abused child and nonabusing family members who can support her or him is a core goal of family therapy. Although data about the effectiveness of family therapy for child maltreatment is largely lacking, empirical studies have supported its efficacy for sexual abuse in boys (Friedrich, Luecke, Beilke, & Place, 1992) and for physical abuse and neglect (Kolko, 1996; Nicol, Smith, & Kay, 1988).

23. Family therapy may be indicated when:
    a. the offender is a family member.
    b. the offender is not a family member.
    c. the family engages in "rigid" patterns of interaction.
    d. all of the above.

24. Treatment of child maltreatment using a family-centered approach is likely to prioritize:
    a. the restructuring of family relationships.
    b. looking for unconscious meaning in the child's play during family sessions.
    c. adjunctive psychopharmacological treatment.
    d. all of the above.

## Family-Based Behavior Therapy or "Parent Training"

Primarily effective in cases of physical abuse, this approach is based on the principles of behavioral psychology in which the occurrence of physically abusive behaviors are understood as the outcome of positive and negative reinforcement. **Behavior therapy** targets high-risk or abusive parents, who may pay attention to their children only when they misbehave, thereby increasing the likelihood that the child will continue to display negative behaviors. Corcoran (2000) describes the child's compliance immediately following physical punishment or abuse as similarly reinforcing for the parent. Behaviorally based parenting skills aim to disrupt the escalating interactional parent–child patterns capable of resulting in physical abuse. Parents are taught how to identify, encourage, and reward positive behaviors in their children while ignoring or punishing negative behaviors (Corcoran). This problem-focused, short-term treatment has amassed substantial empirical support as an effective treatment of physical abuse (Brunk, Henggeler, & Whelan, 1987; Wolfe, Edwards, Manion, & Koverola, 1988).

25. Which of the following interactions would be of interest to a therapist working from a behavioral perspective?
    a. a mother who is frequently frustrated with her children's teachers
    b. a child ignoring another child who is trying to get their attention
    c. a mother ignoring her child when he is behaving appropriately
    d. none of the above

## Cognitive-Behavioral Therapy

Like behavioral therapy, **cognitive-behavioral therapy** (CBT) is often a preventive approach for physical abuse. CBT targets the tendency of abusive parents to attribute negative intentions to their children's behavior (Acton & During, 1992) and who hold unrealistic expectations of what their children are capable of (Kolko, 1996). Enhancing communication and problem-solving skills in dealing with their children's behavior are equally important aspects of parent-focused CBT approaches. For example, a parent who responds only to their child when they are "out-of-control," might feel that even though they are reluctant to use physical force, it is the only thing that will work. Problem-solving skills help the parent identify problems early on (when less coercive interventions are more effective) and consider a range of interventions, as well as their potential impact. These CBT interventions help the parent better understand their child's motivations, delay impulsive responses, and feel that they have choices beyond physical punishment. CBT with physically abusive parents is empirically supported (Corcoran, 2000). Studies have found CBT to improve parenting attitudes, reduce child abuse potential, parenting stress (a risk factor for abuse), and parent aggression (Acton & During).

26. All of the following are goals of cognitive-behavioral therapy (CBT) *except*:
    a. communication skill-building.
    b. working on negative attributions.
    c. increasing problem-solving skills.
    d. pairing a maltreated child with a more resilient peer.

## Resilient Peer Treatment, Therapeutic Day Care, and Residential Treatment

Whereas CBT and behavioral approaches primarily focus on preventing offending parents from engaging in further maltreatment, the developmental and other concerns of child victims are addressed by child-focused treatments. **Resilient peer treatment** (RPT) is a child-focused approach that addresses the developmental problems of maltreated children by pairing withdrawn, maltreated children with outgoing, resilient peers in daycare settings (Fantuzzo et al., 1996). Targeting the cognitive and social–emotional development of child victims, **therapeutic day care** provides intellectual stimulation in the context of child–teacher relationships (Edgeworth & Carr, 2000). Children placed in **residential treatment** programs visit daily with their parents and experience safe, positive parent–child interactions. These child-focused approaches have been found to be "particularly effective" in cases of physical abuse and neglect (Edgeworth & Carr).

27. Child-focused treatments such as therapeutic day care and residential treatment have been found to be primarily effective for:
    a. sexual abuse.
    b. physical abuse.
    c. emotional abuse.
    d. all of the above.

The aforementioned treatments represent the dominant approaches to the treatment and prevention of child maltreatment. Other treatments include: "**social support**" and "**social network**" approaches that target the social isolation that often characterizes abusive and, in particular, neglecting families (Gaudin, Wodarski, Arkinson, & Avery, 1990–1991); **play therapy** which provides children with a safe, nonverbal medium for telling their story of abuse and expressing feelings in the familiar world of play (Gil, 1991); and pharmacological treatments aimed to decrease hyperarousal, distractibility, and other biologically based reactions to maltreatment (Schwarz & Perry, 1994). Future interventions may increasingly integrate a number of these approaches. A recent review (Edgeworth & Carr, 2000) of available treatments indicated that a combination of individual-, parent-, and community-focused approaches are "probably synergistic rather than antagonistic in their effects" (p. 44).

28. Frieda is a young mother who is frustrated with her one-year-old child because he's not yet toilet trained. Which of the following approaches are best suited for Frieda?
    a. family therapy
    b. psychopharmacology
    c. resilient peer therapy (RPT)
    d. cognitive-behavioral therapy (CBT)

29. Offending parents are the focus of all of the following treatment approaches *except*:
    a. family therapy.
    b. behavior therapy.
    c. resilient peer therapy (RPT).
    d. cognitive-behavioral therapy (CBT).

30. A child-focused treatment is indicated when:
    a. a child has developmental or other difficulties.
    b. the offender was not a caretaker or family member of the child.
    c. the offending parent is in adjunctive therapy.
    d. all of the above.

# GENERAL CONSIDERATIONS AND PROCEDURES FOR WORKING WITH FAMILIES AND MALTREATMENT

Although each approach reviewed above offers suggestions about managing the treatment and therapeutic relationship, here we will underscore important issues and procedures you should consider when treating families in which there has been abuse or neglect. It is impossible to do justice to the complexity of these issues and subtlety of these procedures in the space available; we recommend you read Sheinberg and Fraenkel (2001) or our even more detailed manual (Fraenkel, Sheinberg, & True, 1996).

## Forming and Maintaining a Positive Therapeutic Relationship

Most of these families will have had contact with the legal and child welfare systems prior to meeting you, and likely have found these experiences intrusive and unpleasant, even if carried out by well-meaning, sensitive professionals. As a result of the report of maltreatment, children may have been removed from the parents' care and placed in foster care or residential treatment. Many may have been referred by the courts or social services, and some may be legally mandated for treatment. When children have been removed, treatment may be one of the preconditions of children being returned to the parents. In addition, you may be required to file periodic reports to the referring agent, and the family is likely to receive ongoing supervision by these larger systems agencies until it is determined that the child is no longer at risk.

As the therapist, these referral conditions present you with particular challenges to forming a trusting relationship with the offending parent, who is likely now wary of "helping professionals," as well as with the child, who may be afraid that if he or she reveals any further abusive or neglectful incidents, or even any negative feelings about the parent(s) or other family members, he or she will get the family into further trouble. A few procedures help with forming a positive, trusting, and productive therapeutic relationship:

• Distinguish your role as therapist from that of professionals involved in the forensic investigation. Your role is not to collect further information for legal purposes, but rather, to help the child recover from the abuse and ensure that the family has the skills and understanding that will decrease likelihood of further abuse and increase safety and emotional security.

• On the other hand, be clear that you are a mandated reporter and are therefore required to report suspected maltreatment. It is also important that you be open about whatever requirements you have to file progress reports. It is recommended that you co-write such reports with the client family, which usually represents an empowering, collaborative experience for them. Even reports of suspected further abuse can be done with the family, increasing the chance that they will maintain their sense of trust in you through this trying event.

• Invite parents and children to describe the often traumatic events they've experienced since the abuse was reported and respond with empathy. Oftentimes, the disruption experienced by the family following disclosure is more on their minds than the abuse itself, which may have occurred weeks or months—sometimes even years—ago.

• Indicate clearly from the outset that although the focus of your work with them will be to create a safe, abuse-free family context that will benefit both the child and the parents, you invite them to talk about whatever is of concern to them, as the abuse is only one part of their life story. In addition, encourage them to tell you when they feel they've talked about the abuse as much as they feel they "comfortably" can for now (a procedure we've called "talking about talking"). Get used to moving from direct discussion of the abuse to other topics and back again, letting family members take charge of this process as much as possible. Invite the family to be "critical consumers" of the therapy—ask them to give you feedback on your work with them. This encourages a sense of clients' "ownership" of the therapy, especially important when they did not choose to enter therapy.

• Invite family members to talk not only about the story of the abuse, but also about their individual and collective stories of pride (Sheinberg & Fraenkel, 2001)—their strengths, talents, positive coping skills, and the good qualities of their relationships. By helping families locate and build upon these aspects of resilience and strength, they will be better able to look carefully at aspects of individual and family functioning that represent risk factors for abuse. Solely focusing on the abuse creates an overwhelming sense of shame that is likely to reduce family members' ability to stay in treatment.

## Bringing Forth the Complexity in Family Members' Feelings

As we have noted, abuse and neglect challenge the fundamental assumptions and emotions family members hold about themselves and others. The abused child often wonders how someone often loving and protective of her could be abusive towards her (or allow others to abuse her). She may find herself confused by seemingly incommensurate feelings of attachment and love on the one hand, and fear and anger on the other. In turn, she may hold widely different beliefs and feelings about herself: she may on the one hand see herself as a good, intelligent, lovable child, and on the other, as bad, flawed, and deserving of mistreatment. Likewise, the abusive parent may be confused about her capacity to be loving and protective at times, and at others, overly punitive and rageful. The nonoffending parent whose husband sexually abused their daughter may be torn between her feelings of love and attachment for the husband versus her loving and protective feelings for her child. She may have difficulty comprehending how she can simultaneously still care for her husband and at the same time feel anger and disgust about his behavior. Likewise, she may basically support her child yet be upset with her for disclosing the abuse, and may be consumed with guilt for not detecting the abuse sooner, even when it was well hidden from her by the offending family member and the child.

As the therapist, it is crucial that you encourage family members to experience and express the full range of their emotions about themselves and others, rather than focus solely on one set of feelings (for instance, attempting to "empower" the child to feel angry at her abusive father to the neglect of her equally powerful positive feelings). We find it most helpful to adopt a "both–and" rather than an "either–or" frame, and to help family members recognize that they need not *resolve* the conflicts among their various emotions. In other words, abuse results in a *complex story* and therapists need to honor that complexity rather than attempt to reduce it to a simple tale of good and bad, right and wrong.

## Distinguishing Between Moral Clarity and Psychological Explanations

It is important to recognize that in helping abusive parents gain insight into the psychological sources of their behavior, this does not condone or excuse the behavior. Likewise, honoring a nonoffending mother's continued attachment to the sexually offending father and husband does not mean encouraging her to act on those attachments when doing so would put the abused child at risk for continued abuse. It is important for you as the therapist to recognize that by helping parents develop a useful and empathic psychological explanation for the offending behavior toward the goal of preventing such behavior in the future, you encourage rather than undermine parents' capacity to develop greater moral clarity about their behavior and to take full responsibility for it.

---

Significant progress has been made in recent decades in the identification, prevention, and treatment of child maltreatment. Advances in operational definitions have led to improved ability to recognize and report child abuse and neglect. Identification of risk and protective factors, capable of influencing a child's response to maltreatment, has been critical to early prevention of adverse outcomes in child victims. As empirical study has dispelled the myth that most offenders are strangers, preventive interventions have accordingly shifted from "don't talk to strangers" classroom lessons to programs that target at-risk parents, the typical offenders of child abuse and neglect. Finally, though limited in its scope, the empirical study of the treatment of child maltreatment has demonstrated that maltreated children and their families can benefit from therapy. Despite such advances, considerable research is needed to answer remaining questions such as which treatment approaches are most effective and for which types of child maltreatment. Should the current rate of progress be sustained, children will be less likely to be victims of maltreatment and those who do suffer abuse and neglect will be more likely to recover.

## KEY TERMS

**behavior therapy:** A treatment approach based on the principles of behavioral psychology in which abusive or neglectful behaviors are understood as the outcome of positive and negative reinforcement. A core component of this treatment is parent training (see *parent training* below).

**child abuse:** A term which encompasses all forms of abuse including physical, sexual, and emotional.

**child emotional abuse:** Behavior which compromises the psychological health of a child.

**child maltreatment:** A term which encompasses all forms of child abuse and neglect.

**child neglect:** Failure to meet a child's basic needs.

**child physical abuse:** Actual or threatened physical harm to a child.

**child sexual abuse:** Sexual activity with a child when consent is not or cannot be given.

**cognitive-behavioral therapy (CBT):** A preventive treatment approach which aims to restructure maladaptive beliefs and enhance problem-solving skills of abusive or at-risk parents.

**family therapy:** A family-centered approach which aims to restructure family relationships and belief systems which contribute to abuse and neglect.

**mandated reporting/reporters:** Professionals, such as mental health professionals and physicians, mandated by law in most states to report suspected child maltreatment.

**parent training:** A parent-focused, behavioral approach (see behavior therapy above) to physical abuse. To prevent the recurrence of maltreatment, abusive parents are taught basic parenting and problem-solving skills.

**play therapy:** A child-focused approach which allows the child to work through difficult and conflicted feelings associated with experiences of abuse and neglect in the safe world of play.

**protective factors:** Child, parent, family, and community factors which help buffer a child from the effects of child maltreatment. Protective factors also minimize a child's risk of being a victim of maltreatment.

**residential treatment:** A treatment approach involving placing a child on a special unit where he or she can experience structured, positive interactions with his or her parents who visit daily.

**resilient peer therapy (RPT):** A child-focused treatment approach that involves pairing withdrawn, maltreated children with resilient peers.

**risk factors:** Child, parent, family, and community factors which increase the likelihood that the child will be adversely affected by experiences of maltreatment.

**social support/social network treatment:** An approach which aims to decrease the social isolation that often characterizes abusive and, in particular, neglecting families.

**therapeutic day care:** A child-focused treatment approach which addresses the cognitive and social–emotional developmental concerns of maltreated children by offering intellectual stimulation in the context of supportive, child–teacher interactions.


## DISCUSSION QUESTIONS

1. Why is it important to have operational definitions of abuse and neglect that are consistent across professions?
2. How might information about gender differences in the experience of child maltreatment be useful to therapists who work with children?

3. Identify three reasons why "mothers acting alone" represent the most common perpetrators of child maltreatment.
4. You are to evaluate a twelve-year-old boy who has been a victim of ongoing neglect. Based on your knowledge of the potential effects of child maltreatment, identify five questions you might ask to assess the effects of the neglect he has experienced.
5. Frank is to evaluate a family's level of risk for child maltreatment. Applying your knowledge of risk factors for child maltreatment, identify three questions Frank should ask the family.
6. Emily is a seven-year-old girl who has been the victim of ongoing physical abuse. Considering the *protective factors* described in the chapter, identify three treatment goals that would help mitigate the effects of the abuse.
7. Ellen is a therapist whose client has disclosed having "gone too far" while punishing her son with a belt. The client is very upset about the belt marks left on her son's body. The client expresses that she does not want this to happen again and asks Ellen to help her work on controlling her anger. Does Ellen need to report this incident? If she does, how could she maintain her positive relationship with the client? Outline the reasons supporting your decision, and the procedures Ellen could follow to maintain a therapeutic alliance with the client if she did decide to report.
8. Eve, a thirteen-year-old girl, disclosed to her mother that her stepfather has been sexually abusing her over the past year. Her mother wants to help her daughter but feels it is "too much to believe" that her husband "could do such a thing." First, how might a family-centered approach help this family? Second, identify two treatment goals that a family therapist might have for this family.
9. Identify three ways in which problem-solving skills may help a physically abusive parent better relate to his or her child.
10. Identify three ways to form a positive therapeutic relationship with a family that has been legally mandated for treatment.

## SUGGESTED FURTHER READING

Belsky, J. (1993). Etiology of child maltreatment: A developmental–ecological analysis. *Psychological Bulletin, 114*(3), 413–434.

One of the first papers suggesting an "ecological" theory of the cause of maltreatment. The child's family, community, and environment are among the multiple contexts in which abusive and neglectful behaviors are understood from this perspective.

Kempe, C. H., Silverman, F. N., Steele, B. F., Droegemueller, N., & Silver, H. (1962). The battered child syndrome. *Journal of the American Medical Association, 181,* 17–24.

The seminal paper on child physical abuse that marked the beginning of the field of child maltreatment.

Myers, J. E. B., Berliner, L., Briere, J., Hendrix, C. T., Jenny, C., & Reid, T. (Eds.) (2001). *The APSAC handbook on child maltreatment* (2nd ed.). Thousand Oaks, CA: Sage.

An indispensable and comprehensive handbook on the causes, consequences, treatment, and prevention of child maltreatment.

Sedlack, A. J., & Broadhurst, D. D. (1996). *The third national incidence study of child abuse and neglect.* U.S. Department of Health and Human Services. Washington, DC: Government Printing Office.

The National Incidence Study (NIS) bases estimates on information from more than 5,000 professionals who come into contact with abused and neglected children in a variety of settings. The characteristics of victimized children, the relationship of perpetrators to victims, and other informative statistics are presented.

Sheinberg, M., & Fraenkel, P. (2001). *The relational trauma of incest: A family-based approach to treatment.* New York: Guilford Press.

A family-based model focusing on the relational trauma—betrayal of trust, safety, and loyalty—experienced by child victims of sexual abuse. A framework is outlined for engaging all family members to strengthen the child's protective relationships, build family resiliency, and address the child's emotional and behavioral difficulties.

# REFERENCES

Acton, R. G., & During, S. M. (1992). Preliminary results of aggression on management training for aggressive parents. *Journal of Interpersonal Violence, 7,* 410–417.

Belsky, J. (1980). Child maltreatment: An ecological integration. *American Psychologist, 35,* 320–335.

Black, M. (2000). The roots of child neglect. In R. M. Reece (Ed.), *Treatment of child abuse: Common ground for mental health, medical and legal practitioners* (pp. 157–164). Baltimore: Johns Hopkins University Press.

Brunk, M., Henggeler, S. W., & Whelan, J. P. (1987). Comparison of multisystemic therapy and parent training in the brief treatment of child abuse and neglect. *Journal of Consulting and Clinical Psychology, 55,* 171–178.

Carr, A. (2000). Evidence-based practice in family therapy and systemic consultation: I. child-focused problems. *Journal of Family Therapy, 22,* 29–60.

Corcoran, J. (2000). Family interventions with physical abuse and neglect: A critical review. *Children and Youth Services Review, 22,* 563–591.

DeVoe, E. R., & Faller, K. C. (1999). The characteristics of disclosure among children who may have been sexually abused. *Journal of the American Professional Society on the Abuse of Children, 4*(3), 217–227.

Dubowitz, H., Black, M., Starr, R. H., Jr., & Zuravin, S. (1993). A conceptual definition of child neglect. *Criminal Justice and Behavior, 20,* 8–26.

Edgeworth, J., & Carr, A. (2000). Child abuse. In A. Carr (Ed.), *What works with children and adolescents? A critical review of psychological interventions with children, adolescents and their families* (pp. 17–48). London: Routledge.

Emery, R. E., & Laumann-Billings, L. (1998). An overview of the nature, causes, and consequences of abusive family relationships: Toward differentiating maltreatment and violence. *American Psychologist, 53*(2), 121–135.

Erickson, M. F., & Egeland, B. (1996). The quiet assault: A portrait of child neglect. In L. Berliner, J. Briere, S. Bulkley, C. Jenny, & T. Reid (Eds.), *The handbook of child maltreatment* (pp. 4–20). Newbury Park, CA: Sage.

Fantuzzo, J., Sutton-Smith, B., Atkins, M., Meyers, R., Stevenson, H., Coolahan, K., et al. (1996). Community-based resilient peer treatment of withdrawn maltreated preschool children. *Journal of Consulting and Clinical Psychology, 64,* 1377–1386.

Finkelhor, D. (1979). What's wrong with sex between adults and children? Ethics and the problem of sexual abuse. *American Journal of Orthopsychiatry, 49,* 692–697.

Fraenkel, P., Sheinberg, M., & True, F. (1996). *Making families safe for children: Handbook for a family-centered approach to intrafamilial child sexual abuse.* New York: Ackerman Institute for the Family.

Friedrich, W. N., Luecke, W. J., Beilke, R. L., & Place, V. (1992). Psychotherapy outcome of sexually abused boys: An agency study. *Journal of Interpersonal Violence, 7,* 396–409.

Gaudin, J. M., Jr., Wodarski, J. S., Arkinson, M. K., & Avery, L. S. (1990–1991). Remedying child neglect: Effectiveness of social network interventions. *The Journal of Applied Social Sciences, 15,* 97–123.

Gil, E. (1991). *The healing power of play: Working with abused children.* New York: Guilford Press.

Kempe, C. H., Silverman, F. N., Steele, B. F., Droegemueller, N., & Silver, H. (1962). The battered child syndrome. *Journal of the American Medical Association, 181,* 17–24.

Kendall-Tackett, K. A., Williams, L. M., & Finkelhor, D. (1993). Impact of sexual abuse on children: A review and synthesis of recent empirical studies. *Psychological Bulletin, 113,* 164–180.

Kolko, D. J. (1996). Individual cognitive-behavioral treatment and family therapy for physically abused children and their offending parents: A comparison of clinical outcomes. *Child Maltreatment, 1,* 322–342.

National Clearinghouse on Child Abuse and Neglect Information (2002). *Child abuse and neglect state statutes series. Current trends in child maltreatment reporting laws.* Washington, DC: U.S. Department of Health and Human Services.

Nicol, A., Smith, J., & Kay, B. (1988). A focused casework approach to the treatment of child abuse: A controlled comparison. *Journal of Child Psychology & Psychiatry, 29,* 703–711.

Putnam, F. (2003). Ten-year research update review: Child sexual abuse. *Child & Adolescent Psychiatry, 42*(3), 269–278.

Rumm, P. D., Cummings, P., Krauss, M. R., Bell, M. A., & Rivara, F. P. (2000). Identified spouse abuse as a risk factor for child abuse. *Child Abuse & Neglect, 24*, 1372–1381.

Schwarz, E. D., & Perry, B. D. (1994). The post-traumatic response in children and adolescents. *Psychiatric Clinics of North America, 17*(2), 311–327.

Sedlack, A. J., & Broadhurst, D. D. (1996). *The third national incidence study of child abuse and neglect.* U.S. Department of Health and Human Services. Washington, DC: Government Printing Office.

Sheinberg, M., & Fraenkel, P. (2001). *The relational trauma of incest: A family-based approach to treatment.* New York: Guilford Press.

U.S. Department of Health and Human Services, Administration on Children, Youth and Families (2002). *Child maltreatment 2000: Reports from the states to the national child abuse and neglect data system.* Washington, DC: U.S. Government Printing Office.

Westcott, H. L., & Jones, D. P. H. (1999). Annotation: the abuse of disabled children. *Journal of Child Psychology and Psychiatry, 40*, 497–506.

Widom, C. S. (2000). Understanding the consequences of childhood victimization. In R. M. Reece (Ed.), *Treatment of child abuse: Common ground for mental health, medical and legal practitioners* (pp. 157–164). Baltimore: Johns Hopkins University Press.

Wolfe, D. A. (1999). Child abuse: Implications for child development and psychopathology. Newbury Park, CA: Sage.

Wolfe, D. A., Edwards, B., Manion, I., & Koverola, C. (1988). Early interventions for parents at risk for child abuse and neglect. *Journal of Consulting and Clinical Psychology, 56*, 40–47.

Wolock, I., & Horowitz, B. (1984). Child maltreatment as a social problem: The neglect of neglect. *American Journal of Orthopsychiatry, 54*, 530–543.

Zuravin, S. J. (1991). Research definitions of child physical abuse and neglect: Current problems. In R. H. Starr, Jr. & D. A. Wolfe (Eds.), *The effects of child abuse and neglect: Issues and research* (pp. 100–128). New York: Guilford Press.

PART

V

# DIMINISHED HEALTH AND WELL-BEING

# 19

# Care Giving and Grief

Dorothy S. Becvar
*St. Louis University*

## TRUTH OR FICTION?

___ 1. *Those who are dying or mourning the death of a loved one go through predictable stages of grief.*

___ 2. *Grief is a time-limited process.*

___ 3. *Resolution of grief occurs when one has worked through, and thus gotten over, the loss.*

___ 4. *The prognosis for long-term recovery from loss due to sudden death is more negative than recovery from a loss due to anticipated death.*

___ 5. *Anticipatory mourning refers to ideas and expectations regarding how one will feel following the death of a loved one.*

___ 6. *The boundary between life and death has blurred in recent years.*

___ 7. *Therapists should seek legal and professional counsel when euthanasia issues arise while working with dying patients or their loved ones.*

___ 8. *The death of a child usually brings parents closer together.*

___ 9. *The greatest fear of preschool age children whose sibling dies is that they may have said or done something that caused the death.*

___ 10. *The reactions of young children to the death of a parent is similar to those experienced by children when a sibling dies.*

___ 11. *When a spouse or partner dies suddenly, the surviving spouse or partner experiences greater pain than when the death is anticipated.*

___ 12. *The loss of a pet may be as painful as the death of a family member.*

___ 13. *In most states, caring for the body and preparing for burial or cremation requires the involvement of a funeral director or undertaker.*

___ 14. *The last and most difficult aspect of the grief process involves the search for a new relationship to fill the void left by the one who has died.*
___ 15. *Ultimately, the resolution of grief involves finding answers to one's questions.*

This chapter reviews information related to the impact on clients of serious illness, dying, and death, and how you may best help when the focus is dying or grieving. Current approaches to understanding the bereavement process are also considered, along with the various contexts of death and loss.

## WHAT FACTORS INFLUENCE THE IMPACT OF ILLNESS, DEATH, AND LOSS ON FAMILY MEMBERS?

Each **grief** experience must be recognized as unique for each different individual involved. Systemically, all behavior is understood as logical to context (Becvar & Becvar, 2003), with context referring to who is involved, where they are, what is happening, and the perceptions of each person. Thus, to understand client behavior, it is essential to examine the various contexts of illness, death, and grief with a focus on sensitivity to each in all of their complexity (Becvar, 2001). In general, significant factors to consider include type of illness (e.g., acute, long-term, debilitating, one with a stigma associated), cause of death (e.g., illness, accident, murder, suicide), manner in which the death occurred (e.g., anticipated, sudden), and degree of ambiguity (Boss, 1991) involved in the loss (e.g., persons missing in action, persons in a coma, persons with impaired cognitive functioning). Similarly, you cannot assume that losses within a particular category, for example, parental death, have the same impact on the survivors even though they may be members of the same family.

1. The most significant factor(s) influencing the impact of death and loss include:
   a. the cause of the death.
   b. the manner in which the death occurred.
   c. the degree of ambiguity.
   d. all of the above.

Specific factors likely to influence grief reactions include the position of the deceased person in the family, the degree of intensity or closeness of the relationship with that person, the life stages of those involved, family patterns and past experiences related to loss and **bereavement**, spiritual beliefs, ethnicity, and culture. Also influential are interactions between individual differences in illness or death experiences and the persons having the experience. For example, grief may be particularly challenging when the circumstances of the death represent a threat to survivors' world views, especially basic beliefs about such issues as goodness or justice in the world (Nolen-Hoeksema & Larson, 1999). This is also likely to be the case when little social support is available. Those who use the coping mechanisms of avoidance or excessive rumination also may be more challenged by bereavement as are people who tend to be dependent, pessimistic, lack self-control, or are emotionally less stable.

2. Family members each have different reactions to another family member's death because:
   a. the family is dysfunctional.
   b. each individual's experience is unique.
   c. the family rules require these types of responses.
   d. individuals attempt to express their uniqueness during times of crisis.

## HOW HAVE PROFESSIONAL APPROACHES TO GRIEVING CHANGED OVER TIME?

Until recently, most professional approaches to grief were guided by classical models derived from the psychoanalytic perspectives of Sigmund Freud and Erich Lindemann and the attachment theory of Bowlby (1980). Accordingly, all important relationships were assumed to involve an investment of energy; thus when a person died, survivors needed to withdraw that energy in order to be able to form new attachments. An inability to complete this energy withdrawal process in an appropriate, timely manner was indicative of problems, perhaps of pathology. Further assumptions focused on the grieving process as time-limited (Peretz, 1970): During the first two weeks the survivor experienced shock and intense grief; two months of strong grieving followed; then, over a period of two years the grief was expected to decrease and the bereaved individual to recover, regaining by that point full, normal functioning. The grief process was assumed to conclude at the end of two years and if such resolution did not occur within this time, **mourning** was considered to be maladaptive (Raphael, 1983).

3. Classical models of grieving assumed which of the following predictable patterns of grieving?
   a. one week, one, month, one year
   b. two weeks, two months, two years
   c. three weeks, three months, three years
   d. four weeks, four months, four years

While this approach continues to be influential, during the 1980s many studies challenged its fundamental assumptions. Called into question were the beliefs that (a) the bereaved all go through predictable stages of grief, (b) loss inevitably leads to depression and absence of severe distress will result in pathology, and (c) recovery requires working through the loss (Nolen-Hoeksema & Larson, 1999). Based on more recent studies, as well as on stress and coping research, bereavement now tends to be viewed in context, with acknowledgment of the need for sensitivity to individual beliefs and abilities. Further recognized is that the grieving process may have no fixed endpoint, and may even last a lifetime. While bereaved persons may return to normal functioning, they may never "get over" the loss.

In addition, complete detachment is no longer considered to be either desirable or possible. Rather, we understand that the bereaved are able to maintain simultaneously an attachment to both the living and to the one who has died and still function perfectly well. Further, bereavement may take many forms and determination of the degree to which it is adaptive or maladaptive can be made only on an individual basis. Also acknowledged are the challenges to belief systems, to daily life, and to the self-concept that the loss of someone close represents. Given the inevitable need to reorganize on these fronts, acute grief responses may be similar to those of posttraumatic stress disorder (Rando, 1997).

Recent studies also suggest that rather than pathologizing a person's grief process, you must understand each individual's reactions in the context of his or her worldview and unique situation. The goal is to facilitate adaptation (Bernstein, 1997), helping clients learn to live with the loss rather than trying to overcome it. As part of this process, you must acknowledge the degree to which the values, attitudes, beliefs, perceptions, and relationships of survivors will all be affected and altered and that they are likely to be forever changed as a function of the grief experience.

4. According to recent research, a client's grief is determined to be maladaptive:
   a. when the bereaved person fails to work through the loss.
   b. when the bereaved person has withdrawn emotional energy.
   c. on a case by case, individual basis, relative to context.
   d. on the recommendation of other family members.

## WHAT ARE THE CHARACTERISTICS UNIQUE TO THE EXPERIENCE OF UNANTICIPATED DEATH?

The most significant of the many challenges facing clients in the case of sudden or accidental death is the effort required to try to make sense of a traumatic event that has occurred without any warning, one that also may seem both unbelievable and meaningless. In such a situation, survivors are catapulted from normal everyday life into a surreal existence in which it may seem as if the world has gone crazy. One moment they have a relationship with someone; in the next moment that person is gone. And survivors receive an additional blow when violence has been involved, making the death particularly difficult to understand and accept (Nolen-Hoeksema & Larson, 1999).

5. The most significant challenge faced by those bereaved by sudden death is:
   a. the need to make choices about organ donation.
   b. the need to come to terms with what has happened.
   c. the need to inform other family members and friends.
   d. the need to make funeral arrangements.

Survivors of an unanticipated death tend to find their coping ability stressed to the limit (Rando, 1991) as they are confronted with the pain of the loss and also must accommodate shock, disbelief, and extreme disruption in all areas of their lives. At the same time, they must make decisions regarding such issues as organ donation, funeral preparations, and burial arrangements. They must contact family and friends, tell their story endlessly, and hear repeatedly the shock of others. They may need to respond to the grief and needs of other family members. All of this takes place in a context in which, very often, there has been very little or no prior preparation. One of the most typical reactions, therefore, is a sense of complete loss of control. Specific responses may run the gamut from numbness and silence to heartrending wailing and other emotional outbursts (Nurmi & Williams, 1997) as well as a tendency to experience a variety of physical symptoms. These may include high blood pressure, colds and other infections, arthritis, chest pains, and allergies (Kastenbaum, 1986).

Although the grieving process following a sudden death may take longer or be more complicated than in other instances of bereavement, the long-term ability to adapt to a loss under such circumstances tends to be similar to that of survivors of an anticipated death (Bernstein, 1997). To facilitate such adaptation, you must acknowledge the degree to which belief systems may have been challenged. As all assumptions previously held dear are destroyed, survivors may lose both their loved one and their worldview, or frame of reference—the means by which they previously made sense of reality. Your task, therefore, is to help survivors create meaningful stories that enable them to come to terms with the loss and begin to recommit to life, figure out a direction, and acquire the tools to begin heading there. The new worldview may be constructed using old ideas and assumptions that continue to remain meaningful as well as a wide range of alternative perspectives.

To know how best to proceed, you must note how the person died; who, if anyone, was responsible; if it was health related, whether the death might have been prevented; the circumstances if the death occurred as a result of an accident; whether there was negligence on anyone's part; whether it was a violent or wrongful death; whether it was a suicide; whether it falls into the category of **ambiguous loss**; the degree of involvement of the legal justice system; whether an autopsy was required; and whether an inquest or a trial has been or will be necessary. With such information, you will be better equipped to provide support and thus facilitate the grieving processes of clients.

6. Appropriate support for those bereaved by an unanticipated death is best provided by:
   a. ascertaining the circumstances of the death.
   b. offering information regarding support groups.
   c. sharing personal grief and loss experiences.
   d. providing information about books to read.

## WHAT ARE THE CHARACTERISTICS UNIQUE TO THE EXPERIENCE OF AN ANTICIPATED DEATH?

When death is anticipated, the grieving process involves both the survivors and those who are dying. Upon receiving a terminal diagnosis, persons who are ill are confronted with, and ultimately must reconcile themselves to, their own imminent demise. Related challenges include dealing with and perhaps resolving family relationship issues, financial concerns, and personal dreams. Dying persons also must think about the circumstances of their death, an idea likely to be frightening and perhaps overwhelming.

For dying persons as well as for family members and friends, knowledge that the end is near generally initiates a period of **anticipatory mourning**; that is, the grief process begins despite the fact that the person whom one is mourning is still alive (Rolland, 1991) and regardless of whether that person wants to focus on death. Additional stresses arise from the emotional responses and physical responsibilities of caretakers for dying persons. During such periods of increased stress it is likely that problematic family patterns will become more pronounced, particularly in the context of illnesses that have a social stigma, for example, AIDS. A further complicating factor, regardless of type of illness, relates to worries and fears on the part of the dying about becoming a physical or financial burden.

7. In the case of an extended dying process, families are more challenged when:
   a. the person who is ill has unresolved relationship issues and financial concerns.
   b. there are major physical responsibilities.
   c. everyone engages in a process of anticipatory mourning.
   d. there is a social stigma associated with the illness.

Entirely new feelings and reactions may emerge once the death has occurred. Sadness and grief may accompany confusion about the degree of pain experienced given that theoretically the survivors were prepared for the loss. The bereaved also may feel relief that death finally has come, that the dying ordeal is over. There may be guilt about these conflicting emotions despite the fact that they are normal, predictable responses.

On the more positive side, the potential benefits of awareness that death is near include opportunities to complete unfinished business, have input into and perhaps design one's own dying process, participate in decisions regarding acceptable medical intervention, choose someone to make health-related decisions at the point of incapacity, and specify many after-death wishes. There also is time to focus on relationships, perhaps healing old wounds and sharing final thoughts with significant others. Dying persons also have an opportunity to assess their accomplishments and perhaps achieve some final goals or dreams. And others involved also have time to come to terms with what is happening and begin to focus on realigning their own beliefs and meaning systems.

8. When death is anticipated, dying persons:
   a. are faced with the challenge of coming to terms with their own imminent demise.
   b. have the opportunity to tie up loose ends.
   c. worry about becoming a burden to those they love.
   d. all of the above.

## HOW CAN THERAPISTS PROVIDE ASSISTANCE TO THOSE WHO ARE DYING?

When working with dying persons, the goals are to support the potential to live as fully as possible and to facilitate the ability to die well. You also must attend to the needs of caregivers and others likely to be affected by the dying process and the death. For everyone involved, therefore, it may be appropriate to encourage a focus on making the most of each moment of enjoyment, however small. Also important may be the suggestion that being present to the dying process will create the opportunity for a healing experience, one that enables everyone to bear their grief more easily.

Dying persons first face the task of coming to terms with imminent death. Kübler-Ross (1969) describes this as involving five stages: denial, rage, bargaining, depression, and acceptance. Although it is unlikely that all dying persons will go through each stage, or necessarily will follow the same sequence, familiarity with the model may enable you to understand clients' behavior at various points in time. However, there also may be many who have little or no trouble accepting their dying, or may experience it in different ways.

9. Kübler-Ross's stages of death and dying include:
   a. denial, confusion, anger, blaming, and acknowledgment.
   b. anger, confusion, blaming, bargaining, and acceptance.
   c. denial, rage, bargaining, depression, and acceptance.
   d. anger, blaming, depression, bargaining, and acknowledgment.

Once acknowledgment of the inevitability of death has occurred, you must address how the person wishes to die. Is the preference to die at home, and if so, is hospice an option? Advocates of hospice believe that supportive, palliative care until physical death has been medically determined to be the best response to a terminal diagnosis. However, candidates for hospice must meet certain criteria, including the anticipated time until death and the presence of appropriate care givers. When hospice is not an option, the choice may be to die in a hospital, and often to continue treatments aimed at cure until all efforts in that regard have been exhausted. Wherever it takes place, the act of dying also may be seen as an opportunity for growth (Callanan & Kelley, 1992). Foos-Graber (1989) advocates a process of "deathing," in which dying persons actively and consciously engage in dying as a means of supporting soul growth. Involved are various breathing techniques and meditative practices, with dying viewed as one aspect of a spiritual discipline aimed at facilitating transformation to higher states of consciousness.

Whether one chooses to be an active participant as just described as the terminally ill move closer to death, you and other care givers must be sensitive to the many aspects of "nearing death awareness" (Callanan & Kelley, 1992) as dying persons experience visions, sense the presence of departed loved ones, spiritual beings, a bright light, or awareness of being in a particular place. They may feel warmth and love, attempt to communicate, often metaphorically, important messages to family, friends, and other caregivers or engage in a life review. Although little fear may be evident, there often is great concern about those to be left behind.

10. "Nearing death awareness" refers to:
    a. acceptance that one's death is imminent and inevitable.
    b. acceptance that a loved one is dying.
    c. recognition that having visions is normal as one approaches death.
    d. recognition that those close to dying person may have unusual experiences.

Throughout the dying process, a focus on resolving relationship issues and facilitating growth is important. Encouraging caregivers to respond appropriately to the final needs of dying persons demonstrates love and support, enabling them to feel a sense of purpose. Meaningful participation prior to death may help ease the pain once it occurs.

## WHAT HAS BEEN THE IMPACT OF TECHNOLOGY ON THE DYING PROCESS?

In recent years sophisticated technology has greatly enhanced the ability of medical science to prolong life. In addition to various life support systems, advancements in the realm of organ donation and transplantation now enable physicians to prevent what otherwise would be inevitable death. As a result, both the medical and legal communities have struggled around questions regarding when death has occurred and when life-prolonging mechanisms should be discontinued. One of the earliest efforts in this realm focused on delineating the differences between a vegetative state and **brain death**. A set of standards, formulated in 1968 by a group of physicians at the Harvard Medical School, now known as the ***Harvard Criteria***, has become the means for determining that the brain has reached a condition in which it is considered to be irreversibly nonfunctional.

11. Brain death is determined by means of:
    a. the *Yale Criteria*.
    b. the *Cornell Criteria*.
    c. the *Harvard Criteria*.
    d. the *Brown Criteria*.

In addition to these standards, the field of **bioethics**, or biomedical ethics, also has been created. Professionals in this realm attempt to facilitate appropriate institutional responses to dilemmas around the use or withdrawal of medical treatment. The primary goal is making morally and ethically prudent decisions in the face of a biotechnology that has advanced to the point that the boundary between life and death is often blurred. Indeed, when death approaches, family members also may have to make life and death decisions regarding what procedures to allow, when to unplug a machine, or how much suffering to allow. While the dying person's wishes may be known, there may be disagreement on the part of some about following through. And even after decisions have been made, doubt and second thoughts may lead to feelings of guilt.

12. Those in the field of bioethics:
    a. help institutions formulate appropriate responses in the medical realm.
    b. help family members resolve ethical dilemmas related to illness.
    c. help physicians deal with moral dilemmas.
    d. help therapists explain to families what their ethical responsibilities are.

## WHAT DOES THE THERAPIST NEED TO KNOW WHEN QUESTIONS REGARDING EUTHANASIA ARISE?

You must be well informed about euthanasia issues: definitions, legal requirements, and professional limits on potential involvement. Although euthanasia refers to the act of putting to death, in a painless manner, someone with an incurable illness, there are a variety of permutations in meaning. According to one group, ***euthanasia*** refers to "the intentional termination of life by another party at the request of the person concerned" (Final Report, 1987, p. 166) whereas ***assisted suicide*** is "intentionally helping a patient to terminate his or her life at his or her request" (Scheper & Duursma, 1994, p. 4). In the medical realm, distinctions are made between ***voluntary active euthanasia*** (VAE), that is, the physician gives a medication or somehow intervenes to cause death at the request of the patient; ***physician-assisted suicide*** (PAS), that is, the physician provides either information, resources, or direct assistance but the patient terminates her or his own life; and ***physician aid-in-dying***, that is, the physician discontinues treatment at the patient's request. Nevertheless, however construed and implemented, the only state in which PAS is legal is Oregon. You therefore must know the law of your locality before engaging in any euthanasia-related activity and also should seek guidance to avoid violation of professional codes of ethics.

13. Physician aid-in-dying refers to instances in which:
    a. a physician provides assistance and the patient terminates her or his own life.
    b. a physician discontinues treatment at the patient's request.
    c. a physician gives a medication or intervenes to cause death at the request of the patient.
    d. a physician puts to death, in a painless manner, a patient with an incurable illness.

You also should know that according to the Supreme Court, there are two constitutionally permissible means of alleviating dying persons' pain when all other methods fail—when treated either by a *morphine drip* administered at a level to eliminate pain or *terminal sedation* that produces continuous anesthesia, death ultimately will occur (Preston, 2000). Patients become eligible for such procedures via advance directives prepared in compliance with state law and legally witnessed or notarized. Although the validity of advance directives varies by states, many have followed the lead of California, which in 1976, passed the **California Natural Death Act** permitting individuals, in specific situations, to make prior plans for treatment at the end of life. This statute also "protects physicians from being sued for failing to treat incurable illnesses" (Humphrey & Clement, 2000, p. 368). In addition, according to the federal **Patient Self-Determination Act** of 1990, health care providers are required to give information to patients about their right to make advance directives, to have written institutional policies regarding them, and to document their existence.

14. The California Natural Death Act
    a. allows persons to make prior plans for treatment at the end of life.
    b. requires that all persons must die from natural causes.
    c. allows persons to take their own life in certain circumstances.
    d. none of the above.

*Advance directives* are instructions regarding end of life decisions, ideally made prior to serious illness and designed as either a living will or a health care proxy. A *living will* details instructions about desired medical intervention should the person become incapacitated in the future. With a *health care proxy*, created by means of a **durable power of attorney**, an agent is designated to be responsible for making such health care and treatment decisions in the event of future incapacitation. Advance directives may focus on either clinical conditions, for example, the circumstances under which persons would or would not want to live, or a **values history**, for example, the circumstances under which life is not preferred even when further medical treatment is available (Doukas & McCullough, 1991; McLean, 1996). Persons creating an advance directive must be competent, able to understand what they are doing, be fully informed regarding all ramifications, and execute it voluntarily (Beauchamp & Childress, 1994). As you assist with this process, you also must be sensitive to ethnic and cultural variations and values (Young & Jex, 1992), the documents must be internally consistent, and they must focus only on those dimensions included within the scope of standard medical practice (VA Medical Center, 1993).

15. A health care proxy is a document in which a competent adult:
    a. specifies the circumstances under which they would/would not want to live.
    b. describes the circumstances in which continued life would not be preferred.
    c. gives directions regarding medical treatment in the event of future incapacitation.
    d. designates a health care agent to make treatment decisions.

## HOW CAN THERAPISTS HELP PARENTS WHOSE CHILD HAS DIED?

The death of a child seems inconceivable today, thus its occurrence generally pushes parents almost "beyond endurance" (Knapp, 1986). Although mourning processes are likely to vary greatly given the different kinds of relationships parents have with children at different stages of life, no evidence suggests that mourning the loss of a child is any more or less challenging as a function of the age at which the child dies (Rando, 1991). In addition, though often unacknowledged, the loss of a child during pregnancy (Speckhard, 1997) may be equally devastating. Although all parents who lose a child experience the destruction of hopes, dreams, and expectations, there is a cultural disenfranchisement of loss during pregnancy, with less recognition of the pain and less support than is received when a child dies following a live birth.

16. The death of a child is more difficult when:
    a. the child is a baby.
    b. the child is an adult.
    c. the loss occurs during pregnancy.
    d. none of the above.

Regardless of circumstances, the grief following the death of a child is unique as a function of the special bond and distinctive relationship between parents and offspring (Klass, 1988). One's identity as a parent may be compromised, interconnections with others may be lost, and child-focused interactions with grandparents or potential grandparents may cease. You therefore must be sensitive to the need of bereaved parents to talk about what has happened and to tell their story without feeling others will be put off by expressions of their grief. Bereaved parents typically also search for knowledge that their child is okay or may long for communication with their child. They may visit a psychic, hear messages in songs on the radio, see meaning in license plates, or experience more direct contact through dreams, visions, or the sense of a presence in terms of sound, sight, or smell. As they begin exploring in previously avoided areas, they may need validation that their behavior is typical and that they are not crazy.

The relationship between spouses may be particularly vulnerable following the death of a child and help accepting different styles of grieving may be needed (Bernstein, 1997). They may blame each other for some aspect of the death; disagree about spiritual issues or about what to do with the deceased child's room; experience variations in terms of desire for reentry into the world, including a willingness, or not, to interact socially, to return to work, to engage in sexual intimacy, or to do anything just for fun; and feel the other spouse is not present in desired ways. You may suggest that they look to clergy or friends for support and provide assistance in learning patience, tolerance, and forgiveness. Parenting issues also may need attention, including sensitivity to the needs of other children and the impact of the parents' behavior on the children. Parents must maintain some semblance of order, make time to be with their surviving children, and enforce appropriate generational boundaries that allow the children to be children rather than having to take on adult responsibilities.

17. The parental relationship is vulnerable following the death of a child because of :
    a. differences over what to do with the child's room.
    b. differences about spiritual beliefs.
    c. differences in grieving styles.
    d. differences about reentry into life.

## HOW CAN THERAPISTS HELP INDIVIDUALS OF VARIOUS AGES WHO HAVE LOST A SIBLING?

The sibling relationship is the family alliance most likely "to be characterized by ambivalence or conflict" (Nolen-Hoeksema & Larson, 1999, p. 45). Whether such conflicts have been healed, there may be regret for words said or unsaid and things done or undone if a sibling dies. When the relationship was solid, or if the one who died was the only sibling, survivors may be deprived of a close companion, one who shared a similar history. During childhood, surviving children also may find their security threatened as parents act differently, become more inconsistent, or appear vulnerable. Parents may speak too much or too little about the child who has died, may become overprotective, or may withdraw. As they fall short in their ability to help their grieving child(ren), the latter may feel emotionally abandoned, unloved (Bernstein, 1997), or even rejected as the family they once knew is forever lost.

Typical reactions of children of various ages (Aldrich, 1996) are summarized in Table 19.1. Recognizing these different responses will enable you to provide, at appropriate levels, understanding of and support for developmental tasks and issues as well as for various grief reactions. Since the ability of siblings to recover will be influenced by the way in which the loss is handled, allowing for the needed expression of each person is essential. Parents should not hide their grief from young children, who know their parents are sad. Adolescents typically withdraw even under the best of circumstances and may need extra encouragement and permission to speak about what is going on inside. And parents should know that even their best attempts at support may not be perceived as enough.

18. Aggressive behavior following the death of a sibling begins to occur with children:
    a. between the ages of 3 and 5.
    b. between the ages of 6 and 9.
    c. between the ages of 9 and 12.
    d. between the ages of 12 and 20.

19. Bereaved adolescent siblings, but not younger siblings, are likely to experience:
    a. confusion about their parents' behavior.
    b. sadness about the loss of potential.
    c. inability to focus or concentrate.
    d. worry about other family members.

**TABLE 19.1**

Reactions of Children to the Death of a Sibling and the Death of a Parent

|  | Reactions to Sibling Death | Reactions to Parental Death |
|---|---|---|
| *2–5 Years* | crying, fighting, temper tantrums, nightmares, a return to bed-wetting or thumb-sucking | anger, anxiety, behavior disturbances, cognitive difficulties, denial, depression, developmental delays, eating problems, fears for the safety of the surviving parent, feelings of abandonment, guilt, hopelessness, insomnia, loss of trust, phobic reactions, regression, and restlessness |
| *6–9 Years* | crying, fighting, temper tantrums, nightmares, worry about own and parents' vulnerability, difficulty concentrating, poor school performance | guilt about parent's death, acting as if the death has not happened or is not permanent, denial to contain their emotions or avoid looking babyish |
| *9–12 Years* | comprehension of death's finality, fear of its reoccurrence, guilt, avoidance of sibling's friends, feelings of vulnerability, confused, anxious, angry and isolated, aggression, impulsivity, involvement in risky or dangerous situations, nightmares, inability to focus, poor school performance | awareness of finality of death, increased fears for self and surviving parent, anger, irritability, defiance |
| *Teenage* | awareness of finality of death, knowledge that it can and will happen again, worry about having caused the death, need to be stoic, confused, vulnerable, anxious, angry, sad, frightened, lonely, grief for lost potentials | increased focus on relationship issues, feelings of guilt or blame, confused, fearful, concern about self and perceptions of others, intense emotions expressed in intermittent, brief outbursts |

## HOW CAN THERAPISTS HELP CHILDREN OF VARIOUS AGES WHEN A PARENT HAS DIED?

Factors such as age, gender, cognitive and emotional development, and family life-cycle stage all contribute to the fact that the death of a parent is the loss with the greatest diversity of meaning for survivors. For young children the loss of a parent is unthinkable and life changing whereas for mature, older adults it is highly predictable and often assumed to be less disturbing. The death of a mother is not the same as the death of a father and the impact of either is likely to differ for sons and daughters. Similarly, the experience of *orphanhood*, occurring when the last parent dies, varies widely for surviving children.

20. The death of a parent is the loss with the greatest diversity because of:
    a. different levels of intensity in the relationship.
    b. different styles of grieving for females versus males.
    c. different ages, gender, and stages of development of survivers.
    d. different societal perceptions about mothers versus fathers.

The death of a parent is experienced in terms of both the loss and the issues surrounding it. Typical reactions of children of various ages (Nolen-Hoeksema & Larson, 1999; Raphael, 1983; Rando, 1991; Rosen, 1986) are summarized in Table 19.1. Between the ages of 2 and 5, discussion may help children understand the meaning of death (Raphael, 1983) and inclusion in funeral services may alleviate some of their anxiety (Rando, 1991). Encouraging children 6 to 9 to openly acknowledge and express their feelings may help. Those between the ages of 8 and 12, as well as teenagers, need others to be understanding of their diverse reactions, which may include outbursts and withdrawal.

Young adults, whether single or married, may be challenged by competing pressures, on the one hand, to continue to be independent and on the other hand, to return to families of origin (McGoldrick & Walsh, 1991). Given their recent separation from home, guilt about previous negative interactions may occur along with frustration that resolution of conflicts with the deceased parent now is not possible. They also may lose their primary source of emotional support and have few others in their world who can understand what they are experiencing. Their sense of release from parental surveillance may be offset by feelings of abandonment and uncertainty about how to proceed with their lives.

21. Struggles between self versus family responsibilities following parental death typifies:
    a. teenagers.
    b. young adults.
    c. older adults.
    d. none of the above.

Older adults are likely to have achieved a greater sense of acceptance and mutual understanding in relationships with parents and thus the loss may be even more poignant given awareness of their parent's unconditional love and support despite difficulties they may have experienced (Bouvard & Gladu, 1998). A common experience among their peers, much support from friends and family members is likely. However, they may lose a close and intimate relationship and their children also may lose a grandparent who played an important role in the life of their family.

## HOW CAN THERAPISTS HELP FOLLOWING THE DEATH OF A SPOUSE OR PARTNER?

Depending upon the nature of the relationship, the death of a spouse may mean the loss of a companion, a confidante, an advisor, one's date, a person with whom one can share opinions, gossip, secrets, thoughts, feelings, and fears. Also lost is one's sexual partner, the person with whom one experienced intimacy. If there are young children the surviving spouse or partner is deprived of a co-parent, someone with whom to share the joys and trials and tribulations of childrearing as well as daily tasks and chores.

Both widows and widowers tend to have more severe reactions when the death was unexpected. Although the degree of pain is not necessarily greater than when death is anticipated, the impact on the coping ability of survivors is. Women who lose a husband tend to feel abandoned while husbands who lose a wife tend to feel a sense of dismemberment (Kastenbaum, 1986; Zonnebelt-Smeenge & De Vries, 1998). And women have greater permission to cry than do men. Although both may be angry, women are more likely to describe a sense of injustice and men are more likely to experience guilt.

22. Following the death of a spouse or partner, women are more likely than men to:
    a. experience guilt.
    b. experience injustice.
    c. experience grief.
    d. experience confusion.

For young couples and couples in their middle years the death of a spouse is felt as an occurrence "out of time," as it is more to be expected later in life. Thus, although unlikely, when death occurs early, the bereavement process of surviving spouses may be greater (Nolen-Hoeksema & Larson, 1999) and more traumatic than for older persons (Parkes & Wiess, 1983). The younger the couple, the less support there is likely to be from peers or siblings, who may be frightened or unfamiliar with how to respond (McGoldrick & Walsh, 1991). New in-laws also may be confused about their role, further isolating young widows and widowers.

In a family with young children, surviving spouses may find their ability to grieve appropriately is compromised by caretaking and financial responsibilities (McGoldrick & Walsh, 1991). Although fathers may have offers of assistance with domestic duties from friends and families, women may be seen as less needy. In either case, the single parent role is challenging and sensitivity to needs for assistance that allows time for grieving and alleviates family burdens is essential. When the loss of a spouse occurs after the children have reached adolescence, single parents must negotiate alone one of the most overwhelming periods in the life of the family. Additional losses include plans and dreams postponed until responsibilities for children and careers lessen. In later life, the death of a spouse may end one's longest relationship. However, with increased age the challenges of loneliness and of making it alone also become more pronounced, especially for women, as remarriage becomes less likely (Moss & Moss, 1996).

23. When a spouse dies early in the family life cycle, the surviving spouse or partner may:
    a. feel isolated from friends and family members.
    b. feel the ability to grieve appropriately is compromised.
    c. feel cheated of plans to be together in the future.
    d. feel deprived of one's longest relationship.

## HOW CAN THERAPISTS HELP THOSE GRIEVING FOR A FRIEND OR EXTENDED FAMILY MEMBER?

Those who lose a friend or extended family member are most challenged by lack of recognition of or support for their grief as the significance of the event generally is measured in terms of degree of kinship. Even close family members and friends may not be aware of the depth of grief (Smith, 1996), and those who are bereaved may hide it for fear of intruding on immediate family members. When a co-worker dies, colleagues may be confused about how to behave or talk with one another. The parents of a child whose classmate has died may not understand the impact of the loss or take appropriate steps to deal with its ramifications. And when the best friend who died was an animal, there tends to be an even greater lack of understanding of what it can mean to be connected to a pet.

24. The significance of the death of a friend or extended family is a function of:
    a. the degree of kinship between the deceased and the survivor.
    b. the amount of recognition by others of the grief being experienced.
    c. the nature of the relationship between the deceased and the survivor.
    d. the ages of the deceased and the survivor.

With human death, relevant factors to be considered include the role played by the deceased, the ages and degree of emotional dependence of those involved, and the presence of unresolved issues or ambiguity in the relationship. With the death of an animal, the length and depth of the relationship, sources of support in the life of the pet-owner, and sensitivity to the way in which the death occurred require attention.

When called upon to provide assistance following a death in the workplace, you might focus on normalizing the experience by explaining that the reactions being felt are both predictable and understandable. You also might give family members and friends information enabling them to have a more complete sense of what is happening and encouraging their support. And grieving co-workers can be helped to understand the change in context created by the death and its inevitable impact on everyone involved.

When a classmate dies, children need support from within such systems as the school the child attended. You also must alert family members to the need for sensitivity to the potential impact on the children involved. And in some cases, specialized methods of trauma treatment may be required. Following noncatastrophic loss, children typically experience yearning or searching, reminiscing, grief dreams or play, somatic reactions, and distressing thoughts. When the death circumstances are traumatic, they may question why the event occurred, have intrusive and distressing recollections or nightmares, engage in traumatic play, have somatic reactions, and show distress in response to reminders of the event (Nader, 1997). In the case of suicide among young people, surviving classmates also may find themselves confused and conflicted by what has taken place.

25. Bereaved co-workers and bereaved classmates are similar re the need for therapists to:
    a. alert family members about the need for sensitivity.
    b. avoid intruding on the systems involved.
    c. downplay whatever emotions are being experienced.
    d. let them know that there are many losses that are much more severe.

## HOW CAN THERAPISTS HELP CREATE MEANINGFUL FUNERALS, CEREMONIES, AND OTHER RITUALS?

When working with clients needing to make funeral arrangements, you must first ascertain what they would like. You then may provide moral support during meetings with funeral directors and clergy persons, encouraging choices both in the best interests of survivors and consistent with the wishes of the deceased. You may offer information regarding options for burial or cremation, aware that in most states it is legal for family members to care for their own dead (Kreilkamp, 1999) and that all funeral arrangements, end of life documentation, and transportation of the deceased often may be handled by a family member or a person with a durable power of attorney for health care.

26. End of life documentation and transportation of the deceased may be handled by:
    a. a family member who has been asked to do so by the deceased prior to the death.
    b. a family friend who is also a lawyer.
    c. a family member or a person with a durable power of attorney for health care.
    d. none of the above.

You may help clients plan funeral services, listening sensitively, exploring possibilities, and encouraging trust in their intuitive sense about what would be best. You may offer suggestions and information based on experience with others, for example, to celebrate the life of the deceased in addition to mourning the death. If cremation is chosen, you might encourage consideration of some kind of permanent marker or of creating a ritual to accompany the dispersal of the ashes.

Sometimes special ceremonies may be appropriate. Whether small or large, public or private, these may fill a void in the absence of a formal funeral or when what occurred does not seem sufficient. The first step is to ascertain clients' goals—what they hope to accomplish. Keeping the need to be realistic in mind, you may recommend a focus on the positive aspects of the situation. Then, you might discuss who to include, reminding clients of the importance of affirming both survivors and deceased. Throughout, your role is consultant rather than creator, enabling those involved to make the ceremony their own. Similarly, you may act as consultant regarding the creation of healing rituals. Such rituals may involve creating an in-home memorial; writing in a journal or planning time to cry on a regular basis; wearing special articles of clothing or pieces of jewelry; setting a place at the dinner table for the one who has died or lighting a memorial candle; making a scrapbook or a photograph album. Birthdays and holidays also require attention, and the restructuring of old rituals may help survivors get through them more successfully.

27. Therapists helping clients create special ceremonies or healing rituals should:
    a. ascertain the client's goal.
    b. emphasize the positive, growth-producing aspects of the situation.
    c. discuss who is to be included.
    d. all of the above.

Other healing rituals may focus on mending relationships, perhaps writing letters to the deceased and then reading them aloud, or volunteering in a way that would have been meaningful to the deceased person. Involvement in a cause, especially when the death includes an aspect of injustice, may help clients regain a measure of peace. A support group such as the Compassionate Friends may be helpful for bereaved parents. Whatever the choice of ceremony, ritual or activity, the important issue to keep in mind are choices that fit with the needs of the bereaved persons and serve to alleviate their grief.

28. Which of the following is not a ritual appropriate for helping bereaved clients?
    a. writing letters to the deceased and then reading them aloud
    b. practicing denial
    c. getting involved in a cause
    d. volunteering

## HOW CAN THERAPISTS BEST FACILITATE THE SEARCH FOR MEANING?

The search for meaning is perhaps the last and most difficult (Boss, 1991), but also the most important, aspect of learning to live with loss. This search generally evolves slowly, beginning with a questioning of everything and moving into explorations out of which may emerge new ways of making sense of life in general and death in particular. In the immediate aftermath of loss, bereaved persons may focus on finding a cause or, conversely, finding someone to blame. Whether or not there is any culpability, sadness then may become rage. While for some, religion or spirituality may provide comfort, for others this rage may be directed at a supposedly compassionate God/Creator who permitted or was responsible for the death, with once again a great potential for secondary loss.

29. The loss of a client's belief system following the death of a loved one is:
    a. an indicator of pathology.
    b. requires referral to a psychiatrist.
    c. a typical response.
    d. should be the therapist's first focus.

The best help may come from listening carefully, offering questions and reflections that test the logic of various lines of reasoning and enabling clients to become clearer in their thinking. Rather than providing answers, you must present ideas and encourage the process of questioning and searching in relevant ways, perhaps sharing what you have learned from your own experiences or those of others. If there is a dilemma related to the religious/ spiritual arena, you may refer clients to clergy or other spiritual leaders for additional support. You may encourage a wider search, recommending books, use of the Internet, and additional areas on which to focus. Of particular relevance may be the stories of others who have experienced similar types of loss or explorations of the meaning of death in different cultures. For some, meaning also may be forthcoming as a function of involving oneself in a cause or being committed to a larger social issue.

30. Therapist's may best support the search for meaning by:
    a. letting clients know where their logic is faulty.
    b. encouraging as broad a search as seems appropriate.
    c. giving them specific instructions about what to do.
    d. sending clients to support groups.

Sensitivity to the process of recreating belief systems in ways that fit current conditions is essential. Sometimes a complete overhaul is required, sometimes a simple reevaluation will suffice. In either case, it is important to devote time to integrating new information. You also might acknowledge that this is not the end of the story, that the new chapters just written inevitably will require further revisions, and that when it comes to death, there always will be more questions than answers.

# KEY TERMS

**advanced directive:** Instructions regarding end of life issues, generally made prior to serious illness; may focus on either clinical conditions with which a person would or would not want to live or a *values history* (see below).

**ambiguous loss:** Cases in which there is uncertainty either about whether death has occurred or about the cause of death.

**anticipatory mourning:** Period following terminal diagnosis in which dying persons and others begin grieving although the person whom one is mourning is still very much alive.

**assisted suicide:** "Intentionally helping a patient to terminate his or her life at his or her request" (Scheper & Duursma, 1994, p. 4).

**bereavement:** Period following a death during which survivors are faced with the task of coping with loss.

**bioethics:** Also biomedical ethics, the field that focuses on helping institutions to respond appropriately to dilemmas around the use or withdrawal of medical treatment.

**brain death:** Irreversible loss of brain function to the extent that all ability to have conscious experiences or social interactions is lost.

**California Natural Death Act:** Legislation passed in 1976 permitting individuals, in specific situations, to make prior plans for treatment at the end of life, thus legally sanctioning advance directives and also protecting "physicians from being sued for failing to treat incurable illnesses" (Humphrey & Clement, 2000, p. 368).

**durable power of attorney:** The legal mechanism by means of which a person designates another to act in his or her stead, e.g., as *health care proxy* (see below).

**euthanasia:** The act of putting to death, in a painless manner, those who are incurably ill.

**grief:** One response to the experience of bereavement.

**Harvard Criteria:** A set of standards used to determine that the brain has reached a condition in which it is considered to be irreversibly nonfunctional.

**health care proxy:** The designation of a health care agent to make treatment decisions for a person should that person become unable to make such decisions for him- or herself.

**living will:** A document in which a competent adult sets forth directions regarding medical treatment in the event of his or her future incapacitation.

**mourning:** "The culturally patterned expression of the bereaved person's thoughts and feelings" (Kastenbaum, 1986, p. 139).

**Patient Self-Determination Act:** Statute requiring health care providers to give patients information about the right to make advance directives, to have written institutional policies regarding advance directives, and to document their existence.

**physician aid-in-dying:** Instances in which a physician discontinues treatment at the patient's request.

**physician-assisted suicide:** Instances in which the physician provides either information, resources, or direct assistance and the patient terminates her or his own life.

**values history:** An advance directive describing the circumstances in which continued life would not be preferred.

**voluntary active euthanasia:** Instances in which a physician gives a medication or in some way intervenes to cause death at the request of the patient.

# DISCUSSION QUESTIONS

1. Compare and contrast classical models of grieving with current professional approaches to helping clients deal with death, dying, and bereavement.
2. Compare and contrast the differences in impact and ramifications of anticipated versus unanticipated deaths.
3. Describe the issues facing both those who are dying and those who act as care givers for dying persons.
4. Describe and discuss what is meant by "nearing death awareness."
5. Describe and discuss issues that have emerged concurrent with advances in medical technology.
6. Describe and discuss the various forms of advance directives.
7. Compare and contrast the reactions of children at various ages to the death of a sibling versus the death of a parent.
8. Compare and contrast the reactions to loss of a spouse at various stages of the family life cycle.
9. Describe the process of helping clients to create special ceremonies or healing rituals, giving examples of both.
10. Describe what is meant by and involved with the search for meaning following the death of a loved one.

# SUGGESTED FURTHER READING

Becvar, D. S. (2001). *In the presence of grief: Helping family members resolve death, dying and bereavement issues.* New York: Guilford Press.

An overview of the contexts of grief as well as grief in the context of therapy.

Kübler-Ross, E. (1969). *On death and dying.* New York: Macmillan.

The landmark book describing the stages of dying.

Nolen-Hoeksema, S., & Larson, J. (1999). *Coping with loss.* Mahwah, NJ: Lawrence Erlbaum Associates.

A research-based overview of grief reactions.

Rando, T. (1991). *How to go on living when someone you love dies.* New York: Bantam Books.

A classic in the field of death, dying, and bereavement.

# REFERENCES

Aldrich, L. M. (1996, Spring). Understanding sibling grief in children and adolescents. *Thanatos,* pp. 19–21.

Beauchamp T., & Childress J. (1994). *Principles of biomedical ethics* (4th ed.). Oxford, England: Oxford University Press.

Becvar, D. S. (2001). *In the presence of grief: Helping family members resolve death, dying and bereavement issues.* New York: Guilford Press.

Becvar, D., & Becvar, R. (2003). *Family therapy: A systemic integration* (5th ed.). Boston: Allyn & Bacon.

Bernstein, J. (1997). *When the bough breaks: Forever after the death of a son or daughter.* Kansas City, MO: Andrews & McKeel.

Boss, P. (1991). Ambiguous loss. In F. Walsh & M. McGoldrick (Eds.), *Living beyond loss: Death in the family* (pp. 164–175). New York: W. W. Norton.

Bouvard, M., & Gladu, E. (1998). *The path through grief: A compassionate guide.* New York: Prometheus Books.

Bowlby, J. (1980). *Loss, sadness and depression.* New York: Basic Books.

Callanan, M., & Kelley, P. (1992). *Final gifts: Understanding the special awareness, needs, and communications of the dying.* New York: Bantam Books.

Doukas, D., & McCullough, L. (1991). The values history: The evaluation of the patient's values and advance directives. *Journal of Family Practice, 32*(2), 145–150.

Final Report of the Netherlands State Commission on Euthanasia: An English Summary (anonymous translation). (1987). *Bioethics, 1*(2), 163–174.

Foos-Graber, A. (1989). *Deathing: An intelligent alternative for the final moments of life.* York Beach, ME: Nicolas–Hays.

Humphrey, D., & Clement, M. (2000). *People, politics and the right-to-die movement.* New York: St. Martin's Griffin.

Kastenbaum, R. J. (1986). *Death, society, and human experience* (3rd ed.). Columbus, OH: Charles E. Merrill.

Klass, D. (1988). *Parental grief: Solace and resolution.* New York: Springer.

Knapp, R. (1986). *Beyond endurance: When a child dies.* New York: Shocken.

Kreilkamp, A. (1999). Caring for our own dead: Interview with Jerri Lyons, founder and director The National Death Care Project. *Crone Chronicles, 41,* 20–30, 51.

Kübler-Ross, E. (1969). *On death and dying.* New York: Macmillan.

McGoldrick, M., & Walsh, F. (1991). A time to mourn: Death and the family life cycle. In F. Walsh & M. McGoldrick (Eds.), *Living beyond loss: Death in the family* (pp. 30–49). New York: W. W. Norton.

McLean, S. (1996). End-of-life decisions and the law. *Journal of Medical Ethics, 22,* 261–262.

Moss, M. S., & Moss, S. Z. (1996). Remarriage of widowed persons: A triadic relationship. In D. Klass, P. R. Silverman, & S. L. Nickman (Eds.), *Continuing bonds: New understandings of grief* (pp. 163–178). Washington, DC: Taylor & Francis.

Nader, K. O. (1997). Treating traumatic grief in systems. In C. R. Figley, B. E. Bride, & N. Mazza (Eds.), *Death and trauma: The traumatology of grieving* (pp. 159–192). Washington, DC: Taylor & Francis.

Nolen-Hoeksema, S., & Larson, J. (1999). *Coping with loss.* Mahwah, NJ: Lawrence Erlbaum Associates.

Nurmi, L. A., & Williams, M. B. (1997). Death of a co-worker: Conceptual overview. In C. R. Figley, B. E. Bride, & N. Mazza (Eds.). *Death and trauma: The traumatology of grieving* (pp. 43–64). Washington, DC: Taylor & Francis.

Parkes, C. M., & Weiss, R. S. (1983). *Recovery from bereavement.* New York: Basic Books.

Peretz, D. (1970). Reaction to loss. In B. Schoenberg (Ed.), *Loss and grief* (pp. 20–35). New York: Columbia University Press.

Preston, T. A. (2000, May 22). Facing death on your own terms. *Newsweek, 82.*

Rando, T. (1991). *How to go on living when someone you love dies.* New York: Bantam Books.

Rando, T. (1997). Foreword. In C. R. Figley, B. E. Bride, & N. Mazza, (Eds.), *Death and trauma: The traumatology of grieving* (pp. xiv–xix). Washington, DC: Taylor & Francis.

Raphael, B. (1983). *The anatomy of bereavement.* New York: Basic Books.

Rolland, J. (1991). Helping families with anticipatory loss. In F. Walsh & M. McGoldrick (Eds.), *Living beyond loss: Death in the family* (pp. 144–163). New York: W. W. Norton.

Rosen, H. (1986). *Unspoken grief: Coping with childhood sibling loss.* Lexington, MA: Lexington Books.

Scheper, T., & Duursma, S. (1994). Euthanasia: The Dutch experience. *Age and Aging, 23,* 3–8.

Smith, H. I. (1996). *Grieving the death of a friend.* Minneapolis, MN: Augsburg Fortress.

Speckhard, A. (1997). Traumatic death in pregnancy: The significance of meaning and attachment. In C. R. Figley, B. E. Bride, & N. Mazza (Eds.). *Death and trauma: The traumatology of grieving* (pp. 101–121). Washington, DC: Taylor & Francis.

VA Medical Center. (1993). *Advance directives: Making decisions about your health care.* Seattle, WA: Author.

Young, E., & Jex, S. (1992). The Patient Self-Determination Act: Potential ethical quandaries and benefits. *Cambridge Quarterly of Healthcare Ethics, 2,* 107–115.

Zonnebelt-Smeenge, S. J., & De Vries, R. C. (1998). *Getting to the other side of grief: Overcoming the loss of a spouse.* Grand Rapids, MI: Baker Books.

# 20

# Alcohol and Other Drug Dependencies

Edward L. Hendrickson
*Private Practice*

Eric E. McCollum
*Virginia Polytechnic Institute and State University*

## TRUTH OR FICTION?

___ 1. *Most individuals do not use psychoactive substances.*

___ 2. *Alcohol is the most commonly used psychoactive substance.*

___ 3. *A family's belief system is an important factor influencing drug use.*

___ 4. *Psychoactive drug use is considered a problem when it causes difficulty in one or more areas of functioning.*

___ 5. *Tolerance means a family's acceptance of a member's drug use.*

___ 6. *The key to good assessment is developing a trusting relationship with the client.*

___ 7. *Denial and minimization should be confronted vigorously when trying to assess substance use and abuse.*

___ 8. *Other psychiatric disorders often co-occur with substance abuse.*

___ 9. *The continuum of care model suggests that it is important to start with a very intensive form of treatment at the first sign of a substance abuse problem.*

___ 10. *Individual counseling is the most common approach to substance abuse treatment.*

___ 11. *Participating in AA or other self-help groups increase the chances of a positive substance abuse treatment outcome.*

___ 12. *Though family involvement in treatment helps family members deal with stress, it does little to improve outcome for the individual with a substance abuse problem.*

___ 13. *Family members can be an effective force in convincing a drug dependent person to enter treatment.*

___ 14. *Stanton and Todd found the structural family therapy was an effective treatment for young women who were abusing alcohol.*

___ 15. *All family therapists must have the skills to competently assess for substance abuse.*

Substance abuse is a major contributor to many family problems. It is associated with child abuse and neglect, domestic violence, poor school performance, maladaptive emotional development, and economic and health problems, all of which significantly impact family functioning. At the same time, however, the majority of family members use alcohol and other drugs in a nonproblematic manner. The purpose of this chapter is to help you determine when substance use is problematic, provide an overview of effective substance abuse treatment strategies, and discuss the role and functions of family therapists when they encounter families with substance use problems.

Few individuals over the age of 12 do not use a **psychoactive** drug at least once per year. The three most commonly used psychoactive drugs in our society are caffeine, alcohol, and nicotine. It is estimated that over 80% of individuals age 12 or older use caffeine (American Psychiatric Association [APA], 2000; James, 1997), 64% use alcohol, and 35% use nicotine. Additionally, 42% have used other drugs at some point in their life, with marijuana (37%), hallucinogens (13%), cocaine (12%), pain relievers (10%), and stimulants (7%) being the most common (Substance Abuse and Mental Health Services Administration [SAMHSA], 2002). Hence, therapists should assume that almost all families they encounter will have members who are using, or have used, psychoactive drugs.

1. What is the most commonly used psychoactive substance?
   a. alcohol
   b. caffeine
   c. marijuana
   d. nicotine

Family beliefs, values, and traditions affect drug use. For example, some families condone drunkenness while other families expect only moderate alcohol use. Some families prefer to avoid uncomfortable feelings by using substances while other families expect members to express their feelings directly. Such family beliefs can either contribute to problematic use or act as a shield against it. Thus, you should not only gather information about the quantity and frequency of drug use but about also how substance use is viewed in the family, and how any substance use impacts family members.

## DIAGNOSTIC CATEGORIES

When does substance use become a problem? Though many definitions have been proposed for substance use disorders, the most commonly accepted diagnostic criteria today come from the *Diagnostic and Statistical Manual of Mental Disorders, Fourth Edition, Text Revision* (*DSM–IV–TR*) published by the American Psychiatric Association (2000). The *DSM–IV–TR* defines substance use disorders in general as maladaptive patterns of substance use leading to clinically significant impairment or distress. It then classifies such disorders into three categories: **Substance Abuse**, **Substance Dependence**, and **Substance Induced Disorders**. Each of these disorders can be diagnosed for most of the eleven categories of substances included in the *DSM–IV–TR:* alcohol, **amphetamines**, caffeine, cannabis, cocaine, **hallucinogens**, **inhalants**, nicotine, opioids, **phencyclidine** and **sedative–hypnotics**, or **anxiolytics**. The only exceptions are nicotine, which does not have an abuse diagnosis, and caffeine which has neither an abuse nor a dependency diagnosis.

## Substance Abuse Disorders

Use that causes problems in a particular life sphere is considered *substance abuse*. Four criteria are used to diagnose this disorder: substance use that causes problems with work, school or home; use that results in recurrent situations that are physically hazardous (e.g., driving while intoxicated); use that results in recurrent legal problems; or use that results in recurrent social problems. The diagnosis requires multiple recurrences of at least one of these symptoms during a twelve-month period. In other words, if the use continues to cause a problem, then it is a problem.

2. What is *not* a characteristic of a substance dependency disorder?
   a. tolerance
   b. inability to stop using once one starts
   c. having more than 2 drinks per day
   d. continuing to use after knowing that use causes problems

## Substance Dependence Disorders

*Substance dependence* is characterized by loss of control over how much a substance is used once use begins. The seven symptoms of dependence include the presence of tolerance (the need to use more of the substance to get the sought-after effect); withdrawal (occurrence of physical problems when use is discontinued); using more than was intended; unsuccessful efforts to control use; a great deal of time spent obtaining and using the substance; important life activities given up or reduced in order to use the substance; and continued use despite knowing that it causes problems. Substance dependence is diagnosed when at least three of these symptoms are present for a specific substance during a twelve-month period, and is not based only on the amount and frequency of use. Once the diagnosis is made, it is considered a life-long diagnosis. Individuals can have multiple dependence and abuse disorders (such as alcohol dependence, cocaine dependence and cannabis abuse), but not a dependence and abuse disorder of the same substance (i.e., alcohol dependence and alcohol abuse).

## Substance Induced Disorders

Disorders that have the same symptoms as a mental health disorder, but whose symptoms are the direct result of substance use and will cease shortly after use of the substance is discontinued are known as *substance induced disorders*. An example is an individual who experiences significant depression when using alcohol and cocaine but has none of these symptoms when abstinent.

## SCREENING AND ASSESSING

A variety of instruments can be used by family therapists to screen for substance use problems. The five most commonly used tools are the CAGE (Mayfield, McCleod, & Hall, 1974), a four question screening instrument for alcoholism; the Michigan Alcohol Screening Test (MAST; Selzer, 1971), a 24-item screening test for alcoholism; the Alcohol Use Disorders Identification Test (AUDIT; Babor and Grant, 1989), a 10-question screening test for alcohol disorders; the Drug Abuse Screening Test (DAST; Skinner, 1982) a 28-item screening test for drug abuse;

and the Substance Abuse Subtle Screening Inventory (SASSI), a 52-item test designed for adults or adolescents (Miller, 1985). All are in the public domain and can be used at no cost except for the SASSI which can be purchased from the SASSI institute.

3. Which *is not* a commonly used screening tool for substance use problems?
   a. MMPI
   b. CAGE
   c. MAST
   d. DAST

In addition to using structured screening tools, you should ask about substance use during initial assessments with families. There are several principles to follow when asking about substance use. Given that most people underreport their use because of the moral stigma attached to substance use in our society, these principles are designed to increase the accuracy of the information gathered. First, ask about substance use in a way that *assumes a positive response:* "What drugs have you used?" "How old were you when you first began drinking?" If a client reports that they do not use any psychoactive drugs, ask why, as it is quite uncommon not to use at least one substance occasionally. Second, when asking about the frequency and amount used, *start with the highest possible limit.* Clients will usually give only as much information as they think they must in order to satisfy the interviewer, so begin by asking if they use a *significant* amount of a substance *every day.* This both assures them that you are prepared to hear about significant substance use problems and may allow them to report a higher level than they might otherwise. Third, keep your questions *matter of fact and nonjudgmental.* Most people fear others' judgments about our substance use, a fear that may be heightened when clients come to treatment. Do your best to ask substance use questions in the same manner you would use to ask for a client's address or phone number. Fourth, *gently clarify vague responses,* such as, "I use some stuff once in a while." Ask for details persistently but in a respectful manner. However, if a client continues to give vague responses, don't press. What a client is unwilling to tell you often reveals more than what is actually said. Fifth, *use third party information.* The family, other agency's records, and friends often provide more accurate information than the client will. Finally, at the end of the assessment *evaluate the accuracy of the information provided* to determine if the client is denying, minimizing, exaggerating (normally only done by adolescents), or is being accurate about the level of substance use. Remember, however, that it usually takes time to develop an accurate picture of a client's use, so view substance abuse assessment as an ongoing process. Also remember that initial client truthfulness is not as important as developing a relationship that allows the client to trust you. Avoid playing "catch you in a lie" games. Denial and minimization are natural processes associated with substance abuse and dependency and will have to be addressed in treatment, but not necessarily at the start.

4. Screening for substance abuse:
   a. should be left to professional substance abuse counselors.
   b. should be part of a family therapist's assessment of every family or client.
   c. should only be done after a strong therapeutic alliance has been established.
   d. none of the above.

In addition to the problem of getting accurate information, the high **co-occurrence** of other mental disorders with substance use disorders (Kessler et al., 1994) can create a confusing diagnostic picture for the family therapist. Twenty-two psychiatric disorders frequently

**TABLE 20.1**

Mental Disorders That Frequently Co-Occur with Substance Use Disorders

| | |
|---|---|
| *Mood Disorders* | *Psychotic Disorders* |
| Bipolar | Schizophrenia |
| Major Depression | Schizoaffective |
| Dysthymia | *Dissociative Disorders* |
| Cyclothymia | Dissociative Identity Disorder |
| *Anxiety Disorders* | Depersonalization |
| Social Phobia | *Attention-Deficit & Disruptive* |
| Obsessive–Compulsive | *Behavior Disorders* |
| Posttraumatic Stress | Conduct Disorder |
| Generalized Anxiety | Oppositional Defiant |
| *Personality Disorders* | ADHD |
| Antisocial | *Impulse-Control Disorders* |
| Borderline | Pathological Gambling |
| Histrionic | |
| *Eating Disorders* | |
| Bulimia | |
| Anorexia | |

co-occur with substance use disorders (Table 20.1). Each of these disorders produces symptoms that complicate assessment, and are hard to distinguish from substance induced disorders. Four key questions can help the family therapist make this distinction.

1. *Did the psychiatric symptoms predate the onset of the substance use?* Though many clients are poor historians, this information is often available from other family members or long-time friends.
2. *Is there a history of similar mental disorders in the client's biological family?* Many of these disorders have a genetic basis and are more common in biological relatives than in the general population.
3. *Is the onset of the symptoms within the normal age range?* Although there are always exceptions, most mental disorders have a normal age range for symptoms to develop. Significant deviations from these ranges may indicate a substance induced disorder.
4. *Is there a significant change in the psychiatric symptoms after two or more weeks of abstinence?* Though it normally takes an extended period of time for all the symptoms of a substance induced disorder to disappear, a significant reduction of symptoms generally occurs within two weeks of abstinence from most drugs.

A final two-part question to ask clients is *have you ever gone a period of time without using,* and if so, *did your psychiatric symptoms get better or worse?* Although only abstinence or the availability of long-term treatment records can give a clear diagnostic picture, the above questions will serve as a basic screening.

5. Which of the following are common co-occurring disorders with substance abuse?
   a. depression
   b. generalized anxiety
   c. schizophrenia
   d. all of the above

## TREATMENT PLACEMENT AND THE CONTINUUM OF CARE

Once a substance use disorder has been identified, where is the best place to treat it and what treatment modality will be the most effective? The most commonly used client placement criteria are the Patient Placement Criteria for the Treatment of Substance-Related Disorders developed by the American Society of Addiction Medicine (ASAM PPC-2R, 2002). These schemata use six client dimensions (ranging from acute withdrawal to recovery) to determine which of the five levels of care (see following sections) is most appropriate for a client. Additionally, the criteria define a treatment setting as being addiction-only, dual diagnosis capable (for clients whose psychiatric symptoms are mostly stable) and dual diagnosis enhanced (for clients whose psychiatric symptoms are not stable). These levels of care follow closely the traditional substance abuse continuum of care system that includes prevention/early intervention, outpatient treatment, detoxification/residential treatment, and relapse prevention/supportive living. The following is a brief description of each of these traditional treatment components of the substance abuse continuum of care.

> 6. Which *is true* about ASAM Placement Criteria?
>    a. Client dimensions are used for determining treatment placement.
>    b. Levels of care reflect levels of treatment intensity.
>    c. Treatment settings can be defined as addiction only, dual diagnosis capable, or dual diagnosis enhanced.
>    d. All are true about ASAM Placement Criteria.

## Prevention/Early Intervention

The substance abuse profession has a long tradition of providing interventions aimed at preventing substance use problems or intervening with individuals who are engaging in high risk behavior such as driving while intoxicated. Prevention and early intervention activities usually are psychoeducational and are designed to give youth and high risk adults greater knowledge about the risks of substance use in order to help them make more thoughtful decisions. Prevention and early intervention activities may also include brief counseling interventions targeted at problems that might lead to substance abuse, such as depression or family conflict. Among other successes, prevention activities have played an important part in helping reduce adolescent drug use from its high point in 1979 (Johnson, O'Malley, & Bachman, 2002).

> 7. What *is not* a characteristic of psychoeducational approaches?
>    a. providing information about substance abuse
>    b. helping clients discuss how they can apply information about substance abuse to their own lives
>    c. giving clients psychological tests to better educate them about their strengths and weaknesses
>    d. providing a safe environment that allows persons to share what they think and feel about alcohol and drug use

## Outpatient Treatment

Outpatient treatment encompasses a wide range of services in a variety of nonresidential settings. The services range in intensity from once a week groups to daily participation in partial hospitalization programs to opioid maintenance therapy (see "Treatment Modalities"). The majority of individuals in substance abuse treatment at any given time are receiving treatment in outpatient settings. The type and intensity of services normally reflects the individual's treatment history. First-time clients usually have less intense services (e.g., once a week group treatment) while clients with previous treatment failures move to more intensive services (e.g., partial hospitalization).

## Detoxification/Residential Treatment

*Detoxification* is the process of helping an individual manage the immediate physical and psychological symptoms resulting from the discontinuation of a drug. Depending on the extent and the type of drug used, detoxification may take a few hours or several weeks. Detoxification programs focus on stabilizing a client during the period they are experiencing withdrawal symptoms from their drugs of choice. These programs may be hospital based or use a social detoxification format (e.g., a nonmedical residential facility). Most individuals can withdraw from most drugs without intensive medical monitoring (exceptions being withdrawal from certain sedatives and individuals with complicating medical conditions). However, managing the emotional consequences can be more difficult. Substance abuse professionals quickly recognized that medical detoxification alone produced few instances of long-term sobriety, and extended stays in treatment after detoxification has become standard practice. The Minnesota 28-day treatment model is one form of residential treatment and involves an intensive focus on all aspects of the client's life to understand, and begin to change, the causes and consequences of addiction. Another common form of residential treatment is the therapeutic community model that grew out of the Synanon Program begun in California in the 1950s. Therapeutic communities usually involve longer treatment stays (3–6 months or more) and focus on teaching their members new ways of thinking and behaving with an emphasis on self-responsibility.

8. Which *is most true* about detoxification services for substance abuse treatment?
   a. Detoxification services usually occur before outpatient treatment.
   b. Drug detoxification may take a few hours or several weeks depending on the drug and amount used.
   c. Detoxification services must take place in a medical setting.
   d. Withdrawal from most drugs is life threatening.

9. Therapeutic communities usually involve:
   a. longer treatment stays than other residential placements (3 months or more).
   b. clients returning to live in the community where they grew up.
   c. having friends and neighbors monitor a client's activities to prevent relapse.
   d. being held in a locked facility.

## Relapse Prevention/Supportive Housing

Because substance dependence disorders are viewed as lifelong with relapse always a risk, relapse prevention becomes the primary treatment intervention once stable recovery has been achieved. Relapse prevention activities are psychoeducation and skill building in nature and focus on providing the individual with the knowledge and skills necessary to maintain long-term recovery. Relapse prevention skills include such things as managing cravings, learning to socialize without using drugs, or developing anger management skills. Individuals in early recovery also often need a living environment that is drug free and supportive of their recovery.

Such supportive living environments (often called *halfway houses*) may be professionally managed or function as a self-run program managed by the recovering residents themselves. Professionally run recovery homes normally have a resident counselor who monitors the activities of the residents and provides ongoing treatment as needed. Self-run settings rely on residents to set policies and determine house structure. The most common form of self-run house is called Oxford Houses. The first of these houses opened in 1975 and currently there are nearly a 1,000 nationwide found in almost every state. In 1988 the federal government required states to establish a revolving loan fund to provide start-up money for such self-run recovery houses. Most individuals stay from six months to a year in these supportive living environments.

10. Oxford Houses are:
  a. a form of residential treatment.
  b. self-run recovery houses.
  c. very similar to therapeutic communities.
  d. treatment facilities located in jails.

## TREATMENT MODALITIES

Once an individual has entered treatment, a wide variety of modalities are available for the treatment of substance use disorders. Treatment models fall under the categories of medication, group therapy, individual therapy, and case management. It is common for clients to receive more than one of these modalities at a given time.

### Medication Treatments

Medications used in substance abuse treatment include detoxification aids, opioid replacement agents, and symptom management medications. Medications are often used when individuals are detoxifying from alcohol, sedative–hypnotics, and opioids. Some are used to ease the discomfort of the withdrawal symptoms, some are used to speed up the withdrawal process, some are used to begin the repair of body systems damaged by years of drug use, and some are used to reduce life threatening reactions to withdrawal such as seizures. Medications used for detoxification are commonly taken only for the detoxification period and are discontinued when withdrawal symptoms are stabilized.

Opioid replacement therapy involves switching one narcotic drug for another. The first such medication used—Methadone—was introduced in 1963 (Dole & Nyswander, 1965) and is the most common form of opioid replacement therapy in use today. In the 1970s, Levo-Alpha-Acetylmethadol (LAAM), a longer-acting medication than methadone was introduced, and, in 2002, Buprenorphine, which is less likely to cause an overdose or be diverted into illegal channels, was approved as an opioid replacement medication. The advantage of these drugs is that they are much longer acting than heroin and other narcotics, can be taken orally, and are less deterimental to the day to day functioning of the user. Drug replacement therapy is used for individuals with long histories of narcotic dependence who have not done well in other types of treatment. Individuals usually are maintained on these drugs for long periods of time. Another form of drug replacement therapy currently in use is nicotine replacement that comes in the form of a patch, gum, nasal spray, inhaler, or lozenge.

Few medications have been developed specifically for substance dependence symptom management. The first medication introduced in 1948 was Disulfiram (Antabuse). Disulfiram interferes with how alcohol is metabolized in such a way that an individual who drinks alcohol while taking this medication will become acutely ill. Disulfiram can be effective for highly motivated individuals with multiple relapse histories who need additional support to deal with their cravings. Another medication, Naltrexone, introduced in 1984, blocks the euphoric effects of heroin and other opioids. Thus, clients taking Naltrexone will not get high should they choose to use heroin. This medication was also found in the 1990s to be helpful in reducing the frequency and amount of alcohol use for individuals with alcohol dependence disorder. Buproprion (an antidepressant) has also been found to reduce nicotine cravings.

The National Institute on Drug Abuse (NIDA) and the National Institute on Alcohol Abuse and Alcoholism (NIAAA) have vigorous research programs devoted to developing medications that reduce cravings or block the effectiveness of substances, so it seems clear that, in the future, medications will play an important role in the treatment of substance use disorders. Where medications currently play a major part in the treatment of substance use disorders is in the treatment of co-occurring mental disorders. Studies have found that substance disorders are difficult to stabilize when major symptoms of mental disorders are present (Greenfield et al., 1998). Thus, medication effectiveness and compliance are issues that family therapists face when working with families who have members with substance use disorders.

11. Which of the following *is not* a use for medication in the treatment of substance abuse?
    a. reducing the symptoms associated with detoxification
    b. blocking the effects of heroin or other opioids
    c. revealing underlying emotional conflicts that lead to substance use
    d. relieving mental illness symptoms that can lead to substance use

12. Which was the first medication developed for use in treating substance abuse?
    a. Antabuse
    b. LAAM
    c. Naltrexone
    d. Methadone

## Group Treatment

Group treatment is by far the most common treatment modality currently used for substance use disorders. Treatment groups are typically either psychoeducational or cognitive–behavioral in nature. In an effort to motivate clients to change their drug use, *psychoeducation* both provides information about alcohol and drug use and helps clients understand how that information applies to them personally. For example, a group session might focus on the stages of addiction and ask each participant to describe which stage he or she is in. Psychoeducational groups use lectures, written materials, audio-visual aids, discussions guided toward self-disclosure, and skill building exercises to achieve their goals. Such groups are usually time-limited with little if any change in membership.

In contrast to the educational focus of psychoeducation groups, *cognitive–behavioral* therapy groups are designed to provide a safe environment in which participants can share what they think, feel, and do in relationship to alcohol and drug use. The goal for individuals with substance abuse disorders is nonproblematic use and the goal for individuals with dependence or substance induced disorders is abstinence. Such groups focus on overcoming denial; promoting the acknowledgment of substance use problems; making a commitment to change; and planning, implementing, and evaluating new behaviors. Therapy groups may be time-limited or ongoing, and some may have a stable membership while others may have individuals entering and leaving throughout the life of the group.

> 13. Which *is not true* about substance abuse group treatment?
>     a. It is the most common treatment modality for substance abuse.
>     b. It may be held in the form of either psychoeducation or a talk therapy group.
>     c. The group may be time-limited or ongoing.
>     d. All the above are true.

## Individual Treatment

In general, substance abuse treatment views individual therapy as an adjunct to group treatment. It may be used either to prepare individuals for group treatment or to provide extra support for those already in a treatment group. In fact, most individuals do participate effectively in substance abuse group treatment and benefit greatly from peer sharing and feedback, requiring little or no individual attention. However, a few clients with extreme psychiatric symptoms that cannot be stabilized, such as being so paranoid that they are highly uncomfortable around others, will need to receive individual treatment.

In 1991, Miller and Rollnick introduced a brief individual counseling approach called *motivational interviewing* (MI). MI is designed to increase motivation for change and follows five principles: express empathy, develop discrepancy between an individual's goals and their current life situation, avoid arguments, roll with the resistance, and support self-efficacy. MI stands in stark contrast to previous approaches that emphasized a confrontational approach to substance abuse treatment. MI is often used in individual sessions to prepare clients for groups and is also used for individuals who have been sent for a substance abuse evaluation but who will probably not continue in treatment because of limited external leverage. This model has been shown to increase motivation for change as well as treatment engagement and retention. Its use has greatly increased in the last decade and is often integrated into individual substance abuse interventions.

> 14. Motivational interviewing is designed to be given:
>     a. in a group setting.
>     b. in an individual setting.
>     c. through reading and doing worksheets.
>     d. none are true.
>
> 15. One of the ways that motivational interviewing differs from more traditional treatment is that it:
>     a. confronts clients with their lack of motivation to change.
>     b. does not directly confront clients about their drug use.
>     c. is much more confrontational than traditional substance abuse treatment.
>     d. all of the above.

## Case Management

Case management has been given many different meanings, but in general it is considered the professional function of connecting clients with needed services and monitoring both their participation in those services and the effectiveness of those services. The Center for

Substance Abuse Treatment (1998) identified seven principles of effective substance abuse case management: Case management services offer a single point of contact for all services, are driven by client need, are community based, are pragmatic, are anticipatory, are flexible, and are culturally sensitive. For years, individuals with substance use disorders have received case management–like services from a variety of professionals in such places as skid row missions, detoxification centers, halfway houses, and outpatient treatment centers. Case management may be especially important to therapists working with families where one or more family members has a substance abuse problem. Many such families face a variety of treatment, financial, and health needs and often need help in accessing these services. Thus, case management must be considered as one of the family therapist's functions when working with families with substance use problems.

## Self-Help Groups

Though not a treatment modality provided by professionally trained therapists, self-help groups play an important part in the treatment of substance use disorders. Alcoholics Anonymous (AA) is the oldest self-help program currently functioning. It was established in 1935 by two recovering alcoholics to help others attain sobriety. The early groups developed 12 steps and traditions designed to help dependent persons overcome alcohol use. AA has served as a model for many other self-help programs ranging from Narcotics Anonymous to Emotions Anonymous. Support groups also exist for family members, with Al-Anon, Nar-Anon, and Families Anonymous being the most common. Additionally, other self-help programs have been founded as a reaction to the perceived religious or spiritual nature of 12-step programs. SMART and Life Ring Secular Recovery are examples of programs which eschew any mention of religious or spiritual concepts. The advantage of all of these groups is that most are free, they can provide needed support around the clock, and they provide a clear method of dealing with dependence disorders. Research has shown that individuals in treatment who also participate in self-help groups have better treatment outcomes (National Institute on Alcohol Abuse and Alcoholism, 2000). It is important that family therapists be familiar with the functioning of these programs and support family members' participation in them.

16. Alcoholics Anonymous:
    a. was established by two ministers to help alcoholics recover.
    b. began in the 1890s.
    c. improves the outcome for clients in other types of substance abuse treatment.
    d. Is a religious organization.

17. SMART is an example of:
    a. a 12-step program.
    b. a religious-oriented recovery program.
    c. a program that avoids mentioning religious or spiritual concepts.
    d. none of the above.

## EFFECTS OF SUBSTANCE ABUSE ON THE FAMILY

Substance use disorders can significantly impact the functioning and the well-being of the family, and family therapists must be aware of the types of issues that families with substance use problems encounter. The following is an overview of the common child physical and emotional development, abuse and violence, and health and economic issues that such families face.

## Child Physical Development

Adults who use drugs not only affect their own health and relationships, they create the potential for harm to their children as well. Drawing on data from the 1999 and 2000 National Household Survey on Drug Abuse (NHSDA), the Substance Abuse and Mental Health Services Administration (SAMHSA) reported that 3% of pregnant women aged 15 to 44 reported using an illicit drug in the month prior to being interviewed, whereas 12% of pregnant women reported drinking alcohol during the same time period (Substance Abuse and Mental Health Services Administration [SAMHSA], 2002). Women were more likely to report using alcohol or illicit drugs during the first trimester of pregnancy when the effects of the substance on the developing fetus may be more severe. The effects of prenatal exposure to alcohol and other drugs are well documented. Cook, Petersen, and Moore (1990) report that,

> In utero *drug exposure is associated with an increased rate among newborns of (1) low birth weight, with small for gestational age length and head size, (2) central nervous system damage that may delay or impair neurobehavioral development, (3) mild to severe withdrawal effects, and (4) certain congenital physical malformations. (p. 5)*

Low birth-weight babies incur substantially higher medical costs than do normal birth-weight infants. One estimate puts the average cost difference at $59,700 over the first year of life (RAND Corporation, 1998). Finally, drug abuse may disrupt the pregnancy itself resulting in such negative events as spontaneous abortion, precipitous delivery, fetal distress, and hemorrhage.

18. *In utero* drug exposure *is not* associated with:
   a. low birth weight.
   b. missed menstrual periods.
   c. central nervous system damage to the child.
   d. withdrawal symptoms.

## Child Emotional Development

A variety of other ills befall the children of substance-abusing parents including increased risk for depression and conduct disorder (Merikangas, Dierker, & Szatmari, 1998), higher rates of lifetime suicidal ideation (Pfeffer, Normandin, & Kakuma, 1998), and more frequent periods of living outside the nuclear family during childhood (Goldberg, Lex, Mello, Mendelson, & Bower, 1996). Children of substance abusing parents are also at greater risk for substance abuse themselves (Merikangas, et al., 1998) as well as careers as adult criminals (Johnson, Dunlap, & Maher, 1998).

## Abuse and Violence

Child abuse and neglect is often associated with drug and alcohol abuse. Bays (1990) lists a number of factors associated with drug abuse that put substance-abusing parents at greater risk to abuse or neglect their children. These include diverting family resources from meeting the needs of the children to supporting the addiction, criminal activity to support an addiction, mental and physical illness, poor parenting skills, side effects of drugs, and family violence. Additionally, substance abuse is significantly associated with violence between spouses or intimate partners (Greenfeld, 1998), which can have significant impact on the harmed individual or other family members observing the violence.

19. Which of the following are causes of child abuse and neglect when parents are using drugs?
    a. using family money to support a drug habit rather than care of the children
    b. poor parenting skills
    c. mental and physical illness
    d. all of the above

## Economic Costs

The National Institutes of Health estimate that alcohol and drug abuse cost society approximately $246 billion per year in lost productivity, crime, and health care costs (National Institute on Drug Abuse, 1998). This has a direct impact on families who are estimated to absorb 45% of the economic loss that society experiences as a result of drug and alcohol abuse (National Institute on Alcohol Abuse and Alcoholism, 2000).

20. Alcohol and drug use costs to society result from which of the following?
    a. lost productivity
    b. Increased health care costs
    c. Increased crime
    d. all of the above

## FAMILY INTERVENTION MODELS

Family members can play an important role throughout the treatment process. Stanton and Shadish (1997) reviewed all outcome studies available and found that family approaches result in greater engagement of people in treatment, greater treatment completion, and more favorable outcomes than do individual approaches. Therefore, one of the primary advantages of family treatment is that it works. This is not to say, of course, that individual or group approaches don't work or are never appropriate. At times, family members may be unwilling or unable to participate in treatment. Under these circumstances, however, there is some evidence to suggest that a systemic approach with one person (i.e., looking at the interpersonal context of substance abuse and not just individual factors) may be as effective as conjoint therapy (McCollum, Lewis, Nelson, Trepper, & Wetchler, in press). In addition, domestic violence is a common occurrence in couples where one or both partners are using. Although O'Farrell and Murphy (1995) report that couple violence is significantly reduced by couples treatment, care must be taken to screen out couples where the violence is too severe, or the victimized partner wants to end the relationship, in order to ensure safety.

21. Involving families in treatment:
    a. requires the therapist's ability to keep secrets.
    b. should only be done with adolescents who are using drugs.
    c. improves treatment retention and outcome.
    d. requires all family members to be present.

There are challenges for the therapist in conducting treatment for families in which a member is abusing substances. Such families can generate high levels of emotional intensity both in and outside of sessions during treatment that may take therapist time and energy to manage and require that members of the therapy team be available outside of regular office hours. A further challenge is that although family therapy is a clinically- and cost-effective treatment for substance abuse, it still is not widely used in general substance abuse treatment, and may be seen (wrongly, in our view) as interfering with treatment approaches that emphasize individual responsibility and confrontation. Marriage and family therapists who work in substance abuse treatment agencies may have to prove the merit of their approach and establish its usefulness.

In the following sections, we describe several approaches to marriage and family therapy that have empirical support for their effectiveness. We distinguish family therapy approaches from the typical "family night" or "family group" psychoeducational programs that are often part of group treatment. Psychoeducational programs present general principles of substance abuse and recovery in an educational format and family members are encouraged to apply those principles to their own situations. Family therapy approaches, on the other hand, depend on an individual understanding of each family to develop a specific treatment plan. While a family therapy model may have components that are applied to all or most families who are treated with that model, the actual timing and application of each component is tailored to the needs of each family. We will discuss family approaches in three broad categories—treatment engagement, behavioral couple therapy, and family therapy.

## Treatment Engagement

One of the first hurdles that people with substance abuse problems must overcome is their reluctance to admit to a problem and enter treatment or join a self-help group. Family and social network approaches have been used since the 1970s in family therapy (e.g., Speck & Attneave, 1973) and this influence has also been felt in the field of substance abuse treatment where family members and important others in a chemically dependent person's life have worked together to convince the person to enter treatment.

### Johnson Intervention Technique

Perhaps the best-known family-oriented approach to treatment engagement is Vernon Johnson's intervention technique (Johnson, 1986). In a Johnson intervention, family members and important others (for example, an employer or minister) meet with a professional to prepare for the meeting with the substance-abusing family member. Planning involves deciding who should be in the meeting, developing a desired outcome (typically, persuading the family member to enter treatment), and organizing a schedule. These meetings are held without the knowledge of the substance-abusing family member, who comes to the intervention unaware. In its classic form, a Johnson intervention involves each participant sharing both their love and concern for the family member and the emotional effects that the addiction has had on him or her. The family member is urged to accept help and family members often offer an ultimatum if he or she does not do so (e.g., "If you don't enter treatment, I will leave you."). Part of the planning process is to make sure that a treatment plan and resources are already in place with the hope that the family member will leave the intervention meeting to immediately begin treatment.

There is evidence to suggest that the intervention approach works when families carry through. Logan (1983) reported a 90% success rate with 60 families and Loneck, Garrett, and Banks (1996) found intervention to be more effective at getting a chemically dependent person

(CDP) to enter treatment than was coerced entry (e.g., court order)—and better at getting them to complete treatment. Despite its widespread use, Johnson's approach has raised concerns. Families must carry out the intervention for it to be effective. Liepman, Nirenberg, and Begin (1989) found that only 7 of 25 families who began the intervention planning process actually carried through, resulting in only 6 family members beginning treatment—a 25% success rate. Why the reluctance to follow through? Lewis (1991) contends that the confrontational nature of an intervention meeting may frighten family members who may fear giving their family member an ultimatum. In fact, many family members, especially women, are reluctant to carry out the intervention plan because of its confrontational nature (Barber & Gilbertson, 1997).

22. One problem with the Johnson Intervention technique is:
    a. it requires too much time for most families.
    b. it limits involvement to only one or two family members.
    c. many families are reluctant to follow through with the plan because it is confrontational.
    d. it is not very effective at getting family members to stay in treatment.

## A Relational Intervention Sequence for Engagement (ARISE)

In an effort to remedy some of the difficulties with the Johnson method, Garrett, Landau, and Stanton developed ARISE (Garrett et al., 1998). There are several differences between ARISE and the Johnson approach. First, there is no secrecy. The substance-abusing family member is told from the beginning that the family is meeting to talk about his or her problem and how to help. They are invited to attend all meetings. Second, an array of options is offered to the family ranging from intervening with their family member themselves with telephone support from the professional to a full-scale Johnson intervention. The decision about what level of effort to expend is based on the professional's assessment of the substance-abusing family member's readiness for change (Prochaska & DiClemente, 1986). Chemically dependent people who are already feeling ambivalent about their substance abuse may need little effort on the part of the professional while a CDP who is still firmly entrenched in denial may require several network meetings over 2 to 3 months. Thus, ARISE does not use a "one size fits all" approach but tailors the work to the needs of each individual and his or her family.

Finally, ARISE is based on a model of family strengths that differs from the pathology-oriented view of other approaches. Both family members and the CDP are reminded that they all bring resources to the process and that all can contribute to a solution to what is a *family* problem. Both the intervention continuum and the focus on strengths appear to decrease family and CDP resistance.

Garrett, Landau-Stanton, Stanton, Stellato-Kabat, and Stellato-Kabat (1997) report that ARISE is as effective at treatment engagement as is coercion by the courts or an employer or self-referral. By definition, CDPs brought by their families represent a highly resistant group so the equivalence between these groups is important. In addition, nearly 90% of the CDPs whose families used the ARISE method completed a 16-week intensive outpatient program compared to the same proportion of the coerced group and only 48% of the self-referred group. Again, since family members may be able to intervene before a CDP has reached the point at which legal or employment consequences are in place, the equivalence of the coerced and ARISE groups is important. Finally, the staged method used by ARISE interventionists appears to be useful. Landau and Garrett (2002) report that 83% of 110 CDPs became involved in treatment via the ARISE approach and 55% became engaged after only one telephone call from a concerned family member.

23. The ARISE family intervention model differs from the Johnson Intervention model in that:
    a. the substance-abusing member is told from the beginning that the family is concerned about the substance use.
    b. family members can choose a wide variety of intervention options.
    c. it is not nearly as effective as the Johnson intervention model.
    d. a and b are both correct.

## Behavioral Couple Therapy

There is a growing body of evidence supporting the usefulness of couple therapy in the treatment of addiction. Much of this research has been done by O'Farrell and associates at the Harvard Medical School who use a cognitive–behavioral approach. Behavioral couple therapy (BCT) involves several components. First, the CDP negotiates a *sobriety contract* with his or her partner. The couple meets daily and the CDP uses this meeting to pledge abstinence for that day, following the "one-day-at-a-time" tradition of AA. The partner records the CDP's success at keeping the contract daily. Attendance at 12-step meetings and urine screens are also recorded if they are part of the CDP's overall treatment plan. Other studies have used contracting to ensure that the alcoholic patient takes Disulfiram (Antabuse) daily (see, for instance, Rotunda & O'Farrell, 1997). The partner witnesses and records the alcoholic patient taking the medication and the partner then thanks the patient for his or her willingness to take medication to conquer the alcohol problem.

In addition to sobriety contracting, BCT typically prescribes a variety of assignments to change couple interactions. "Catch Your Partner Doing Something Nice" and "Caring Days" interventions are used to increase positive feelings between partners. In the former, partners are asked to notice one positive thing their partner does each day; in the latter, partners plan a special day with activities designed to demonstrate their caring for their partner. "Shared Positive Activities" result in couples spending time together in enjoyable activities, which have often been abandoned given the conflict surrounding the addiction. Finally, "Communication Skills" are taught to help clients manage conflict in a productive manner.

24. Behavioral couple therapy:
    a. often involves a sobriety contract.
    b. requires sufficient communication skills to negotiate successfully.
    c. requires couples meet on a monthly basis.
    d. all of the above.

Several research studies (summarized in O'Farrell & Fals-Stewart, 2000) have shown the efficacy of behavioral marital therapy with male alcoholic patients. O'Farrell and Fals-Stewart conclude that the studies demonstrate a pattern of "more abstinence and fewer alcohol-related problems, happier relationships, and lower risk of marital separation for alcoholic patients who receive BCT than for patients who receive only individual treatment" (p. 52). Similar findings are reported for drug problems and for women who are drug or alcohol dependent (Winters, Fals-Stewart, O'Farrell, Hirchler, & Kelley, 2002).

While a number of attempts have been made to design couples treatment models based on systems theory concepts, the outcome findings on such models are equivocal at best about their efficacy. Some studies show family systems approaches are superior to individual treatment (McCollum et al., in press) or a control group (Orchen as cited in O'Farrell & Fals-Stewart, 2002), whereas Grigg (as cited in O'Farrell & Fals-Stewart, 2002) found no difference. In addition, there is little evidence that one form of systems intervention differs from another. This area of the field needs continuing development both in terms of developing systemic models of treatment and in rigorously evaluating them.

## Family Therapy

Family therapy for substance abuse has focused primarily on the treatment of adolescents and young adults in the context of their families of origin. Because of the family's influence on all aspects of substance abuse and treatment—from initiation of substance use to treatment outcome—researchers and clinicians have been interested in family approaches to treatment for more than 20 years, beginning with Stanton and Todd's (1982) work with heroin addicts and their families. Stanton and Todd found that young heroin addicts had much more frequent contact with their families of origin than the societal image of the "loner" drug addict would suggest. The research literature suggests that 80% to 95% of addicts under the age of 35 have at least weekly contact with one or both parents (Stanton & Shadish, 1997), a finding that lends credence to the use of family approaches with young adults.

### *Structural Family Therapy*

Stanton and Todd used structural family therapy in their work and found that family therapy was significantly better than nonfamily therapy approaches. Structural family therapy has continued to be the basis for most of the family therapy work being done in the field, probably as a result of the generally chaotic nature of families in which one or more members are abusing drugs or alcohol.

Stanton and Todd focused first on the client–parent (or adult caregiver) triad and worked to disentangle the CDP from his[1] parents' relationship. Developmentally, this model assumes that the CDP and his parents are stuck in a "launching phase" and that drug abuse serves, in part at least, to maintain the position of the CDP as not yet emancipated from the family. Reframing (described by Stanton and Todd as making "noble ascriptions" about family members' intentions) is also part of this model. Seemingly negative acts are placed in a context of adapting to a difficult context. For instance, parents might be told that their "codependent" behavior with a young adult is evidence of their love in a situation where there are few good choices available to them. Similarly, a CDP might be told that he is sacrificing his independence through drug use and continued reliance on his parents as a way to make sure his family is not faced with the problems his emancipation would unmask. Finally, typical structural work is undertaken to establish boundaries between the CDP and his parents and to strengthen the parental/marital relationship. Goals of treatment include drug and alcohol abstinence on the part of the CDP, productive use of time (school or work), and living independently from parents.

Stanton and Todd were the first to produce evidence that family therapy might be an effective treatment for substance abuse. They found that their two family therapy conditions (family therapy where families were paid to attend, and family therapy where they were

---

[1] We use the male pronoun because all of the participants in Stanton and Todd's study were male.

not paid) were better able to reduce drug and alcohol abuse than were the two comparison conditions—nonfamily treatment (group therapy for the CDP only) and family movies, a group where families watched educational movies about families in various cultures. This condition served as a placebo treatment.

25. In Stanton and Todd's early work with heroin users:
    a. methadone was used for all clients.
    b. clients were required to work or go to school.
    c. clients were encouraged to live with their parents for support to prevent relapse.
    d. clients were encouraged to avoid contact with their families for the first 90 days of their treatment.

26. Stanton and Todd found that:
    a. family therapy was more effective than nonfamily treatment.
    b. group treatment was more effective than family treatment.
    c. both were equally effective.
    d. it was absolutely necessary to pay families if they were to participate in treatment.

## Multiple System Approaches

In true systemic fashion, recently the focus of intervention for adolescent substance abusers has moved from the family to encompass larger systems that are thought to influence substance abuse and other antisocial behaviors—peer group, school, and the general community. Thus, family therapy becomes part of a larger treatment effort that attempts to make changes in many areas of an adolescent's life in order to construct a social network that supports sobriety and prosocial behavior. Henggeler's multisystemic therapy (MST) is one example of a multiple system approach. MST therapists work intensively (usually several hours a week) with an adolescent and his or her family to create a new environment for the adolescent. Adolescents are removed from deviant peer groups, encouraged to focus on school or work success, and their families are involved in supportive relationships with community resources that will help them help their child. Family interventions are largely structural in nature and emphasize putting parents in charge of their children, providing clear consequences for the child's behavior, and increasing positive interactions. This work often involves some attention to the marital and parental subsystem since conflict between parents may keep them from communicating effectively with one another about the child's needs. MST has been shown to be effective on a variety of outcome measures for substance-abusing youth, including reducing substance abuse (Henggeler et al., 1991), and improving school performance and family functioning (Brown, Henggeler, Schoenwald, Brondino, & Pickerel, 1999). MST is also successful at retaining families in treatment. Henggeler, Pickerel, Brondino, & Crouch (1996), for example, reported that 98% of 60 families completed a full course of treatment averaging 130 days. A similar model—multidimensional family therapy (Liddle, 2002)—is aimed specifically at adolescent substance abuse. It also has been demonstrated to help youth reduce their use of drugs and alcohol.

27. Multisystemic approaches to treatment:
    a. use multiple systems theories to create change.
    b. can be delivered in only one or two hours a week.
    c. intervene in many areas of an adolescent's life.
    d. has not been a very effective approach.

## TREATMENT RETENTION, READMISSION, AND OUTCOME

Treatment for substance use disorders has been found to be overwhelmingly more effective than no treatment. A variety of factors appear to contribute to positive treatment outcomes. The seven variables that are linked to positive treatment outcomes are as follows: longer treatment stays, being older, being employed, being married, family involvement in treatment, participation in self-help groups and, for narcotic addicts, having the proper methadone dosage (Hartel et al., 1995; Hoffman, Harrison and Belille, 1983; Hubbard et al., 1989; Mammo & Weinbaum, 1993; O'Farrel, Cutter, Choquette, Floyd, & Bayog, 1992; Simpson and Sells, 1982; Vallant, 1983). Similar factors have been found to contribute to positive treatment outcomes for individuals with co-occurring mental disorders (Bond, McDonel, Miller, & Pensec, 1991; Hendrickson, Stith, Schmal, 1995; Maisto, Carey, Carey, Purnine, & Barnes, 1999). Two of these variables—being married and family involvement in treatment—are factors on which family therapists traditionally have direct impact.

Of these variables, the key outcome predictor for individuals with a substance use disorder appears to be *retention in treatment*. In general, the longer individuals stay in treatment, the better they do in the long run. Several large-scale substance abuse treatment outcome studies (Hubbard et al., 1989; Hubbard, Craddock, Flynn, Anderson, & Etherridge, 1997; Simpson & Sells, 1982), found that 90 days' retention in treatment is a critical threshold that predicts long-term substance abuse changes for both outpatient and residential treatment. The critical threshold for methadone maintenance is one-year retention. A study of adolescents in substance abuse treatment also found the same 90 days threshold for significantly increased positive outcomes for outpatient and residential treatments. Additionally, a study by Hendrickson and Schmal (2000) found that 90 days' retention is also a critical threshold for predicting positive treatment outcome for individuals with co-occurring serious mental illness and substance use disorders. Treatment stays of at least 90 days appear to be a critical variable in predicting long-term treatment outcomes for substance use disorders.

Though readmission rates are often viewed as a negative treatment outcome, several substance abuse studies (Hubbard et al., 1989; Simpson and Sells, 1982) find that accumulative treatment time can be as effective as a single treatment episode. Thus readmission can ultimately contribute to a positive treatment outcome. Major substance abuse studies have found that 54% to 59% of clients entering substance abuse treatment had been in some form of substance abuse treatment prior to that admission (Hubbard et al., 1989, Hubbard et al., 1997; SAMHSA, 1994). Treatment Episode Data (TED; SAMHSA, 1998) that maintains information on substance abuse treatment programs receiving federal funding reports that the more intensive the treatment service, the more likely that it is not the client's first admission. Thirty percent of clients admitted to outpatient programs had prior substance abuse treatment services, and 50% of clients admitted to residential programs and 70% of individuals admitted to methadone programs had prior treatment admissions. Thus, it is important that family therapists promote family involvement in the treatment process and completion of substance abuse treatment.

28. Which *is not* a variable that predicts successful substance abuse treatment?
    a. being older
    b. having the proper methadone dose
    c. volunteering for treatment
    d. being employed

29. The *most important* variable that predicts treatment success is:
    a. being employed at the time of discharge.
    b. participation in AA or other 12-step groups.
    c. completing at least 90 days of treatment in an outpatient or residential facility.
    d. having the family involved in the treatment process.

30. Which statement *is most* true about substance abuse treatment?
    a. Substance use disorders are very treatable conditions.
    b. Most individuals in substance abuse treatment have been in similar treatment before.
    c. The family plays a very important role in promoting successful treatment outcomes for individuals with substance use disorders.
    d. All are equally true.

Substance use disorders are common and very treatable conditions. Family involvement in the treatment process greatly increases the chances of a positive treatment outcome. It is critical that you be able to identify substance use disorders, be aware of how to promote the family's participation in the treatment process of these disorders, and be aware of how their actions may either concur or conflict with current best practices for the treatment of these disorders. It is not necessary for therapists working with a family to provide any needed substance abuse treatment, however it is critical that they understand the nature of these disorders, the nature of effective treatment and their role in promoting and supporting this treatment.

## KEY TERMS

**amphetamine:** A central nervous system stimulant; "speed."
**anxiolytic:** A drug that relieves anxiety; "Valium," "Xanax," "tranquilizers."
**co-occurring disorders:** When an individual has both a substance use and another mental health disorder.
**hallucinogen:** A substance that induces the perception of things that don't exist, e.g., seeing things or hearing things that aren't there.
**inhalant:** A gas or vapor people inhale to get high.
**phencyclidine:** A veterinary anesthetic sometimes used as an allucinogen; "angel dust," "PCP."
**psychoactive substance:** Any substance that affects mood, cognition, or behavior.
**sedative–hypnotic:** A central nervous system depressant; "sleeping pills" or "downers."
**substance abuse:** Use of a psychoactive substance that causes a problem in any life sphere.
**substance dependence:** The inability to control one's substance use once it has begun.

## DISCUSSION QUESTIONS

1. What are the differences between a diagnosis of substance abuse and substance dependence?
2. Describe the principles of interviewing clients about their substance use.
3. Briefly describe the levels of treatment for substance abuse.
4. Pick three types of medications used in substance abuse and describe their use.
5. What are the primary principles of motivational interviewing?

6. How do you think involving families in treatment contributes to better treatment outcome?
7. Contrast the Johnson Intervention and ARISE treatment engagement models.
8. Describe two interventions used in behavioral couples therapy.
9. What areas might a multisystemic approach focus on in working with a drug-abusing adolescent?
10. Several factors are associated with better treatment outcome. What are they and how can family therapists promote them?

## SUGGESTED FURTHER READING

Inaba, D. (2000). *Uppers, downers, all arounders: Physical and mental effects of psychoactive drugs* (4th ed.). Ashland, OR: CNS Productions.

Written in an accessible style, this book describes the physical and psychological effects of a host of drugs and medications.

Kaufman, E., & Kaufman, P. (1992). *Family therapy of drug and alcohol abuse* (2nd ed.). Boston: Allyn & Bacon.

This book describes the major approaches to the family treatment of drug and alcohol abuse.

National Institute on Drug Abuse. (2000). *Approaches to drug abuse counseling.* Available online at: http://165.112.78.61/ADAC/ADAC1.html

This free publication from NIDA describes and summarizies the many approaches to group and individual treatment for substance abuse. Each chapter is written by a major proponent of the approach described.

NIAAA Web site: www.niaaa.nih.gov
NIDA Web site: www.drugabuse.gov

Both the National Institute on Drug Abuse (NIDA) and National Institute on Alcohol Abuse and Alcoholism (NIAAA) Web sites provide a wealth of online information about substance abuse and its treatment.

Robert, L. J., & McCrady, B. S. (in press). *Alcohol problems in intimate relationships: Identification and intervention. A guide for marriage and family therapists (NIH Publication No. 03-5284)*. Rockville, MD: National Institute on Alcohol Abuse and Alcoholism.

## REFERENCES

American Psychiatric Association (2000). *Diagnostic and statistical manual of mental disorders* (4th ed., test revision). Washington, DC: Author.

American Society of Addiction Medicine (2001). *Patient placement criteria for the treatment of substance-related disorders* (2nd ed., rev.). Chevy Chase, MD: Author.

Babor, T. F., & Grant, M. (1989). From clinical research to secondary prevention: International collaboration in the development of the Alcohol Use Disorders Identification Test (AUDIT). *Alcohol Health and Research World, 13*, 371–374.

Barber, J. G., & Gilbertson, R. (1997). Unilateral interventions for women living with heavy drinkers. *Social Work, 42*, 69–77

Bays, J. (1990). Substance abuse and child abuse: Impact of addiction on the child. *Pediatric Clinics of North America, 37*, 881–904.

Bond, G. R., McDonel, E. C., Miller, L. D., & Pensec, M. (1991). Assertive community treatment and reference groups: An evaluation of their effectiveness for young adults with serious mental illness and substance abuse problems. *Psychosocial Rehabilitation Journal, 15*, 31–43.

Brown, T. L., Henggeler, S. W., Schoenwald, S. K., Brondino, M. J., & Pickerel, S. G. (1999). Multisystemic treatment of substance abusing and dependent juvenile offenders: Effects on school performance at posttreatment and 6-month follow-up. *Children's Services: Social Policy, Research and Practice, 2*, 81–93.

Center for Substance Abuse Treatment (1998). *Comprehensive case management for substance abuse treatment: Treatment improvement protocol 27*. Rockville, MD: Author.

Cook, P. S., Petersen, R. C., & Moore, D. T. (1990). *Alcohol, tobacco and other drugs may harm the unborn* (DHHS Publication No. ADM 90-1711). Washington, DC: U.S. Government Printing Office.

Dole, V. P, & Nyswander, M. E (1965). A medical treatment for diacetylmorphine addiction. *Journal of the American Medical Association, 193*, 646.

Garrett, J. A., Landau, J., Shea, R., Stanton, M. D., Baciewicz, G., & Brinkman-Sull, D. (1998). The ARISE intervention: Using family and network links to engage addicted persons in treatment. *Journal of Substance Abuse Treatment, 15*, 333–343.

Garrett, J. A., Landau-Stanton, J., Stanton, M. D., Stellato-Kabat, J., & Stellato-Kabat, D. (1997). ARISE: A method for engaging reluctant alcohol- and drug-dependent individuals in treatment. *Journal of Substance Abuse Treatment, 14*, 235–248.

Goldberg, M. E., Lex, B. W., Mello, N. K., Mendelson, J. H., & Bower, T. A. (1996). Impact of maternal alcoholism on separation of children from their mothers: Findings from a sample of incarcerated women. *American Journal of Orthopsychiatry, 66*, 228–238.

Greenfeld, L. A. (1998). *An analysis of national data on the prevalence of alcohol involvement in crime*. Report prepared for Assistant Attorney General's National Symposium on Alcohol Abuse and Crime. Washington, DC: U.S. Department of Justice.

Greenfield, S. F., Weiss, R. D., Muenz, L., Vagge, L. M., Kelly, J. F., Bello, L. R., & Michael, J. (1998). The effect of depression on return to drinking. *Archives of General Psychiatry, 55*, 259–265.

Hartel, D. M., Schoenbaum, E. E., Selwyn, P. A., Kline, J., Davenny, K., Klein, R. S., et al. (1995). Heroin use during methadone maintenance treatment: The importance of methadone dose and cocaine use. *American Journal of Public Health, 85*, 83–88.

Hendrickson, E. L., & Schmal, M. S. (2000). Dual diagnosis treatment: An 18-year perspective. Paper presented at MISA Conference sponsored by MCP-Hahnemann University, Philadelphia, PA.

Hendrickson, E. L., Stith, S. M., & Schmal, M. S. (1995). Predicting treatment outcome for seriously mentally ill substance abusers in an outpatient dual diagnosis group. *Continuum: Developments In Ambulatory Mental Health Care, 2*, 271–289.

Henggeler, S. W., Borduin, C. M., Melton, G. B., Mann, B. J., Smith, L. A., Hall, J. A., et al. (1991). Effects of multisystemic therapy on drug use and abuse in serious juvenile offenders: A progress report from two outcome studies. *Family Dynamics of Addiction Quarterly, 1*, 40–51.

Henggeler, S. W., Pickerel, S. G., Brondino, M. J., & Crouch, J. L. (1996). Eliminating (almost) treatment dropout of substance abusing or dependent delinquents through home-based multisystemic therapy. *American Journal of Psychiatry, 153*, 427–428.

Hoffman, N. G., Harrison, P. A., & Belille, C. A. (1983). Alcoholic anonymous after treatment: Attendance and abstinence. *International Journal of Addictions, 18*, 311–318.

Hubbard, R. L., Craddock, S. G., Flynn, P. M., Anderson, J., & Etheridge, R. M. (1997). Overview of 1-year follow-up outcomes in the drug abuse treatment outcome study (DATOS). *Psychology of Addictive Behaviors, 11*, 261–278.

Hubbard, R. L., Marsden, M. E., Rachal, J. V., Harwood, H. J., Cavanaugh, E. R., & Ginsburg, H. M. (1989). *Drug abuse treatment: A national study of effectiveness*. University of North Carolina Press: Chapel Hill.

James, J. E. (1997). *Understanding caffeine: A biobehavior analysis*. Thousand Oaks, California: Sage.

Johnson, B. D., Dunlap, E., & Maher, L. (1998). Nurturing for careers in drug use and crime: Conduct norms for children and juveniles in crack-using households. *Substance Use and Misuse, 33*, 1511–1546.

Johnson, L. D., O'Malley, P. M., & Bachman, J. G. (2002). *Monitoring the future: National results on adolescent drug use*. Bethesda, MD: National Institute on Drug Abuse.

Johnson, V. E. (1986). *Intervention: How to help someone who doesn't want help*. Minneapolis, MN: Johnson Institute Books.

Kessler, R. C., Nelson, C. B., McGonagle, K. A., Edlund, M. J., Frank, R. G., & Leaf, P. J. (1994). The epidemiology of co-occurring addictive and mental disorders: Implications for prevention and service utilization. *American Journal of Orthopsychiatry, 66*, 17–31.

Landau, J., & Garrett, J. A. (2002, October). Families can make a difference: Family motivation to change. Paper presented at the annual meeting of the American Association for Marriage and Family Therapy, Cincinnati, OH.

Lewis, J. A. (1991). Change and the alcohol-affected family: Limitations of the "intervention." *The Family Psychologist, 7*, 43–44.

Liddle, H. A. (2002). Multidimensional family therapy for adolescent cannabis users. *Cannabis Youth Treatment Series* (Vol. 5). Rockville, MD: Center for Substance Abuse Treatment.

Liepman, M. R., Nirenberg, T. D., & Begin, A. M. (1989). Evaluation of a program designed to help family and significant others to motivate resistant alcoholics into recovery. *American Journal of Drug and Alcohol Abuse, 15*, 209–221.

Logan, D. G. (1983). Getting alcoholics to treatment by social network intervention. *Hospital and Community Psychiatry, 34*, 360–361.

Loneck, B., Garrett, J. A., & Banks, S. M. (1996). A comparison of the Johnson intervention with four other methods of referral to outpatient treatment. *American Journal of Drug and Alcohol Abuse, 22*, 233–246.

Maisto, S. A., Carey, K. B., Carey, M. P., Purnine, D. M., & Barnes, K. L. (1999). Methods of changing patterns of substance use among individuals with co-occurring schizophrenia and substance use disorder. *Journal of Substance Abuse Treatment, 17*, 221–227.

Mammo, A., & Weinbaum, D. F. (1993). Some factors that influence dropping out from outpatient alcoholism treatment facilities. *Journal of Studies of Alcohol, 45*, 359–362.

Mayfield, D., McCleod, G., & Hall, P. (1974). The CAGE Questionnaire: Validation of a new alcoholism screening instrument. *American Journal of Psychiatry, 131*, 1121–1123.

McCollum, E. E., Lewis, R. A., Nelson, T. S., Trepper, T. S., & Wetchler, J. L. (in press). Couple treatment for drug abusing women: Effects on drug use and need for treatment. *Journal of Couple and Relationship Therapy.*

Merikangas, K. R., Dierker, L. C., & Szatmari, P. (1998). Psychopathology among offspring of parents with substance abuse and/or anxiety disorders: A high-risk study. *Journal of Child Psychology and Psychiatry, 39*, 711–720.

Merikangas, K. R., Stolar, M., Stevens, D. E., Goulet, J., Preisig, M. A., Fenton, B., et al. (1998). Familial transmission of substance use disorders. *Archives of General Psychiatry, 55*, 973–979.

Miller, G. A. (1985). *Substance Abuse Subtle Screening Inventory (SASSI) manual.* Bloomington, IN: Spencer Evening World.

Miller, W. R., & Rollnick, S. (1991). *Motivational interviewing: Preparing people to change addictive behavior.* New York: Guilford Press.

National Institute on Alcohol Abuse and Alcoholism. (2000). *Tenth special report to the U.S. Congress on alcohol and health.* Bethesda, MD: Author.

National Institute on Drug Abuse. (1998). *NIDA media advisory: Economic costs of alcohol and drug abuse estimated at $246 billion in the United States.* Retrieved March 22, 2003, from http://www.drugabuse.gov/MedAdv/98/MA-513.html

O'Farrel, T. J., Cutter, H. S. G., Choquette, K. A., Floyd, F. J., & Bayog, R. D. (1992). Behavioral marital therapy for male alcoholics: Marital and drinking adjustment during the two years after treatment. *Behavior Therapy, 23*, 529–549.

O'Farrell, T. J., & Fals-Stewart, W. (2000). Behavioral couples therapy for alcoholism and drug abuse. *Journal of Substance Abuse Treatment, 18*, 51–54.

O'Farrell, T. J., & Fals-Stewart, W. (2002). Alcohol abuse. In D. H. Sprenkle (Ed.), *Effectiveness research in marriage and family therapy* (pp. 123–161). Alexandria, VA: American Association for Marriage and Family Therapy.

O'Farrell, T. J., & Murphy, C. M. (1995). Marital violence before and after alcoholism treatment. *Journal of Consulting and Clinical Psychology, 63*, 256–262.

Prochaska, J. O., & DiClemente, C. C. (1986). Toward a comprehensive model of change. In W. R. Miller & N. Heather (Eds.), *Treating addictive behaviors: Processes of change* (pp. 3–27). New York: Plenum.

RAND Corporation. (1998). *RAND health research highlights: Preventing very low birthweight births: Saving a bundle.* Retrieved January 14, 2003, from www.rand.org/publications/RB/RB4514

Rotunda, R., & O'Farrell, T. J. (1997). Marital and family therapy of alcohol use disorders: Bridging the gap between research and practice. *Professional Psychology, 28*, 246–252.

Selzer, M. L. (1971). The Michigan Alcoholism Screening Test: The quest for a new diagnostic instrument. *American Journal of Psychiatry, 127*, 89–94.

Simpson, D. D., & Sells, S. B. (1982): Effectiveness of treatment for drug abuse: An overview of the DARO research program. *Advances in Alcohol and Substance Abuse, 2*, 7–29.

Skinner, H. A. (1982). The drug abuse screening test. *Journal on Addictive Behaviors, 7*, 363–371.

Speck, R. V., & Attneave, C. (1973). *Family networks.* New York: Pantheon Books.

Stanton, M. D., & Shadish, W. R. (1997). Outcome, attrition, and family-couples treatment: A meta-analysis and review of the controlled, comparative studies. *Psychological Bulletin, 122*, 170–191.

Stanton, M. D., & Todd, T. C. (1982). *Family therapy for drug abuse and addiction.* New York: Guilford Press.

Substance Abuse and Mental Health Services Administration. (1994). *The national treatment improvement study (NTIES).* Rockville, MD: Author.

Substance Abuse and Mental Health Services Administration. (1998). *Treatment episode data (TED): National admissions to substance abuse treatment services.* Rockville, MD: Author.

Substance Abuse and Mental Health Services Administration. (2002). *2001 National Household Survey on Drug Abuse (NHSDA).* Rockville, MD: Author.

Substance Abuse and Mental Health Services Administration. (2002). *Substance use among pregnant women during 1999 and 2000*. Retrieved January 14, 2003, from http://www.samhsa.gov/oas/2k2/preg/preg.pdf

Vallant, G. E. (1983). *The natural history of alcoholism: Causes, patterns, and paths to recovery.* Cambridge, MA: Harvard University Press.

Winters, J., Fals-Stewart, W., O'Farrell, T. J., Hirchler, G. R., & Kelley, L. K. (2002). Behavioral couples therapy for female substance-abusing patients: Effects on substance use and relationship adjustment. *Journal of Consulting and Clinical Psychology, 70*, 344–355.

# 21

# Nonpharmacological Addictions

## William G. McCown
### *Louisiana University Monroe*

## TRUTH OR FICTION?

___ 1. Many behavioral excesses are extremely similar to drug or alcohol dependence in their capacity to disrupt an individual and her or his family system.

___ 2. It is necessary to ingest a substance to develop an addiction.

___ 3. Nonpharmacological addictions usually only appear in the context of a family system.

___ 4. The present diagnostic systems employed by mental health professionals recognize nonpharmacological addictions as being similar to pharmacological addictions.

___ 5. Addiction can be described as a condition when a single reward or categories of rewards tends to dominate a person's thinking, feelings, thoughts, and interactions.

___ 6. It is rare for people with addictions to feel superior to the nonaddict.

___ 7. Physical dependence is always necessary for addictions.

___ 8. Nonpharmacological addictions are usually quite rare.

___ 9. Pharmacological addictions differ from nonpharmacological addictions because the latter are easy to stop.

___ 10. Families can both foster and limit addictive behavior.

___ 11. If treatment is to be successful, it is often necessary to address the way the family reorganizes in response to the addicted person's behaviors.

___ 12. Family therapy is generally not a good opportunity for educating the family about addictions.

___ 13. It is often important that the family be able to find a meaning for an addictive person's behaviors.

The author is grateful for the contribution of Kimberly Zimmerman, MD.

___ 14. *The role of families in the development of nonpharmacological addictions is important.*

___ 15. *In addition to being invaluable for treatment, families are often the most accurate source of information about their members' nonpharmacological addictions.*

The concept that people can be addicted to behaviors or experiences fits many of our observations from life. Most of us know someone who spends too much time on the Internet, perhaps exercises too much, or is perpetually spending all his or her time watching "trashy" or campy movies. We may have already even labeled them, perhaps part humorously, as "addicts." However, as therapists and counselors, we need to know if these apparent behavioral excesses really are a variety of addictions. Can people be addicted to an experience, person, place, or object? Or, perhaps, should we reserve this emotionally-laden term for someone who ingests particular classes of substances, as traditional psychiatry suggests?

The following case study presents an overview for four arguments advanced in this chapter: First, *nonpharmacological addictions,* as my colleagues and I refer to this class of behaviors, are not only possible, but are common. Second, these addictions are often as serious in their consequences as any substance dependence. Third, nonpharmacological addictions are usually encountered within a family context and often seem to be fostered by family processes. Therefore, fourth, and as this chapter will argue in greater detail, family therapy is usually the first choice for treating the variety of nonpharmacological addictions that clinicians encounter.

## CASE EXAMPLE

John is a forty-six-year-old, married man living with three children. Two years ago, he began jogging at the suggestion of his physician. John went from barely being able to walk a few blocks to his present daily routine—a regimen that most people, including his health care professionals, regard as massively excessive.

John regularly wakes up *four hours* before any of the other family members. He calls this period his "quiet time—a time I can concentrate on my performance." He warms up for half an hour and then runs approximately 15 to 25 miles each day regardless of the weather or family commitments. John then unwinds for another half hour.

By the time he is finished, John is naturally exhausted. He has also taken five or six hours out of his day, time that is during the most hectic period in his household. His family has gotten up, gone to school or work or about their activities without him. "I kind of like it with Dad's running craze," said John's fifteen-year-old stepdaughter. "He used to be such a jerk in the mornings, cranky for no reason. Now, I just wave to him when he comes jogging by. I don't care if he is a jerk. He isn't here!"

On John's last visit to his physician, the doctor was concerned that John might be anorexic. John's body fat was exceptionally low and his weight was very low for his six-foot frame. When asked about this possibility John was aghast: "No way! I just like the feeling. It's a natural tranquilizer that you should try." He went on to state that he ate normally, did not count calories, and did not deny himself any desserts or rich foods. "You try that at my age without running and see what your cholesterol does. I dare you!"

His physician initially just shrugged his shoulders, knowing that there were many worse things that John could be doing. However, his physician recalled thinking that he usually only saw such adamant denial about health issues from people who were hiding an addiction. Maybe John was using amphetamines? No, his physician reasoned, it just wasn't like John to use illegal drugs. For a brief few seconds he thought about referring John to a mental health professional, based on a clinical hunch that "something wasn't right." However, he soon forgot about this as John continued extolling the virtues of running a marathon.

Then John injured his ankle. His doctor told him he should not run for two to five weeks. John panicked at the thought of all of this idle morning time. He subsequently reported that he felt edgy, anxious, depressed, and "utterly explosive around my family." His physician could not explain the intensity of John's feelings and referred him to a therapist. John was not happy with the referral but he agreed to comply in order to "make my wife happy, I guess."

John told the therapist that he "constantly craved" running. He later noted, "I spent the whole time I was [previously] injured thinking about running, reading running magazines, looking at different shoes, glued to the running pages on the Internet. Not running was like a disease or something."

John's therapist realized that her client might be experiencing some type of physiologically based withdrawal from his demanding physical regimen. She had read that major neurotransmitters responsible for feelings of well-being—serotonin and neurohormones from the endorphin family—were increased when people exercised strenuously. She also had read that running was occasionally recommended as an antidepressant. Her hypothesis was that John was running to self-medicate for depression. At this time, she reasoned, he was experiencing an abrupt withdrawal, perhaps akin to the sensation smokers experience when they quit.

However, the therapist also had some training in family systems theory. She politely asked John about the quality of his interactions with his family. They were absolutely fine, he noted. However, on even a cursory inquiry, she soon realized that running had allowed John to abdicate from a number of parental responsibilities. For example, he timed his exercise to avoid contact with his wife and children. When confronted by the therapist that this could be a motive for his running, John laughed incredulously, declaring his love and devotion to his family: "Hey, they are my life! Why would I avoid them?"

Curiously, John's injury failed to heal as quickly as the physician first thought. The longer he was injured, the more the level of his family's tension increased. During one session with his therapist, John appeared especially agitated, almost as if he were withdrawing from a drug of abuse. Finally, he exclaimed to the therapist that he "really hated" many aspects of his family life. For example, he could not stand being around his family in the morning "when there is all this confusion and tension." Furthermore, he detested the idea of getting up with his wife. "We never did before we had kids. She was the first one up and it just went smoother. Two people fighting over one bathroom—struggling to find what to wear during the day—I tell you she is a real witch in the morning, just impossibly demanding."

By the end of the session the therapist surmised that John was "addicted" to running, even though she knew that there was no official nomenclature in psychiatry for this type of addiction. However, she could see that John's addiction was as real as that to any drug. Furthermore, the effects on his family were as disrupting as those from alcohol, cocaine, or heroin addiction. John's intense running damaged his family. They felt abandoned and disliked. Family members became angry and tensions mounted. John responded to this increased tension by running even more often. This behavioral pattern created a vicious cycle of avoidance, with the family system reorganizing to meet the losses of its major authority figure. Simply, John had a *nonpharmacological addiction*, a class of related behaviors that my colleagues and I believe frequently benefit from family therapy.

1. The case of John, described in the opening section of this chapter suggests:
    a. All addictions must have a pharmacological component to them.
    b. Often people will use exercise or other means to hide addictions to substances.
    c. It is possible to be addicted to an experience, as well as to a substance.
    d. Many behaviors seem like addictions, even though they are not.

2. John's behavior was probably puzzling to his physician because:
    a. Most people think of addiction as a disease that affects the young.
    b. Most people think of addiction as a disease that does not affect productive people.
    c. Most people think of addiction as a voluntary choice of behaviors.
    d. Most people think addiction has to involve the use of an outside substance, such as alcohol or amphetamines.

## NONPHARMACOLOGICAL ADDICTIONS: AN INTRODUCTION TO A SILENT EPIDEMIC

Family therapists who limit their treatment to people with chemical addictions ignore another class of addictive behaviors that I call *nonpharmacological addictive disorders*. These behaviors occur when individuals are addicted to an *experience, person,* or *situation,* rather than to a specific chemical of abuse. Gambling, an example of addition to an experience and situation, is perhaps the best known of these. Internet and sexual addictions are close seconds. Combined, between 12% and 20% of the population have one or more of these three nonpharmacological addictions (McCown & Chamberlain, 2004). Additional evidence suggests that these numbers are increasing yearly.

Addictive behavior involving *people* as the object of addiction frequently occurs in unhealthy romantic relationships. This facet of addiction is also common in dysfunctional relationships between family and friends. A *person-specific* addiction may even involve people we do not know. For example, the author recently evaluated a woman name "Mary," who had imaginary love affairs with famous musicians and actors. When confronted with the fact that she did not know any of these people, Mary admitted that these relationships were entirely fanciful. However, she continues to travel several thousand miles a year, hoping to become acquainted with one of her "loves" in person. In the meantime, Mary has quit her job and left her family, so that she can spend more time trying to meet the objects of her affection.

People may also be addicted to specific classes of behaviors, such as thrill seeking or falling in love. Often, their addictive behavior is assumed to be a long-standing personality trait and the addictive aspects of the behavior may be overlooked by others. For example, J'Wan is a thirty-two-year-old lawyer who routinely procrastinates major work assignments, making her difficult to work with and unpopular with coworkers. J'Wan noted that, "This is the only way I can function. I know deadlines are imminent. But getting things done at the last minute is an unbelievable feeling. And besides, I don't hurt anyone."

J'Wan illustrates a characteristic lack of insight regarding the harmfulness of her behavior. Denial is common in both nonpharmacologic and other addictions. On the other hand, some people strongly identify with their addictions and eventually define themselves by their behavioral excesses. Robert, another individual with habitual problems meeting deadlines recently noted, "I'm just the kind of person who can get things done under pressure. That's my talent—that's who I am."

3. Regarding nonpharmacological addictions:
   a. They are so rare that even if they exist they are not of interest to the clinician.
   b. Gambling, excessive Internet use, and inappropriate involvement in pornography probably fall under this definition.
   c. Evidence clearly indicates that nonpharmacological addictions are simply problems of self-control.
   d. With exposure to so many different stimuli these days, nonpharmacological addictions are probably decreasing.

4. People who are addicted to nonpharmacological substances:
   a. never show denial commonly found in substance abusers.
   b. occasionally show denial commonly found in substance abusers.
   c. often show denial similar to that found in substance abusers.
   d. show denial only if they have a substance abuse problem.

# NONPHARMACOLOGICAL ADDICTIONS AS "GENUINE" ADDICTIONS

According to official nomenclature of the American Psychiatric Association (APA, 2000), addictions are only possible when *substances* are *ingested*. This contrasts with clinicians and researchers who believe that addictions are best defined by the *behaviors that they produce*. This group of clinicians and researchers argues that the actions of people who work too hard, attend religious services beyond a functional level, or engage in sexual behavior that is considered excessive, are often indistinguishable from people who are addicted to an ingested drug. Every addiction has behavioral components. We use the term *nonpharmacological* to delineate "substance-less" addictions. Table 21.1 shows some of the similarities and differences between **pharmacological** and **nonpharmacological addictions**.

Practitioners often realize that some people can "manage" potential addictive stimuli, while others cannot. Some people drink abusively and heavily for years before the toll becomes obvious. Similarly, some people are able to hold on to a fanatical following of a particular sports team and still be employed and fulfill other obligations. However, the odds are that eventually, the addiction will overpower the individual. This occurs when rewards associated with the addicted behavior are more important than other aspects of the person's life. Basically, a person loses capacity to enjoy anything but a single experience. This is a key component or the process of addiction.

Later, under the influence of this single reward, the individual often neglects personal responsibilities. This occurs in pharmacological and nonpharmacological addictions alike. For example, the problem gambler might neglect eating or feeding his family, just as the cocaine user will forget food and drink while on a cocaine binge. The sports fanatic may "forget" to go to work during a critical playoff, just as the alcoholic misses work because of a hangover.

Another phenomenon common to pharmacological and nonpharmacological addictions is that the addicted person tends to view people who do not share his or her addiction with a quite cynical perspective. People who are rewarded primarily by a single reinforcer tend to demeaningly label others with more normal reward functioning as "straight." This does not refer to sexual orientation, but to a shared definition of the community of people who have similar behavioral excesses. The concept of *straight* implies that the world can be organized

**TABLE 21.1**

Similarities and Differences between Pharmacological and Nonpharmacological Addictions

| Addiction Properties | Pharmacological Addictions | Nonpharmacological Addictions |
|---|---|---|
| Common in contemporary society | Yes | Yes, more than realized |
| Progressive | Yes | Yes |
| Behaviorally toxic | Yes | Yes |
| Tolerance | Often | Often |
| Addicted person excludes others not involved in addiction | Yes | Yes |
| Characterized by secrecy and denial | Usually | Usually |
| Negative effects on addicted person's health | Usually | Often |
| Addiction involves family system | Practically always | Practically always |
| Addiction involves ingestion of a specific substance | Yes | No |
| Classified as impulse control disorder or obsessive compulsive disorder | No | Yes |
| Recognized by traditional accounts as a "true addiction" | Yes | No |

into two opposing groups, with the only interesting people being those who are rewarded by the particular experience that the addict especially enjoys. This concrete thinking soon generates an "us against them" mentality that makes it even harder for the addicted individual to function in "straight" society or in his or her family system.

The behaviors of people who become rewarded primarily by a single reinforcement have increasingly negative effects on their families. McCown and Johnson (1993) have argued that the body and the family system both follow the same pattern when confronted with novel stressors. Any complex system eventually learns to go beyond a return to homeostasis and subsequently overcompensates from such deviations. Often this produces addiction as a side effect.

Smoking, for example, is initially disrupting and stressful to multiple physical systems. If a person continues smoking, countermanding physiological stimuli neutralize the nauseating and aversive feelings. The body tries to return to a state of homeostasis, which is eventually reached. However, if a person continues to smoke, the body's mechanisms that strive for a return to homeostasis are actually disproportionately greater than the stimulus of the cigarette. As a result, the body's overcompensation produces a source of reward, which in this case is very addicting.

This same pattern helps explain "positive addictions." Exercise is initially very painful until the body develops a capacity for homeostasis under physical stress, perhaps weeks later.

If exercise is continued for longer periods, the body's attempts to return vital systems to homeostasis flood the brain with chemicals that produce the well known "runner's high."

McCown and Johnson (1993) have theorized that family systems respond to addiction or other stressors the way the body reacts to smoking or exercise. The stress of a family member's addiction at first severely disrupts the system. However, with increasing experience, the family learns to overcompensate in its quest for a rapid return to its previous functioning (homeostasis). However, instead of returning to homeostasis, in time, families learn to move past it, to a point of rigidity. Families may even encourage addicted members to "slip" in order to strengthen or empower other members. The results, however, are almost always a tendency to stifle healthy family growth and adaptation.

5. The author believes that both pharmacologically and nonpharmacologically addicted people:
   a. avoid associating with people who share their addiction.
   b. form strong associations primarily with people who share their addiction.
   c. keep their addiction a secret, except to their families.
   d. form strong bonds with non addicted people so that they may conceal their addictions.

6. The author and his associates believe that much of the family pathology that accompanies addiction:
   a. is due to the family's pressures which cause a person to become addicted.
   b. is due to the family's attempts to forgive the actively addicted individual.
   c. is due to the family's efforts to maintain a homeostasis, despite the activities of the addicted individual.
   d. is unrelated to the primary problem of the addiction in any of its members.

Generally, as McCown and Chamberlain (2004) note, two features distinguish addictions—regardless of whether they are pharmacological or nonpharmacological—from other behaviors. First is the concept of motivational strength; a second is motivational toxicity. *Motivational strength* indicates how hard individuals will work to perform behaviors or obtain substances that they abuse. *Motivational toxicity* is a slightly more complex phenomenon. It describes the manner in which an excessive experience or drug disrupts the hierarchy of normal motivations that we all possess. This latter characteristic invariably involves families, because they are slighted in favor of the drug or experience of abuse.

How common are nonpharmacological addictions? My colleagues and I have estimated that they may be several times more common than biological addictions. We base this on client self-reports, as well as known incidences of gambling disorders, sexual attraction to nonsexual objects, and the fact we have recorded over two hundred phenomena that some people have had an addiction to at some time in their lives. Table 21.2 illustrates some of the many experiences or noningested substances to which people can show addiction.

7. Motivational toxicity is best thought of as:
   a. how hard individuals will work to perform behaviors or obtain substances that they abuse.
   b. the way in which an excessive experience or drug disrupts the hierarchy of normal motivations.
   c. toxic effects of drugs on the brain.
   d. poisonous effects of drugs on family members.

**TABLE 21.2**

Common Nonpharmacological Addictions

---

- Aerobic exercise
- Arguing
- Bargain hunting
- Body piercing
- Collecting items in excess
- Community or institutional leadership (that interferes with other duties)
- Counseling or therapy
- Craft making
- Creating art or poetry
- Creating crises
- Dating
- Day dreaming
- Dependency on children for major reward
- Dieting
- Disrupting existing institutions (e.g., constantly creating disagreement in churches, schools, or similar groups that previously functioned satisfactorily)
- E-mailing
- Excessive fan behavior (sports, movies, music, etc.)
- Excessive planning (when little or nothing is implemented)
- Excessive religious involvement
- Fantasizing
- Fantasy sports leagues
- Fishing
- Flirting
- Gambling
- Gardening
- Golf
- Helping others (co-dependency)
- Home repair
- Internet

- Making money
- Motorcycle riding
- Music acquisition (e.g., collecting various genres)
- Music listening
- Music playing
- Online auctions
- Organizing or cleaning (which may also be due to obsessive compulsive disorder)
- Parachuting or other thrill-sports
- Perfectionism (needing to appear to give full effort to everything)
- Photography
- Political involvement
- Pornography
- Procrastination
- Reading (when it interferes with other life goals)
- Self-help meeting attendance (beyond the level necessary for personal growth and abstinence)
- Self-improvement reading and related activities
- Sex
- Shoplifting
- Speeding
- Sports
- Studying (beyond that required to reach a goal)
- Tattooing
- Television
- Weight training
- White water rafting or similar sports
- Work or work-related behaviors

---

My colleagues and I define an **addiction** as a *continuum* where a single reward increasingly dominates an individual's thoughts, behavior, social milieu, and intentions. This occurs so profoundly that it impairs the individual's functioning or hurts those around them. A major departure from the medical model is the departure from the view that addiction is an all-or-nothing phenomena. As an example, I recently treated a woman who gambles to excess—but only on rainy days when her children are fighting. Using strict psychiatric criteria, it would be difficult to say which diagnosis, if any, she meets. However, despite official terminology, she finds it useful to conceptualize her behaviors as a "situational" addiction, intensified by certain environmental factors. She recognizes that risk factors make her behave "more like an addict sometimes, less like an addict other times."

8. The author and his associates believe that addictions are best described as:
   a. an "all or nothing" phenomena, where a person either has an addiction or does not.
   b. an artificial concept that only exists in fiction or due to social labeling.
   c. a continuum, that develops gradually.
   d. a sudden onset disease that is impossible to hide.

## Confusion Regarding Physical Dependency and Addictions

The most common misunderstanding among traditional addiction treatment providers is that addiction refers to a state of physical **dependence** on a drug. In this case, discontinuing the drug's intake produces a **withdrawal** syndrome consisting of various somatic disturbances. A more contemporary definition recognizes addiction as a behavioral syndrome where drug use or excessive experiences dominate the individual's motivation and where the normal constraints on behavior are largely ineffective. The distinguishing feature of addiction is the ability of anything to dominate the individual's or system's behaviors, regardless of whether physical dependence exists (Johnson & McCown, 1997).

These conditions may or may not be accompanied by the development of physical dependence. In some situations, addictions to experience show tolerance, such as with gambling (McCown & Chamberlain, 2000). Similar tolerance may also be seen in people with addictions to other people or to specific situations.

9. The chapter argues that:
   a. A Physical dependence is necessary for addiction.
   b. Physical dependence sometimes accompanies addiction and sometimes does not.
   c. Physical dependence is always independent of addiction.
   d. Physical dependence is always the most complicating factor in addictions.

## Confusion Regarding Psychological Dependence

Once a practitioner understands that addiction is not restricted to physical tolerance and withdrawal, he or she escapes a common and dangerous misperception. The practitioner no longer divides addictive behaviors into being "real" and "merely psychologically addicting." This latter phrase has no place in contemporary understandings of addictions treatment and management. In fact, the concept is dangerous. For example, during the late seventies, a number of researchers argued that cocaine was merely "psychologically addicting." Presumably, they meant that cocaine causes no physical tolerance. Nevertheless, cocaine is an incredibly powerful behavioral motivator, one with profound motivational toxicity, and one that fosters extraordinary addictive behaviors. As a result, many people exposed themselves to cocaine and a percentage of them became profoundly impaired by this "merely psychologically addicting" drug.

10. The author argues that if a more satisfactory definition of addiction were used in the past:
    a. No one would be defined as an addict.
    b. Many drugs that are now thought to be addicting would be recognized as harmless.
    c. Families would be spared problems from their addicted members.
    d. The danger of drugs such as cocaine would have been recognized much earlier.

## PHARMACOLOGICAL AND NONPHARMACOLOGICAL ADDICTIONS: COMMON PATHWAYS IN COMPLEX BIOLOGICAL SYSTEMS

Too often, family therapists seem reticent to discuss the biological factors associated with addiction. A few therapists still deny that biology is important. On the other hand, an emerging consensus is that biological factors are necessary but not usually sufficient to cause addiction. Furthermore, the neurobiology of nonpharmacological addictions is quite similar to pharmacological addictions.

A very brief summary of the neurobiology of addiction may be helpful. The brain has specialized reinforcement systems which have evolved to ensure survival. These "reward" systems direct future behavior by reinforcing actions that generally have promoted survival in the past. For example, intake of food and reproduction are controlled by specific brain systems associated with pleasure. However, some chemicals or excessive experiences activate brain reward systems directly and dramatically. Essentially, they provide too much reward for an individual's neurobiology to handle.

For example, ingestion of certain chemicals is accompanied by massive mood elevations and other affective changes. These changes may lead to a reduction in other activities previously considered rewarding. Similarly, excessive behavior that activates brain reward mechanisms alter normal functioning. This also results in a potentially addictive state. Several models explain nonpharmacological addiction and are reviewed by McCown and Chamberlain (2000, 2004).

> 11. From this discussion we may infer that the author believes that:
>     a. All addictions probably have distinctive pathways in the brain.
>     b. Nonpharmacological and pharmacological addictions may share similar brain pathways and probably have a similar underlying biological connection.
>     c. Speculation about the biology of addiction is unimportant.
>     d. Pharmacological and nonpharmacological addictions clearly change different parts of the brain.

## Obsessive Compulsive Disorder and Nonpharmacological Addictions: The Critical Distinctions

Proponents of the pharmacological definition of addictions respond by saying that the sexual addict or the person addicted to shopping for fabrics is not *really* an addict. These people, it is argued, have **obsessive compulsive disorders** (OCD), an anxiety condition that fosters their bizarre behaviors. This clinical concept and its language are so ingrained that the clinician can hardly avoid using it in routine descriptions. For example, a clinician may discuss clients who spend massive time reading gothic novels, making extremely expensive purchases on a shopping channel, or endlessly watching reruns of a popular science fiction show. They almost "naturally" refer to these people as being "obsessed." By our more behavioral definition, however, they are clearly *addicted*.

OCD is not really similar to most aspects of addictions. Instead, OCD is an anxiety disorder, where obsessive thoughts lead to behaviors that the individuals realize are illogical and inappropriate. Still, the individual feels compelled to perform these actions. When the patient with OCD resists compulsive behaviors, he or she feels extreme anxiety. There are no rewards associated with OCD behaviors, except for the overwhelming reduction in anxiety. On the other hand, addictions are initially extremely pleasant experiences. This contrasts with OCD, which plagues people with intrusive, unwanted thoughts or obsessions and is inherently distasteful.

Furthermore, nonpharmacological addictions frequently involve the psychological-systemic processes of "denial." People with OCD recognize that their obsessions are illogical. But people with a nonpharmacological addictions are often clueless regarding their specific irrationalities and are consequently highly resistant to treatments. The person with OCD almost always wants to get better. People with a nonpharmacological addiction usually want the world to stop punishing them for acting as they please. This is a critical distinction.

Another manner in which OCD differs from nonpharmacological addictions is in the treatment options that are commonly employed. OCD is much more likely to be successfully treated by pharmacological agents. Research indicates that, like depression and bipolar disorder, OCD is caused by an imbalance of neurotransmitters, most likely *serotonin*. This brain chemical regulates mood and sleeping patterns, among other behaviors. Researchers have found that certain antidepressant medications may help alleviate obsessive behaviors. Their apparent action involves increasing the amount of available serotonin at key receptors in the brain. This improves communication between the nerve cells necessary to suppress unnecessary worry.

Behavior therapy has also proven successful in helping people with OCD overcome anxiety. In behavior therapy, a patient is exposed to the feared object or obsession, but prevented from completing the compulsive behavior. For example, people who fear contamination may be encouraged to touch dirty laundry and be denied the chance to wash their hands for a specified period of time. Most often, behavior therapy includes guidelines or a "contract" in which the patient and treatment team agree on certain goals.

On the other hand, classic behavioral therapy involving exposure or response prevention is usually considered ineffective for the treatment of addictions. This is true for both nonpharmacological addictions and substance dependence. However, family therapy is usually more helpful in the treatment of nonpharmacological addictions than in OCD. Family therapy may be valuable in treating obsessive compulsive disorder, but it is not generally considered the major component of treatment.

12. Whereas family therapy is extremely helpful in addictions treatment:
    a. It is equally helpful in the treatment of OCD.
    b. It is actually more helpful in the treatment of OCD.
    c. It is not yet as helpful in the treatment of OCD.
    d. It is never used for patients or clients with OCD.

Table 21.3 indicates differences between OCD and common nonpharmacological addictions. Where there is doubt, however, referral to a person with expertise in discriminating between OCD and addictions is good clinical practice. Usually, competent psychologists are able to test to numerically quantify addictive behaviors and OCD. This may be necessary when it is suspected that OCD and addictions co-exist, which rarely but occasionally occurs.

## FAMILY THERAPY AND NONPHARMACOLOGICAL ADDICTIONS

Several years ago, colleagues and I were examining factors that influenced the development and outcome of a variety of addictive behaviors. We had treated a number of cases in which the identified patient (IP) presented with vague symptoms that resembled classically defined

**TABLE 21.3**

Differences between Obsessive Compulsive Disorders and Nonpharmacological Addictions

| Specific Symptoms | Obsessive Compulsive Disorder (OCD) | NonPharmacological Addictions |
|---|---|---|
| Specific behaviors interfere with quality of life | Yes | Yes |
| Behaviors overwhelm other rewards in life | No | Yes |
| Primarily related to reduction in immediate anxiety | Yes | No |
| Effectively treated with selective serotonergic reuptake inhibitors (SSRIs) | Yes, somewhat | No |
| Effectively treated by behavioral therapies | Yes, somewhat | No |
| Behavior is often "ritualized" and subjectively recognized as irrational | Yes | No |
| Behavior is specifically pleasurable | No | Yes |
| Behavior generates extensive fantasies and "secondary reinforcers" | No | Yes |
| Behavior prompted by overwhelmingly negative cognitions (obsessions) | Yes | No |
| Behavior seen as harmless leisure activity | No | Yes |
| Tendency for persons with behaviors to scorn those without it | No | Yes |

addictive behaviors. However, it was not clear whether chemical addiction was involved. For example, many of these cases involved people whose only complaint was that their spouse expressed excessive concern that they watched too much television or perhaps were "obsessed" with finding bargains. Most of these cases had been labeled as OCD or "impulse control disorders," although they failed to meet true criteria for these diagnoses.

We began to collect data on these cases because we realized that we were failing in their treatment. After applying appropriate statistical tests (e.g., discriminant analysis), we concluded that clients whose initial problems reflected habits involving spending time away from their families were very similar to drug abusers. These results contrasted with families of clients without addictions, as well as families from a community sample of demographically matched nonclients.

By this time, we were using the term *nonpharmacological addictions* as an alternative to the term *obsessions* or *impulse control problems* for these clients. What was confusing, though, was how common apparent nonphysiological addictions were. Many people seemed to have evidence of them. Few, however, sought treatment. We had no idea why, but could generate numerous case histories. At this point, we were baffled. Our concept of nonpharmacological addictions simply seemed to be a measure of eccentric excesses. We could not figure why some people sought treatment, often miserable and without a clue to their dysfunctions, while others were seemingly happy and aware of their behavioral overindulgences.

Eventually, with the help of statistical procedures and the enthusiasm of some graduate students, we were able to see a clear pattern: The overwhelming factor in determining whether an individual was seen by a mental health professional for "obsessive" behaviors was whether he or she had a nuclear family with whom they dwelled. Apparently, living with your family turns an excessive and eccentric behavior into an addiction! Initially this seems to make little sense. How could a family make someone worse? Aren't families supposed to buffer against stressors?

13. The author and his associates began researching nonpharmacological addictions because:
    a. There were many treatments readily available for people with the correct diagnosis.
    b. Many patients seem to be "falling through the cracks" and not receiving appropriate treatment and were baffling to their treatment providers.
    c. The symptoms of nonpharmacological addictions were identical to OCD.
    d. The symptoms of nonpharmacological addictions were totally unlike anything seen before.

We later hypothesized that one of two conditions are likely to be occurring with the development of nonpharmacological addicts. One was that the family was actually making the IP more pathological. This is congruent with traditional systems theory and is often a "best guess" in working with these families. A second hypothesis is that the family is the force behind securing treatment for these people, who otherwise would not be noticed. People without families continue to write operas in dead languages or to learn the Latin names of hundreds of thousands of birds and no one complains. Data suggests that sometimes, both answers are true. However, the first hypothesis is usually more commonly descriptively accurate.

Additional data suggests that a well-functioning family can also prevent the development of nonpharmacological addictions. It can do this by providing satisfactory alternative sources of rewards. Typical families perform this function effortlessly. However, for some reason, the family of the nonpharmacologically addicted patient fails in this area.

A question we are now considering is whether families are necessary for the development of nonpharmacological addictions. We estimate that people are about four times more likely to develop nonpharmacological addictions if they are living with families that they consider problematic or dysfunctional. On the other hand, people who view their families as supportive are only 30% as likely to develop a nonpharmacological addiction as is a "random control," or typical person chosen off of the streets. With these findings, we began to focus on treatments involving the family system. Here we found an abundance of literature regarding pharmacological addictions. We believe that many of these techniques are directly applicable to nonpharmacological addictions as well.

14. The author and his colleagues demonstrate how:
    a. Research must always come before careful practice.
    b. Research ideas are often generated by scientific questions from other theories.
    c. Clinical problems can successfully generate research questions.
    d. Research must be kept separate from the clinic to avoid extraneous theories.

15. The author and his associates believe that families can:
    a. often change a behavioral excess to a nonpharmacological addiction.
    b. often act to bring people with behavioral excesses into treatment.
    c. often prevent the occurrence of a behavioral excess becoming an addiction.
    d. all of these are true.

16. For reasons that are not clear to the author and his associates, most families act to control behavioral excesses by:
    a. instituting rigid social controls.
    b. isolating or condemning the member who engages in excesses.
    c. offering a variety of rewards to compete with any behaviors that a person may be engaging in excessively.
    d. secretly deny the severity of all forms of addiction.

## Learning From Family Therapies for Pharmacologically Dependent Systems

Our next step involved examining the literature and clinical experiences regarding family therapy of well-recognized pharmacological addictions. Most current sophisticated models of substance abuse do not endorse biology as the complete cause of addictive behaviors. These models recognize that addictions do not develop in social isolation. For many individuals with substance abuse disorders, interactions with the family of origin, as well as with the current family, set the patterns and dynamics for their problems with substances. Furthermore, family member interactions with the substance abuser can perpetuate and aggravate problems. On the other hand, families may also assist in controlling chronic addictions.

Extrapolating from the pharmacological literature, we argue that family therapy for non-pharmacological addictions offers a number of advantages over individual therapies. Family therapy offers an opportunity to focus on the expectation of change within the family (which may involve multiple adjustments). It can allow the system to test new patterns of behavior and is an excellent venue to teach family members how the concept of a family *system* works. Family treatment is a unique opportunity to educate families that nonpharmacological disorders are strikingly similar to pharmacological addictions. Furthermore, it is instrumental in allowing families to understand that addicted people need the strengths of every family member.

Finally, it allows the family to focus on the meaning of the symptoms. In a safe environment it allows the family to come to their own conclusions why the IP and the family both fell into addictive patterns. Families can experiment with alternative explanations and eventually endorse a narrative about the addiction that provides them with hope and meaning.

17. A crucial question not answered by the author's work at this time is:
    a. How do some families fail at providing a variety of natural rewards?
    b. How does a family decide to offer only one reward to its members?
    c. How are addictions possible in dysfunctional families?
    d. How do families communicate to the addicted person that the addiction is acceptable?

18. Based on what the author tells us about the treatment of nonpharmacological addictions:
    a. It is an inefficient use of time to let the family try to understand the meaning of the addictive behavior.
    b. It is wrong to have families try to figure out the meaning of an addiction within their family system because they usually will be wrong.
    c. It is often very helpful when the family develops their own meaning of the process of addiction and how it affected their lives.
    d. Understanding the meaning of addiction is always the first step in family therapy of addictions.

## Using the Family as an Assessment Tool for Nonpharmacological Addictions

Early in our work, we floundered over whether we could reliably and validly determine the existence of a nonpharmacological addiction. Now, we know you will usually find out nothing from the suspected addicted person. They usually display a distorted perspective common in pharmacological addictions—denial. Families, however, do not necessarily participate in this denial and even when they do, there are usually strong contrary opinions. Often, if a spouse has a nonpharmacological addiction, the other spouse may be in denial as well. However, the children are usually an uncensored source of less biased observations.

The Single Interest Assessment Inventory (SIAI; Table 21.4) was developed to determine whether a person in a family system has a nonpharmacological addiction. Note that in the questionnaire we deliberately avoid the term *addiction* because of the associated stigma. Our research suggests that people who have an addiction, whether pharmacological or otherwise, will generally score low on this inventory. In the case of a married couple, the spouse may also score low if he or she is in denial. At the present, we believe that the best assessors for nonpharmacological intervention are family members that are siblings, children, or parents.

19. The Single Interest Assessment Inventory was developed to be administered to:
    a. the addicted person alone.
    b. the spouse of the addicted person.
    c. the children of the addicted person.
    d. the entire family system.

20. The Single Interest Assessment Inventory was not developed to be accurate when administered alone to:
    a. the addicted person by him- or herself.
    b. the spouse of the addicted person.
    c. the children of the addicted person.
    d. the entire family system.

21. Data obtained with the Single Interest Assessment Inventory suggest:
    a. Addicted people give the best information about their addiction of anyone in the family system.
    b. The addicted person and his or her spouse give the best information about the extent of the addicted person's addictions.
    c. It is impossible to assess addiction accurately in a family context.
    d. Often, different family members will furnish very valuable information about another family member's problems with addictions.

## HARD AND SOFT FAMILY THERAPIES

Over a decade ago, an associate and I (McCown & Johnson, 1993) argued that brief, crisis-oriented therapy was most appropriate for families who probably did not have the resources to commit to deeper levels of change. Our concern was a trend that suggested too many family therapists were upsetting family systems of clients who likely would terminate treatment prematurely. When the clients failed to follow through with treatment, this left whatever dysfunctional system they had previously maintained in tatters. The results were a vicious

**TABLE 21.4**

Single Interest Assessment Inventory

---

Please answer these questions based on the following scale:

1. I very strongly disagree that this statement describes the person.
2. I strongly disagree that this statement describes the person.
3. I somewhat disagree that this statement describes the person.
4. I am neutral or just do not know.
5. I somewhat agree that this statement describes the person.
6. I strongly agree that this statement describes the person.
7. I very strongly agree that this statement describes the person.

Please circle the person you are answering this question about: myself, my spouse, my parent, my older brother or sister, my younger brother or sister, another family member (please specify_____), my friend

When you answer the questions below, they will be about the person you have circled above and involve their behavior and thinking during the *last month*.

1. This person spends most of his or her time on one or two activities in life.
2. This person manages to meet most of his or her obligations successfully. (-)
3. This person has an interest in something that others sometimes might think is excessive or even fanatical.
4. It seems like fewer and fewer things make this person happy.
5. This person is interested in a variety of experiences in life and most people recognize this quickly. (-)
6. Some people might say this person's interests are too narrow or focused.
7. This person spends a lot of time fantasizing or talking about their favorite activity in life.
8. Only one or two things in life really make this person happy.
9. This person can usually find reward or pleasure in most activities that they are required to do. (-)
10. This person needs to broaden their experiences and do more in life than the one or two activities that seem to make them happy.
11. There are one or two things in life that if this person does not do, he or she will simply be miserable.
12. This person probably would not give up what they do for fun, even if you paid them.
13. At times it seems that this person spends too much energy, money, or time on one or two things that seem to make them the happiest.
14. There are some things this individual is so enthusiastic about that I can't see them ever quitting, even if they had to for health reasons.

Items with "(-)" are reverse scored, meaning their number is subtracted from the total.

---

cycle of crisis proneness on the part of the client or IP and the development of a pattern of treatment resistance on the part of the system.

This phenomena was explored in greater depth by Bütz, Chamberlain, and McCown (1997), using new terminology from the branch of science loosely labeled as "chaos theory." Bütz et al. were interested in whether findings in the science of nonlinear dynamical systems theory paralleled developments in family therapy. Their conclusion was that physics and family therapy were both realizing that the maximum likelihood for deep change in a system occurs when a system is about to break down. Technically, it occurs when a system "borders the chaotic." Furthermore, as both family therapists and physicists know, systems on the verge of chaos can "self-organize" or develop increasing complexity to better meet the environmental demands on them. Two decades ago this was a fanciful thought. Now, it is accepted as a part of orthodox physics and chemistry and is taught in introductory text books in the "hard sciences." Family therapists have known it for much longer, however. It has influenced practice for many years.

22. The work of Bütz, Chamberlain, and McCown has demonstrated that:
   a. A great deal of what family therapists have been doing for years now parallels recent discoveries in physics and mathematics.
   b. It is irrelevant to learn from disciplines such as physics and mathematics.
   c. Family systems change in unique ways compared to other systems.
   d. Only families in chaos are likely to change.

McCown and Chamberlain (2000) differentiate between "hard" and "soft" approaches to family therapy. The former argues that a disorder will not be successfully treated unless serious fundamental changes occur in a family. These changes disturb the homeostasis of the existing family order and allow a new degree of *self-organization* or enhanced functioning following a crisis, a phenomena that is now commonly recognized in a variety of complex systems throughout nature. On the other hand, softer approaches are useful for clients who are not necessarily committed to family therapy or where family therapy is adjunctive, rather than central to treatment. Table 21.5 highlights some of these differences in intervention techniques and intentions between soft and hard interventions.

## Applications of Soft and Hard Therapy Techniques

For the treatment of nonpharmacological addictions, soft family therapy techniques are largely characterized as supportive. Some of my colleagues and I have reached a tentative conclusion that soft therapies are generally ineffective for changing the IP with a nonpharmacological

**TABLE 21.5**

Differences between "Soft" and "Hard" Therapies

| Therapy Characteristics and Uses | Soft Family Therapy | Hard Family Therapy |
|---|---|---|
| Primarily educational and alliance building | Often | Never |
| Helpful if a system is "slightly" off course | Yes | No–too disruptive |
| Useful where families are crisis prone and treatment resistant | No | Yes |
| Causes substantial change in family functioning | Occasionally or sometimes | Yes |
| Useful where recovery of addicted person makes another component of system more dysfunctional | No | Yes |
| Examines behaviors of previous generations | Not usually | Frequently |
| Risks having a system deteriorate and function more poorly | No | Yes, sometimes |
| Helpful for severely pathological family | Not likely | Yes |
| Length of treatment | Usually short | Usually longer |

addiction. At best, they may encourage the family to continue to "hang in there" and may help other family members to differentiate themselves from the IP. This type of therapy may be helpful in reducing the stress of individual members of the family system or even in reducing enabling. However, they rarely are substantial enough to result in the deeper level of change that is necessary to break individuals away from nonpharmacological addictions.

We do not have sufficient empirical support regarding this position and await a more organized research effort to expand our conclusions. However, we have a collaborative effort of several hundred hours of transcripts, as well as case studies and follow-up data. The results suggest that if family therapy is going to be effective with advanced cases of nonpharmacological addictions, it must be disruptive to the pathological family system. Borrowing a term from physics, it must provide for *catastrophic* changes. The therapist, after observing the family, is in a position to determine whether the system can withstand the rigors of this type of intervention, which usually follows techniques from structural or strategic family therapists. These interventions are designed to restore the identified patient to their appropriate family role, strengthen generational boundaries, and thereby allow the nonpharmacologically addicted person to experience additional rewards in their lives. In the process, they compete with the addiction and allow the addicted person to reexperience his or her previous lifestyle.

Eventually, if therapy is successful, these rediscovered rewards can act to crowd out the single rewarding property associated with the addiction because other events, thoughts, feelings, and experiences are once again pleasurable and rewarding. This allows an addicted person to exist with the possibility of being free from what one client called "the insanity of addiction to something you really do not like." As in other areas of family therapy, advances in physics and mathematics are neatly mirroring successful clinical practice. For example, the recent volume by Wolfram (2002), though lengthy and at times somewhat technical, nicely summarizes how almost identical processes occur throughout all facets of nature, including the brain. Physicists and family therapists, it seems, have much more in common than they realize.

23. By restoring the capacity of an addicted individual to be rewarded from other events:
    a. It is likely that the addiction will lose much of its attractiveness.
    b. An individual may return to a more normal lifestyle.
    c. Family therapists are practicing phenomena that occur throughout nature.
    d. All of the above are true.


# THE SUCCESSFUL FAMILY TREATMENT OF NONPHARMACOLOGICAL ADDICTIONS: A CASE EXAMPLE OF HARD FAMILY INTERVENTION

Exactly how do hard family therapy interventions work? This class of interventions is more a philosophy about what is necessary in family therapy, rather than a specific set of techniques. This will be illustrated in an ongoing case from a colleague, where the therapist applied what we now label "hard" techniques to produce dramatic changes in an otherwise resistant system.

Jenna, a pseudonym, was an executive at an internationally known company. Her husband, "Ron," a carpenter and building contractor with less formal education, was a cause of embarrassment for her in her world of executive travel. Because she was frequently out of town, her husband single-handedly ran the home, took care of the three teenage children, managed household finances, and performed almost as a single parent.

Jenna began spending whatever time she had in her area following a local sports team, the Chicago Cubs (again a pseudonym), the popular baseball team. She became a season ticket holder and when the Cubs were out of the area, she watched them at a local sports bar. Ron and the children were not included in these activities. At the end of the baseball season, Jenna sunk into a depressive agitation, often behaving rudely toward her family. Her daughter recalls that Jenna was "traveling, at a game, watching a game at a bar, or trying to avoid us." By her own account, Jenna spent 30 or more hours of time with fellow Cubs fans.

By now her family had learned to function well without her. The oldest child had assumed many parental responsibilities. Ron worked and lovingly attended to his children and their needs in adolescence. Jenna was generous with her large check, which was four times what her husband made. Ron did not care about the money, but wanted Jenna back, at least occasionally "so that we can do things as a family again."

The children were less sanguine. "Mom has gone off and become a Cubs fanatic," the youngest noted. "Between that and her work, it was her way of telling us that she didn't care about the family. Not only that, but the Cubs always lost. Go figure. . . ."

Jenna might have tried to continue this life, at least as long as the children were living at home. She was committed to the notion of a two-parent life for her children, despite the fact that she steadfastly avoided the necessary commitments. However, her work performance began to suffer slightly, especially when her team lost. Furthermore, she presented her boss with a rather irrational vacation schedule, based on seeing the Cubs play out of town. The vice president, who was relying on her for completion of an important project, was stymied. He too liked the Cubs. Yet he had seen addiction before, having a son with a cocaine problem. He believed that Jenna must be experiencing a substance abuse disorder and that the Cubs attraction was a ruse to hide her chemical dependencies. He notified an employee assistance counselor, as was the company policy.

While talking to the counselor, Jenna's behavior was polite but inappropriate. She constantly made references to sports and the Cubs and avoided conversations about stress at work or home. The counselor found no evidence that Jenna was abusing drugs or alcohol. Nor was there evidence of any major psychopathology. What was clear was that Jenna was "obsessed" with the Cubs. The counselor had no explanation and suggested that Jenna see a psychiatrist, thinking Jenna might be bipolar (manic depressive) or perhaps even have early signs of a brain tumor.

The psychiatrist was not helpful. He tried Jenna on several drugs that are useful for obsessive compulsive behaviors. These had no effect. He then tried her on drugs to control bipolar disorder, thinking she might have an undiagnosed manic depressive illness. This was no help either. Eventually, he recommended that Jenna consult a family therapist, a procedure he usually employed when he had abandoned all other hope!

Jenna was reluctant to participate further. However, she was aware of a potential vice presidency position if she could get a "clean bill of health."

The therapist met with Jenna for a single session and formulated a clear plan. The therapist hypothesized that Jenna's actions were a nonpharmacological addiction that was "fueled" by her desire to escape marriage to a partner she considered socially inferior. Furthermore, Jenna's fast-paced life style left little interest for the routine tasks of child rearing. The therapist agreed to meet with Jenna again, but only if she brought her husband.

The therapist, trained in strategic and structural approaches to therapy, realized that it would take a tremendous amount of stress to the family system to dislodge it from its comfortable but dysfunctional moorings. In a style that would be dangerous in the hands of a less skilled professional, the therapist started the next session with a question.

"Tell me, Jenna, are you happy with your affair?"

Jenna was incredulous. She denied any extramarital infidelities. "Believe me, if I had wanted to mess around, I would have had plenty of opportunities on any of my business trips."

The therapist did not miss a beat in her response.

"I didn't say you had or were having an affair with a person. Instead you are having an affair with an entire sports team, something that is far more harmful to your family than any sexual involvement." The therapist then recited the history that Jenna had gleefully told her the previous week, about her thousands of dollars spent on sports tickets, thousands more in out of town trips, and hundreds of hours in the company of people she had almost nothing in common with, except for mutual fanaticism of the Chicago Cubs.

"Jenna," the therapist prescribed, "I want you to move out for a week. I think you are addicted to the Cubs. When you move out, I want you to have no contact with your family, unless it is an emergency, or have anything having to do with the Cubs, for that matter. At the end of the week we will reschedule another session. If you want to stay married you will have to give up your interest in the Cubs. It is that simple."

In the meantime, Jenna was instructed to work regular hours and to keep a diary of her feelings and thoughts. This included several scales designed to measure her anxiety, depression, and craving for sports each day, as well as her ability to concentrate and a subjective assessment of her work performance.

Needless to say, Ron was astounded. However, he realized that he had somehow lost his wife and had in a strange way intuitively understood that he had played a role that facilitated her leaving home. They both departed sadly, though without a commitment.

At the end of the week the couple met again. The therapist asked Jenna what her week had been like.

"It was hell. I missed my family. I realized that something was wrong with me. I was tense, angry, the same feelings I get when I am at home but ten times worse. At work, I was worthless. Good Lord, it was like when I quit smoking before I was pregnant. I was just like a caged animal. For a couple of days all I could think about was turning on the TV and watching Cubs. It was a real craving, just amazing.

"A couple of days into my 'exile,' something changed. Maybe three days, I don't know. I just realized how lucky I had it. I mean, I have a wonderful, loving husband, good kids, and great kids really. I'm doing fine at my job. This whole thing of following the Cubs, it is confusing. I don't understand why I am such a fan. But I do know it's crazy, it's like a drug addiction or something.

"All I know is I want back in the family."

Therapy was not finished. Additional phases involved allowing Ron to understand the nature of nonpharmacological addictions, reintegrating the family, re-establishing appropriate boundaries, and then finally exploring what the addiction meant to the IP and the family. Anger and resentment surfaced among family members. As soon as the IP became more functional and decreased her nonpharmacological addiction, the oldest daughter developed a dangerous experimentation with drinking alcohol. Ron, relinquishing some of his complete autonomy and authority in the family system, developed anxiety and began to acquire habits that he knew would be bothersome to his wife. For example, he left the kitchen messy, a situation she abhorred.

Within six months, the family was functioning better than it had in years. Jenna continued her success in work. Her boss ascribed her "strange behavior" to exhaustion. She and her husband again had a normal relationship and she even brought him to company functions! The irony is that the corporate head and founder genuinely appreciated Ron's lack of pretentiousness and entrepreneurial spirit.

Not every case ends this smoothly. Ron and Jenna remained happily married. The children eventually left for college. Jenna lost her fanaticism for the Cubs, though she still reads the sports pages daily. The therapist and her colleagues learned a valuable lesson regarding how a master clinician can treat nonpharmacological addictions in a family context.

24. In the case study with Jenna, one factor that seemed to accelerate her excessive sports involvement was:
    a. positive involvement with her family.
    b. an attempt to reject her family for her career.
    c. job stresses that encouraged her to develop a drinking problem.
    d. personal issues related to her religious beliefs.

25. As is often common in a variety of nonpharmacological addictions:
    a. The family was the last group to recognize that Jenna had a problem.
    b. The family recognized that Jenna had a problem long before Jenna did.
    c. The family reorganized itself and ignored Jenna's problem.
    d. The family was primarily responsible for Jenna's fanaticism about sports but not her addiction.

26. Jenna's therapist most likely performed a "radical" family intervention because:
    a. She realized that Jenna was at risk not to return.
    b. She realized that a fresh interpretation of the problem would keep Jenna interested in therapy.
    c. She was not trained in any other more appropriate therapies.
    d. She realized that only a radical intervention could dislodge Jenna's addictive fanaticism and save her marriage.

27. From what has been presented in this chapter we can speculate that:
    a. The treatment of nonpharmacological addictions is far from mastered and needs the attention of creative therapists.
    b. Additional research is urgently needed to further understand the processes involved in nonpharmacological addictions.
    c. Many of the advances in family therapy and family systems theory closely parallel revolutionary progress in physics, mathematics, and other sciences that are not usually associated with family therapy.
    d. All of these are true.

---

Behaviors can be just as severely addicting as pharmacological substances. The impact of nonpharmacological addiction can be disastrous to the individual who has the addiction, as well as that person's social system and to society. The addicted person's family is intimately involved in the skein of reciprocal causality that causes such addictions to develop. We hope further clinical work and research can help potentially millions of patients who are presently missing the opportunity for meaningful treatment. The frontiers of treatment of nonpharmacological addictions are just now being explored. My colleagues and I welcome the energy, creativity, ideas, and tenacity of the next generation of family therapists.

## KEY TERMS

**addiction:** (As used in this chapter.) The process by which one reward or class of rewards becomes the most important aspect of an individual's thinking, behaving, and feeling.

**dependence:** Needing more of a drug or experience to obtain a previous level of the same pleasurable feeling. Dependence is not the same as addiction and is not confined to pharmacological addictions.

**motivational strength:** This indicates how hard individuals will work to perform behaviors or obtain substances that they abuse.

**motivational toxicity:** The manner in which an excessive experience or drug disrupts the hierarchy of normal motivations that we all possess.

**nonpharmacological addiction:** A situation where individuals are addicted to an *experience, person, or situation,* rather than to a specific chemical of abuse.

**obsessive compulsive disorder:** An anxiety disorder characterized by obsessions, which are recurrent, distressing thoughts, or impulses experienced as unwanted and irrational. Compulsions are repetitive behaviors, usually performed in response to the obsession to reduce anxiety or distress.

**pharmacological addictions:** Addictive behaviors that involve ingesting drugs or alcohol. Most people think that all addictions have to involve substances that are ingested.

**self-organization:** The capacity of a complex system undergoing a critical period to rearrange itself for superior functioning. This phenomenon is seen throughout nature, from the behaviors of molecules to that of galaxies and arguably occurs in family systems as well.

**withdrawal:** Condition where the body seems to respond to the absence of an addictive substance or experience by initiating a process of instituting a "mirror image" of the drugs' or experience's initial effects. As the homeostatic changes slowly reverse, withdrawal symptoms gradually decline.

## DISCUSSION QUESTIONS

1. Why does it seem that society has been slow to recognize that addiction to behaviors is also possible?
2. The sheer amount of stimulation around us is increasing at a rapid rate. Do you believe that this has any implications for nonpharmacological addictions? If so, is there any type of preventive strategy? Where should prevention begin?
3. How might individual or family stress influence the acquisition or treatment of nonpharmacological addictions?
4. Are there other techniques from family therapy that you believe might be especially effective with families where there is a member with a nonpharmacological addiction?

## SUGGESTED FURTHER READING

Haly, J. (1987). *Problem solving therapy* (2nd ed.). San Francisco: Josey Bass.

This is a classic in strategic therapy that forms the basis of much of the "hard" interventions that are often necessary for nonpharmacological addictions.

Orford, J. (2001). *Excessive appetites: A psychological view of addictions* (2nd ed.). New York: Wiley.

This book is the classic presentation that addictions are not a product of biology alone but are related to complex psychosocial factors. The newer edition includes revisions in basic science discovered since the first edition, in 1984. Orford probably did more to popularize the concept of addictions, both pharmacological and nonpharmacological, as "excessive appetitive behavior."

Stanton, M. D., & Todd, T. (Eds.). (1982). *Family therapy of drug abuse and addiction.* New York: Guilford Press.

This book is a classic, the first solid demonstration of the effectiveness of family therapy for substance abusers. It is must reading!

## Valuable Web Sites:

www.biopsychiatry.com.

This Web site, which goes by a variety of names, has a strong agenda suggesting that neuropharmacology will provide better living. However, its well-organized links and constantly updated research make it an outstanding reference for people interested in the biology of addictions, as well as other disorders.

www.strengtheningfamilies.org/html/ programs_1999/10_MDFT.html

This Web site explores *multidimensional family therapy.* Multidimensional family therapy (MDFT) is a family-based treatment developed for adolescents with drug and behavior problems and for substance abuse prevention. The technique has also proven useful for people with nonpharmacological addictions as well.

www.peele.net

*The Stanton Peele Addiction Web Site.* Stanton Peele, PhD, is a social/clinical psychologist who has greatly influenced the addiction field by attempting to argue that addiction is a choice, not a disease. This is a very interesting site for traditional "disease model" advocates.

www.habitsmart.com

*HabitSmart Home Page.* This Web site was launched in early 1995, and was among the first sites dedicated to not only providing alternative theories of addictive behavior and change but also to expanding the concept of what addiction is and how to effectively manage it.

## REFERENCES

American Psychiatric Association. (2000). *Diagnostic and statistical manual of mental disorders* (4th ed., text revised). Washington, DC: Author.

Bütz, M., Chamberlain, L., & McCown W. (1996). *Strange attractors: Chaos, complexity, and the art of family therapy.* New York: Wiley.

Johnson, J., & McCown, W. (1997). *Family therapy of neurobehavioral disorders.* New York: Haworth.

McCown, W., & Chamberlain, L. (2004). *Gambling disorders: Experimental and empirical research.* Victoria, British Columbia: Trafford Publish House.

McCown, W., & Chamberlain, L. (2000). *Best possible odds: Innovative theory and treatment of gambling disorders.* New York: Wiley.

McCown, W., & Johnson, J. (1993). *Therapy with treatment resistant families: A consultation/crisis intervention approach.* New York: Haworth.

Wolfram, S. (2002). *A new kind of science.* Cambridge, MA: Wolfram Press.

# 22

# Depression and Anxiety

## Frank M. Dattilio
*Harvard Medical School and*
*University of Pennsylvania School of Medicine*

## TRUTH OR FICTION?

___ 1. *A couple or family in crisis is one of the most volatile situations that a mental health professional is likely to encounter during his or her career.*

___ 2. *The mental health therapist should never be concerned with covert diagnoses in the relationships when treating depression or anxiety.*

___ 3. *ICD-10 is the preferred diagnostic system used in North America over the DSM–IV.*

___ 4. *Bipolar disorders are the most commonly seen disorders in couples.*

___ 5. *A cyclothymic disorder is characterized by a prominent and persistent disturbance of mood judged to be a direct physiological consequence of drug abuse and medication.*

___ 6. *The terms severity, psychotic, remission, chronic are just a few of the specifiers used with depressive diagnosis.*

___ 7. *There is very little research on the co-occurring relationships between marital and family distress.*

___ 8. *When depression and marital problems are concomitant, the treatment of choice is marital therapy.*

___ 9. *It has been found that the risk of depressive symptoms increases ten-fold in individuals when marital distress exists.*

___ 10. *Depression in couples tends to be acute rather than chronic.*

___ 11. *One of the focal points of disorder-specific couples intervention for both depression and anxiety is to identify secondary gain.*

___ 12. *Pharmacotherapy has proven to be an effective adjunct to the treatment of both depression and anxiety among couples.*

___ 13. *Social phobia is the most common type of anxiety disorder found with couples in distress.*

___ 14. *One finding in the professional literature is that a nonagoraphobic or panic-disordered spouse may consequently experience some level of threat in response to the amelioration of the problem or autonomy of the identified patient during treatment.*

___ 15. In vivo *exposure and interoceptive techniques have been deemed to be the least efficacious treatments for anxiety and marital problems.*

One of the most volatile situations a mental health practitioner will encounter during the course of his or her professional career is a couple or family in the midst of a crisis. In some respects, this scenario surpasses other types of circumstances in terms of volatility because the **system** involves more than one set of personality dynamics.

Add to this that the most commonly reported complaints in the mental health arena fall within one of the subcategories of anxiety and depressive disorders, and you have a most challenging mix. In fact, in a comprehensive survey of primary care physicians, **anxiety** and **depression** were identified as two of the six most common conditions encountered in family practice (Orleans, George, & Houpt, 1985).

1. Primary care physicians have identified which two disorders as among the six most common conditions encountered in family practice?
   a. schizophrenia and bipolar disorder
   b. anxiety and depression
   c. eating disorders and sleep disorders
   d. drug and alcohol disorders

## WHAT SHOULD I KNOW ABOUT DEPRESSION AND ANXIETY IN RELATIONSHIPS?

This chapter focuses on providing a comprehensive understanding about treating anxiety and depression, specifically within the context of couples and family therapy. Although the basic tenets of treating these disorders with individuals are similar to working from a couple or family perspective, they are not the same, particularly with regard to the techniques used and the manner in which the treatment process unfolds. The differences take on great importance, especially in light of covert dynamics that serve to perpetuate each disorder and how they affect the couple and family relationship.

2. Anxiety and depressive disorders differ to what degree when working with couples and families as opposed to individually?
   a. significantly
   b. moderately
   c. slightly
   d. not at all

The initial overview presents various diagnoses for both depression and anxiety and at times what are reported to be the most efficacious modes of treatment. The discussion then shifts to how these treatment approaches are adapted for a couple or family given that within this context, anxiety or depression are seen as co-occurring with marital or family distress. Treatment then must take into account the potential for multiple diagnoses and also the dynamic interplay that occurs between spouses or among family members.

# DEPRESSION

According to the *Diagnostic and Statistical Manual of Mental Disorders,* 4th Edition, Text Revision (*DSM–IV–TR;* American Psychiatric Association [APA], 2000), which is the most widely used diagnostic classification for mental disorders, five areas of depression are listed under the general category of mood disorders. These include major depressive disorder; dysthymia; bipolar disorder I and II; cyclothymic, mood disorders due to medical conditions; and substance induced mood disorders. A broader classification divides these diagnoses into either **unipolar** or **bipolar** illnesses. Unipolar depression has been classified into three subcategories, namely, major depressive disorder, dysthymic disorder, and depressive disorders not otherwise specified (NOS). One of the main features of unipolar depression is a category of manifestations referred to as *negative signs and symptoms,* which includes flattened mood, loss of interest, and **vegetative signs** such as sleep disturbances, decreased or increased appetite, psychomotor agitation, fatigue, difficulty concentrating, and thoughts of worthlessness or guilt (APA, 2000). The following is a brief overview of the categories of depression most commonly seen with couples who present for treatment. While any one of the subclassifications of depression may be found among couples and family members, the most frequent diagnoses are adjustment disorder with depressed mood and dysthymic disorder. The reader is referred to chapter 4 of this text, "Psychopathology," which explains all of the disorders in much greater detail.

3. Of the five depressive disorders in the *DSM–IV–TR,* which of the following is not included as a category of the new disorders?
   a. refractory depression
   b. cyclothymic disorder
   c. bipolar disorder
   d. dysthymia

## Major Depressive Disorder

Major depressive disorder is characterized by one or more major depressive episodes (at least two weeks of depressed mood or loss of interest accompanied by at least four additional symptoms of depression must be present). Major depressive disorder may be qualified as being a single or recurrent episodes.

## Dysthymic Disorder

Dysthymic disorder is characterized by at least two years of depressed mood for more days than not, accompanied by additional depressive symptoms that do not meet criteria for the major depressive disorder or a depressive episode.

## Adjustment Disorder With Depressed Mood

This subtype of adjustment disorder is designated when the predominant manifestations include symptoms such as flattened mood, tearfulness, or feelings of hopelessness during a situation in which an individual experienced significant emotional behavioral symptoms in response to one or multiple identifiable psychosocial stressors. This is one of the more frequently encountered mood disorders found among couples in conflict or with family members who are in a crisis. These symptoms usually develop within three months after the onset of the stressor, such as the elevation of infidelity or marital tension, and then remain for a limited time. They are also classified as either being in an **acute phase**, which involves persistent symptoms of less than six months, or a **chronic phase**, in which the specifier can be used to indicate six months or more in duration.

It is clear that the diagnosis of depression can be quite complex given the many potential variables involved. To complicate matters further, depression may co-occur with other disorders such as any of the personality disorders outlined on Axis II of the *DSM*.

---

4. Which disorder is characterized by at least two years of depressed mood for more days than not?
   a. major depressive disorder
   b. bipolar II disorder
   c. substance induced mood disorder
   d. dysthymic disorder

5. In major depressive disorders, which of the following is not a symptom?
   a. sleep disturbance
   b. flattened mood
   c. syncope
   d. fatigue

---

## Comorbidity

The co-occurring relationship between marital and family distress and depression has been well documented in the professional literature (Beach, 2001; Dattilio & Jongsma, 2000; Fincham, Beach, Harold, & Osborne, 1997). Actually, the identification of this combination dates to the early 1970s with the work of Weissman and Paykel (1974), in which a population of women diagnosed with unipolar depression also reported accompanying marital problems. Subsequent results corroborated Weissman and Paykel's findings, lending support to the idea that a lack of a confiding intimate relationship served as a substantial risk factor for depression in women. Weissman (1987) later found that "unhappy marriages" served as a firm risk factor for the onset of major depression (p. 455). Since that time, depression has been recognized as a public health problem along with marital distress, which has recently been acknowledged as a public health problem (Miller, 2000). Both are noted for affecting physical health as well as causing distressing behaviors, thoughts, and emotions that clearly disrupt marital and family functioning and other aspects of an individual's life (Mead, 2002). What is more, the potential for depression to contaminate within marital and family situations is very high, particularly because of the proximity and the depth of the interaction that exists in the relationship. Such disturbances in functioning are manifested in issues related to communication, problem solving, and tolerance of stress (Jacobson & Christensen, 1996). Clearly, the association between depression and marital dissatisfaction is significant, and meta-analytic studies suggest that the link between depressive symptoms and marital dissatisfaction is greater for women than for men (Whisman, 2001). Weissman (1987) further reported that married women and men who were "not getting along" with their spouses were 25 times more likely to experience depression than married spouses who were getting along. Being in a "troubled" spousal relationship is said to increase a couple's odds of experiencing an affective disorder by approximately four-fold.

There is some debate in the professional literature as to the advantage of treating depressive disorders within the context of marital and family therapy as opposed to separately in individual psychotherapy. Typically, marital and family therapy has been designated as the treatment of choice when the two are concomitant—that is, when marital or family problems are intertwined with depression and one or more family members are involved (Mead, 2002). An example of this might be a wife's depression that is due in part to her husband's infidelity. This issue is compounded by the fact that the husband claims that he has strayed outside of the marriage because his wife has been unresponsive to him emotionally and has shown no interest in sexual relations. The reciprocal relationship may render it difficult for a therapist to discern which problem occurred first and how each affects the other. Beach, Sandeen, and O'Leary (1990) strongly suggested that marital dissatisfaction most often predates depression. Marital dissatisfaction is likely to lead to an increased risk of depression by reducing available support and therefore contributing to the further alienation and isolation of the depressed spouse.

On the other hand, Coyne (1976) proposed that depression is most likely to predate marital dissatisfaction with the depressive condition serving as an aversive stimulus in the marital relationship. This theory has been supported by other researchers as well (Davila, 2001).

A clinician might legitimately question which should be treated first, the dysfunction in the marital relationship or the depression. Even more confusing, a clinician might be challenged by a patient to address the depression as a way to "distract" treatment and avoid dealing with marital or family issues. Like the two sides of a coin, the pictures are separate but inextricably connected. Hence, they must be treated concomitantly. Couples therapy is also supported in the professional literature as the most efficacious mode of treatment for depression when it coexists with marital problems (Beach, 2001).

## Depressive Symptoms

Interestingly, researchers O'Leary, Christian, and Mendell (1994) found that the risk of depressive symptoms increased tenfold in an individual when marital distress existed. The risk of major depressive disorder increased twenty-five-fold for unhappy marriages compared with untroubled marriages (Weissman, 1987). Unfortunately, there is very little research reported to explain how marital distress moderates depression or what effect depression has on marital and family relationships. Whisman (2001) suggested that the relationship that exists between depression and marital distress and other variables may well be bidirectional, each influencing the other. Depression has also been known to precipitate marital problems (Whisman, 2001). Consequently, there is a reciprocal effect that is almost always negative. It is no surprise then that a history of depression in a relationship greatly increases the probability of divorce (Kessler, Walters, & Forthofer, 1998). This is likely due to the fact that living with an individual who is suffering from any form of depression can be very taxing, and the strain will almost certainly increase the distress in a relationship (Benazon & Coyne, 2000). Depression also appears to be more prominent among female spouses than males according to a more recent study (Dudek et al., 2001).

Significantly, in a series of research studies conducted with depressed couples, the investigators found that the depressive symptoms of one spouse influenced the depressive symptoms of the other. These results were applied to both males and females in both cross sectional and longitudinal analyses (Tower & Kasl, 1995). Proximity was also found to be a factor in depression when the couple reported maintaining a close relationship. The symptoms of depression tended to moderate their interaction more than in cases in which couples reported being alienated from each other. It is no surprise that depressive symptoms and marital dissatisfaction tend to be powerful predictors of each other.

Depression in couples is usually chronic rather than acute and thus has been likened to a physical illness in its course (Mead, 2002; Benazon & Coyne, 2000). Further research has indicated that in a study of 400 outpatients over 12 years, many couples were found to have some symptoms of depression approximately 59% of the time (Judd, 1998). Nine out of ten patients fluctuated between mild, moderate, and full syndrome diagnosis of depression. They also were reported to experience two changes in symptom level per year. Clearly, depression, like marital distress, needs to be conceptualized in a manner similar to an individual diagnosed with a medical illness. Therefore, both the family members and the identified patient need to acquire skills to aid in overcoming depression throughout the patient's lifetime. It is when the condition is exacerbated that the crisis usually takes hold. Treatment is typically aimed at helping couples adapt to the depressed individual's symptoms and to developing coping strategies and ways to anticipate periods of accelerated depressive behavior.

## Patterns of Interaction

With regard to patterns of interaction during marital and family distress and depression, depressive symptoms and marital dissatisfaction have been shown to be powerful predictors of couple conflict resolution strategies. Different predictors have been associated with attacking and avoiding strategies and conflict resolution. Less marital satisfaction is related to attacking conflict resolution strategies for male partners. The fact that men tend to experience an increase in depressive symptoms more readily than do women according to some studies might be related to why men withdraw from marital conflict much more than do women (Gottman, 1994).

It has also been determined that in relationships in which one spouse is depressed, there are more negative communications exchanged than with relationships in which there is no depression present (Nelson & Beach, 1990; Schmaling & Jacobson, 1990). Negative exchanges no doubt are connected to the depression to an extent, but they may also encompass aspects that are unrelated to the depression.

Levkowitz, Fennig, Horesch, Barak, and Treves (2000) found that depression is associated with marital distress, even during periods of symptom remission. The constant negativity of the depressed spouse becomes aversive to the partner. If the nondepressed spouse then follows a natural inclination to either counterattack or withdraw, the positive attributions from the nondepressed spouse may no longer be effective antidotes. The depressed spouse is likely to interpret the partner's defense response as rejection. In addition, the counterattack or withdrawal may reinforce the depressed spouse's negative views of the world, thus contributing to the vicious cycle of depression. See Table 22.1 for a summary of the aspects of marital and family relationships and depression.

**TABLE 22.1**

Aspects of Relationships and Depression

- System—involving more than one set of personality dynamics
- Two most commonly reported complaints are anxiety and depression
- Anxiety and depression co-occur with marital and family distress
- *DSM-IV* is the most commonly used diagnostic classification system
- Negative signs and symptoms are one of the most common aspects of depression
- Comorbidity is an important aspect of treating anxiety and depression

6. The term comorbidity refers to which of the following?
   a. the death of the patient and spouse
   b. how depression causes marital problems
   c. how marital problems cause depression
   d. the relationship between individual psychopathology and marital and family distress occurring simultaneously

7. According to researchers Jacobson and Christensen, difficulties with depression in marital relationships manifest most often through what combination of problems?
   a. communication, problem solving, and tolerance of stress
   b. skill building, sexual relations, and eating habits
   c. sleep difficulties, work-related issues, and child rearing
   d. interpersonal relationships, extended family relationships, and physical illness

8. The majority of research on marital problems and depression suggests which of the following?
   a. marital dissatisfaction is most often likely to predate depression.
   b. depression is most often likely to predate marital dissatisfaction.
   c. the research literature is mixed.
   d. none of the above.

## Attributions

Bradbury and Fincham's (1990) review of the literature on **attributions** suggests that negative attributions, such as criticism and blaming between marital partners, are strongly associated with marital distress. Epstein and Baucom (2002) have conducted further studies with regard to this issue, finding that the depressed spouse's negativity and impact on the partners' interactions are likely to be very wearing on the relationship as time goes on. Consequently, inferences about the spouse's depression may be used to make inferences to explain problems in the relationship.

Numerous empirical studies indicate that distressed partners tend to blame each other for problems and attribute negative actions and unchangeable traits to each other more than do the nondistressed partners (Epstein & Baucom, 2002). Holtzworth-Munroe and Jacobson (1985) labeled this **attributional bias** on the part of unhappy couples **distress maintaining**. Such interpretations on the part of partners leaves very little room for optimism that one's spouse will behave in a more affirmative manner in other situations or in the future. When depression is part of the mix, the problems become magnified. Epstein (1985) described how the attributions of distressed spouses are similar to those of depressed individuals in that the attributions foster a sense of helplessness about positive change. Distressed partners tend to view the other person's negative behaviors as being due to enduring traits. They then explain and justify their own behavior as a response to those negative traits. In addition, when spouses make negative attributions to relationship problems, especially in the case of depression, they are also more likely to have ineffective problem-solving discussions and to behave more negatively toward each other (Bradbury & Fincham, 1992; Miller & Bradbury, 1995).

## Couple-Based Interventions in the Presence of Individual Psychopathology

The challenge in considering how to balance individual and couples problems in treatment cannot be overstated. We may ask ourselves what types of interventions are appropriate in various situations and how to implement couples and family interventions in cases where individual psychopathology is present. Baucom, Shoham, Mueser, Daiuto, and Stickle (1998) suggested that there are several efficacious couple- and family-based interventions that have been developed for various disorders including depression, anxiety, and bipolar disorder. In most cases, these interventions were developed initially for treatment of individual problems and did not include the assumption that a couple was experiencing significant relationship distress as a result of them. However, over time, couples-based interventions have gained recognition as being efficacious in the treatment of individual psychopathology, whether or not relationship distress is present. Baucom et al. presented three types of couple-based interventions that couple therapists can use when individual psychopathology exists. These include **partner-assisted interventions, disorder-specific couples intervention**, and regular couple therapy.

9. Much of the professional research has found that depression in couples tends to be which of the following?
   a. diffuse and slow acting.
   b. chronic rather than acute.
   c. intermittent and acute.
   d. inconsistent across time.

10. In relationships in which one spouse is depressed, _____ is more likely than in cases where no depression is present
    a. clear communication exchanged
    b. positive communications exchanged
    c. improved communication exchanged
    d. negative communication exchange

11. Researchers have found attributions to be important issues in marital discord because of which of the following?
    a. They develop as a result of longstanding depression.
    b. They include criticism and blaming between marital partners, which is strongly associated with marital distress.
    c. Outsiders attribute depression to marital problems.
    d. Attribution is just a matter of people blaming each other.

## Partner-Assisted Interventions

In this particular approach, the nondepressed partner is used as a surrogate therapist or a coach in assisting the spouse who has the disorder. This is in addition to addressing individual problems. Partner-assisted interventions seem to be the most potent when the spouse with the illness has specific therapy homework assignments that must be followed outside of the session. Specific homework exercises can be found in more detail in Dattilio (2002). In this intervention, the nondepressed partner helps to coach the depressed spouse as he or she carries out the homework assignment. Outcomes with this technique depend solely on the dynamics that exist in the relationship. In some cases, placing the nondepressed partner in the role of the coach may add a new level of control, which is diametrically opposed to the goals of treatment. If control is an issue in the relationship, this is probably not the best method to use. This approach can also prove to be difficult if part of the relationship problem involves an inability to work together.

## Disorder-Specific Couples Intervention

This intervention focuses specifically on the interaction patterns of the couple and roles that might contribute to the precipitation or maintenance of symptoms and marital difficulty. The focus here is on how the relationship influences the individual partner's disorder, directly or indirectly. Enabling behaviors are the highlight, specifically those that may be unknown to the assisting spouse. Also considered are the nondepressed spouse's family members and the possibility of engaging alternative means of interaction. The trick here is also to look at some of the secondary gains that the nondepressed spouse may be obtaining as a result of the partner remaining weak and dependent. This dynamic may be more subtle but no less relevant than the depressed spouse's need to develop greater self-reliance.

## Couples Therapy (CT)

Couples therapy is probably the most popular intervention at this level, and it assumes that the overall dysfunction in the relationship is a contributory factor in the maintenance of the individual's depressive symptoms, despite the fact that one partner may be predisposed to depression because of his or her own personality dynamics. Further, the distress in the relationship clearly exacerbates or brings the depressive symptoms to the surface; it is this precipitation that is the focus of treatment (in addition to the lack of support). The following modalities of couples therapy tend to be some of the more effective in the treatment of depression and relationship dysfunction.

*Behavioral Marital Therapy.* Behavioral marital therapy (BMT) has been well documented in its efficacy for dysfunctional marital relationships (Baucom, Shoham, Mueser, Daiuto, & Stickle, 1998), especially in cases in which one of the spouses is depressed (Beach & O'Leary, 1992; Jacobson, Fruzzetti, Dobson, Whisman, & Hops, 1993). Beach (2001) stated that BMT for depression is a safe intervention with proven efficacy in relieving marital discord and that it appears to enhance marital functioning and relieve depressive symptoms (p. 209). Beach went on to say that if one of the partners states or suggests that marital problems are related to the depression, his treatment of choice would be BMT, particularly if the partner is experiencing dysthymia or depression. The severity of depression is not viewed as being a factor that would inhibit the effectiveness of BMT. In fact, in an earlier study, no differences were found in recovery rates for spouses with different levels of severity of depression (Beach, 1996), unless one of the depressed spouses was experiencing suicidal ideation (Beach et al., 1990). Treatment interventions typically involve **quid pro quo exchanges** as well as the exchange of positive behaviors. The exchange of positive behaviors tends to be more effective than the exchange of negative behaviors. The couples concomitantly learn to increase their rate of communication and, with communications training, they improve their exchange. They typically learn coping skills for becoming more tolerant of depressive episodes and behaviors. Improving self-esteem and the formation of mutual exchange in the relationship are also emphasized. The final component of treatment reinforces coping strategies to help couples weather relapses of marital difficulties and depressive episodes.

*Cognitive–Behavioral Therapy With Couples and Families.* Cognitive therapy has been the premiere treatment for depression in individuals, but it has also recently been utilized successfully with couples and family members experiencing depression (Dattilio, 1998, 2001; Dattilio & Padesky, 1990; Teichman, Bar-El, Shore, & Elizur, 1998; Teichman, Bar-El,

Shore, & Sirota, 1995). It was specifically found in a pre- posttreatment study that marital cognitive therapy outperformed individual cognitive therapy as a treatment for depression. Kung (2000) published an excellent article discussing the intertwined relationship among depression and marital distress and those elements of therapy that are most effective as a treatment outcome. Cognitive therapy was found to have a significant impact on patients' cognitions in relationships. Whereas behavioral marital therapy has traditionally focused on the association between marital satisfaction and the exchange of pleasing versus aversive behavior between partners, cognitive–behavioral therapy (CBT) with couples expands this aspect to consider the cognitive dynamics as well. CBT with couples has its roots in behavioral approaches to relationship problems, cognitive psychology, and cognitive therapy. In other cognitive approaches especially, emphasis is primarily on partners' cognitions and, more recently, on emotions. Initial outcome studies have demonstrated the efficacy of CBT in modifying couples' negative relationship cognitions (Baucom & Epstein, 1990; Baucom, Epstein, Rankin, & Burnett, 1996). The cognitive–behavioral approach is designed to address the interrelations among partners' behaviors, cognitions, and affects as they influence the quality of marriages and other intimate relationships, including the level of depression. Unlike behavioral marital therapy, CBT with couples combines cognitive–behavioral interventions, even if from session to session there may be more attention on one than the other. With cases of depression, issues such as cognitive distortion, biased interpretation of interactions, and automatic thoughts are highlighted while communications training, problem-solving training, and behavioral change agreements are utilized. Much of the work involves training clients to identify automatic thoughts and develop strategies for dealing with dysfunctional cognitions. It is regarded as an educational and skill-building approach that emphasizes collaboration between the therapist and the couple or family member in identifying and modifying factors that contribute to conflict, distress, and depression in daily interactions. Cognitive-behavior therapists conduct careful assessments of couples and families to identify severe psychopathology and they give careful attention to recognizing strong influences of family interaction processes on the functioning of each member (Dattilio, 2001; Dattilio, Epstein, & Baucom, 1998).

## Pharmacotherapy

Pharmacological treatments are among the most promoted treatment modalities for depression. Antidepressant medication is clearly on the rise in this context (Mead, 2002). More commonly, however, pharmacotherapy is used as an adjunct to marital treatment of depression, particularly when there are accompanying problems with the marital relationship. In some cases, however, therapy is considered a *psychosocial intervention* and an adjunct to pharmacotherapy, especially with bipolar disorder (Miklowitz et al., 2003). Here, medication is not the sole treatment primarily because pharmacology has not been demonstrated to be as effective as marital therapies are in treating marital distress with depression (Teichman, Bar-El, Shore, & Elizur, 1998), even though some researchers feel that medication, or a combination of medications, is effective in reducing the depression itself. According to the literature, when treating marital distress and concommitant depression, medication may be needed for various depressive disorders, particularly when they are debilitating (Winters, 2000), but otherwise, the treatment should be augmented with marital therapy to work toward remission of both the depression and marital distress.

When medications are used, the prescriptive palette usually includes antidepressant medications such as **selective serotonin reuptake inhibitors (SSRIs)**, tricyclic antidepressants, and in extreme cases, antimanic compounds or monoamine oxidase inhibitors (MAOIs). In the end, medication may be helpful for alleviating symptoms of depression, particularly when the depression is severe, but, alone, it does not appear to improve the quality of couples' marital relationships. To do that, medication needs to be combined with marital psychotherapy. Unless the etiology of a depression is clinical, as in the case of bipolar disorders, then medication is not likely to produce a cure by itself and psychotherapy is necessary.

## Interpersonal Psychotherapy and Emotionally Focused Couples Therapy

There are also two other treatment modalities with marital and family cases that have demonstrated some effectiveness for depression. *Interpersonal psychotherapy* has reported some reduction in depressive symptomatology and an increase in social skills. In addition, *emotionally focused couples therapy* has shown to be effective for marital distress and depression (Johnson & Williams-Keeler, 1998). In another study, Dessaulles (1991) compared pharmacotherapy and emotionally focused couples therapy with marital distressed couples in which the wife reported depression. The results indicate that emotionally focused therapy is only somewhat effective for marital distress and co-occurring depression because the impact of the depression on the female spouse is that the marital adjustment was not affected. Husbands of depressed patients did not improve with regard to their report of marital readjustment either.

## Marital Treatments for Depression

There are myriad treatments that have proven effective in treating dysfunctional relationships with couples (Table 22.2; Dattilio, 1998; Dattilio & Bevilacqua, 2000). However, when depression is part of the picture, treatment may become more complicated. Marital distress has been shown to reoccur even after various types of treatment supported by the literature (Christensen & Heavey, 1999) have been applied. Even with communications training, problem-solving skills, and improved interpersonal skills in place, couples have shown that they still experience difficulty, particularly when one or both spouses are depressed (Judd, 1998). It appears that specific treatments that focus on remediation of depressive symptomatology may be more efficacious than marital treatment in this context than those that do not (Beach, 2001; Dattilio, 1990; Dattilio & Jongsma, 2000; Epstein & Baucom, 2002; O'Leary, Heyman, & Jongsma, 1998).

TABLE 22.2

Highlights of Treatment

- Partner-assisted intervention
- Disorder-specific couples intervention
- Couples therapy
- Behavioral marital therapy (BMT)
- Cognitive–behavioral therapy (CBT) with couples and families
- Pharmacotherapy
- Interpersonal psychotherapy
- Emotionally focused couples therapy

12. Which interventions seem to be the most efficacious when the spouse with depression
    has specific therapy homework assignments that must be followed outside of the session?
    a. partner-assisted interventions
    b. individual interventions
    c. group interventions
    d. therapist interventions

13. Which of the following interventions focus specifically on the interactional patterns of
    couples and roles that might contribute to the precipitation or maintenance of symptoms
    in marital difficulty?
    a. partner-assisted interventions
    b. disorder-specific couples interventions
    c. individual interventions
    d. group interventions

14. Which modality in therapy is dedicated to improving self-esteem and the formation of
    a mutual exchange in the relationship?
    a. cognitive therapy with couples
    b. emotionally focused therapy
    c. interpersonal psychotherapy
    d. behavioral marital therapy

## ANXIETY

The *DSM–IV–TR* provides several subclassifications of anxiety disorder. These subclassifications include panic attacks, panic disorder without agoraphobia, panic disorder with agoraphobia, agoraphobia without a history of panic disorder, specific phobia, social phobia,
obsessive-compulsive disorder, posttraumatic stress disorder, acute stress disorder, generalized anxiety disorder, anxiety disorder due to a general medical condition, substance induced
anxiety disorder, and anxiety disorder not otherwise specified. The various subclassifications
that are found most frequently in marital couples presenting for treatment include panic disorder, agoraphobia, and generalized anxiety disorder.

### Panic Attacks

*Panic attacks* are defined as a discrete period of intense fear or discomfort in which four or
more of the following symptoms occur abruptly and escalate to a peak within ten minutes.

#### Symptoms of Anxiety and Panic Disorder

1. Palpitations, pounding heart, or accelerated heart rate.
2. Sweating
3. Trembling or shaking
4. Sensations of shortness of breath or smothering
5. Feelings of choking
6. Chest pain or discomfort
7. Nausea or abdominal distress
8. Feeling dizzy, unsteady, lightheaded, or faint
9. Derealization (feelings of unreality) or depersonalization (being detached from oneself)

10. Fear of losing control or going crazy
11. Fear of dying
12. Paresthesias (numbness or tingling sensations)
13. Chills or hot flashes

## Agoraphobia

**Agorophobia**—literally, fear of public places—refers to anxiety brought on by being in places or situations from which escape might be difficult or prove embarrassing or in which help may not be available in the event of an unexpected or situationally predisposed panic attack or panic-like symptoms. Agoraphobics tend to avoid being outside of the home alone, especially in a crowd, standing in line, riding public transportation, or being anywhere they may anticipate disabling anxiety and fear, causing them to make a fool of themselves or become immobilized. Individuals usually experience marked distress or anxiety in any of these situations and if they remain in one, it is with great difficulty.

## Panic Disorder Without Agoraphobia

This specific disorder involves recurrent and unexpectant panic attacks (see criteria under panic attacks). At least one of the attacks has been followed by one month or more of one or more of the following: persistent concern about having additional attacks; worry about the implications of the attacks or its consequences, such as losing control, going crazy, or having a heart attack; or a significant change in behavior related to the attacks. The clear absence of agoraphobic symptoms (which include avoidance of certain public situations) must be present.

## Panic Disorder With Agoraphobia

This category describes recurrent, unexpected panic attacks (see panic symptoms). In addition, at least one of the attacks has been followed by one month or more of one or more of the following: persistent concern about having additional attacks, worry about the implication of an attack or its consequences, and a significant change in behavior due to the attacks. The difference between this disorder and the previous is the presence of agoraphobic avoidance.

## Agoraphobia Without History of Panic Disorder

Under this heading we find the presence of agoraphobia related to fear of developing panic-like symptoms, however, the criteria has not been met for a diagnosis of panic disorder. The distinguishing characteristic here is the experience of phobic avoidance but with very few anxiety symptoms, and the fact that a full panic disorder never occurs.

## Generalized Anxiety Disorder

The following factors characterize **generalized anxiety disorder:**

1. Excessive anxiety and worry (apprehensive expectation), occurring more days than not for at least 6 months, about a number of events or activities (such as work or school performance).
2. The person finds it difficult to control the worry.
3. The anxiety and worry are associated with three (or more) of the following six symptoms (with at least some symptoms present for more days than not for the past 6 months).

   a. restlessness or feeling keyed up or on edge

   b. being easily fatigued

   c. difficulty concentrating or mind going blank

   d. irritability

   e. muscle tension

   f. sleep disturbance (difficulty falling or staying asleep, or restless unsatisfying sleep)

4. The focus of the anxiety and worry is not confined to features of an **Axis I** disorder, e.g., the anxiety or worry is not about having a panic attack (as in panic disorder), being embarrassed in public (as in social phobia), being contaminated (as in obsessive-compulsive disorder), being away from home or close relatives (as in separation anxiety disorder), gaining weight (as in anorexia nervosa), having multiple physical complaints (as in somatization disorder), or having a serious illness (as in hypochondriasis), and the anxiety and worry do not occur exclusively during posttraumatic stress disorder.

5. The anxiety, worry, or physical symptoms cause clinically significant distress or impairment in social, occupational, or other important areas of functioning.

6. The disturbance is not due to the direct physiological effects of a substance (e.g., a drug of abuse or a medication) or a general medical condition (e.g., hyperthyroidism) and does not occur exclusively during a mood disorder, a psychotic disorder, or a pervasive developmental disorder.

In addition to the aforementioned disorders, one that may be encountered frequently in treating couples and families is adjustment disorder with anxiety. This subtype **adjustment disorder** is designated when the predominant manifestations include symptoms such as nervousness, worry, or jitteriness. Often found among couples in conflict or in families in crisis, subtype symptoms usually develop within three months after the onset of a stressor or remain for a limited amount of time. They are also classified as either being in an acute phase, which involves persistent symptoms of less than six months, or in a chronic phase in which the specifier can be used to indicate six months or more in duration.

15. According to the professional literature, when treating marital distress and accompanying depression, pharmacotherapy may be needed for various depressive disorders, particularly when they are _____.
   a. debilitating
   b. beginning to reduce
   c. just starting
   d. none of the above

16. Which of the following is not a subclassification of the anxiety disorders outlined in the *DSM–IV–TR*?
   a. panic attacks
   b. panic disorder with or without agoraphobia
   c. anticipatory anxiety
   d. posttraumatic stress disorder

17. Two of the most common anxiety disorders found in marital distress are _____.
   a. specific phobia and social phobia
   b. obsessive-compulsive disorder and posttraumatic stress disorder
   c. panic and agoraphobia
   d. substance induced anxiety and anxiety disorder due to general medical condition

## Comorbidity

The co-occurring relationship between marital and family distress and anxiety is not as well documented in the professional literature as is depression. Specifically, panic disorder and agoraphobia seem to be the two anxiety subtypes that have more of a profound effect on relationships, particularly marriages and family (Barlow, O'Brien, & Last, 1984; Baucom, Stanton, & Epstein, 2003).

In this regard, working with couples when there is anxiety present may be particularly difficult for clinicians because there is more of a need to develop a comprehensive understanding of the disorder itself rather than of the vast array of treatments available. Specifically, the therapist must understand how these individual symptoms are exacerbated or maintained within an intimate relationship because anxiety may produce unusual effects that range from somatic symptoms to dissociation. Of course, any of the anxiety disorders can affect a marital relationship, but the subcategories addressed in this chapter are panic disorder, agoraphobia, and generalized anxiety disorder, which are the most commonly seen in this context.

Early treatments centering on couples therapy for agoraphobia were introduced in the literature in the early 1980s. Unlike simple phobias, which tend to be equally distributed across gender, approximately 75% of agoraphobics have been reported to be female (Agras, Sylvester, & Oliveau, 1969; Marks, 1969). Emmelkamp (1974) noted that in a number of cases, the client's agoraphobia appeared to play an important part in the marital relationship. Further, it interfered with the treatment. In such cases, conjoint marital therapy was required after treatment was completed. Earlier studies have addressed the topic of phobias, particularly of agoraphobia, directly and their impact on marital factors in the relationship. Agulnik (1970) interviewed 50 agoraphobics and their spouses and concluded that the phobic patient was dependent on the spouse who, while not neurotic himself, was "spuriously fortified by such dependence" (p. 63). Hafner (1977a) replicated the study and supported what he called a form of mating in which husbands were found to be emboldened by dependency behaviors in their wives who were agoraphobic. Liotti and Guidano (1976) observed a similar pattern of reinforcement among reports of anxiety and panic from wives of agoraphobic husbands. These findings suggest that there is a strong interplay between these dynamics that needs to be addressed during the treatment process.

## Marital Relations and Satisfaction

In examining marital adjustment in relation to treatment, Hafner (1977b) interviewed a large group of spouses of agoraphobics, obtaining satisfaction ratings both with spouses and with overall marital adjustment after a certain period. A one-year follow-up showed those reporting the poorest marriages also demonstrated the most symptom re-emergence of anxiety, with a significant number of subjects actually becoming worse. Interpersonal relationships and particularly marital relationships have been considered important in the maintenance of certain anxiety disorders, specifically agoraphobia. Barlow, O'Brien, and Last (1984) have noted that observations during treatment have partially confirmed speculations about anxiety and marital relationships. At least two phenomena were seen: First, many clinicians and investigators report that husbands and marriages deteriorated with increased independence of the agoraphobic woman. Problems such as suicide attempts by husbands and extreme pressure on wives to return to dependent roles emerged. Second, evidence exists to support the idea that the state of marital relationships prior to treatment is a good predictor of treatment outcome (Bland & Hallman, 1981). Milton and Hafner (1979) reported that agoraphobics with unsatisfactory marriages, defined as those couples in the lower half of the median split on a measure of overall marital adjustment, were less likely than clients with satisfactory marriages to improve following intensive, prolonged *in vivo* exposure treatment. Couples with unsatisfactory marriages were also more likely to relapse during the six-month follow-up period. The results of Barlow, O'Brien, and Last's study suggests that including the husbands directly in the treatment of agoraphobic women provides a substantial clinical advantage based on their comparison as 12 out of the 14 clients responded to treatment. Women treated without their husbands did not do as well in treatment. Further research suggests that agoraphobic spouses benefit psychologically from their enhanced caretaking role and are likely to react negatively if therapy for the agoraphobic partner leads to improved functioning and less dependence (Daiuto, Baucom, Epstein, & Dutton, 1998).

## Model of Anxiety Disorders

An excellent article by Marcaurelle, Bélanger, and Marchand (2003) in which they provide a clinical review of marital relationships and the treatment of panic disorder with agoraphobia, indicates that there are approximately four models of panic and agoraphobic disorders that are proposed in the literature.

The first model is one that espouses the concept that the spouse of the individual who is suffering from panic disorder or agoraphobia is himself or herself subject to psychological disorders and is obtaining secondary gain or psychological reward from the role of caretaker. The nonagoraphobic or panic-disordered spouse may consequently experience some level of threat by the amelioration of symptoms or the growing autonomy of the identified patient during the course of treatment. The second model is based on the hypothesis of what is known as the *complimentary union* in which it is anticipated that both spouses maintain a secondary gain from the dynamics that exist around agoraphobia or panic. In this model, the dynamic has to do with a dependency, particularly on the part of the individual with the anxiety disorder, who may be seeking parental protection from the domineering spouse or who feels valued by maintaining control in the relationship (Hafner, 1977a). Once again, amelioration of such a disorder may disrupt the homeostasis of the relationship as increased autonomy may be experienced by the non-anxiety–disordered spouse as threatening.

The third model holds that agoraphobia, in particular, may be serving as a way to reduce or avoid marital conflict in the short term. As Symonds (1971) proposed decades ago, agoraphobic avoidance may be how a dissatisfied spouse, who is dependent and anxious about being alone, may cope with the conflicts that exist between the dissolution or maintenance of marital problems. This may be a means of drawing attention to a situation in which the individual feels trapped or immobile in a relationship.

The last model considers *interpersonal problems* as central and suggests that relationship problems of individuals who suffer from panic disorder or agoraphobia are the result of agoraphobic situations or a "state" (Hoffart, 1997, p. 151). This theory purports that interpersonal problems, including marital difficulties, result from pathological states rather than contribute to them. The agoraphobic or panic-disordered individual may tend to be more dependent on individuals close to him or her because of the disorder. Consequently, tension develops in intimate or interpersonal relationships. This tension may be further exacerbated by depressive or anxious affects that are often secondary to the disorder. Therefore, general symptoms such as interpersonal or marital difficulties are likely to decrease along with the decrease of any anxiety symptoms. See Table 22.3 for a summary of anxiety subtypes and their characteristics.

**TABLE 22.3**

Anxiety Subtypes and Characteristics

- Agoraphobia—avoidance of public places and of being alone; fear of fear
- Panic disorder—interoceptive disturbances and uncomfortable body sensations
- Generalized anxiety—excessive worry and apprehension
- Adjustment disorder—usually in reaction to a specific stressor
- Comorbidity—in this context, co-occurring relationship between anxiety and marital/family distress

## Treatment

Many significant studies have made the point that the quality of the marital relationship prior to treatment dictates the most effective treatment outcome. Certainly, better marital satisfaction and/or marital adjustment prior to treatment should lead to greater reduction of anxiety symptoms subsequent to treatment.

### *Cognitive–Behavioral Treatment*

According to the literature, the cognitive–behavioral therapies combined with pharmacotherapy appear to be the most efficacious. Regardless of the subtype of anxiety disorder, the use of interventions such as systematic desensitization, cognitive restructuring, *in vivo* exposure, and interoceptive exposure therapy has been documented with success. *In vivo* exposure treatments clearly appear capable of improving marital adjustment as well as marital communication and interpersonal relations. Many of the cognitive–behavioral treatments enlist the help of a spouse as a cotherapist based on the idea that the patient's compliance with **exposure homework assignments** will be greater and his or her general level of distress from marital conflict will be lower if he or she is actively supported by the spouse (Barlow, O'Brien, & Last, 1984).

The major empirically supported treatment for panic disorder with agoraphobia involves exposure to feared stimuli on two levels. One level is **interoceptive exposure** which involves focusing on feared body sensations internally, and the second level is *in vivo* **exposure**, which requires focusing on fears related to stimuli outside of the body (i.e., external spaces, distance from home, etc.). Central to both is the perception of danger related to either internal or external situations. Often, the individual's response to the perceived threat involves bodily sensations connected to physiological arousal, which may include involuntary stimuli such as accelerated heart rate, rapid breathing, etc. In turn, these sensations may cause individuals to feel as though they may be going to have a heart attack or die or go crazy. Individuals may subsequently engage in maladaptive escape or avoidance behaviors in the hope of evading a far less catastrophic event. Obviously, this cycle can greatly disrupt both the individual's and the couple's or family's life.

The exposure techniques have been used to allow individuals to gradually confront that which they fear and learn to restructure their response internally as well as externally. That is, the cognitive restructuring helps them to reframe catastrophically interpreted body sensations and learn that in fact no harm will come to them as a result of their sensations. It also helps them to confront the feared stimuli in eternal situations while remaining there until the anxiety subsides. The goal of treatment is in part to break the false connection in the individual's mind between escape or avoidance and anxiety reduction. To do this, we show clients that the catastrophic results that they anticipate actually do not occur and that what they experience is anxiety, whether it be generalized anxiety or a specific phobia, and that the symptoms may cause unpleasant feelings but are not fatal or harmful. Craske and Barlow (2002) have pioneered many of the approaches on which interoceptive and *in vivo* exposure techniques for individuals with anxiety are built. The same interventions that are used on an individual basis are also adapted in couples and family therapy. The difference, however, is that a spouse or family member is enlisted to assist in the process of intervention.

## Partner- or Family Member-Assisted Intervention

Typically, the partner or family members are present for all phases of the treatment, particularly with panic and agoraphobia. The family is then educated with respect to the basic elements of the anxiety and how they manifest as panic or agoraphobia or even generalized anxiety. The idea behind this is not only to treat the individual within the family context, but also to help family members and partners understand their role in attributions that may contribute to the patient avoiding or becoming overly dependent on them. Couples and family members are also asked to participate during the process of interoceptive and *in vivo* exposure. Whether it be through breathing exercises or **induced hyperventilation** or **prolonged exposure** in circumstances that produce anxiety, a partner or family member is involved in helping the individual understand that the symptoms are limited and benign. The restructuring of thoughts and diminishing of avoidance behaviors are extremely important. A partner or family member excessively reassuring the patient is an area of concern in the assisted interventions. The role typically shifts across time. Individuals have a tendency to rely on signals or individuals or objects that indicate that they are safe from any danger. These variables have to be identified by the therapist and attempts need to be made to reduce their availability.

Once the individual has successfully reduced their anxiety or phobic avoidance and is reportedly experiencing less anxiety or managing it better with less avoidance, then the marital or family relationship becomes the area of focus. The purpose is twofold, not only to maintain treatment gains, but also to prevent relapse and to identify what might have been the underlying issue spawning the symptoms of anxiety. This is the point of therapy in which individual spouses or family members begin to rearrange or alter their roles in order to accommodate the newly acquired positive behaviors of the identified patient. Markers are made by the therapist for couples and family members to become cognizant of their own behaviors that facilitate regression and bolster the anxiety disorder.

18. The majority of research in anxiety disorders and marital problems indicates that the nonanxiety disordered spouse tends to be _____.
    a. depressed by the patient's dependence
    b. unmoved by the patient's dependence
    c. improved by the patient's dependence
    d. fortified by the patient's dependence

19. Much of the research has found that marriages tend to _____ with increased independence of agoraphobic patients.
    a. improve
    b. deteriorate
    c. remain the same
    d. improve first then deteriorate later

20. A treatment of choice for anxiety disorders and marital problems combined includes _____.
    a. pharmacotherapy alone
    b. cognitive therapy alone
    c. cognitive-behavior therapy combined with pharmacotherapy
    d. none of the above

## *Pharmacotherapy*

Many of the pharmacological treatments that are used with depression in couples and family relationships also are useful for anxiety. Although antidepressant medication continues to be utilized for treating anxiety, anxiolytic medications such as benzodiazepines have become the treatment of choice. Most typically, these medications are used as an adjunct to other types of treatment such as psychotherapy. Treatment should be augmented with marital therapy to work toward remission of both anxiety and marital distress.

Some of the SSRIs, or tricyclic antidepressants, have been used in combination with benzodiazepines to treat anxiety disorders. In addition, MAOIs have also been used, particularly with panic disorders or when anxiety co-occurs with depression. See Table 22.4 for a summary of treatments of anxiety and relationships.

As with depressive disorders, unless the etiology of the disorder is clearly rooted in a chemical dysregulation, the medication alone will not serve as a cure. Psychotherapy is necessary to ensure permanent change.

21. Which symptom is *not* found among individuals diagnosed with panic disorder?
    a. feelings of choking
    b. headaches
    c. sweating
    d. chills or hot flashes

22. One of the primary differences between panic disorder and agoraphobia is in the degree of _____.
    a. avoidance
    b. discomfort
    c. fatigue
    d. heart palpitations

23. Approximately what percentage of agoraphobics are women?
    a. 50%
    b. 25%
    c. 75%
    d. 100%

**TABLE 22.4**

Treatments of Anxiety and Relationships

- Cognitive-behavior treatment—exposure therapy, desensitization
- Partner- or family member-assisted intervention
- Pharmacotherapy and combined individual and family treatment

24. Barlow and O'Brien's 1984 study concluded which of the following?
    a. Marital happiness had no bearing on treatment outcome.
    b. Couples with unhappy marriages are more likely to relapse during the six-month follow-up period.
    c. Relapse in couples occurs no less than one year posttreatment.
    d. None of the above.

25. Which theory contends that both spouses maintain a secondary gain from the dynamics that exist around agoraphobia and panic?
    a. circulanty
    b. the Double Bind theory
    c. follé à deaux
    d. complimentary union

26. With anxiety disorders, particularly panic and agoraphobia, amelioration of the disorder in treatment may disrupt _____ of the relationship and increase _____, which may be observed by the non-anxiety disordered spouse as threatening.
    a. metabolism, stamina
    b. homeostasis, autonomy
    c. focus, anxiety
    d. balance, frustration

27. In generalized anxiety disorder, which is *not* a common criteria found with the diagnosis?
    a. panic
    b. irritability
    c. sleep disturbance
    d. muscle tension

28. The diagnosis of adjustment disorder with anxiety is assigned when the predominant manifestations include which symptoms?
    a. nervousness, worry, or jitteriness
    b. dissociation, depression, or dysthymia
    c. body dysmorphia, anxiety, or insomnia
    d. hypomania, hypervigilance, or paranoia

29. Which of the anxiety disordered sybtypes avoid being outside of the home alone or being in a crowd?
    a. panic disorder
    b. generalized anxiety disorder
    c. agoraphobia
    d. social phobia

30. Which treatment intervention is *not* found among those used in the treatment of anxiety disorders?
    a. *in vivo* exposure
    b. desensitization
    c. physical therapy
    d. programmed muscle relaxation

## KEY TERMS

**acute phase:** A specifier that indicates involvement of symptoms that persist for less than six months.

**adjustment disorder:** A temporary disorder of varying severity that occurs as an acute reaction to overwhelming stress.

**agoraphobia:** An anxiety disorder characterized by a fear of being in open, crowded, or public places or of being left alone or in a place where help is unavailable.

**anxiety:** A diffuse, objectless apprehension or a vague, uneasy feeling.

**attributional bias:** Interpretations that leave little room for optimism that a partner will change.

**attributions:** The ascribing of negative action or blame to a partner.

**Axis I:** The initial category of disorders listed in the *Diagnostic and Statistical Manual of Mental Disorders* (*DSM-IV*) that includes all the various disorders or conditions in the classification, except for the personality disorders and mental retardation, which are found on Axis II.

**bipolar depression:** A major mental disorder characterized by episodes of mania, depression, or mixed moods.

**chronic phase:** A specifier that indicates involvement of symptoms that persist for six months or more.

**comorbidity:** The co-occurring relationship of two or more disorders.

**complimentary union:** A model of marital anxiety disorders based on the hypothesis that both spouses maintain a secondary gain from the dynamics that exist around agoraphobia and panic.

**depression:** A mood disturbance characterized by feelings of sadness, despair, and discouragement, resulting from a situation or condition.

**disorder-specific couples interventions:** An intervention that focuses specifically on the interaction patterns of the couple and roles that might contribute to the precipitation or maintenance of symptoms.

**exposure homework assignments:** Out-of-office assignments that are used to reduce anxiety by repeated contact over a specified period of time.

**generalized anxiety:** An anxiety reaction characterized by persistent apprehension, producing symptoms that range from mild chronic tenseness to more intense states of restlessness and irritability.

**induced hyperventilation:** A technique involving deliberate rapid breathing that is used to disrupt the balance of carbon dioxide and oxygen in order to produce hyperventilation.

**interoceptive exposure:** Exposing one to internal body sensations that have been known to produce anxiety in the individual previously, such as monitoring accelerated heart or respiration rates.

**interpersonal problems:** A model of anxiety disorder that suggests that relationship problems of individuals who suffer from panic disorder or agoraphobia are the result of agoraphobic situations or "states."

*in vivo* **exposure:** "In vivo" meaning, in life, or live exposure to an anxiety-producing object or situation as opposed to one that is imaginal.

**negative signs:** A term used to describe symptoms of depression, such as flattened mood and loss of interest.

**panic attack:** An intense, sudden, and overwhelming fear or feeling of anxiety that produces terror and immediate physiological changes that involve autonomic activity.

**partner-assisted interventions:** When a less disordered partner is used as a surrogate therapist or a coach in assisting the spouse who has the disorder.

**prolonged exposure (imaginally or *in vivo*):** Prolonged contact with a phobic stimulus that will clearly produce varying levels of anxiety, whether imaginally or *in vivo*.

**quid pro quo exchanges:** A little of this for a little of that.

**Selective Serotonin Reuptake Inhibitors (SSRIs):** Antidepressant compounds that directly affect the serotonergic system of neurotransmission in the brain.

**system:** A unit involving more than one individual or set of personality dynamics.

**unipolar depression:** A major disorder of mood that is characterized by depression.

**vegetative signs:** A term used to describe depressive symptoms, which include more physical symptoms such as sleep disturbance, decreased or increased appetite, and those that sustain basic life function.

## DISCUSSION QUESTIONS

1. What are some of the main benefits for treating depression in couples therapy as opposed to individual therapy?
2. In what ways would a dysfunctional marital or family relationship make a depressive condition worse for one or both spouses?
3. How would you go about determining if a spouse has an adjustment disorder with depression as opposed to a dysthymic disorder? What differences in criteria would you look for?
4. Why is it likely that a comorbid disorder may exist with marital or family problems? What are the mechanics that correlates them?
5. Compare and contrast partner-assisted intervention with disorder-specific couples intervention. Why do you believe that one would be better than the other?
6. What is the likely reason that behavioral marital therapy has been documented as being so much more efficacious than other modalities of treatment? What does it appear to have going for it that the others do not?
7. Trace how an individual spouse might develop an anxiety disorder as a result of an unhappy marital relationship? What might account for the development of symptoms?
8. In what ways might individual psychotherapy be superior to partner- or family member-assisted interventions for panic or agoraphobia?
9. What are the likely benefits of treating an anxiety disorder in couples therapy without the use of medications as an adjunct?
10. What would be your best approach if a couple came to you for marital therapy, and both partners complained of symptoms of anxiety and depression? What would be your first step following the assessment phase?

## SUGGESTED FURTHER READING

Barlow, D. H. (2002). *Anxiety and its disorders: The nature and treatment of anxiety and panic.* New York: Guilford Press.

> Many consider this book the bible for anxiety disorders—Barlow is a leader in the field. The best referenced text on the market, it also includes an excellent section on couple and family treatment.

Beach, S. R. H. (Ed.). (2001). *Marital and family processes in depression: A scientific foundation for clinical practice.* Washington, DC: American Psychological Association.

This is probably the finest book on the market addressing depression and marital problems. Up to date and informative, it is edited by the world's top authority on the subject.

Dattilio, F. M. (Ed.). (1998). *Case studies in couple and family therapy: A systemic and cognitive perspective.* New York: Guilford Press.

A case study overview of different treatment for couples and families, many of which involve depressive disorders. Chapters are authored by leaders in the field of marriage and family therapy on 19 different modalities of treatment. This comprehensive text is used by many marriage and family therapy training programs.

Epstein, N. B., & Baucom, D. H. (2002). *Enhanced cognitive-behavior therapy for couples.* Washington, DC: American Psychological Association.

An impressive reference on cognitive–behavioral techniques with couples by two of the top authorities in the field. It offers detailed documentation of research and several case vignettes, which will prove invaluable to readers.

Mead, D. E. (2002). Marital distress, co-occurring depression, and marital therapy: A review. *Journal of Marital and Family Therapy, 28*(3), 299–314.

An up-to-date article on the topic of depression and couple and family treatment.

# REFERENCES

Agras, S., Sylvester, D., & Oliveau, D. (1969). The epidemiology of common fears and phobias. *Comprehensive Psychiatry, 10,* 151–156.

Agulnik, P. L. (1970). The spouse of the phobic patient. *British Journal of Psychiatry, 117,* 59–67.

American Psychiatric Association. (2000). *Diagnostic and statistical manual of mental disorders* (4th ed., text revision). Washington, DC: Author.

Barlow, D. H., O'Brien, G. T., & Last, C. G. (1984). Couples treatment of agoraphobia. *Behavior Therapy, 15,* 41–58.

Baucom, D. H., & Epstein, N. B. (1990). *Cognitive–behavioral marital therapy.* New York: Brunner/Mazel.

Baucom, D. H., Epstein, N. B., Rankin, L. A., & Burnett, C. K. (1996). Assessing relationship standards: The Inventory of Specific Relationship Standards. *Journal of Family Psychology, 10,* 72–88.

Baucom, D. H., Shoham, V., Mueser, K. T., Daiuto, A. D., & Stickle, T. R. (1998). Empirically supported couples and family therapies for adult problems. *Journal of Consulting and Clinical Psychology, 66,* 53–88.

Baucom, D. H., Stanton, S., & Epstein, N. (2003). Anxiety. In D. K. Snyder & M. A. Whisman (Eds.), *Treating difficult couples* (pp. 13–30). New York: Guilford Press.

Beach, S. R. H. (1996). Marital therapy in the treatment of depression. In C. Mundt, M. J. Goldstein, K. Hahleweg, & P. Fiedler (Eds.), *Interpersonal factors in the origin and course of affective disorders* (pp. 341–361). London: Gaskell.

Beach, S. R. H. (2001). *Marital and family processes in depression: A scientific foundation for clinical practice.* Washington, DC: American Psychological Association.

Beach, S. R. H., & O'Leary, K. D. (1992). Treating depression in the context of marital discord: Outcome and predictors of response of marital therapy versus cognitive therapy. *Behavior Therapy, 23,* 507–528.

Beach, S. R. H., Sandeen, E. E., & O'Leary, K. D. (1990). *Depression in marriage: A model for etiology and treatment.* New York: Guilford Press.

Benazon, N. R. (2000). Predicting negative spousal attitudes toward depressed persons: A test of Coyne's Interpersonal Model. *Journal of Abnormal Psychology, 109,* 550–554.

Benazon, N. R., & Coyne, J. C. (2000). Living with a depressed spouse. *Journal of Family Psychology, 14,* 71–79.

Bland, K., & Hallman, R. S. (1981). Relationship between response to graded exposure and marital satisfaction in agoraphobics. *Behavior Research and Therapy, 19,* 335–338.

Bradbury, T. N., & Fincham, F. D. (1990). Attributions in marriage: Review and critique. *Psychological Bulletin, 107,* 3–33.

Bradbury, T. N., & Fincham, F. D. (1992). Attributions and behavior in marital interaction. *Journal of Personality and Social Psychology, 63,* 613–628.

Christensen, A., & Heavey, C. L. (1999). Interventions for couples. In *Annual Review of Psychology* (pp. 165–190). Stanford, CA: Annual Reviews.

Coyne, J. C. (1976). Toward an interactional description of depression. *Psychiatry, 39,* 28–40.

Craske, M. G., & Barlow, D. H. (2002). Panic disorder and agoraphobia. In D. H. Barlow (Ed.) *Clinical handbook of psychological disorders: A step-by-step treatment manual* (3rd ed.). New York: Guilford Press.

Daiuto, A. D., Baucom, D. H., Epstein, N. B., & Dutton, S. S. (1998). The application of behavioral couples therapy to the assessment and treatment of agoraphobia: implications of empirical research. *Clinical Psychology Review*, *18*, 663–687.

Dattilio, F. M. (1990). Cognitive marital therapy: A case study. *Journal of Family Psychotherapy*, *1*(1), 15–31.

Dattilio, F. M. (Ed.). (1998). *Case studies in couples and family therapy: Systemic and cognitive perspectives*. New York: Guilford.

Dattilio, F. M. (2001). Cognitive-behavior family therapy: Contemporary myths and misconceptions. *Contemporary Family Therapy*, *23*(1), 3–18.

Dattilio, F. M. (2002). Homework assignments in couple and family therapy. *Journal of Clinical Psychology*, *58*(5), 570–583.

Dattilio, F. M., & Bevilacqua, L. J. (Eds.). (2000). *Comparative treatments for relationship dysfunction*. New York: Springer.

Dattilio, F. M., Epstein, N. B., & Baucom, D. H. (1998). An introduction to cognitive-behavior therapy with couples and families. In F. M. Dattilio (Ed.), *Case studies in couples and family therapy: Systemic and cognitive perspectives* (pp. 1–36). New York: Guilford Press.

Dattilio, F. M., & Jongsma, A. E. (2000). *The family therapy treatment planner*. New York: Wiley.

Dattilio, F. M., & Padesky, C. (1990). *Cognitive therapy with couples*. Sarasota, FL: Professional Resource Exchange.

Davila., J. (2001). Paths to unhappiness: The overlapping causes of depression and romantic dysfunction. In S. R. H. Beach (Ed.), *Marital and family processes in depression: A scientific foundation for clinical practice* (pp. 71–87). Washington, DC: American Psychological Association.

Dessaulles, A. (1991). *The treatment of clinical depression in the context of marital distress*. Unpublished doctoral dissertation, Ottawa, Canada: University of Ottawa.

Dudek, D., Zieba, A., Jawor, M., Szymaczek, M., Opila, J., & Dattilio, F. M. (2001). The impact of depressive illness on spouses of depressed patients. *Journal of Cognitive Psychotherapy*, *15*(1), 49–57.

Emmelkamp, P. M. G. (1974). Self-observation versus flooding in the treatment of agoraphobia. *Behavior Research and Therapy*, *12*, 229–237.

Epstein, N. B. (1985). Depression and marital dysfunction: Cognitive and behavioral linkages. *International Journal of Mental Health*, *13*, 86–104.

Epstein, N. B., & Baucom, D. H. (2002). *Enhanced cognitive-behavior therapy for couples: A contextual approach*. Washington, DC: American Psychological Association.

Fincham, F. D., Beach, S. R. H., Harold, G. T., & Osborne, L. N. (1997). Marital satisfaction and depression: Different causal relationships for men and women? *Psychological Science*, *8*, 351–357.

Gottman, J. M. (1994). *What predicts divorce? The relationship between marital processes and marital outcomes*. Hillsdale, NJ: Lawrence Erlbaum Associates.

Hafner, R. J. (1977a). The husbands of agoraphobic women: Assortative mating or pathogenic interaction? *British Journal of Psychiatry*, *130*, 233–239.

Hafner, R. J. (1977b). The husbands of agoraphobia women and their influence on treatment outcome. *British Journal of Psychiatry*, *131*, 289–294.

Hoffart, A. (1997). Interpersonal problems among patients suffering from panic disorder with agoraphobia before and after treatment. *British Journal of Medical Psychology*, *70*, 149–157.

Holtzworth-Munroe, A., & Jacobson, N. S. (1985). Causal attributions of married couples: When do they search for causes? What do they conclude when they do? *Journal of Personality and Social Psychology*, *48*, 1398–1412.

Jacobson, N. S., & Christensen, A. (1996). *Integrative couple therapy: Promoting acceptance and change*. New York: Norton.

Jacobson, N. S., Fruzzetti, A. E., Dobson, K. S., Whisman, M., & Hops, H. (1993). Couple therapy as a treatment for depression: II. The effects of relationship quality and therapy on depressive relapse. *Journal of Consulting and Clinical Psychology*, *61*, 516–519.

Johnson, S. M., & Williams-Keeler, L. (1998). Creating healing relationships for couples dealing with trauma: The use of emotionally focused marital therapy. *Journal of Marital and Family Therapy*, *27*, 145–155.

Judd, L. L. (1998). The clinical course of unipolar major depressive disorders. *Archives of General Psychiatry*, *54*, 989–991.

Kessler, R. C., Walters, E. E., & Forthofer, M. S. (1998). The social consequences of psychiatric disorders, III: Probability of marital stability. *American Journal of Psychiatry*, *155*, 1092–1096.

Kung, W. W. (2000). The intertwined relationship between depression and marital distress: Elements of marital therapy conducive to effective treatment outcome. *Journal of Marital and Family Therapy*, *26*, 51–63.

Levkowitz, V., Fennig, S., Horesch, N., Barak, V., & Treves, I. (2000). Perception of ill spouse and dyadic relationship in couples with affective disorder and those without. *Journal of Affective Disorders*, *58*, 237–240.

Liotti, G., & Guidano, V. (1976). Behavioral analysis of marital interaction in agoraphobic male patients. *Behaviour Research and Therapy*, *14*, 161–162.

Marcaurelle, R., Bélanger, C., & Marchand, A. (2003). Marital relationship and the treatment of panic disorder with agoraphobia: A critical review. *Clinical Psychology Review, 23*(2), 247–276.

Marks, I. M. (1969). *Fears and Phobia.* Heinemann: London.

Mead, D. E. (2002). Marital distress, co-occurring depression and marital therapy: A review *Journal of Marital and Family Therapy, 28*(3), 299–314.

Miklowitz, D. J., Richards, J. A., George, E. L., Frank, E., Suddath, R. L., Powell, K. B., et al. (2003). Integrated family and individual therapy for bipolar disorder: Results of a treatment development study. *Journal of Clinical Psychiatry, 64*(2), 182–191.

Miller, G. E., & Bradbury, T. N. (1995). Refining the association between attributions and behavior in marital interaction. *Journal of Family Psychology, 9,* 196–208.

Miller, R. B. (2000). The case for marital distress as a public health problem: *Revitalizing the Institution of Marriage for the 21st century.* Brigham Young University: Provo, UT.

Milton, F., & Hafner, J. (1979). The outcome of behavior therapy for agoraphobia in relation to marital adjustment. *Archives of General Psychiatry, 36,* 807–811.

Nelson, G. M., & Beach, S. R. H. (1990). Sequential interaction in depression: Effects of depressive behavior on spousal aggression. *Behavior Therapy, 21,* 167–182.

O'Leary, D. A., Christian, J. L., & Mendell, N. R. (1994). A closer look at the link between marital discord and depressive symptomatology. *Journal of Social and Clinical Psychology, 13,* 33–41.

O'Leary, D. A., Heyman, R. F., & Jongsma, A. E. (1998). *The couples psychotherapy treatment planner.* New York: Wiley.

Orleans, C. T., George. L. K., & Houpt J. L. (1985). How primary care physicians treat psychiatric disorders: A material survey of family practitioners. *American Journal of Psychiatry, 142,* 52–57.

Schmaling, K. B., & Jacobson, N. S. (1990). Marital interaction and depression. *Journal of Abnormal Psychology, 99,* 229–236.

Symonds, A. (1971). Phobias after marriage: Women's declaration of independence. *American Journal of Psychoanalysis, 31,* 144–152.

Teichman, Y., Bar-El, Z., Shor, H., & Elizur, A. (1998). Changes in cognitions, emotions, and behaviors in depressed patients and their spouses following marital cognitive therapy, traditional cognitive therapy, pharmacotherapy, and no intervention. *Journal of Psychotherapy Integration, 8,* 27–53.

Teichman, Y., Bar-El, Z., Shor, H., & Sirota, P. (1995). A comparison of two modalities of cognitive therapy (individual and marital) in treating depression. *Psychiatry: Interpersonal and Biological Processes, 58,* 136–148.

Tower, R. B., & Kasl, S. V. (1995). Depressive symptoms across older spouses and the moderating effect of marital closeness. *Psychology and Aging, 10,* 625–638.

Weissman, M. M. (1987). Advances in psychiatric epidemiology: Rates and risks for major depression. *American Journal of Public Health, 77,* 445–451.

Weissman, M. M., & Paykel, E. S. (1974). *The depressed women: A study of social relationships.* Chicago: University of Chicago Press.

Whisman, M. A. (2001). The association between depression and marital dissatisfaction. In S. R. H. Beach (Ed.), *Marital and family processes in depression: A scientific foundation for clinical practice* (3–24). Washington, DC: American Psychological Association.

Winters, K. (2000). Why patients should take psychotropic medications. *Perspectives in Psychiatric Care, 36,* 38–52.

# 23

# HIV/AIDS

Julianne M. Serovich
Shonda M. Craft
*The Ohio State University*

## TRUTH OR FICTION?

___ 1. *Confidential HIV testing means that the results may be available to anyone with access to a person's medical information, such as doctors or insurance companies.*

___ 2. *The HIV virus may remain dormant for no more than five years.*

___ 3. *A serodiscordant couple refers to a couple in which there is one HIV-positive person and one person who is not positive.*

___ 4. *An at-risk other refers to persons deemed by the therapist to be in imminent danger of contracting HIV from a client.*

___ 5. *In areas in which it is illegal for an HIV-positive individual to choose not to disclose, it is the therapist's duty to warn any individuals who might be at significant risk of transmission.*

___ 6. *Mood and physical fluctuations are very common for people who are HIV-positive, thus need not be addressed by the therapist.*

___ 7. *Persons living with HIV can find it very therapeutic to plan their funeral, wake or memorial service.*

___ 8. *Group therapy for HIV-positive children has revealed themes such as feelings of loss, social isolation, anger, and relational ambivalence were uncommon, especially in the beginning stages of therapy.*

___ 9. *The stigma associated with HIV/AIDS has been identified as being relevant to people living with the disease.*

___ 10. *Issues pertaining to HIV specifically need not cause tremendous burden on professionals as materials can be obtained utilizing local libraries, health departments, community agencies, and consumer groups.*

___ 11. *African American men and women have been significantly impacted by HIV. However, men contract HIV more often from heterosexual contact and women from homosexual contact.*

___ 12. *Studies suggest the possibility that homophobic therapists may be less comfortable working with HIV-positive clients, even when such individuals are heterosexual.*

___ 13. *If a client grants verbal permission for a therapist to disclose his or her status to an at-risk other, other documentation of consent to release this information is not required.*

___ 14. *In the event of physical decline, family therapy can be continued at alterative sites, such as a family home, hospice, or hospital if the client's condition permits.*

___ 15. *The death of the HIV-positive family member typically terminates therapy.*

The AIDS epidemic is not over. Over the past several years there has been a steady decline in the number of reported AIDS cases, yet the rates of newly diagnosed HIV infections remain steady. As of June 2001, more than 793,000 cases of AIDS and 145,000 cases of HIV infection in the United States have been reported to the Centers for Disease Control (CDC, 2002). In 1996, the CDC estimated that as many as one in every 250 Americans may be infected with HIV. These figures represent a significant rise in infection rates in very diverse populations in the United States. As the rate of HIV infection continues to escalate, so do the chances that you will be treating an individual infected with, or a family affected by, HIV/AIDS. The purpose of this chapter is to address the special issues and considerations therapists might face with the increasing HIV/AIDS epidemic. More specifically we will (a) introduce you to the basic terms and concepts related to HIV/AIDS, (b) increase your awareness of who is infected with HIV and how infection occurs, and (c) address issues marriage and family therapists should consider before working with HIV-infected individuals and their families. Table 23.1 summarizes these issues and considerations.

1. Which of the following is true of the AIDS epidemic over the past several years?
   a. There has been a steady decline in the number of reported AIDS cases.
   b. The rates of newly diagnosed HIV infections remain steady.
   c. One in every 250 Americans is infected with HIV.
   d. All of the above.

## WHAT IS AIDS? WHAT IS HIV? HOW ARE THE TWO RELATED?

HIV stands for **Human Immunodeficiency Virus**. HIV weakens the immune system by replicating itself in a certain type of white blood cell (CD4 cells). Over time, the immune system is overtaken by these HIV replicates, rendering an infected person more susceptible to other infections. These other infections are referred to as *opportunistic infections* and can include such illnesses as pneumonia, influenza, lymphoma, or Kaposi's sarcoma. AIDS stands for **Acquired Immunodeficiency Syndrome** (CDC, 2003a) and is the result of prolonged HIV infection. According to the CDC, a person may receive an AIDS diagnosis when their CD4 cell count drops below 200 cells per cubic millimeter of blood or they have been diagnosed with at least one opportunistic infection (CDC, 2003b). It is important to note that a person with AIDS also has HIV but when someone receives an HIV-positive diagnosis, they may not necessarily have AIDS.

**TABLE 23.1**

Issues and Considerations for Treating HIV-Positive Clients

| Topic | Information |
|---|---|
| Methods of HIV transmission | Bodily fluids: blood, semen, vaginal secretions, and breast milk |
| Affected groups | Gender: gay men, heterosexual women<br>   Age: adolescents<br>   Race/Ethnicity: African Americans |
| Methods of protection | Avoid sharing needles<br>Abstinence<br>Use of latex barriers (condoms, dental dams).<br>Those who may have come in contact with bodily fluids should be tested for HIV. |
| Important issues to address in therapy with the family | Confidentiality: disclosure to at-risk others<br>   Client concerns about illness, death, sexuality, and stigma<br>   Changes in client's physical and/or mental capabilities<br>   Frank discussions about death and dying<br>   Consideration of family's cultural and religious norms<br>   Children's living arrangements, as well as feelings of loss, anger, social isolation, and relational ambivalence |
| Important self of the therapist issues to address | Education regarding myths and facts of HIV/AIDS<br>   Attitudes toward homosexuality, drug use/abuse, prostitution<br>   Values, biases, or prejudices toward marginalized groups (i.e., drug users, prostitutes, homosexuals, racial/ethnic minorities<br>Attitudes about death and illness |

2. A person who is HIV-positive:
   a. will also have a diagnosis of AIDS.
   b. will not be more susceptible to common infections.
   c. will develop AIDS after contracting certain opportunistic infections.
   d. will experience no change in his/her immune system.

# WHAT GROUPS ARE PRIMARILY INFECTED WITH HIV/AIDS?

## Gay Men

Men still constitute the largest group of infected individuals; however, over the past few years, the demographic profile of these men has been changing. Historically, gay men have constituted a majority of AIDS cases; yet currently, gay men represent 46% of all HIV infections and 56% of all AIDS cases (CDC, 2002). HIV and AIDS cases for men involving injection drug usage (13% and 22% respectively) have increased over the years but currently remain steady (CDC, 2002). Although 6% of gay men with HIV report both sex and IV drug usage as risk factors, HIV-positive injection drug users are predominantly heterosexual Hispanic (18%) and African-American (17%) men (CDC, 1998a). Among young men, 52% of all 13- to 19-year-olds and 56% of 20- to 24-year-olds reported contracting HIV from having sex with other men (CDC, 2002). Five percent of the 13- to 19-year-olds and 7% of the 20- to 24-year-olds contracted HIV from heterosexual contact while 3% of the 13- to 19-year-olds and 6% of the 20- to 24-year-olds contracted HIV from injection drug use (CDC, 2002). Furthermore, since 1994, AIDS has been the leading killer of males between the ages of 25 and 44 in the United States (National Center for Health Statistics, 1994). These figures suggest a changing demographic profile of men with HIV/AIDS.

3. Which group still constitutes the largest group of infected individuals?
   a. men
   b. women
   c. adolescents
   d. none of the above

## Heterosexual Women

The fastest rising at-risk group for HIV infection is heterosexual women (CDC, 2002). Currently, women constitute only 17% of AIDS cases; however it has been rising steadily over the years. The CDC (2002) reports that reported cases of HIV infection in adolescent and adult women results primarily from heterosexual contact (42%) and injection drug usage (19%). The modes of contraction for AIDS cases in adult and adolescent women are different from men. Infections in women have resulted primarily from heterosexual contact (41%) and injection drug usage (40%) (CDC, 2002). The discrepancies between rates of HIV infection and reported AIDS cases are interesting to note and reflect a significant change in women's risk patterns. It is unlikely the elevated infection rates of HIV in women will decline anytime soon, as more than 10,000 cases of new HIV infections were reported to the CDC between 2000 and 2001 representing 25% of all new HIV infections (CDC, 2002). Seventy-nine percent of these new HIV infections were diagnosed in women between the childbearing ages of 20 and 44 (CDC, 2002). These figures are twice as high as what was reported between 1997 and 1998 (CDC, 1998a).

4. Which population is the fastest rising at-risk group for HIV infection?
   a. gay men
   b. heterosexual women
   c. African American men
   d. adolescents

5. The CDC (2002) reports that HIV infection in adolescent and adult women results primarily from which of the following?
   a. heterosexual contact and injection and drug use
   b. homosexual contact and injection drug use
   c. blood transfusions
   d. it is impossible to tell how adolescent and adult women contract HIV

## African Americans

Besides severely affecting women, HIV has significantly impacted the African American community. African American adolescent and adult men account for 34% of all AIDS and 44% of all new HIV infection cases (CDC, 2002). These men are contracting HIV from either homosexual contact (32%) or IV drug use (17%). This same phenomenon is also occurring in African American adolescent and adult women, who accounted for 57% of all AIDS and 67% of all new HIV infection cases (CDC, 2002). Modes of contraction for African American women are slightly different from men, however, with 41% of HIV and 39% of AIDS cases originating from heterosexual contact.

6. The modes of HIV contraction for African American women:
   a. are primarily from homosexual contact.
   b. include sex with intravenous drug users.
   c. are mainly from heterosexual contact.
   d. have not been clearly identified.

## Adolescents

Young children and adolescents currently account for a very small percentage of the AIDS cases in the United States; however, young men and women between the ages of 13 and 24 are at an increased risk for HIV infection because youth are engaging in risky sexual behaviors at younger ages (CDC, 1995; Rosenberg, 1995). As of June 2001, 4% of all new HIV infections were diagnosed in adolescents ages 13 to 19; however, 11% of the total HIV infection cases were in persons between the ages of 20 and 24, reflecting the likelihood of contraction occurring during adolescence (CDC, 2002). The number of adolescents infected is probably far greater than these figures indicate, considering the virus may remain dormant an average of five to ten years.

7. Adolescents currently account for what percent of all HIV cases in the United States?
   a. 1%
   b. 4%
   c. 11%
   d. 14%

## HOW IS HIV TRANSMITTED?

HIV is primarily transmitted by direct contact with an infected person's bodily fluids, specifically blood, semen, and vaginal secretions. These fluids, however, must have a pathway to a person's bloodstream for infection to occur. In the past, researchers have concluded that the possibility exists of transmitting the virus orally, such as through sexual contact or kissing. Open wounds or sores in the mouth could provide the requisite pathway necessary for transmission of the virus (CDC, 2003c). However, recent studies have questioned the viability of such transmission. According to the CDC (2003c), there have been few documented cases of HIV transmission during oral sex. Open wounds or sores in the mouth could provide the requisite pathway necessary for transmission of the virus (CDC, 2003c) but the risk of transmitting the virus orally may be lessened with the use of barriers such as dental dams and condoms. One exception to the oral transmission rule is breast milk where infants can contract the virus via breastfeeding. The virus may also be present in other fluids, such as urine, saliva, or tears; however, the quantity is often not enough to produce a threat. Although there is fear that HIV might be transmitted in other ways (e.g. mosquitoes or toilet seats); these claims have never been substantiated scientifically.

8. Which bodily fluid could potentially transmit HIV by direct contact?
   a. saliva
   b. urine
   c. blood
   d. tears

According to the CDC (2003d), since the beginning of the HIV epidemic there has been concern about biting and bloodsucking insects, such as mosquitoes, transmitting the virus to humans. Scientific studies conducted by the CDC and other researchers have not produced evidence to support insect transmission, even in areas where there are many cases of AIDS and large populations of insects. According to the CDC (2003d), when a mosquito bites it does not inject the consumed blood into the person bitten. In addition, HIV has not been shown to reproduce or survive within the bloodstreams of insects (CDC, 2003d). Given this information, the risk of contracting HIV from a mosquito or other insect bite appears to be extremely low and, most likely, nonexistent.

9. The risk of contracting HIV from a mosquito bite is very low because:
   a. mosquitoes die immediately once they are infected with HIV.
   b. the virus is unable to reproduce or survive within insects.
   c. there has not been enough research to determine the risk.
   d. none of the above.

## IS THERE A CURE FOR HIV/AIDS?

There are many different drugs available now for treating HIV/AIDS, but there is no cure. According to the U. S. Food and Drug Administration (USFDA, 2003), twenty-four drugs have been approved for the treatment of HIV infection. These drugs, best known as *antiretrovirals*, inhibit the replication of the virus. Antiviral drugs used to treat HIV can delay the progression to AIDS by slowing down the destruction of the immune system. While none of these drugs is a cure for the disease, they have been effective in prolonging the lives of infected people. HIV patients can eventually develop AIDS, despite treatment. Much of the medical therapy involves treating the opportunistic infections that signal the progression to AIDS. One bit of good news is that infected pregnant women can take an anti-HIV drug which will decrease the chance of them transmitting HIV to their baby. In fact, according to one study, only 8% of infants born to an infected woman taking medications developed HIV, versus 25% of infants born to untreated women (CDC, 1994).

10. Which of the following statements are true concerning anti-HIV drugs?
    a. Antiretrovirals are ineffective in prolonging the lives of infected individuals.
    b. Pregnant women can take an anti-HIV drug which will decrease the chance of them transmitting HIV to their baby.
    c. Due to advances in research, many of the side effects of antiretroviral drugs have been eliminated.
    d. None of the above.

Antiretroviral drugs have many side effects, such as metabolic changes, muscle wasting, heart failure, numbness, pain, bone degeneration, and depression (USFDA, 2003). Because of the severity of these complications, some people stop taking the drugs. Antiretroviral drugs are also very expensive. This is a problem for many people who do not have health insurance and cannot afford the thousands of dollars that these drugs can cost each year.

11. Which of the following present a common reason for individuals to stop taking their antiretroviral drug?
    a. negative side effects such as numbness, pain, heart failure and muscle wasting
    b. depression
    c. high cost
    d. all of the above

## HOW DOES A PERSON PROTECT HIM- OR HERSELF FROM BECOMING INFECTED?

An important step in the prevention effort is to be tested for HIV. People who know they are HIV infected can seek immediate treatment and potentially reduce transmission to others. There are two ways of testing for the virus; anonymously or confidentially. *Anonymous testing* means no personal information will be used to identify your test results. *Confidential testing* means the results may be available to anyone with access to a person's medical information, such as doctors or insurance companies. Commonly, a person will be tested for the presence of HIV antibodies. A positive test result indicates that a person has been exposed to HIV and that his/her body has begun producing antibodies to combat the virus. A negative test result may indicate that either the individual has not been exposed to HIV or that their immune system may still be in the window period of infection; the latter may be disconfirmed by retesting in three to six months.

12. A negative HIV test result:
    a. indicates that the person has HIV.
    b. should be reconfirmed within three to six months.
    c. can only be obtained through anonymous testing.
    d. means the person will never need another HIV test.

The best way to prevent HIV is to minimize exposure to bodily fluids, particularly blood and semen. This means avoiding the sharing of needles used to inject drugs and tattoos, practicing sexual abstinence, or engaging in safe sex procedures. Safe sex includes the use of latex barriers (such as condoms) during each act of sexual intercourse to protect both partners from infection. Condoms should be used when performing vaginal, anal, and oral sex.

13. Which option is the most effective means of preventing the transmission of HIV/AIDS?
    a. oral contraceptives
    b. spermicide
    c. intrauterine device (IUD)
    d. condom

14. Latex barriers should be used during which of the following?
   a. each act of sexual intercourse
   b. vaginal and anal sex
   c. oral sex
   d. all of the above

The use of latex or polyurethane (a type of plastic) condoms when engaging in sexual intercourse—vaginal, anal, or oral—can greatly reduce a person's risk of acquiring or transmitting sexually transmitted diseases, including HIV infection, through the exchange of semen or vaginal secretions. Condoms are most effective when they are used consistently and correctly. Failure rates for condoms are relatively high (12%) compared to other common contraceptive methods (Planned Parenthood, 1998). However, it is important to remember that latex and/or polyurethane condoms are the only contraceptives effective against the transmission of HIV and other sexually transmitted diseases. Two studies of **serodiscordant couples** (one HIV-positive person, one person who is not positive) demonstrated that the probability of cross-infection could be significantly reduced with correct and consistent condom usage, as about 2% of un-infected partners in couples who practiced consistent and correct use of condoms experienced HIV infection, compared to 10% to 15% in those couples that did not use condoms (CDC, 1993). Thin sheets of latex, known as dental dams, can also be used during oral sex to prevent the possible transmission of infected bodily fluids.

15. Research has shown that serodiscordant couples reduced their risk of HIV transmission by:
   a. not engaging in sexual intercourse.
   b. using condoms correctly and consistently.
   c. not changing their sexual behaviors in any way.
   d. using condoms only for oral sex.

## HOW PREPARED ARE MARRIAGE AND FAMILY THERAPISTS FOR TREATING PERSONS WITH HIV/AIDS?

Studies conducted with clinicians from allied disciplines suggest that discrimination by mental health professionals has been pervasive (Crawford, Humfleet, Ribordy, Ho, & Vickers, 1991; Dhooper, Royse & Tran, 1988; Diaz & Kelly, 1991; Peterson, 1989). Studies have suggested that mental health professionals are well-informed about HIV (Bor, Elford, Perry & Miller, 1988), yet others concluded that a significant majority of social workers would not provide services to HIV-positive persons (Dhooper et al., 1988). You should note that these studies were conducted in the 1980s and may not be representative of the current attitudes of helping professionals.

It is very important to assess your attitudes toward HIV-infected persons. Very few studies have been conducted specifically on marriage and family therapists' attitudes toward HIV-positive persons or their knowledge of HIV. Those which have been done also suffer from being dated and potentially unreliable. Bor and colleagues (1988) surveyed marriage and family therapy trainees at the Tavistock Clinic in London and found that these therapists were educated about the transmission of HIV and rejected the notion that HIV-positive clients need to be isolated from the community. In addition, though over half (51%) had dealt with some AIDS-related issues on the job, even more (78%) anticipated that they would be having to handle AIDS-related issues in the future. In these early studies, AIDS was often investigated in terms of how it correlated with attitudes towards homosexuality. For example, Preston and her colleagues, in the development of an AIDS attitude scale, found that a single homosexuality factor explained 53% of the variance within their measure (Preston, Young, Koch, & Forti, 1995). This may reflect the association often made between being gay and living with HIV; that is, people have a tendency to think about HIV when they think about gays or lesbians.

16. According to research by Bor and colleagues (1988), marriage and family therapists:
    a. reported having no education about how HIV was transmitted.
    b. anticipated that AIDS would not be relevant in the future.
    c. rejected the notion of isolating HIV-positive clients from the community.
    d. had little experience dealing with AIDS.

There does appear to be a beneficial effect for therapists to have personal friendships with gays and lesbians. In one study, Green and Bobele (1994) found that marriage and family therapists who had more contact with people with AIDS, gay men, or lesbians were less likely to express phobic attitudes about HIV-positive people. In fact, both having gay or lesbian friends and the percentage of gays/lesbians and persons with AIDS in a marriage and family therapist's practice were predictive of reduced AIDS phobia. Therapists with higher levels of HIV knowledge were also less likely to have negative attitudes about people living with the disease. Although the relationship among level of HIV knowledge, attitude, and degree of contact with gays, lesbians, and those infected seem to be complex, there appears to be a general indication that empathy and consideration may result from a greater understanding of HIV.

These studies suggest the possibility that homophobic therapists may be less comfortable working with HIV-positive clients. For example, Pais, Piercy, and Miller (1998) found that marriage and family therapists were much more likely to break confidentiality based on unsafe sexual practices when the clients were male, gay, young, African American, and when the therapists had little previous experience working with gay or lesbian clients. In addition, therapists who were female, religiously conservative, and had fewer experiences with gays and lesbians were more likely to disclose than others. Marriage and family therapists were most likely to report willingness to disclose directly to the sexual partner (59.2%), clinical supervisor (50.2%), their lawyer (36%) and immediate family members of the HIV-infected patient (30.4%). In a similar study, psychologists indicated that they held heterosexual clients more responsible for protecting their partners from contracting HIV than they did homosexuals (Kozlowski, Rupert, & Crawford, 1998). In fact, psychologists attributed greatest responsibility to the partner of homosexuals for self-protection. Finally, among African American social work students, it has been found that lack of knowledge about HIV and AIDS was related to apprehension with working with HIV-positive individuals (Owens, 1995).

17. Which of the following statements is true?
    a. Marriage and family therapists who had more contact with people with AIDS, gay men, or lesbians were more likely to express phobic attitudes about HIV-positive people.
    b. Therapists with higher levels of HIV knowledge were more likely to have negative attitudes about people living with the disease.
    c. One study found that marriage and family therapists were much more likely to break confidentiality based on unsafe sexual practices when the clients were gay.
    d. None of the above.

18. Marriage and family therapists were most likely to report their willingness to disclose to:
    a. immediate family members.
    b. no one in particular.
    c. lawyers.
    d. sexual partners.

## HOW SHOULD ISSUES SURROUNDING HIV/AIDS BE TREATED IN THE THERAPY ROOM?

Systemic models of treatment and intervention are typically not comprehensive enough to cover the unique situations you might face in therapy with HIV-positive persons or their families. Therapeutic models provide guidelines for interventions and should be supplemented with specific information about various presenting problems garnered from research and clinical case studies. Given the trends in the clinical literature, it becomes crucial for you to be knowledgeable about, and able to address and possibly educate others about, issues regarding HIV/AIDS.

Three primary areas will be addressed in this section. First, the importance of being educated regarding various aspects of the disease process and its transmission will be discussed. Then, we will discuss the ethical and legal considerations that may need monitoring. Finally, specific therapeutic considerations regarding working with HIV-positive person and their families will be provided.

19. Which of the following models are most effective for individuals in therapy?
    a. therapeutic models supplemented with specific information from research and clinical case studies
    b. systemic models
    c. cognitive–behavioral model
    d. solution focused model

## HOW WILL BEING EDUCATED ABOUT HIV/AIDS HELP ME AS A CLINICIAN?

Among marriage and family therapists, education about HIV and its treatment has been found to dispel myths and improve attitudes toward individuals who are HIV positive (Green & Bobele, 1994). Likewise, education has been demonstrated to reduce stigma and discrimination against persons living with HIV/AIDS and increase the comfort level of mental health providers working with this population (Weiner & Siegel, 1990). Because information concerning HIV prevention and disease progression changes rapidly, it is important for you to stay abreast of current education and training on treatment or prevention issues. Besides basic HIV education, you should also be educated on how the development of the disease might affect the process of therapy. For example, dementia is often caused by HIV progression and can produce mental impairment and confusion, thereby affecting the therapeutic process. In addition, individuals often experience painful opportunistic infections and side effects from drug therapies. Psychological effects of disease progression can include changes in sexual desire; fears of death; and worry over the loss of self, partner, family, and friends. Essentially, working with HIV positive persons entails not only a basic medical understanding of the disease, but also an understanding of the implications it has on other life processes.

20. Psychological effects of HIV/AIDS progression can include which of the following?
    a. changes in sexual desire
    b. fears of death
    c. worry over the loss of self, partner, family, and friends
    d. all of the above

Treatment of HIV-related illnesses can be complex and involve numerous medical specialists. While it is perhaps impossible and unnecessary for you to understand the intricacies of current medical treatments, it is important to note that treatment protocols become an integral part of an HIV-positive person's life. Treatment regimes can be complicated, involving the timing of numerous doses of medication throughout the day and night. It is important, therefore, for you to be sensitive to medical burdens and encourage clients to teach you about relevant medical terminology, treatment modalities, side effects, and repercussions of medical treatments.

21. Therapists should encourage their HIV-positive clients to provide education regarding:
    a. treatment modalities and side effects.
    b. the cost of medical treatment.
    c. the intricacies of their current medical treatment.
    d. none of the above.

Talking about safer sex practices is an integral part of working with HIV-positive individuals but should also be integrated in work with other populations as well. It is especially important that you identify persons who would benefit from safer sex information. These persons might be sexually active adolescents or adults of any sexual orientation, those in sexually polygamous relationships, those sharing needles, persons who are divorcing or newly separated, or who are contemplating having sex or sharing needles with anyone in the above categories. Possible sources of updated information include community-based HIV/AIDS organizations, local health departments, or university health clinics near you. These organizations or departments typically can dispense information to professionals or can recommend relevant trainings or reading materials.

22. Individuals that would benefit from safer sex information include:
    a. sexually active adolescents or adults of any sexual orientation.
    b. persons who are divorcing or newly separated.
    c. those sharing needles.
    d. all of the above.

## WHAT ETHICAL CONSIDERATIONS SHOULD I BE AWARE OF WHEN TREATING A FAMILY WITH A MEMBER WHO HAS HIV/AIDS?

There are no federal laws or policies which can protect or help direct you in regard to the ethical considerations faced when working with HIV-positive clients. In fact, most legislation resides at the state level and is not specifically written for mental health professionals. When working with HIV-positive clients and their families, numerous situations might call for a particular ethical or lawful response. One of the most pressing issues relates to disclosure to an at-risk other. These are persons deemed by you to be in imminent danger of contracting HIV from a client. Typically, these persons are sexual or intravenous drug-sharing partners who have not been told of the diagnosis with whom high risk activities are occurring.

23. Legislation regarding the ethical considerations faced when working with HIV-positive clients:
    a. defines those persons who should be deemed as at-risk others.
    b. specifically addresses mental health professionals.
    c. is mainly found at the state level.
    d. provides direct assistance and protection to therapists.

Few researchers have examined the disclosure process of HIV-positive individuals to sexual or intravenous drug-sharing partners and most studies have been conducted with men. Rates of reported disclosure to sexual partners have been varied and in some studies, rates have been remarkably low. For example, although Hays and colleagues (1993) reported 98% of their sample disclosed to lovers/partners, other studies have reported disclosure rates to sexual partners of 89% (Schnell et al., 1992); 76.9% (Marks et al., 1992); 66% (Perry, Ryan, Fogel, Fishman, & Jacobsberg, 1990); 65% (Marks et al., 1991) and 48% (Marks, Richardson, & Maldonado, 1991). More recent studies suggest similar trends. Niccolai, Dorst, Myers, and Kissinger (1999) reported that 75.7% of their sample disclosed to their last sexual partner and Stein et al. (1998) reported a disclosure rate of 60% to all sexual partners. For example, researchers have reported the likelihood of disclosure decreased in direct proportion to the number of partners (Marks et al., 1991). Perry and colleagues (1994) reported individuals were less likely to inform casual partners than steady partners of their HIV status.

24. Which of the following statements is false?
    a. The likelihood of disclosure decreased in direct proportion to the number of partners.
    b. Individuals are more likely to inform casual partners than steady partners of their HIV status.
    c. Rates of reported disclosure to sexual partners have been varied.
    d. None of the above.

## What Do I Do if My HIV-Positive Client Tells Me They Are Engaging in Unsafe Sexual Behaviors?

One of the few organizations to define a policy in regard to HIV and disclosure is the American Medical Association (AMA). The AMA (2003) suggests that if physicians have an identifiable person who is at risk for infection, the physician is required to persuade the patient to disclose to those people who may be at significant risk of transmission. If the patient does not disclose, the physician must notify the local health department. If the health department does not follow through, the physician is required to notify the at-risk person him or herself. In some states, however, physicians are not held liable whether they either choose to disclose or not disclose a patient's HIV-positive status to an at-risk individual.

25. If physicians have an identifiable person who is at risk for infection, the physician is to first:
   a. notify the local health department.
   b. notify the at-risk person him or herself.
   c. persuade the patient to disclose to those people who may be at significant risk of transmission.
   d. none of the above.

The American Counseling Association (ACA) has also addressed infectious diseases in terms of confidentiality. According to the ACA, counselors who know that a client has a communicable and fatal disease is justified in disclosing information to an identifiable third party who is at a high risk of contracting the disease (ACA, 1999). Thus a counselor working with HIV-positive clients would be in a position to breach confidentiality if he or she believed that a particular identifiable person was unwittingly at risk for HIV transmission.

Many organizations, such as the American Association for Marriage and Family Therapy (AAMFT), the American Psychological Association (APA), and the American Psychiatric Association (also APA), have not established such policies. Indeed, their task is arduous in the face of variable state laws. For example, states often vary on which information should be reported to health departments (e.g., names, addresses, mode of contraction), who should report this information (e.g., doctors, heath departments), and what penalties should be levied, if any, for not reporting. Subsequently, ethical ambiguities may create confusion for you. Legal complications also play a role in the confusion about whether or not a client should have the right to choose whether to disclose his or her seropositive status. In a familiar 1976 landmark ruling, *Tarasoff v. Regents of University of California*, the courts decided that a therapist was liable for the murder of a woman his client had threatened to kill (Gostin, 2002). Traditionally, this ruling has been used as the benchmark from which to judge whether the duty to warn outweighs a client's right to confidentiality. Typically the *duty to warn* has applied to situations in which a clearly identifiable person is at significant risk for personal harm (Lamb, Clark, Drumheller, Frizzel, & Surrey, 1989). With HIV, however, identifying a particular potential victim may be more difficult. The HIV-positive individual may not disclose the names of sexual partners; he or she might not be able to recall all sexual partners; or, he or she might not anticipate future sexual encounters. You should make proactive attempts to assess such possible situations with your clients.

26. Therapists may not be able to clearly identify individuals potentially at risk for HIV because:
   a. mental health organizations have not developed policies that address this issue.
   b. that is the role of the local health department.
   c. duty to warn does not apply to HIV/AIDS.
   d. clients may not be willing and/or able to provide adequate information.

Some work has been done in regard to this difficulty as it relates to the field of marriage and family therapy (e. g., Landau & Clements, 1997; Schlossberger & Hecker, 1996). Landau and Clements proposed that the duty to warn in AIDS-related cases depends upon prevailing law. That is, in areas in which it is illegal for an HIV-positive individual to choose not to disclose, it is the therapist's duty to warn any individuals who might be at significant risk of transmission. This includes past or current sexual partners and IV drug users with whom the client shares needles. In many states, however, such disclosures may be illegal and could bring you litigation for breach of confidentiality. In states where there are no laws regarding an HIV-positive individual's legal responsibility to inform significant others, you clearly have no legal duty to warn. Certainly, however, all therapists must struggle with this decision ethically, even if the law does not suggest that you have an ethical duty to the possible victim.

In order to assess legal concerns and make good clinical and legal decisions, it is imperative that you become familiar with state and local procedures and policies regarding HIV-testing and disclosure. Some states have mandatory partner notification programs that will anonymously notify individuals that they may have been in contact with an HIV-infected person. These programs, often associated with local health departments, also provide testing and counseling for partners. Such a program could be of tremendous assistance to you and your clients when clients are fearful or unwilling to disclose their diagnosis to an at-risk other. If provided with sufficient information, most health departments can track down partners for testing and counseling.

27. Therapists should be familiar with state and local policies regarding HIV disclosure because:
    a. they must participate in mandatory partner identification programs.
    b. the duty to warn often depends on the prevailing law.
    c. a breach of client confidentiality never results in litigation.
    d. none of the above.

We encourage you to have procedures to be followed regarding notification or confidentiality. For example, you should have a protocol established for addressing client requests to help notify a sexual partner regarding his or her possible risk of HIV infection. As stated previously, community agencies often offer this type of assistance. You must also be sure to make clear to clients their legal or ethical duties regarding the duty to warn. Regardless, although cases may be handled on an individual basis, attorneys should be contacted regarding the development of such policies and procedures in order to maintain legal compliance.

28. Which practices should be observed regarding notification or confidentiality?
    a. Clients do not need to be made clear of their legal or ethical duties regarding the duty to warn.
    b. Attorneys should be contacted regarding the development of policies and procedures on notification and confidentiality.
    c. The client must provide written consent, thereby waiving his or her right to confidentiality.
    d. Both B and C.

## How Do I Protect My Client and Myself?

As with any highly sensitive case, appropriate documentation of conversations concerning disclosure to at-risk others is imperative and you should be versed as to how such case notes should be written. In addition, you should assess if the HIV-positive diagnosis should be documented in case notes. If a client grants permission for a therapist to disclose his or her status to an at-risk other, proper documentation of consent to release this information is required. That is, if contact is to be made between the therapist and an at-risk other or an agency equipped to handle AIDS disclosure issues, the client must provide written consent of these communications, thereby waiving his or her right to confidentiality.

Finally, you must assess your ethical responsibility to your client in terms of confidentiality and the right to treatment. In addition, you should address questions of how your sexual orientation, attitude toward homosexual orientation, or your value judgment about AIDS or HIV-positive persons affects your ability to help people living with HIV/AIDS. Given the reality that educational, employment, medical, and housing discrimination readily occur based on public knowledge of a person's seropositive status, confidentiality for clients who are HIV-positive is imperative. Your negative attitude about AIDS or people living with the disease might compromise your commitment to this principle. You should be reminded that the AAMFT Code of Ethics (2001) indicates that therapists cannot discriminate against clients on the basis of certain personal characteristics, such as sexual orientation, gender, or race. In fact, Principle 1.1.states "Marriage and family therapists provide professional assistance to persons without discrimination on the basis of race, age, ethnicity, socioeconomic status, disability, gender, health status, religion, national origin, or sexual orientation" (p. 2). Clients with HIV and their families have a right to mental health services. A basic knowledge of HIV and AIDS should allay any fears you may have of disease contraction. However, if you have negative beliefs about HIV-positive persons this might sabotage the therapeutic process by you willfully choosing not to become educated. Examining perceptions of people living with HIV will serve to improve your ability to deal with sensitive issues as well as avoid a tenuous situation in which the client may be ultimately harmed by ignorance or bigotry.

## ARE THERE TREATMENT ISSUES I SHOULD BE AWARE OF IN WORKING WITH HIV-POSITIVE PERSONS?

Working with clients and sensitive issues can be emotionally draining for even the most seasoned therapist. Frequently, persons with HIV and their families present in therapy with very emotionally laden concerns about illness, death, sexuality, stigma, and discrimination. Because of the delicate nature of the concerns, you need to be sensitive to a number of issues.

First, you should address any fears or concerns you have of working with persons living with HIV and their families. Such concerns might include fear of contraction of HIV, discomfort with discussing death, negative reactions to a family's grief or a client's physical decline, and possibly your own denial of your or your client's possible death. HIV is a chronic illness in which patients may experience fluctuations in their physical health. That is, HIV-positive clients can report feeling physically strong one session and weak and frail the next. You should be aware that such mood and physical fluctuations are common and personal reactions to these changing conditions should be monitored and addressed.

Talking about death with clients is another difficult topic with which many therapists need to grapple. Persons living with HIV can find it very therapeutic to plan their funeral, wake, or memorial service. It is important then, for you to talk directly about death and dying issues such as a living will or other legal document preparation, wake and funeral arrangements and preferences, the possibility of writing one's own eulogy, and the choice of whether to have an open or closed casket service. It is particularly important to predetermine how you will handle absences related to hospital visits, illnesses, or death of a friend or family member.

Considering HIV is becoming a chronic versus terminal illness, it is not unusual for therapy to be interrupted by frequent hospitalizations. In the event of physical decline, family therapy can be continued at alternative sites such as a family home, hospice, or hospital if the client's condition permits.

The death of the HIV-positive family member does not necessitate the termination of therapy. Families might, however, request the suspension of therapy immediately after death to handle more pressing needs. If you work with families of HIV-positive individuals you might also need to assess your value system in regards to working with marginalized populations. This may be the first time you knowingly work with prostitutes, drug users, or homosexuals. You should incorporate opportunities for yourself to reflect on your values, biases, or prejudices with regard to such populations. Moreover, given the disproportionately high incidence of HIV among racial and ethnic minorities, it is imperative that you be sensitive to diverse cultural norms. The stigma associated with the disease, still often associated with homosexuality, may have an impact on how well an individual, or his family is able to deal with the disease. In addition, cultural or religious traditions may affect how a family expresses their feelings toward the loss associated with HIV (Landau-Stanton, Clements, & Stanton, 1993). Finally, the willingness of the family to be open about the disease and to accept traditional medical interventions might vary depending upon particular cultural or religious influences (Boyd-Franklin, Aleman, Jean-Gilles, & Lewis, 1995).

29. Which issues should *not* be addressed with families in therapy?
    a. planning of a funeral or memorial service
    b. if the HIV-infected client would like to write his or her own eulogy
    c. creation of a living will or other legal documents
    d. none of the above

## What Issues Should I Be Aware of When Working With Children?

Children are an important population that requires careful clinical consideration. Children may be either HIV-positive, or affected by HIV-positive family members. In either case, they may be in foster care or some other type of surrogate care, especially if the parent is abusing drugs or is unable to care for them for other reasons (Carten & Fennoy, 1997). These types of situations can create confusion and chaos in children's lives and the embedded systems in which they live. An analysis of group therapy for HIV-positive children revealed that themes such as feelings of loss, social isolation, and anger, along with relational ambivalence were quite common, especially in the beginning stages of therapy (Gomez, Haiken, & Lewis, 1995). Additionally, caretakers might experience guilt, especially if the child was infected through sexual abuse or maternal transmission (Gomez, et al., 1995).

30. When working with children in therapy it is important to assess which of the following?
    a. if they are HIV-positive as well
    b. who is caring for their physical and emotional needs
    c. feelings of loss, social isolation, anger, and relational ambivalence
    d. all of the above

As the progression of HIV infection continues to creep its way into the lives of millions of families, you will be increasingly faced with the task of working with individuals and families affected by HIV/AIDS. The stressors and demands appear to only be proportionate to the degree you are educated, prepared, and have assessed your personal qualifications and ability to work with these cases. That is, the more you know and understand about HIV as well as the potential ethical dilemmas and special concerns these cases present, the better prepared you will be to treat such individuals and families. Although the job of being a therapist continues to become more challenging as the field is faced with more complex social issues, the call for improved competency will not diminish. Issues specifically pertaining to HIV need not cause tremendous burden on professionals as materials can be obtained utilizing local libraries, health departments, community agencies, and consumer groups. Being educated is the key.

## KEY TERMS

**Acquired Immune Deficiency Syndrome (AIDS):** The result of prolonged HIV infection that is diagnosed when CD4 cell count of the infected person drops below 200 cells per cubic millimeter of blood or they have been diagnosed with at least one opportunistic infection.

**anonymous testing:** No personal information will be used to identify your test results.

**antiretrovirals:** A classification of drugs that inhibit the replication of HIV and delay the progression to AIDS by slowing down the destruction of the immune system.

**confidential testing:** The results may be available to anyone with access to a person's medical information, such as doctors or insurance companies.

**Human Immunodeficiency Virus (HIV):** A virus that weakens the immune system by replicating itself in CD4 cells, making a person more susceptible to other infections.

**opportunistic infections:** Illnesses such as pneumonia, influenza, lymphoma, or Kaposi's sarcoma.

**serodiscordant couples:** Couples composed of one partner that is HIV-positive and one partner who is not HIV-positive.

## DISCUSSION QUESTIONS

1. How has the presence of HIV/AIDS affected your personal or professional life?
2. What do you think are your strengths and weaknesses in being able to treat individuals, families, or couples affected by HIV/AIDS?
3. What are the most important *clinical issues* to consider when working with individuals, families or couples affected by HIV/AIDS?
4. What are the most important *ethical issues* to consider when working with individuals, families, or couples affected by HIV/AIDS?
5. What would you do if a client told you they were HIV-positive and having unsafe sex or needle sharing?
6. How will your religious or moral values affect your work with individuals, families, or couples affected by HIV/AIDS?
7. What are the major issues to contend with when treating children of HIV-infected persons?
8. What experiences have you had treating marginalized populations such as drug users, prostitutes, gays, lesbians, bisexuals, and transsexuals?
9. What are the best ways to prevent the spread of HIV/AIDS?
10. How will emerging trends in the epidemic possibly influence your work with individuals, families, or couples affected by HIV/AIDS?

## SUGGESTED FURTHER READING

Island, D., & Letellier, P. (1991). *Men who beat the men who love them: Battered gay men and domestic violence.* New York: Harrington Park Press.

Highlights research on violence and HIV in these relationships.

Murphy, D. A., Marelich, W. D., Dello Stritto, M. E., Swendeman, D., & Witkin, A. (2002). Mothers living with HIV/AIDS: Mental, physical, and family functioning. *AIDS Care, 14*(5), 633–644.

A study of 135 HIV-infected mothers.

Nichols, J. E., Speer, D. C., Watson, B. J., Watson, M. R., Vergon, T. L., Vallee, C. M., et al. (2002). *Aging with HIV: Psychological, social, and health issues.* San Diego, CA: Academic Press.

Presents information on an often-ignored segment of HIV-infected individuals.

Ritter, K. Y., & Terndrup, A. I. (2002). *Handbook of affirmative psychotherapy with lesbians and gay men.* New York: Guilford Press.

Aims to increase sensitivity to gay and lesbian client needs.

Tate, D., Paul, R. H., Flanigan, T. P., Tahima, K., Nash, J., Adair, C., et al. (2003). The impact of apathy and depression on quality of life in patients infected with HIV. *AIDS Patient Care & STD's, 17*(3), 115–120.

Discusses the impact of apathy on mental health and quality of life.

## REFERENCES

American Association for Marriage and Family Therapy. (2001). *AAMFT Code of Ethics.* Access: http://www.aamft.org/resources/LRMPlan/Ethics/ethicscode2001.asp

American Counseling Association. (1999). *ACA Code of Ethics and Standards of Practice.* Access: http://www.counseling.org/resources/codeofethics.htm

American Medical Association. (2003). H-20915 HIV/AIDS reporting, confidentiality, and notification. *AMA Policy Finder*, A-03. Access: http://www.ama-assn.org/ama/noindex/category/11760.html

Bor, R., Elford, J., Perry, J., & Miller, R. (1988). AIDS/HIV in the work of family therapy trainees. *Journal of Family Therapy, 10*, 375–382.

Boyd-Franklin, N., Aleman, J. C., Jean-Gilles, M. M., & Lewis, S. Y. (1995). Cultural sensitivity and competence: African-American, Latino, and Haitian families with HIV/AIDS. In N. Boyd-Franklin, G. L. Steiner, & M.G. Boland (Eds.), *Children, families and HIV: Psychosocial and therapeutic issues* (pp. 115–126). New York: Guilford Press.

Carten, A. J. & Fennoy, I. (1997). African American Families and HIV/AIDS: Caring for surviving children. *Child Welfare, 76*, 107–125.

Centers for Disease Control. (1993). Update: Barrier protection against HIV infection and other sexually transmitted diseases. *Morbidity and Mortality Weekly Report, 42.* (USGPO Publication No. 1993-799-131). Atlanta, GA.

Centers for Disease Control. (1994). Recommendations of the U.S. Public Health Service Task Force on the Use of Zidovudine to Reduce Perinatal Transmission of Human Immunodeficiency Virus. *Morbidity and Mortality Weekly Report, 43* (USGPO Publication No. 1994-533-178). Atlanta, GA.

Centers for Disease Control. (1995). *HIV/AIDS Surveillance Report, 7*(2), 1–38.

Centers for Disease Control. (1996). *HIV/AIDS Surveillance Report, 8*(2), 1–40.

Centers for Disease Control. (1998a). *HIV/AIDS Surveillance Report, 10*(2), 1–43.

Centers for Disease Control. (1998b). *What is AIDS? What causes AIDS?*

Centers for Disease Control. (2000). *HIV/AIDS Surveillance Report, 12*(2), 1–44.

Centers for Disease Control. (2002). *HIV/AIDS Surveillance Report, 14*, 1–48.

Centers for Disease Control. (2003a). *What is AIDS?* Access: http://www.cdc.gov/hiv/pubs/faq/faq2.html

Centers for Disease Control. (2003b). *What causes AIDS?* Access: http://www.cdc.gov/his/pubs/faq/faq36.html

Centers for Disease Control. (2003c). *Can I get HIV from oral sex?* Access: http://www.cdc.gov/hiv/pubs/faq/faq19.htm

Centers for Disease Control. (2003d). *Can I get HIV from mosquitoes?* Access: http://www.cdc.gov/hiv/pubs/faq/faq32.htm

Crawford, I., Humfleet, G., Ribordy, S. C., Ho, F. C., & Vickers, V. L. (1991). Stigmatization of AIDS patients by mental health professionals. *Professional Psychology: Research and Practice, 22*, 357–361.

Dhooper, S. S., Royse, D. D., & Tran, T. V. (1988). Social worker practioner's attitudes toward AIDS victims. *Journal of Applied Social Sciences, 12*, 108–123.

Diaz, Y. E., & Kelly, J. A. (1991). AIDS-related training in U.S. schools of social work. *Social Work, 36*, 38–42.

Gomez, K. A., Haiken, H. J., & Lewis, S. Y. (1995). Support group for children with HIV/AIDS. In N. Boyd-Franklin, G. L. Steiner, & M. G. Boland (Eds.), *Children, families and HIV: Psychosocial and therapeutic issues* (pp. 156–166). New York: Guilford Press.

Gostin, L. O. (2002). Surveillance and public health research: Privacy and the "right to know." In L. Gostin (Ed.), *Public health law and ethics: A reader* (pp. 295–334). Berkeley: University of California Press.

Green, S. K., & Bobele, M. (1994). Family therapists' response to AIDS: An examination of attitudes, knowledge, and contact. *Journal of Marital and Family Therapy, 20*, 349–367.

Hays, R. B., McKusick, L., Pollack, L., Hilliard, R., Hoff, C., & Coates, T. J. (1993). Disclosing HIV seropositivity to significant others. *AIDS, 7*, 425–431.

Kozlowski, N. F., Rupert, P. A., & Crawford, I. (1998). Psychotherapy with HIV-infected clients: Factors influencing notification of third parties. *Psychotherapy: Theory, Research & Practice, 35*, 105–115.

Lamb, D. H., Clark, C., Drumheller, P., Frizzel, K., & Surrely, L. (1989). Applying Tarasoff to AIDS-related psychotherapy issues. *Professional Psychology, Research and Practice, 20*, 37–43.

Landau, J., & Clements, C. D. (1997). AIDS update for family therapists. *Family Therapy News, 28*, 16–26.

Landau-Stanton, J., Clements, C. D., & Stanton, M. D. (1993). Psychotherapeutic intervention: From individual through group to extended network. In J. Landau-Stanton & C. D. Clements (Eds.), *AIDS, health and mental health: A primary sourcebook* (pp. 24–26). New York: Brunner/Mazel.

Marks, G., Richardson, J. L., & Maldonado, N. (1991). Self-disclosure of HIV infection to sexual partners. *American Journal of Public Health, 81*, 1321–1322.

Marks, G., Richardson, J. L., Ruiz, M. S., & Maldonado, N. (1992). HIV-infected men's practices in notifying past sexual partners of infection risk. *Public Health Reports, 107*, 100–105.

National Center for Health Statistics. (1994). Annual summary of births, marriages, divorces, and deaths: United States, 1993. *Monthly Vital Statistics Report, 42*. (DHHS Publication No. 95–1120). Hyattsville, MD: Public Health Service.

Niccolai, L. M., Dorst, D., Myers, L., & Kissinger, P. J. (1999). Disclosure of HIV status to sexual partners: Predictors and temporal patterns. *Sexually Transmitted Diseases 26*, 281–285.

Owens, S. (1995). Attitudes toward and knowledge of AIDS among African American social work students. *Health and Social Work, 20*, 110–115.

Pais, S., Piercy, F., & Miller, J. (1998). Factors related to family therapists' breaking confidence when clients disclose high-risks-to-HIV/AIDS sexual behaviors. *Journal of Marital and Family Therapy, 24*, 457–472.

Perry, S., Card, A. L., Moffatt, M., Ashman, T., Fishman, B., & Jacobsberg, L. (1994). Self-disclosure of HIV infection to sexual partners after repeated counseling. *AIDS Education and Prevention, 6*, 403–411.

Perry, S., Ryan, J., Fogel, K., Fishman, B., & Jacobsberg, L. (1990). Voluntarily informing others of positive HIV test results: Patterns of notification by infected gay men. *Hospital & Community Psychiatry, 41*, 549–551.

Peterson, K. J. (1989). Social workers' knowledge about AIDS: A national survey. Unpublished manuscript, University of Kansas, School of social Welfare, Lawrence, KS.

Preston, D. B., Young, E. W., Koch, P. B., & Forti, E. M. (1995). The Nurses' Attitudes About AIDS Scale (NAAS): Development and psychometric analysis. *AIDS Education & Prevention, 7*, 443–454.

Planned Parenthood of Wisconsin, Inc. (1998). *Basics of birth control.* (Publication No. 2-603-66). Milwauke, WI.

Rosenberg, P. S. (1995). Scope of the AIDS epidemic in the United States. *Science, 270*, 1372–1375.

Schlossberger, E., & Hecker, L. (1996). HIV and family therapists' duty to warn: A legal and ethical analysis. *Journal of Marital and Family Therapy, 22*, 27–40.

Schnell, D. J., Higgins, D. L., Wilson, R. M., Goldbaum, G., Cohn, D. L., & Wolitski, R. J. (1992). Men's disclosure of HIV test results to make primary sex partners. *American Journal of Public Health, 82*, 1675–1676.

Stein, M. D., Freedberg, K. A., Sullivan, L. M., Savetsky, J., Levenson, S. M., Hingson, R., et al. (1998). Disclosure of HIV-positive status to partners. *Archives of Internal Medicine, 158*, 253–257.

U.S. Food & Drug Administration (2003). Drugs used in the treatment of HIV infection. Access: http://www.fda.gov/oashi/aids/virals.html

Weiner, L. S., & Siegel, K. (1990). Social worker's comfort in providing services to AIDS patients. *Social Work, 35*, 18–25.

PART

# VI

# PROFESSIONAL DEVELOPMENT

# 24

# Ethical and Legal Issues
# in Family Therapy

Samuel T. Gladding
*Wake Forest University*

## TRUTH OR FICTION?

___ 1. Ethics and morality are basically the same.

___ 2. Ethical and legal opinions are usually in agreement.

___ 3. Prior to 1962, there was not an ethical code for the practice of marriage and family therapy.

___ 4. Codes of ethics protect family practitioners from the public and help increase public trust in the integrity of the profession of marital and family therapy.

___ 5. Confidentiality is the cornerstone of professional ethics in marriage and family therapy.

___ 6. Autonomy is the ethical principle that all human beings have the right to make decisions and act on them in an independent fashion.

___ 7. The gender of a family therapist and those within a family does not play a role in what issues are addressed in therapy and how they are addressed.

___ 8. The right of privileged communication rests with the client not the therapist.

___ 9. Your primary responsibility as a family therapist is to your client family.

___ 10. The law is cut and dried, as well as clear and precise, when it comes to matters dealing with family therapy.

___ 11. There is no general body of law covering the helping professions such as marriage and family therapy.

___ 12. If family therapists act in good faith, they are not likely to be found responsible for a client family's lack of progress or a mistake in judgment.

___ 13. If you are careful in working with families, you do not have to worry about ever being sued.

___ 14. *Family therapists can, and should, release any information they have on a family to a court of law when so ordered, even if they did not obtain this information first-hand.*

___ 15. *In marriage and family therapy, the concept of liability is directly connected with malpractice.*

The overall goal of this chapter is to give you a better understanding of ethical and legal issues in family therapy.

In regard to ethics, I want to: (a) introduce you to what ethics and morality are, (b) help you understand what codes of ethics are and how they work, (c) make you aware of some of the limitations of codes of ethics and some of the most common ethical violations in family therapy, (d) give you guidelines on how to make an ethical decision, (e) provide you with an overview of the AAMFT Code of Ethics, and (f) answer frequently asked ethical questions concerning such topics as confidentiality and client welfare.

In regard to legal issues, I want to help you understand: (a) what the law is and what is considered legal, (b) what liability and malpractice are and the difference between civil and criminal liability, (c) how to honor client rights and handle client records, (d) proper ways to act as a family therapist in court, (e) legal situations that involve family therapists, and (f) how a family therapist can best work in a litigious society.

## ETHICS AND FAMILY THERAPY

### What Are Ethics and How Do They Differ From Morality?

*Ethics* involves making decisions of a moral nature about people and their interactions in society. The term is often used synonymously with *morality,* and in some cases the two terms overlap. Both deal with what is good and bad or the study of human conduct and values. Yet each has a different meaning.

"Ethics is generally defined as a philosophical discipline that is concerned with human conduct and moral decision making" (Van Hoose & Kottler, 1985, p. 3). Ethics are normative in nature and focus on principles and standards that govern relationships between individuals, such as those between family members and therapists and families.

Two principles underlie relationship ethics found in families. They are:

1. *Equitability,* which is the proposition that everyone is entitled to have his or her welfare considered in a way that is fair from multiple perspectives
2. *Caring,* which is the idea that moral development and principles are centered in the social context of relationships and interdependency

Morality, on the other hand, involves judgment or evaluation of action. It is associated with such words as *good, bad, right, wrong, ought,* and *should*. Family therapists have morals. The theories we employ in working with families have embedded within them moral presuppositions about human nature and family life (Gladding, Remley, & Huber, 2001).

1. Ethics differs from morality in its emphasis on:
   a. what is good and what is bad.
   b. human conduct and moral decision making.

c.  esoteric philosophical concepts.

d.  the codes of behavior embedded within the discipline.

2.  The principle of *equitability*, which is one of the two principles underlying relationship ethics, is the proposition that:

a.  everyone is entitled to have his or her welfare considered in a way that is fair from multiple perspectives.

b.  moral development and principles are centered in the social context of relationships and interdependency.

c.  words such as *good, bad, right, wrong, ought*, and *should* are the basis for human interactions.

d.  personal interactions should be governed by moral principles.

## What Do Codes of Ethics Do?

A **code of ethics** for a profession is meant to enhance, inform, expand, and improve members of the profession's abilities to serve as effectively as possible those clients seeking their help. In addition, a code of ethics informs you of what is expected of you as a family therapy practitioner. Codes of ethics guide your professional, and sometimes your personal, behavior. Another reason for ethical codes is that without a code of established ethics, a group of people with similar interests cannot be considered a professional organization. Three other reasons for the existence of ethical codes according to Van Hoose and Kottler (1985) are as follows:

1.  Ethical codes protect the profession from government. They allow the profession to regulate itself and function autonomously instead of being controlled by legislation.

2.  Ethical codes help control internal disagreements and bickering, thus promoting stability within the profession.

3.  Ethical codes protect practitioners from the public, especially in regard to malpractice suits, and protect the public from charlatans and incompetent therapists. If you, as a family therapist, behave according to ethical guidelines, the behavior is judged to be in compliance with accepted standards. Thus, ethical codes help increase public trust in the integrity of the profession of marital and family therapy.

3.  Without a code of ethics, a group of people with similar interests, such as family therapists, would:

a.  be unruly.

b.  not be considered a profession.

c.  be ill defined.

d.  be governed by special interests.

4.  Ethical codes are instrumental in doing all of the following *except:*

a.  protecting a profession from government interference.

b.  controlling internal bickering among members of a professional group.

c.  protecting a profession from the public, especially in regard to malpractice law suits.

d.  promoting a mental picture of what a profession is.

## What Are the Limitations of Codes of Ethics?

Codes of ethics offer only general philosophical guidance for conceptualizing and responding to conflicts. It is not their purpose to recommend specific behaviors in limited situations. If it were, codes would become voluminous, lack broad-based support, and infringe upon the role of the individual professional in ethical decision making.

A number of specific limitations exist in any code of ethics. The following points are some of the limitations most frequently mentioned:

- Some issues cannot be resolved by a code of ethics.
- Enforcing ethical codes is difficult.
- There may be conflicts within the standards delineated by the code.
- Some legal and ethical issues are not covered in codes.
- Ethical codes are historical documents. Thus, what may be acceptable practice at one time may be considered unethical later.
- Sometimes conflicts arise between ethical and legal codes.
- Ethical codes do not address cross-cultural issues.
- Ethical codes do not address every possible situation.
- There is often difficulty in bringing the interests of all parties involved in an ethical dispute together systematically.
- Ethical codes are not proactive documents for helping therapists decide what to do in new situations.

Thus, ethical codes are useful in many ways, but they do have their limitations.

If sued for malpractice, a therapist will be judged in terms of actions appropriate to other therapists with similar qualifications and duties. Ethical standards of the profession will be a probable basis for comparison (Corey, Corey, & Callanan, 2003). If therapists act in good faith, they are not likely to be found responsible for a client's lack of progress or mistake in judgment on their part if the mistakes were the type a careful and skillful therapist could make.

5. Specific limitations on codes of ethics include the fact that:
   a. some ethical issues are not covered in codes of ethics.
   b. enforcing ethical codes is difficult.
   c. some issues cannot be resolved by codes of ethics.
   d. all of the above.

6. If sued for malpractice, a family therapist will be judged by:
   a. whether his or her actions were appropriate compared to other therapists with similar qualifications and duties.
   b. the American Association for Marriage and Family Therapy.
   c. a jury picked from peers who are also therapists.
   d. a judge in a civil court of law.

## What Are the Most Common Unethical Behaviors in Family Therapy?

Unethical behaviors in family therapy can take many forms. The temptations common to people everywhere exist for you as a therapist. Some forms of unethical behavior are obvious and willful, whereas others are more subtle and unintentional. Regardless, the harmful outcome is the same. The following list summarizes the most prevalent forms of unethical behaviors in family therapy:

- Violating confidentiality
- Exceeding one's level of professional competence
- Negligent practice
- Claiming expertise one does not possess
- Imposing one's values on a client
- Creating dependency in a client
- Sexual activity with a client
- Certain conflicts of interest, such as dual relationships
- Questionable financial arrangements, such as charging excessive fees
- Improper advertising

Some of these actions, such as negligent practice and questionable financial arrangements, are also illegal (Gladding et al., 2001).

7. All of the following are prevalent forms of unethical behavior in family therapy *except:*
   a. accepting a referral from a therapist you do not know well.
   b. claiming expertise you do not possess.
   c. sexual activity with a client.
   d. improper advertising.

## What Are the Basic Guidelines for Ethical Decision Making?

Ethical decision making demands proficiency in four processes. The first process involves interpreting a situation as requiring an ethical decision. This process involves the ability to perceive the effect of one's actions on the welfare of others. Individuals differ in their ability to be sensitive to the needs and welfare of others with some mental health practitioners being substantially insensitive to the ethical dimensions of their work.

The second process is formulating an ethical course of action. Ethical action does not always feel good, nor does it always lead to choices that are "good" in an absolute sense. In proposing a model for ethical reasoning, Kitchener (1984) distinguished between the *intuitive level* and the *critical-evaluative level* of ethical justification. The first level involves doing what you subjectively believe is right while the next level is based on a more objective evaluation of circumstances.

The third process includes integrating personal and professional values. It is possible for you to know what you "should" do ethically but decide against taking ethical action because of competing values and motives. This process recognizes that how individuals decide to act is heavily influenced by factors such as ambition, money, and self-interest. Research and ordinary observation have consistently shown that persons do not always do what they think they "should" do but rather respond to personal values and practical considerations in determining what they actually "would" do (Smith, McGuire, Abbott, & Blau, 1991). For example, a therapist who knows that a colleague is acting unethically may, because of friendship or loyalty, decide not to intervene.

The final process involves implementing a plan of action. An important aspect of assuming responsibility is the ability to tolerate the ambiguity that accompanies ethical decision making.

As a family therapist, you must understand that few absolute answers exist and certainty is frequently impossible.

8. The third step in the four-step process of making an ethical decision is:
   a. interpreting a situation as requiring an ethical decision.
   b. formulating an ethical course of action.
   c. integrating personal and professional values.
   d. implementing a plan for action.

## What Are the AAMFT Ethical Guidelines?

The establishment of ethical guidelines is relatively new to the helping professions. The first American Association for Marriage and Family Therapy (AAMFT) code of ethics was approved by the membership in 1962. The latest revision occurred in 2001.

The AAMFT Code of Ethics (2001) contains the following eight sectional topics:

1. Responsibility to clients, including the avoidance of dual relationships, sexual intimacy, and dependence
2. Confidentiality, including making sure clients understand the limitations of confidentiality and that therapists act in ways that protect client confidentiality
3. Professional competence and integrity, including an emphasis that therapists not practice new techniques or specialties unless they have been properly educated and a reminder that therapists have an ethical obligation to stay up to date on new developments in the field
4. Responsibility to students, employees, and supervisees, including the prohibition of providing therapy to students and supervisees or having sexually intimate relationships with them
5. Responsibility to research participants, including an emphasis on informed consent and protection of research subjects
6. Responsibility to the profession, including using adherence to the code of ethics as a way of resolving any employer requirements that conflict with the code and avoiding plagiarism or failure to cite authorship when due
7. Financial arrangements, including making sure that clients are well informed about the cost of therapy and what will happen if they are unable or unwilling to pay
8. Advertising, including the basic idea that advertising should be honest and not misleading

9. The first AAMFT Code of Ethics was approved by members in 1962. The latest AAMFT Code was approved in _____.
   a. 1995
   b. 1997
   c. 2001
   d. 2003

10. The AAMFT Code of Ethics is comprised of _____ sections.
    a. 6
    b. 8
    c. 10
    d. 12

## What Are Some of the Most Common Ethical Concerns?

All ethical concerns are important but some occur more frequently than others. Among these are the following.

*Client Welfare.* The codes of ethics of all major professional associations affirm that as a therapist your primary responsibility is to your clients. The needs of clients, not therapists, take first priority in the therapeutic relationship. Also implied is that therapeutic relationships should be maintained only as long as clients are benefiting from them.

Five principles applied by Beauchamp and Childress (1994) to biomedical ethics have been recommended as specifically relevant to issues of client welfare in psychotherapy, including family therapy: autonomy, beneficence, nonmaleficence, justice, and fidelity (Kitchener, 1984). *Autonomy* is the principle that all human beings have the right to make decisions and act on them in an independent fashion. *Beneficence* is the principle that one must actively attempt to benefit another in a positive manner. The principle that one must avoid causing harm to another is *nonmaleficence*. *Justice* is the principle that all individuals should be treated fairly; equals must be treated as equals and unequals must be treated in a way most beneficial to their specific circumstances. *Fidelity* is the principle of commitment to keep promises, uphold truth, and maintain loyalty.

Some experts identify nonmaleficence as the primary ethical responsibility in the field of therapy. Nonmaleficence not only involves the "removal of present harm" but the "prevention of future harm, and passive avoidance of harm" (Thompson, 1990, p. 105). It is the basis on which therapists respond to clients who may endanger themselves or others and why they respond to colleagues' unethical behavior.

11. Of the five principles recommended as specifically relevant to issues of client welfare in psychotherapy, the one some experts identify as primary is _____.
    a. autonomy
    b. nonmaleficence
    c. justice
    d. fidelity

12. The ethical principle that states a person must actively attempt to benefit another person in a positive manner is known as _____.
    a. fidelity
    b. justice
    c. beneficence
    d. nonmaleficence

*Confidentiality.* The single most widely recognized ethical issue in the practice of psychotherapy is *confidentiality* which is "often referred to as the cornerstone of ethics" (Kaplan & Culkin, 1995, p. 336). Confidentiality had its genesis in the physician–patient relationship in the 16th century, when physicians began to realize that contagious diseases were being spread by persons who feared that if they told anyone of their affliction including their physician, they would be condemned to social isolation. Today, there are two primary reasons for maintaining confidentiality in psychotherapy:

1. Confidentiality protects clients from the social stigma frequently associated with therapy.
2. Confidentiality promotes vital client rights, integral to therapists' professed concern for the welfare of clients.

Confidentiality is maintained as a standard by the ethical codes of all professional therapy organizations.

> 13. The single most widely recognized ethical issue in the practice of psychotherapy, including family therapy, is _____.
>     a. confidentiality
>     b. competence
>     c. sexuality
>     d. cultural insensitivity

*Competence.*   Family therapists are expected to be competent in working with families. Competency means knowing what options are open and likely to produce the best possible results. Competency also means eschewing theoretical practices that are controversial and not grounded in research.

> 14. Competence as a family therapist means:
>     a. knowing what options are open and likely to produce the best possible results.
>     b. eschewing theoretical practices that are controversial and not grounded in research.
>     c. both a and b.
>     d. doing the right thing in the right way with families every time.

*Gender Issues.*   Gender can be an important ethical issue in conducting family therapy. The gender of the therapist and of those within the family can play an important part in what issues are addressed during treatment and how they are addressed. In working with families, therapists need to be attuned to such ethical and practical issues as the following:

- The balance of power between spouses both financially and physically
- The rules and roles played by members of different genders and how they are rewarded
- What a shift in a family's way of operating will mean to the functionality of the family as a whole (McGoldrick, 1999).

> 15. In addressing gender issues in family therapy, a clinician should be attuned to:
>     a. the balance of power between spouses.
>     b. the rules and roles played by members of different genders and their rewards.
>     c. what a shift in a family's way of operating will mean to the functionality of the family as a whole.
>     d. all of the above.

*Multicultural Issues.*   Another area in which ethical issues commonly arise is in the multicultural domain. In working with minority culture families, Pedersen (1996) proposes that there are three serious errors, all of which have ethical implications that should be avoided. These errors have a tendency to:

- Overemphasize similarities
- Overemphasize differences
- Make assumptions that either similarities or differences must be emphasized.

Instead, family therapists need to take a "culturally relevant perspective that attempts to identify cultural significance from the family's own perspective rather than a prescribed set of cultural characteristics that may or may not be relevant to a family" (Kurilla, 1998, p. 210).

16. When a family therapist attempts to identify cultural significance from a family's own perspective, he or she is:
    a. emphasizing similarities in cultures.
    b. emphasizing differences in cultures.
    c. emphasizing both similarities and differences in cultures.
    d. being culturally relevant.

## THE LAW AND FAMILY THERAPY

### What Is Law?

*Law* is the precise codification of governing standards that is established to ensure legal and moral justice. Law is created by legislation, court decision, and tradition, as in English common law (Anderson & Hopkins, 1996). The law does not dictate what is ethical in a given situation but what is legal. Sometimes what is legal at a given time (e.g., matters pertaining to race, age, or sex) is considered unethical or immoral by some significant segments of society. Thus, there may be a wide gap between law and ethics.

Family therapy is governed by legal standards. *Legal* refers to law or the state of being lawful, whereas law refers to a body of rules recognized by a state or community as binding on its members (Gladding et al., 2001). Contrary to popular opinion, "law is not cut and dried, definite and certain, or clear and precise" (Van Hoose & Kottler, 1985, p. 44). Rather, it always seeks compromise between individuals and parties. It offers few definite answers, and there are always notable exceptions to any legal precedent.

There is no general body of law covering the helping professions. Another major difficulty with any law governing client and therapist communication is that laws vary from state to state. However, there are a number of court decisions and statutes that influence legal opinion on family therapy and therapists need to keep updated.

17. In general, the law:
    a. is cut and dried, definite and clear.
    b. frequently seeks compromises between individuals and parties.
    c. dictates what is ethical in most situations.
    d. does not make room for many exceptions.

18. The only time the law overrides a professional code of ethics is:
    a. the law always overrides a professional code of ethics.
    b. to protect the public's health, safety, and welfare.
    c. when an ethics code or principle in the code is illegal.
    d. when a profession does not have sufficiently strong standards.

In most cases, the law is generally supportive or neutral toward professional codes of ethics and therapy in general. It supports licensure or certification of family therapists and other helping specialists as a means of ensuring that those who enter professions attain at least minimal standards. In addition, the law is neutral in that it allows professionals to police themselves and govern therapeutic relations with their clients and fellow therapists. The only time the law overrides a professional code of ethics is when it is necessary to protect the public health, safety, and welfare. This necessity is most likely to occur in situations concerning confidentiality, when disclosure of information is necessary to prevent harm. In such cases, you, as a family therapist, have a duty to warn potential victims about the possibility of a client's violent behavior.

## What Is Liability?

*Liability* in family therapy involves issues concerned with whether therapists have caused harm to couples or families. The concept of liability is directly connected with malpractice. *Malpractice* in therapy is defined as a failure to render proper service resulting from professional **negligence** or ignorance and resulting in harm to a client (Corey et al., 2003). Until recently, there were relatively few family therapy malpractice lawsuits. But with the increased number of licensed, certified, and practicing therapists, malpractice suits have become more common. Therefore, family therapists need to make sure they protect themselves from such possibilities.

Two ways you can protect yourself from malpractice are (a) to follow professional codes of ethics, and (b) to follow normal practice standards. Regardless of how careful you are, however, malpractice lawsuits can still occur. Therefore, carrying liability insurance is a must.

Liability can be classified under two main headings: civil and criminal. *Civil liability* means you can be sued for acting wrongly toward another or for failing to act when there is a recognized duty to do so. *Criminal liability,* on the other hand, involves you working with a client in a way the law does not allow.

The concept of civil liability rests on the idea of a *tort,* a wrong that legal action is designed to set right (Anderson & Hopkins, 1996). The legal wrong can be against a person, property, or even someone's reputation and may be unintentional or direct. Family therapists are most likely to face civil liability suits for malpractice in the following situations: (a) malpractice in particular situations (birth control, abortion, prescribing and administering drugs, treatment), (b) illegal search, (c) defamation, (d) invasion of privacy, and (e) breach of contract (Anderson & Hopkins). Three situations in which family therapists risk criminal liability are (a) accessory to a crime, (b) civil disobedience, and (c) contribution to the delinquency of a minor (Anderson & Hopkins, 1996; Gladding et al., 2001).

19. Liability in family therapy is:
    a. concerned with whether therapists have caused harm to couples or families.
    b. directly connected with malpractice.
    c. both a and b.
    d. a rare occurrence that only happens to clinicians who are not well prepared.

20. Family therapists can protect themselves from malpractice if:
    a. they follow professional codes of ethics.
    b. they follow normal practice standards.
    c. they carry maximum coverage of liability insurance.
    d. both a and b.

21. Family therapists face criminal liability suits for malpractice in the following situations *except*_____.
    a. defamation
    b. accessory to a crime
    c. civil disobedience
    d. contribution to the delinquency of a minor

## What Is Privileged Communication?

*Privileged communication* is a legal right which exists by statute and which protects clients, such as families, from having their confidences revealed publicly from the witness stand during legal proceedings without their permission (Gladding et al., 2001). Where privileged communication laws apply, therapists are prevented from testifying in court about clients without their consent. If a client waives this privilege, a therapist has no grounds for withholding information. The privilege belongs to the client and is meant for the protection of the client, not the therapist (Corey et al., 2003). It is important to note that privileged communication for the therapist–client relationship is not legally supported in a large number of states.

Gumper and Sprenkle (1981) have examined the potential repercussions of privileged communication laws for psychotherapy. They report a wide variation in legal statutes, and this variation presents particular problems for marriage and family therapists. Dominant among the problems that arise is the question, "Who owns the right to waive privilege in marriage and family therapy?" Gumper and Sprenkle specifically reemphasized that ownership of this privilege—and therefore the right to waive it—resides with the client, not the therapist.

22. The legal right of privileged communication belongs to and is meant to protect the_____.
    a. client
    b. therapist
    c. both the client and therapist
    d. attorney

## What Rights Do Clients Have in Family Therapy?

There are two main types of client rights: implied and explicit. Both relate to due process. *Implied rights* are linked to substantive due process. When a rule is made that arbitrarily limits an individual (i.e., deprives the person of his or her constitutional rights), he or she has been denied substantive due process. *Explicit rights* focus on procedural due process (the steps necessary to initiate or complete an action when an explicit rule is broken). An individual's procedural due process is violated when an explicit rule is broken and the person is not informed about how to remedy the matter. A couple or family has a right to know what recourse they have when either of these two types of rights is violated.

23. A client's implied rights are linked to _____ while a client's explicit rights focus on _____.
    a. procedural due process; substantive due process
    b. substantive due process; procedural due process
    c. steps necessary to complete an action; important information
    d. clients have explicit but not implied rights

## What Is the Best Way to Protect Clients' Records?

The records of all clients are legally protected except under special circumstances. For example, in some instances, such as those provided by the Buckley Amendment, an individual has the legal right to inspect his or her record. In the vast majority of cases, therapists are legally required to protect clients of all ages by keeping records under lock and key, separate from any required business records, and not disclosing any information about a client without that person's written permission (Mitchell, 2001). The best method to use in meeting a request for disclosing information is a release-of-information form, which can be drawn up by an attorney. Therapists should not release client information they have not obtained firsthand.

Because record keeping is one of the top areas pertaining to legal liability of therapists, the question often arises about what should go into records. Basically, records should contain all information about the couple or family necessary for treatment. The number and types of forms in a record vary with the agency and practitioner, but six categories of documents are usually included:

1. *Identifying or intake information:* name, address, telephone number(s), date of birth, sex, occupation, and so on
2. *Assessment information:* psychological evaluations, social/family history, health history, and so on
3. *Treatment plan:* presenting problem, plan of action, steps to be taken to reach targeted behavior, and so on
4. *Case notes:* for example, documentation of progress in each session toward the stated goal
5. *Termination summary:* outcome of treatment, final diagnosis (if any), after-care plan, and so on
6. *Other data:* client's signed consent for treatment, copies of correspondence, notations about rationale for any unusual client interventions, administrative problems, and so on.

It is vital for therapists to check their state legal codes for exact guidelines about record keeping. It is critical for those who receive third-party reimbursement to make sure that their client records refer to progress in terms of a treatment plan and a diagnosis (if required). In no case, however, should confidential information about a family or family member be given over the telephone. Therapists are also ethically and legally bound to ensure that a client's rights are protected by not discussing clinical cases in public.

24. All but which of the following are actions family therapists should take to protect client records?
    a. keep records under lock and key
    b. separate client records from business records
    c. do not give out client information without written permission
    d. do not keep client information on a computer

25. Client records should contain all of the following types of information *except* _____.
    a. assessment data
    b. credit records
    c. case notes
    d. treatment plan

26. It is acceptable for a family therapist to discuss a clinical case as long as it:
    a. is not in public.
    b. is not over the telephone.
    c. is with another professional in a confidential setting.
    d. is interesting and informative.

## What Is It Like to Go to Court as a Family Therapist?

The court system in the United States is divided into federal and state courts. Each is similarly patterned with "trial courts, a middle-level appellate court, and a supreme court" (Anderson & Hopkins, 1996, p. 7). Most family therapists who appear in court do so on the state level because the federal courts deal with cases arising primarily under the laws of the United States or those involving citizens of different states where the amount of controversy exceeds $50,000.

Most family therapists wind up in court in two main ways. One is voluntary and professional: when the therapist serves as an expert witness. An *expert witness* is an objective and unbiased person with specialized knowledge, skills, or information, who can assist a judge or jury in reaching an appropriate legal decision (Gladding et al., 2001). A therapist who serves as an expert witness is compensated financially for his or her time.

The other way a family therapist may appear in court is through a ***court order*** (a *subpoena* to appear in court at a certain time in regard to a specific case). Such a summons is issued with the intent of having the therapist testify on behalf of or against a present or former family member or a family. Because the legal system is adversarial, family therapists are wise to seek the advice of attorneys before responding to court orders (Gladding et al., 2001). By so doing, therapists may come to understand law, court proceedings, and options they have in response to legal requests. You may also find that role playing possible situations before appearing in court may help you function better in these situations.

Overall, in preparing for legal encounters, family therapists should read about important legal issues such as preparing for court appearances, documenting counseling records, counseling minors, understanding confidentiality and privileged communication, receiving third-party payments, and managing a counseling agency.

27. Most family therapists who appear in court do so at the _____ level.
    a. state
    b. federal
    c. appellate
    d. supreme

28. When a family therapist is given a subpoena, he or she should:
    a. appear in court.
    b. complain to the court.
    c. consult an attorney.
    d. ignore the subpoena and continue seeing clients.

## What Are Common Legal Situations Involving Family Therapists?

There are a number of legal situations that involve family therapists. However, some are more common than others. Among these are those involving a therapist as an expert witness, a child custody evaluator, and a court ordered witness.

An ***expert witness*** is a family therapist who is asked to give testimony about probable causes and recommendations in regard to family members, such as juveniles who are acting out behaviorally. Because courts are adversarial, an expert witness must be schooled in the ways of courtroom protocol. They must be specific, stay objective, and speak from authoritative sources when making their points.

A ***child custody evaluator*** is a family therapist who is asked to determine what is in the best interest of a child in a custody arrangement. In these cases, the family therapist represents the child and the court, not the parents. If you become a child custody evaluator, you must have an extensive background in child development, family systems theory, parenting skills, and psychometry among other things, and be willing to make home visits, conduct psychological testing, and have conversations with the child involved.

A final frequent way a family therapist can work with the legal system is as a **court ordered witness**. In this role, the therapist appears before a court to testify on behalf of or against a family or family member. It is unusual for a family therapist to function in such a role because it is adversarial and not systemic.

29. When a family therapist appears in court to determine the best interest of a child in a custody arrangement, he or she is appearing as a(n) _____.
    a. expert witness
    b. child custody evaluator
    c. court ordered witness
    d. friend of the court

## How Can a Family Therapist Best Work in a Litigious Society?

Attorneys and family therapists tend to think in different ways. The professionals in these specialties live for the most part in two different cultures and base their practices on unique worldviews. For this reason, there is a strong rationale for considering therapy and the legal system from a cross-cultural perspective (Rowley & MacDonald, 2001).

To become successful in a litigious society, family therapists, who are part of a minority culture, must become acculturated into the majority culture, the law. There are several ways you, as a therapist, can accomplish this goal, including:

- Becoming "knowledgeable with those elements that are common to both mental health and the law"
- Understanding and being prepared to "work with those elements of the law that differ from the culture of mental health," such as seeking information from a family therapist without an appropriate release
- Reviewing the AAMFT *Code of Ethics* and other relevant ethical codes annually
- Participating in continuing education programs that review laws pertinent to family therapy
- Learning more about the legal system through "organizations and publications that interface with the mental health and legal system," for example, *American Psychology–Law Society News* or *The Forensic Examiner*
- Creating a collaborative relationship with a lawyer, a judge, or other legal practitioner
- Developing a relationship with a family therapist who is knowledgeable about the world of law
- Consulting and receiving feedback on possible decisions when there is an ethical–legal dilemma (Rowley & MacDonald, 2001, pp. 427–428)

30. To become successful in a litigious society, especially in court, family therapists should:
    a. learn more about the legal system.
    b. review the AAMFT Code of Ethics and other relevant ethical codes.
    c. become more acculturated into the majority culture of the legal profession.
    d. all of the above.

# KEY TERMS

**autonomy:** The principle that all human beings have the right to make decisions and act on them in an independent fashion.

**beneficence:** The principle that one must actively attempt to benefit another in a positive manner.

**caring:** One of the propositions underlying relationship ethics is that moral development and principles are centered in the social context of relationships and interdependency.

**child custody evaluator:** A family therapist who is asked to determine what is in the best interest of a child in a custody arrangement.

**civil liability:** Being sued for acting wrongly toward another or for failing to act when there [is] a recognized duty to do so.

**code of ethics:** A formal document for a profession that informs its members what is expected of them as practitioners and thus allows them to serve their clients and the public better.

**court order:** A subpoena to appear in court at a certain time in regard to a specific case.

**court ordered witness:** A therapist who appears before a court to testify on behalf of or against a family or family member.

**criminal liability:** Working with a client in a way the law does not allow.

**equitability:** One of the propositions underlying relationship ethics is that everyone is entitled to have his or her welfare considered in a way that is fair from multiple perspectives.

**ethics:** A philosophical discipline that is concerned with human conduct and moral decision making.

**expert witness:** A family therapist who gives testimony about probable causes and recommendations in regard to family members.

**fidelity:** The principle of commitment to keep promises, uphold truth, and maintain loyalty.

**justice:** The principle that all individuals should be treated fairly; equals must be treated as equals and unequals must be treated in a way most beneficial to their specific circumstances.

**law:** The precise codification of governing standards that is established to ensure legal and moral justice; a body of rules recognized by a state or community as binding on its members.

**legal:** Matters pertaining to the law or the state of being lawful.

**liability:** Involves issues concerned with whether therapists have caused harm to couples or families.

**malpractice:** Harm to a client resulting from professional negligence.

**morality:** The judgment or evaluation of action through words such as *good, bad, right, wrong, ought,* and *should.*

**negligence:** The departure in therapy from acceptable professional standards.

**nonmaleficence:** The principle that one must avoid causing harm to another.

**privileged communication:** A legal right which exists by statute and which protects clients from having their confidences revealed publicly from the witness stand during legal proceedings without their permission.

**tort:** A wrong that legal action is designed to set right.

# DISCUSSION QUESTIONS

1. How would you explain to the public the difference in acting in an ethical as opposed to a moral way when working with a family in therapy?

2.  When you consider the many reasons for codes of ethics, which do you consider the most important? Justify your answer by ranking the reasons for codes of ethics according to their relative importance.
3.  Which of the many limitations in a code of ethics do you consider to be most significant? Justify your answer.
4.  Find out some common forms of dual relationships. Discuss at least four of them and the potential harm associated with each.
5.  Which of the eight sections of the AAMFT Code of Ethics do you think is most difficult for family therapists to deal with? Which do you think is easiest? Give reasons for your opinions and, if you have time, investigate the correctness of your answer with the AAMFT.
6.  Compare and contrast the ethical implications of violating client welfare as opposed to breaking confidentiality. Where do these two ethical principals overlap and where do they differ?
7.  How are the law and ethics similar? How do they differ? Give examples in each case.
8.  Explain the differences between civil and criminal liabilities. What are some common examples of family therapists and others becoming liable for their actions as professional helpers?
9.  What do you see as the advantages and disadvantages of having privileged communication in a therapeutic situation such as family therapy?
10. Pretend you are a family therapist. Draw a map of your office and describe how you would ensure the safety of its records.
11. Describe what you think it would be like to function in court as a family therapist. Of the possible roles therapists can fill in court, which one do you find most appealing? Why?
12. Do you think the concept of family therapy as a minority culture is a helpful one in contrasting it to the majority culture of the law? What other comparisons might be helpful in distinguishing between these two ways of working with families?

## SUGGESTED FURTHER READING

Wall, J., Post, S., Browning, D., & Doherty, W. J. (Eds.). (2002). *Marriage, health, and the professions: If marriage is good for you, what does this mean for law, medicine, ministry, therapy, and business?* Grand Rapids, MI: Eerdmans.

This book examines ethically responsible ways for the professions of law, medicine, therapy, business, and ministry to handle information about the positive contributions of marriage to the health and well-being of men and women.

Woody, R. H., & Woody, J. D. (2001). *Ethics in marriage and family therapy.* Washington, DC: American Association for Marriage and Family Therapy.

This book explores contemporary ethical issues in marriage and family therapy such as multiple relationships, violence, abuse and neglect, morality, spirituality, and sexuality.

## REFERENCES

American Association for Marriage and Family Therapy. (2001). *Code of ethics.* Washington, DC: Author.
Anderson, B. S., & Hopkins, B. R. (1996). *The counselor and the law* (4th ed.). Alexandria, VA: American Counseling Association.
Beauchamp, T. L., & Childress, J. F. (1994). *Principles of biomedical ethics* (4th ed.). New York: Oxford University Press.

Corey, G., Corey, M. S., & Callanan, P. M. (2003). *Issues and ethics in the helping professions* (6th ed.). Pacific Grove, CA: Brooks/Cole.

Gladding, S. T., Remley, T. P., Jr., & Huber, C. H. (2001). *Ethical, legal, and professional issues in the practice of marriage and family therapy* (3rd ed.). Upper Saddle River, NJ: Prentice Hall.

Gumper, L. L., & Sprenkle, D. H. (1981). Privileged communication in therapy: Special problems for the family and couples therapist. *Family Process, 20,* 11–23.

Kaplan, D., & Culkin, M. (1995). Family ethics: Lessons learned. *The Family Journal: Counseling and Therapy for Couples and Families, 3,* 335–338.

Kitchener, K. S. (1984). Ethics in counseling psychology: Distinctions and directions. *The Counseling Psychologist, 12,* 15–18.

Kurilla, V. (1998). Multicultural counseling perspective: Culture specificity and implications in family therapy. *The Family Journal: Counseling and Therapy for Couples and Families, 6,* 207–211.

McGoldrick, M. (1999). Women and the family life cycle. In B. Carter & M. McGoldrick (Eds.), *The expanded family life cycle* (3rd ed., pp. 106–123). Boston: Allyn & Bacon.

Mitchell, R. (2001). *Documentation in counseling records* (2nd ed.). Alexandria, VA: American Counseling Association.

Pedersen, P. (1996). The importance of similarities and differences in multicultural counseling: Reaction to C. H. Patterson. *Journal of Counseling & Development, 74,* 236–237.

Rowley, W. J., & MacDonald, D. (2001). Counseling and the law: A cross-cultural perspective. *Journal of Counseling and Development, 79,* 422–429.

Smith, T. S., McGuire, J. M., Abbott, D. W., & Blau, B. I. (1991). Clinical ethical decision making: An investigation of the rationales used to justify doing less than one believes one should. *Professional Psychology: Research and Practice, 22,* 235–239.

Thompson, A. (1990). *Guide to ethical practice in psychotherapy.* New York: Wiley.

Van Hoose, W. H., & Kottler, J. A. (1985). *Ethical and legal issues in counseling and psychotherapy* (2nd ed.). San Francisco: Jossey Bass.

# 25

# Preparing for Licensing Examinations

Kinly Sturkie
*Clemson University*

## TRUTH OR FICTION?

___ 1. *From the viewpoint of the state, licensure examinations are regarded as a primary measure of practitioner competence.*

___ 2. *Licensure examinations target the knowledge and skills that should have been mastered by the minimally competent practitioner.*

___ 3. *State MFT licenses, and the exams upon which they are issued, are primarily intended to enhance the status, visibility, and billing prerogatives of MFT practitioners.*

___ 4. *Licensure examinations attempt to measure both knowledge and the practical application of knowledge.*

___ 5. *Because of family therapy's unique systemic orientation, the California and National Examinations in MFT had to be developed using different processes than most other examinations in the mental health field.*

___ 6. *Twenty-five percent of states currently require an oral examination for marital and family therapy licensure.*

___ 7. *Licensure examinations in family therapy focus solely on the clinical aspects of practice.*

___ 8. *A number of states require two different written examinations in marital and family therapy.*

___ 9. *The goal of professional examination construction is to operationalize what MFTs do and what they need to know to do, so that specific exam items relating to these tasks and bodies of knowledge can be developed.*

___ 10. *Candidates sitting for the National Examination in MFT should guess at answers about which they are not sure, because there is no mathematical penalty for doing so.*

_____ 11. *Professional exams in the MFT field have a pass-rate of approximately 90%.*
_____ 12. *After examination administration, statistics for each item are reviewed to be sure that it has performed in accordance with exam specifications.*
_____ 13. *A critical part of examination preparation is becoming familiar with one's respective state licensure laws and important national legal issues in the mental health field.*
_____ 14. *The pass-point for licensure examinations in the MFT field are generally set at the average score, minus one standard deviation.*
_____ 15. *The format for most academic qualifying examinations in MFT parallels the format of the National Examination.*

This chapter describes why professional examinations are an important part of the licensure process for marital and family therapists, how these examinations have been developed and are maintained, and how you might best prepare for them. This chapter also briefly explores the nature of the qualifying (i.e., preliminary and comprehensive) exams that are a part of many graduate programs.

## MARITAL AND FAMILY THERAPY EXAMINATIONS IN CONTEXT

The 1980s and 1990s were pivotal for the development of the marital and family therapy (MFT) field as it attempted to honor its persona of cutting edge formulations and nonconventionality, while simultaneously attempting to be recognized and embraced by consumers, insurers, and other professionals as a part of the mainstream in the mental health treatment community. This involved a tightwire walk of sorts between the progressive forces of therapeutic vitality, innovation, and latitude on the one hand (see, for example, Hoffman, 2002), and the very conservative forces of professional licensure, third-party payers, and interprofessional rivalries on the other (Sturkie, 2001). Family therapy had emerged several decades earlier as a method of treatment rooted in the (occasionally radical) rejection of traditional psychiatric epistemologies, diagnostic systems, and treatment approaches (Haley, 1971). However, it became increasingly clear over time that the very characteristics which had been a source of family therapy's initial strength and appeal were threatening to marginalize it as a growing profession in the ever-changing practice environment (Shields, McDaniel, Wynne, & Gawinski, 1994). For example, though many marital and family therapists (MFTs) had stringently objected to the approach to diagnosis and treatment planning embodied in the American Psychiatric Association's (2000) *Diagnostic and Statistical Manual of Mental Disorders* (*DSM*) through its many iterations (see chapter 4 of this text), full participation in the mental health field was becoming increasingly tied to these practitioners having the professional education, competence, willingness, and, particularly, formal authority to diagnose and treat mental disorders using this individual-focused system (Sturkie & Bergen, 2001). Despite the myriad philosophical and practical objections directed toward it, by the late 1980s the *DSM* almost hegemonically defined the language and conceptual frames for practice, and the ability to participate in managed care and other third-party payment programs required the use of this language and these frames. In short, marital and family therapy *as a profession* began experiencing significant pressure to move closer to the conventional center of the mental health field in terms of its language, treatment models, and, perhaps most notably, public relations. Though viewed by many practitioners as unwelcome, the profession's viability depended on this move toward center, and licensure and formal examinations would become two of the vehicles by which this move would be accomplished.

1. Changes in the practice environment during the 1980s pressured marital and family therapy as a profession to:
   a. give up its radical identity in the mental health field.
   b. move more toward the center of the mental health field in terms of its language and treatment models.
   c. decline, for ethical reasons, to participate in third-party payment programs.
   d. resist efforts toward licensure and external control by state boards.

2. Marital and family therapy's reputation for therapeutic innovation and experimental interventions:
   a. threatened to marginalize it in the mental health field.
   b. increased its broad appeal to both consumers and other professionals.
   c. made the use of examination-based measures of competency irrelevant.
   d. remained its strongest asset when it was threatened by other professions.

3. The use of the *DSM–IV* and its earlier editions:
   a. is irrelevant given the epistemology of the MFT field.
   b. experienced broad support from family therapists.
   c. has administrative, but not clinical relevance, for MFTs.
   d. became a necessity in the field, regardless of how MFTs may have felt about it.

## LICENSING EXAMINATIONS AND PROFESSIONAL COMPETENCY

Two of the more powerful influences toward more conventional practice involved the interrelated issues of independent practice and third-party payments. As third-party payments for mental health treatment became increasingly available during the 1970s, more and more practitioners moved to independent practice. However, the move away from agency-based practice often stripped away the protective layers of supervision, agency accreditation, and peer consultation that helped safeguard agency clients. This vacuum of protection had to be filled somehow, and increasingly it was through the use of individual credentials such as state **licenses** (Sturkie, 2001). Though controversial, licensure laws were seen as providing some level of protection for clients in independent practice settings through: (a) their expanding lists of ethical guidelines and legal mandates, (b) the reference points they established for prudent practice, (c) the assurance of basic competency demonstrated by the use of licensing examinations, and (d) the additional avenues of recourse they provided for aggrieved clients (Lee, 1993; Sturkie & Bergen, 2001; Lee & Sturkie, 1997). However, only eight states had any kind of MFT licensure or **certification** laws in 1980 and these were, by and large, relatively weak (Sporakowski & Staniszewski, 1980).[1] In particular, virtually none provided the formal authority in their scopes of practice for MFTs to make the increasingly indispensable *DSM* diagnosis. Therefore, more and more MFT practitioners aspired to achieve strengthened licensure status that would serve both to protect their clients *and* to support their desire for independent practice and the use of third-party payments.

By 2002, forty-six states had passed MFT licensure and certification laws. In the majority of these states, a license had also been made a formal requirement for independent practice, with passing an examination being a primary requirement for licensure.[2] Though some states had developed their own exam programs when licensure or certification was first achieved (for example, North Carolina, Georgia, and Texas), by 2002 there were only two major MFT licensing examination programs nationwide: the California Board of Behavioral Sciences' (CBSE) MFT Exam, which was entering its fourth decade, and the Association of Marital and Family Therapy Regulatory Boards (AMFTRB) National Examination in Marital and Family Therapy (hereafter referred to as *the National Examination*). For the most part, most individual states found the prospect of developing and maintaining an individual, legally defensible exam program too complex and expensive. As is elaborated below, there were a number of other compelling reasons for moving toward a national examination program.

4. The primary purpose for MFT licensure is to:
   a. provide practitioners with a means for billing third-party payers.
   b. reinforce the public legitimacy of their chosen profession.
   c. protect consumers from inept and ill-prepared practitioners.
   d. enhance the professional identity and quality of practitioners.

5. The importance of state licensure was greatly increased by:
   a. the growth of independent practice and third-party payments.
   b. lawsuits against unethical practitioners.
   c. competition among different professional groups for clients.
   d. a surge in the use of questionable treatment approaches.

6. The National Examination in MFT was developed and is maintained by:
   a. the American Association for Marital and Family Therapy.
   b. the Commission on Accreditation for Marital and Family Therapy Education.
   c. the Association of Marital and Family Therapy Regulatory Boards.
   d. the International Association of Marital and Family Counselors.

## THE ADDITIONAL PURPOSES FOR PROFESSIONAL EXAMS

As much distress as they generate for persons preparing to take them, there are a number of reasons why professional examinations are important. First, as a part of a licensure program, they provide a practical means for assessing whether or not persons seeking to enter the field have mastered the basic knowledge and skills deemed by their professional colleagues as indicating at least a minimal level of competence. As has been suggested, in the broadest sense, licensing boards and examination programs exist primarily to safeguard the public, not to enhance the status or to broaden the prerogatives of practitioners (though they do the latter as well). State boards are therefore concerned with being able to discriminate the ill-prepared or inept practitioner from one who is at least minimally competent. Licensing examinations are one of the principal ways (along with measures of "good moral character" and personal competency, educational attainment, and supervised clinical experience) by which this discrimination is made.

Second, as has also been noted, professional licensure (and the requirements supporting it) are also employed by many third-party payers who use licensure status as evidence of clinical capability and general professional standing. Prior to MFT licensure in most states, clinical membership in the American Association for Marital and Family Therapy was the primary professional credential available to MFTs. Though critically important, this private certification did not afford the ability to bill third-party payers that exam-based licensure status has afforded. As Sturkie and Bergen (2001) put it:

> *The development of an examination [was a critical step for the MFT] profession in its efforts to achieve full recognition by potential consumers, as well as by the health care companies and governmental agencies which insure and support them. Without a national exam program comparable to those of other mental health disciplines, marital and family therapists would never gain professional or economic parity as service providers. (p. 92)*

A third important reason for licensure examinations involves family therapy's own developmental history. Marital and family therapy has had a unique, multidisciplinary history, enriched by many varied intellectual traditions and streams. The requirement for an examination helps to ensure that potential practitioners have mastered a fundamental body of basic knowledge and skills, regardless of their professional background, education, or identity (AMFTRB, 1989; Lee, 1993). Almost half the persons taking the National Examination have a degree in something other than marital and family therapy (Lee, 1998), two separate organizations (COAMFTE and CACREP)[3] accredit MFT training programs (Stevens-Smith, Hinkle, & Stahmann, 1993), and many persons have earned their qualifying coursework in free-standing, postgraduate training institutes rather than through traditional academic programs. The presence of these myriad pathways into the profession greatly increases the importance of a relatively uniform examination process by which the mastery of knowledge of persons from different backgrounds can be reliably measured and compared.

Finally, in our highly mobile society, the existence of a relatively common, shared exam program helps State boards to gauge the relative comparability of licensure requirements for the purposes of allowing licensure through endorsement as practitioners move from one jurisdiction to another (Sturkie & Johnson, 1994). For example, a practitioner from Minnesota who moves to Florida will have already taken the appropriate exam to apply for licensure by endorsement in Florida. It should be noted, however, that most other states do not accept the California exam for endorsement purposes, and California does not accept the National Examination, because the comparability of these exams has never been formally evaluated.

7. Examinations have been particularly important in the MFT field because:
   a. MFTs are far more likely than other professionals to engage in conjoint treatment.
   b. their models of intervention have less proven efficacy than those of other professions.
   c. MFTs are often involved in legal actions, such as custody disputes.
   d. MFTs have included practitioners from many different educational and professional backgrounds.

8. A licensure examination score:
   a. is rarely recognized outside of one's own state.
   b. provides a standard means of comparing practitioners moving from one jurisdiction to another.
   c. is not valid after three years.
   d. from one jurisdiction is relevant and acceptable in most others.

9. A national examination was important for the MFT profession because:
   a. educational requirements for MFTs are typically lower than for other professions.
   b. there is more diversity in treatment approaches than in other professions.
   c. MFTs, proportionately, have more ethical complaints lodged against them.
   d. it helped establish MFTs parity with other professional groups.

## FORMS OF PROFESSIONAL EXAMINATIONS

To this point, this discussion has implicitly focused on the primary form of professional examinations: written examinations. However, there are a variety of exams associated with licensure in the marital and family therapy field. Several states, including California, Minnesota, and Tennessee, have or have had, an oral examination that supplements the written exam, and many others have the legal prerogative of requiring an oral examination if they so choose (see below). Six states also employ their own supplemental written examination that is taken in addition to the National Examination. These supplemental exams typically focus on the content of the respective statutes and regulations that are applicable to MFT practitioners in that state, as well as other aspects of the state's broader mental health laws and other civil and criminal matters. You should clarify what supplemental exams you must take with your respective state boards which will typically provide a study guide for you. Colorado also requires licensure applicants to attend a one-day workshop relating to ethics and the legal requirements in that state, for which they must take pre- and post-workshop tests (Sturkie & Bergen, 2001).

## EXAM AND ITEM CONSTRUCTION

An important consideration in preparing for professional examinations is to understand the processes by which they are developed, administered, and graded. Though there are some rather significant differences between the California and the National Examinations, the processes by which they and most other exams in the mental health field have been developed are the same. Understanding the logic of examination development should inform your study strategy.

First, examinations are typically connected to a licensing or certification statute that includes a *scope of practice* for the profession. Scopes of practice in the current MFT statutes vary from a few sentences to more than a dozen pages long, depending on the level of detail with which the respective legislature decided to define what the relevant practitioners are formally sanctioned to do. Scopes of practice are critically important in that they both allow and prohibit practitioners from engaging in certain professional activities such as treating persons with major mental illness, performing standardized testing, and practicing hypnosis or sex therapy, to note but a few examples. Considerable progress has been made in the past decade in strengthening the scopes of practice in MFT statutes (in part, making them true licensure laws), but both licensure candidates and active practitioners must be aware of what professional activities their respective laws prescribe and proscribe.

The process by which the conceptual matrix for exam content is developed is usually referred to as a **role delineation study** or **occupational analysis**. The purpose of the occupational analysis is to operationalize: (a) the major areas of *responsibility* of the profession (which are sometimes referred to as **practice domains**), (b) the *tasks* that are associated with each domain, and (c) the *knowledge* and skills necessary to competently accomplish each task (Lee, 1993; Lee & Sturkie, 1997). An initial occupational analysis is usually performed by a panel of recognized experts in the field who develop a broad, three-level conceptual model including every potentially relevant set of responsibilities, tasks, and bodies of knowledge and skill for practitioners. For example, in its most recent occupational analysis, the National Examination program identified eight major areas of professional responsibility (practice domains) for MFTs (see AMFTRB, 1999):[4]

1. Thinking about practice: Epistemological issues/professional paradigm
2. Incorporating awareness of the larger system
3. Addressing interpersonal and family processes
4. Attending to therapeutic relationships
5. Assessing and diagnosing
6. Designing and conducting treatment
7. Evaluating ongoing processes, outcomes, and terminations
8. Maintaining professional ethics and standards of practice

As will be elaborated, these areas of responsibility were then operationalized into sixty-one task and fifty-two knowledge statements (AMFTRB, 1999, 2002).

The California Examination plan (test matrix) has been revised a number of times, most recently in 1997 and again in 2002. The 2002 matrix contained six major practice domains:

1. Clinical evaluation
2. Crisis management
3. Treatment planning
4. Treatment
5. Law
6. Ethics

These domains included over one hundred component task statements and over one hundred related knowledge and skill statements (CBBS, 2004d).[5]

Once the basic areas of professional responsibility are determined, the tasks and the bodies of knowledge and skill associated with these tasks are defined. For example, as mentioned above, the National Examination has a domain related to *assessing and diagnosing*. This domain involves "an awareness of the various dimensions of the client/therapist system that must be evaluated in order to form the basis for effective therapy" (AMFTRB, 2002). This domain is elaborated through a dozen task statements that include the following three that were chosen for illustrative purposes.

1. Assess the strengths and resources of the individual/couple/family and therapist by observation, inquiry, or use of a structured instrument or technique (i.e., a genogram) in order to expand knowledge of family process.
2. Assess the level of mental or physical risk or danger to the individual/couple/family and others by observation and inquiry in order to enable the therapist to take appropriate action to ensure the safety of clients and others.
3. Assess the individual/couple/family in terms of formal diagnostic criteria in order to satisfy third-party requirements. (AMFTRB, 2002)

You will note that these different tasks are supported by very different bodies of knowledge. For example, the first task statement relates to what might be considered assessment in family therapy. In the National Examination matrix, these tasks are supported by knowledge statements relating to "family diagnosis" and "major couples/family assessment tools." The question for you, then, is: What family assessment tools are particularly recognized in the family field?" A review of a basic compendium on marital and family therapy such as Becvar and Becvar (2000) will help clarify this issue for you.

The second task statement included above relies on knowledge of the ethical and legal requirements of practice, presumably including Tarasoff, child abuse and elder abuse reporting laws, laws relating to confidentiality, and others (see chapter 24 in this volume). In the National Examination matrix, these knowledge statements include "professional/ethical standards in couples and family therapy" and "statutes and case law relevant to clinical practice."

The third task statement noted above speaks to the need for an understanding of the *DSM*, although this is couched more as an administrative matter than as a clinical concern. The relevant knowledge statements in the exam matrix include "individual psychopathology" and "individual diagnostic systems (*DSM/ICD*)" (AMFTRB, 2002).

The California Examination plan includes similar practice domains, therapeutic tasks, and bodies of knowledge and skill, though much of this information is presented in a more detailed format. For example, the practice domain *clinical evaluation* in the California matrix includes task statements relating to "initial assessment," "clinical assessment," and "diagnosis," all of which are elaborated and operationalized. Each set of therapeutic tasks is also explicitly connected to specific bodies of knowledge and skill.

10. State licensure laws prescribe and define:
    a. what practitioners can and cannot do.
    b. what practitioners may and may not do.
    c. whatever the practitioner believes he or she is trained to do.
    d. the ethical, but not the clinical, aspects of practice.

11. Occupational analyses contain all but which of the following?
    a. areas of professional responsibilities
    b. tasks typically associated with the professional activity
    c. strategies for managing the business aspects of the profession
    d. bodies of knowledge relevant to the professional responsibility

12. Examination matrices are:
    a. updated regularly to track changes in the profession.
    b. too obscure to help in the study process.
    c. are poor representations of what the profession is really about.
    d. are deemed confidential and are unavailable to exam candidates.

## FROM CONCEPTUAL MODEL TO EMPIRICAL VALIDATION

For both the National and California Examinations, the major practice domains, component tasks, and knowledge statements which had been identified by groups of experts were subsequently validated by samples of active practitioners. For the National Examination, practitioners from eleven states were involved in an initial validation study in 1989 (AMFTRB, 1990), and practitioners from forty-two states were surveyed for the 1998 validation study (AMFTRB, 1999). The most recent California Examination validation study involved a survey of more than 2,000 California practitioners (CBBS, 2004b).

The validation process has several important functions: (a) estimating the relative amount of time a practitioner would normally devote to engaging in a particular therapeutic task, (b) assessing the relative importance ascribed to the task for demonstrating basic clinical competence, and (c) assessing the relative importance of the therapeutic task for protecting the public. Therefore, if a task or knowledge statement is rated as relatively unimportant to the examination's critical function of consumer protection, or if a task or knowledge statement is rated as being more relevant for an experienced practitioner, it is assigned a diminished value or it is dropped from the matrix altogether.

After all the task and knowledge statements have been assessed in the three validation areas, the conceptual matrix then has an empirical basis for specifying the number and kinds of content areas that ultimately have to be addressed by the individual test items (Lee, 1993; Lee & Sturkie, 1997). An advantage of doing a series of occupational analyses over time is that evolving areas of emphasis and professional concern may be reflected in the newer exam specifications. For example, based on the then-current test specifications for the California Examination in 1997, 7.1% of the items related to the law and 10.2% related to ethics. However, the specifications changed with the 2002 study, resulting in 13% of the items relating to the law and 13% to ethics (CBBS, 2004d). In a relative sense, then, these two areas are of growing importance. As another example, there are twice as many items relating to clinical evaluation as compared with crisis management on the California Examination. The time committed to the study of these areas might appropriately reflect these differences. Familiarity with the test matrices in general will help you to identify those areas in the treatment literature with which you are most and least familiar.

13. Empirical validation of the test matrix is performed by:
    a. large samples of active practitioners.
    b. a panel of experts in psychometrics.
    c. approved supervisors in AAMFT.
    d. members of the American Family Therapy Academy.

14. The tasks associated with the test matrix are evaluated for all but which of the following qualities?
    a. relevance to practice
    b. importance for public protection
    c. degree of therapeutic innovation
    d. level of practitioner competency

15. Validation studies are repeated over time to:
    a. make the examination harder as candidates become better prepared.
    b. assess the changing relevance of each task for day-to-day practice.
    c. operationalize new skills.
    d. focus on cutting edge ideas.

## EXAM ITEMS

For the most part, individual items are developed through a process very similar to the test matrix as a whole. Practitioners and educators (*subject matter experts*) who are particularly knowledgeable in each of the areas of the matrix are asked to develop working items relating to that area. These items are anchored in the professional literature with an explicit reference.

A panel of experts then reviews each working item and rates its content for both its clinical relevance for the minimally competent practitioner and for its relative importance to the public protection function of the exam. Items are also edited for their format, clarity, and grammar. Each item also has a subsequent review by a psycho-metrician (test development expert) and another review panel made up of practitioners not involved in the item's original development (Lee, 1993; Lee & Sturkie, 1997).[6]

Once an item has been approved through this process, it is placed in the test bank under an appropriate rubric. It is then available for selection for use in any form of the exam which is subsequently constructed based on the test specifications. Then, following administration, but prior to final scoring, the statistical performance of each item is evaluated using a number of recognized psychometric procedures to ensure that the item "behaved" appropriately. If an item is too difficult or otherwise fails to fall within the recognized empirical standards for item performance, it is reviewed again and may be eliminated from the test bank with a correction made to scoring. Both exam programs also have a mechanism by which candidates can comment (following administration) on individual test items or on the examination as a whole.

The National Examination has two hundred multiple choice items with four response options. The California Standard Written Examination has 175 regular multiple choice items and up to twenty-five more items that are having their conceptual and empirical qualities evaluated for possible inclusion on a future form of the exam. The performance on these latter twenty-five items is not a consideration in determining the candidate's final test score. Candidates have four hours to complete each of these examinations. There is also no guessing penalty so candidates should answer every item. Both are now administered employing a computer-based testing format. Each state board serves as the gatekeeper for the exam. You can only schedule to take the exam with the permission of your respective state board.

The National Examination was originally conceptualized as the capstone requirement for licensure (Lee & Sturkie, 1997). The basic premise was that much of the knowledge necessary for competent practice, and—by extension—the ability to pass the examination, would derive from the supervisory experience during the internship. Again, the exam was conceived as providing a measure of practitioner judgment, not simply the ability to recount facts, and it was believed that clinical judgment would be developed in supervisory experience as well as in the classroom. However, the requirement that the exam be the last step in the credentialing process was altered for a number of practical and political reasons. First, though each of the states which had contracted to use the exam pledged to authorize candidates to sit for it only at the end of the licensure process, in actuality many candidates were allowed to take the exam earlier. Second, an analysis of exam pass-rates performed by Lee (1998) indicated that there was no real advantage in making candidates wait. Third, with the proliferation of mental health licenses in general and third-party payments in particular, it became advantageous for agencies to hire only those persons who had attained some kind of formal credential, even if it was just an "intern's" license. For example, many states have a tiered licensure system for social workers. Immediately upon finishing their formal education, social workers are allowed to sit for a Licensed Master Social Worker (LMSW) exam and achieve initial licensure. Then, after a prescribed period of supervision and clinical contact hours, they are authorized to sit for a second examination that provides for a higher level of licensure—for example, as a licensed clinical or licensed independent social worker. Many novice practitioners argued that requiring them to wait to sit for the marital and family therapy examination put them at a disadvantage in the job market as compared with their other professional colleagues who were allowed to sit for a basic licensure exam more quickly. Finally, as will be elaborated below, both the California and National Examinations also have a significant percentage of candidates who fail them.

Taking the exam earlier protects against the expense of supervision for persons who may not be licensable anyway.

16. The National Examination contains:
    a. 150 multiple choice items which the candidate has three hours to complete.
    b. 250 multiple choice items which the candidate has four hours to complete.
    c. 200 multiple choice items which the candidate has four hours to complete.
    d. 250 multiple choice items which the candidate has three hours to complete.

17. The candidate applies to take the National Examination through:
    a. the American Association for Marital and Family Therapy.
    b. the Association of Marital and Family Therapy Regulatory Boards.
    c. his or her respective state board.
    d. a private online testing agency

18. The exam is usually taken:
    a. as soon as the qualifying academic courses have been taken.
    b. at the completion of the first one hundred hours of supervised practice.
    c. before one enters his or her graduate practicum.
    d. at the completion of all other licensure requirements.

## ITEM FORMATS

In addition to varied areas of content, examinations also employ items at different levels of abstraction in an attempt to explore different kinds of competencies. These include items that focus on the basic recollection of facts and knowledge, the application of knowledge, and the synthesis of knowledge and skills from multiple sources. For example, the following items tap the practitioner's familiarity with major writers or basic treatment concepts.[7]

## Exemplar 25-1

19. In whose model of couples therapy is one most likely to address feelings?
    a. Murray Bowen
    b. Jay Haley
    c. Susan Johnson
    d. Salvador Minuchin

The best answer is "c," which refers to Susan Johnson's emotionally focused therapy.

## Exemplar 25-2

20. In which model of therapy is one most likely to use the "exceptions frame"?
    a. structural
    b. strategic
    c. solution focused
    d. narrative

The best answer to this question is response option "c," solution focused (see, for example, Becvar & Becvar, 2000). Concept or knowledge items like these tap basic information that has been judged during the development and validation of the exam matrix as being essential to competent family therapy practice. That is not to say that every minimally competent practitioner knows the principles underlying solution focused or emotionally focused therapy. To be sure, the National Examination matrix includes sixteen different models of therapy, each of which may have its own permutations, and the California Examination includes many different theoretical frameworks (including solution focused). However, it is being suggested that this type of item samples the *kind* of information deemed appropriate for the minimally competent practitioner.

Of course, the same concept can be examined using a clinical vignette, scenario, or exhibit.

## Exemplar 25-3

21. During an interview with a depressed client, the therapist says: "Please tell me what you are doing when you are *not* feeling depressed." This therapist's intervention is based on which model of therapy?
    a. structural
    b. strategic
    c. solution focused
    d. narrative

Response option "c" is best because solution-focused therapists emphasize the "exceptions frame"—what is happening when the symptom is not evident.

The same information can be also employed to focus more on differential intervention strategies. In the following item, for example, different therapeutic responses based on different models of therapy make up the response options.

## Exemplar 25-4

22. A male client enters therapy complaining of depression, with a lack of energy, a loss of motivation, and constant self-criticism. If his therapist is solution focused, which of the following questions would best illustrate this treatment approach?
    a. "When and how do you think you developed the belief that you are not as capable as other persons?"
    b. "Were either of your parents depressed when you were growing up or is either experiencing any depression now?"
    c. "Please tell me what is happening when you are not feeling depressed."
    d. "When did you first begin to use the word *depression* to describe what you have been experiencing, or did some else give it that name?"

The following item represents a somewhat longer scenario.

## Exemplar 25-5

A 24-year-old male client enters therapy at the behest of his spouse. The client has undergone a discernible change in his behavior in recent weeks, is having difficulty sleeping, has been making inappropriate comments to co-workers for which he has been sanctioned, and has been uncharacteristically charging hundreds of dollars on his credit cards. The couple dated for six months and has been married for one year. The client previously disclosed to his wife that he was a heavy marijuana smoker in his teens, but has not used marijuana in years.

> 23. The therapist should first consider the possibility that the client is:
>     a. experiencing a late onset substance-induced psychotic disorder.
>     b. having a manic episode.
>     c. cyclothymic.
>     d. suffering from bipolar II disorder.

Response option "b" represents the best answer because the symptoms detailed in the vignette are consistent with a manic episode as it is defined in the *DSM*.

Obviously, not all questions are related to therapy, per se.

## Exemplar 25-6

> 24. The primary method of assessing the quality of attachment between a caregiver and a young child involves:
>     a. observing the levels of aggression in a group of small children playing away from their caregivers.
>     b. watching how a child responds to an absent parent when the parent reenters a room.
>     c. measuring the physiological reactivity of a parent listening to a tape of his or her child crying.
>     d. interviewing the parents about any developmental problems the child may have experienced.

The best answer is found in response option "b" which is an allusion to the "Strange Situation Test," a primary research tool in the attachment literature (Karen, 1994).

You should also anticipate encountering problem-solving questions in serial form, that is, multiple items based on the same clinical vignette or scenario in the National Examination. However, the ability to answer one of the questions in a set of serial items is not contingent upon being able to answer any other item related to the scenario.

## Exemplar 25-7

Ms. Brown enters therapy with her 16-year-old daughter, Sheila, because of "constant bickering which makes us both miserable." Ms. Brown is divorced from Sheila's father (who Sheila has not seen in years), and Sheila's stepfather (with whom Sheila had been very close, but now sees very infrequently). Ms. Brown's parents are both dead, as is her only sibling who was killed in a car accident. Sheila has an older sister, Suzanne, who is away at college, but calls her mother regularly "to check on her." Sheila also became pregnant by her boyfriend last year, and had an abortion. Sheila has not seen her boyfriend since she announced she was pregnant. These latter events created even more conflict in Sheila and her mother's relationship. Ms. Brown's desire for therapy is to "make our lives together livable." Sheila's desire is that her mother "get a life and leave me alone."

25. According to family systems theory, Sheila's abortion may be particularly significant for mother because it reactivated feelings of:
    a. loss.
    b. anger.
    c. abandonment.
    d. guilt.

26. A structural family therapist might explore the possibility that the conflict between Sheila and her mother is primarily related to:
    a. normal developmental stressors.
    b. sibling competition and favoritism.
    c. loneliness and overdependence.
    d. a fatherless home.

27. A therapist endeavoring to reframe their conflict might suggest:
    a. "Sheila, it seems as if your mom is losing her "baby," and you have tried to give her another one."
    b. "You are two strong women who have managed despite the unreliable men in your lives.
    c. "Sheila, your mother has had a difficult time, and I appreciate how you have attempted to protect her from depression."
    d. "Sheila, you don't need to have a baby to remain at home."

In the fall of 2003, the California Board of Behavioral Sciences voted to discontinue the use of its oral examination program (see below). Instead, the Board moved to the use of a second written examination which can only be taken after a candidate has successfully passed the first ("standard") examination (CBBS, 2004b). This "Written Clinical Vignette Examination" is based on the same test matrix as the standard examination, but has only thirty graded items. These items include rather lengthy vignettes (or exhibits) which employ a multiple choice format, though each response option can have a number of component parts (CBBS, 2004c). This exhibit-based examination format attempts to better explore the integration of knowledge that had previously been the focus of the oral examination program, while simultaneously increasing the reliability of examination scoring.

## PASS-POINTS AND MINIMAL COMPETENCE

As has been emphasized, the principal purpose of licensure and licensure examinations is to protect consumers from ill-prepared and inept practitioners. At the same time, states also don't want to restrict free trade by arbitrarily prohibiting appropriately trained and skilled persons from being able to practice (thereby earning a living). As Sturkie and Bergen have noted, "this dilemma inevitably leads to a very difficult question: how much (or little) does one need to know to be regarded as minimally competent?" (2001, p. 98). Therefore, one of the most critical elements in examination construction and maintenance is the formulation and ongoing evaluation of an examination pass-point.

There are a variety of ways by which pass-points can be established (Kane, 1985), but the preferred method in the mental health field is through the use of an Angoff study or panel (Angoff, 1971; see also AMFTRB, 1989, 1996a; Lee, 1993). In an Angoff study, the members of a panel of experts individually review every item on an exam. Each panel member is then asked to make an estimate of the percentage of minimally competent practitioners he or she believes could answer each item correctly. The panel members' estimates are then averaged across each item. After an average estimate is derived for each item, the item estimates are averaged for the whole exam. This overall average-estimate is what constitutes the pass-point.

Since the Angoff procedure is commonly recognized as being the best method for establishing pass-points,[8] individual boards are discouraged from developing their own pass-points for the National Examination. It is recommended instead, that they use the Angoff-based national pass-point. This pass-point is both fairer to candidates (than, for example, a norm-based pass-point) and more defensible for the Board as compared with other methods.

Based on their current, respective pass-points, approximately 70% of the persons sitting the National Examination pass it (AMFTRB, 1998a, whereas approximately 55% to 60% of candidates for the California exam do (CBBS, 2004a).

## ORAL EXAMINATIONS

Given the nature of what marital and family therapists do, it is remarkable that so few states require oral examinations. The rationale for an oral exam has been clearly articulated by the California Board of Behavioral Science Examiners, one of the few boards that has historically required them.

> *The purpose of an oral examination is to assess job-related knowledge and skills that cannot be assessed in any other format. Oral examinations are a necessary requirement for professions that require practitioners to interact verbally with clients, assess a problem in real time (for which additional research or consultations is usually not available) and solve problems that pose an immediate threat to the safety or welfare public. (CBBS, 1998, p. 4)*

Oral examinations are based on the same test matrix as written exams. The same areas of responsibility, bodies of knowledge, and skills are tested by evaluating the candidate's response in real time to different clinical scenarios. These responses are then assessed by a panel of judges using the following anchor points (CBBS, 1998, p. 9):

1. *Exceptional*—responses that are "subtle, integrated, sophisticated, comprehensive, insightful, creative"
2. *Skilled*—responses that are "complete, inclusive, thorough, in-depth, confident"
3. *Sufficient*—responses that are "consistent, relevant, basic, sound, realistic, accurate, appropriate, essential"
4. *Deficient*—responses that are "vague, superficial, incomplete, irrelevant, jargon"
5. *Unqualified*—responses that are "confused, omissive, incorrect, lacking skill, inexperienced, insufficient, erroneous, contrary"
6. *Very Unqualified*—responses that are "harmful, dangerous to client, discredit to profession, unprofessional"

Oral examinations are controversial for a variety of reasons. Despite these explicit anchor points, California pass-rates were substantially lower than on written exams, raising questions of reliability and fairness. As imperfect as multiple choice questions are, they only have one correct answer and a number of empirical procedures are used to evaluate each item's quality and reliability. However, the line between, for example, "sufficient" and "deficient" on an oral examination is inevitably more vague. That is to say, what may be gained by using the more realistic problem-solving format may also be lost in lowered scoring reliability as compared with written exams. Oral examinations are also more expensive to administer and evaluate. The cost factor, along with reliability issues, seems to have resulted in most states eschewing them, as important as they seem to be, and has been noted, California recently discontinued its program. Minnesota does require an oral examination, but it focuses primarily on a knowledge of legal requirements for practice in that state. This oral exam format focuses on the critical function of consumer protection, without entering into the murkier area of clinical judgment.

## COMPREHENSIVE EXAMINATIONS

As the terminology implies, graduate programs use a variety of test formats to explore both the breadth and depth of knowledge of persons entering the clinical component of their programs, as well as their readiness to be conferred an advanced degree. There is substantial variation in the specific testing formats, but they include the following:

1. *Traditional Comprehensive Exams.* Candidates are required to sit for one or two days of written examinations, covering a broad variety of topics. This testing is usually accomplished by responding to complex essay questions, writing one's answers on a laptop computer. Some programs allow "take-home" examinations; others do not. Candidates are usually provided with a reading list and sample questions.

2. *Video-Based Comprehensive Exams.* This approach to testing uses the traditional "comps" format for part of the exam, but an additional component involves the student's essay response to a segment from a movie or an actual video-taped therapy session to which a specific body of knowledge must be applied. For example, a candidate may be required to use an assessment model from the family literature to describe the structure, form, or interactional patterns within the family evidenced on the tape.

3. *Position Papers or Declarations.* In position papers, the candidate articulates his or her own philosophy of therapy, grounding it in the professional literature as a whole. Candidates are generally required to include content from as many as a dozen areas of epistemology, theory, and therapy. A self-assessment of their own personal qualities that support the development of their model must also be included.

4. *Comprehensive Case Presentations With Both Written and Oral Components.* The most common approach seems to be some variation on a multi-format case presentation in which the candidate develops a position paper, presents the model using a "workshop" format, presents video-taped segments that illustrate the model, and has an oral examination of his or her work.

5. *Multiple Choice Exams.* A minority of programs require students to sit for a relatively brief (for example, 50-item) multiple-choice exam that follows the National Examination format.

In summary, there is substantial variation in the comprehensive models employed in graduate programs. Given the different testing formats they employ, and the unique content they address, they represent an important component to holistic evaluation of the candidate. Furthermore, they should provide invaluable practice for impending licensure exams.

## PREPARATION FOR EXAMINATIONS

In addition to the sets of questions related to the major practice domains, the National Examination program also regularly asks a number of questions about the demographics of the candidates, their academic and clinical training, and their opinions about the items' fairness and their relevance to their clinical practice. Lee (1998, 2000) examined the responses to these items for several candidates who sat for the National Examination during a series of administrations. You will be pleased to know that most candidates regarded the items as being representative of the kinds of situations normally encountered in practice, and the majority thought they had enough time to complete the exam. However, about half rated the overall exam as "moderately difficult," and 70% of the respondents thought 25% to 50% of the items were beyond entry level. These candidates obviously disagreed with the members of the Angoff panels.

Those who were most likely to pass took the exam relatively soon after graduation from their degree program and used multiple preparation methods. Preparation methods included individual study, participation in study groups, and examination workshops and home study courses. The particular combination of methods did not seem to be as important as the fact that multiple methods had been used. (The important message here is don't rely solely on self-study.) Also, though from a variety of educational backgrounds, most of the candidates had had substantial experience working with multiclient systems.

In summary, you are urged to become familiar with the knowledge and task domains of the exam matrix, review your accumulated graduate educational materials relative to the matrix, consult with one or more of the major marital and family therapy compendia to "back-fill" areas with which you are less familiar, and be involved in some form of review that involves other candidates as well (Lee, 1998; Lee & Sturkie, 1997).

Several private organizations with no formal ties to the relevant exam programs offer in-home and workshop-based test preparation programs, though according to Lee (1998), only about 5% of candidates participate in them. However, you are encouraged to use a home-study course, even if you cannot attend a workshop. These courses may help you improve your overall test-taking strategy, allow you to complete a number of practice items that should help diminish your test anxiety, and help you get in the rhythm of using the multiple-choice format for accessing what you know. Group presentations and supervision are valuable forums for practicing the skills associated with oral examinations including problem formulation, relevant treatment strategies, and the legal and ethical aspects of treatment. As has been suggested, you have probably experienced a number of "oral examinations" while a graduate student, but learning to think on one's feet is an acquired skill that is mastered only through constant repetition.

Finally, both written exam programs provide reasonable accommodations to candidates who require them, though you should let your respective board know as soon as you apply to take the exam.

28. Pass-points on professional examinations are usually set by:
   a. determining a "floating score" that allows 80% of those taking it to pass.
   b. the state board which sets its own threshold, such as 70%.
   c. calculating the average score for everyone taking it, and then setting the pass-point one standard deviation below the average score.
   d. a panel that estimates the number of minimally competent practitioners it believes would be expected to answer each item correctly.

29. Which is *not* a reason that oral examinations are controversial?
   a. They often have lower pass-rates than written exams.
   b. It is more difficult to reliably score them.
   c. They are expensive to implement.
   d. They fail to duplicate the conditions of therapy as well as written exams do.

30. Comprehensive exams, as compared with licensure exams, have a greater emphasis on:
   a. basic theory.
   b. models of therapy.
   c. ethical aspects of practice.
   d. the candidate's personal therapy model.

## ENDNOTES

1. Though these terms are used in a variety of ways, *licensure* typically refers to a formal credential, issued by the state, that is a requirement to engage in the professional activity. *Certification* typically connotes a credential, issued by the state or a private organization, that represents professional achievement, but which is not a requirement to practice. Certification is often referred to as *title protection*.
2. As of the summer of 2003, the only states without MFT licensure or certification laws were Delaware, Montana, North Dakota, and West Virginia (AMFTRB, 2003).
3. Commission on Accreditation for Marital and Family Therapy Education and The Council on Accreditation for Counseling and Related Educational Programs.
4. Another role delineation study is being undertaken for the National Examination during 2003. (Personal communication with Lois Paff Bergen, Executive Director of AMFTRB, July, 2003).
5. For the latest and most complete specifications for each exam, go to www.amftrb.org and www.bbs.ca.gov, respectively.
6. AMFTRB develops items for the National Examination under the direction and supervision of Professional Examination Services (PES) of New York (see www.professionalexam.org).
7. These items have been created by the chapter author and have not been evaluated using the demanding development process for items that ultimately make it to the exam. See the *Candidate's Handbook* (AMFTRB, 2002) for actual practice items for the National Examination, and the *California Board's Handbook* (CBBS, 2004b,c).
8. Lee (1993) has described all the national psychometric standards that had to be met during the initial development of the exam.

## KEY TERMS

**certification:** A formal credential, issued by a state or a private organization, that denotes specialized education and training. When issued by states, persons typically must be certified to use a specific professional title (for example, "certified marriage and family therapist"), though noncertificate holders may still practice marital and family therapy.

**license:** A formal credential, issued by a state, that is a requirement for engaging in professional practice. Licenses are primarily issued to safeguard consumers. In the marital and family therapy field, some states have issued "licenses" that were actually certifications.

**occupational analysis:** A process through which the various components (knowledge, skills, and areas of responsibility) of a profession are developed conceptually by panels of experts. These components and their professional relevance are then are validated empirically by large samples of practicing members of the profession. An occupational analysis is used to create an empricially-derived matrix from which individual exam items can be developed.

**practice domain:** An area of responsibility which is integral to the competent performance of a professional activity.

**role delineation study:** (See "occupational analysis" above).

## DISCUSSION QUESTIONS

1. What are the principal reasons professional examinations are used as a component of the licensure process in the mental health field? What are the weaknesses of examinations, and how are these weaknesses addressed in other components of the licensure process?
2. What is the logic upon which licensure exams are developed? How can a knowledge of this process help one organize a study strategy?
3. What are the criteria by which the quality of an exam item is evaluated? Given the mission of state licensure boards, do you believe the criteria to be adequate?
4. What is the purpose of the oral component of state licensure exams? What kind of information regarding the candidate do oral exams provide that written exams do not? Why are oral exams controversial? Do you think they are appropriate in the licensure process? Why or why not?
5. What are the principal differences in the kinds of candidate evaluations afforded by licensure and comprehensive exams? How do comprehensive exams help in the study process for licensure exams?
6. What is the primary model or theoretical framework that guides your practice? Write two practice items that would reflect this approach.
7. Imagine you were taking an oral examination and were given the vignette included in Exemplar 25-5. How would you articulate the diagnostic and treatment planning issues associated with this case study?
8. What are the principal ethical and legal issues implicitly reflected in Exemplars 25-4 and 25-5? Write a series of practice items that reflect these major dimensions.
9. What components of your respective state statute do you *not* see reflected in the two exam matrices? (For example, some states have very explicit requirements relating to professional disclosure, and how, and how long, professional records need to be maintained.) How can your state statute and regulations help you to become a more prudent practitioner?
10. If you were creating a formal credentialing process to safeguard both the rights of consumers and practitioners, how would you structure it? What kinds of exams would you employ, if any, and why?

## SUGGESTED FURTHER READING

Becvar, D. S., & Becvar, R. (2000). *Family therapy: A systemic integration*. Needham Heights: Allyn & Bacon.

This is an excellent overview of the entire marital and family field that should aid you in studying for licensure exams.

Piercy, F., Sprenkle, D., & Wetchler, J. (1996). *Family therapy source book* (2nd Ed.). New York: Guilford Press.

This is another invaluable text for organizing the review of a large body of literature.

Sturkie, K., & Bergen, L. (2001). *Professional regulation in marital and family therapy*. Needham Heights: Allyn & Bacon.

This book will tell you more than you want to know about the various aspects of regulation and the requirements for and the pursuit of licensure.

# REFERENCES

American Psychiatric Association. (2000). *Diagnostic and statistical manual of mental disorders* (4th ed., text rev.). Washington, DC: Author.

Angoff, W. H. (1971). Scales, norms, and equivalent scores. In R. L. Thorndike (Ed.), *Educational measurement* (pp. 508–600). Washington, DC: American Council on Education.

Association of Marital and Family Therapy Regulatory Boards. (1989). *Development of a criterion-referenced test standard for the examination in marital and family therapy.* New York: Professional Examination Service.

Association of Marital and Family Therapy Regulatory Boards. (1990). *Role delineation validation study for the marital and family therapy examination program.* New York: Professional Examination Service.

Association of Marital and Family Therapy Regulatory Boards. (1996a). *Development of a criterion-referenced test standard for the examination in marital and family therapy.* New York: Professional Examination Service.

Association of Marital and Family Therapy Regulatory Boards. (1996b). *Role delineation validation study for the marital and family therapy examination program.* New York: Professional Examination Service.

Association of Marital and Family Therapy Regulatory Boards. (1998a). *Annual report for the marital and family therapy examination program.* New York: Professional Examination Service.

Association of Marital and Family Therapy Regulatory Boards. (1998b). *Role delineation: Validation survey.* New York: Professional Examination Service.

Association of Marital and Family Therapy Regulatory Boards. (1999). *Report on the conduct and results of the practice analysis validation study for the AMFTRB marital and family therapy examination program.* New York: Professional Examination Service.

Association of Marital and Family Therapy Regulatory Boards. "MFT National Exam: Information for candidates. 'AMFTRB.org' (2002).

Becvar, D. S., & Becvar, R. (2000). *Family therapy: A systemic integration.* Needham Heights: Allyn & Bacon.

California Board of Behavioral Sciences. (1998). *Candidate handbook: marriage, family, and child counselors oral examination.* Sacramento: BBS.

California Board of Behavioral Sciences. (2004a). Examinations: Exam statistics. [http://www.bbs.ca.gov/].

California Board of Behavioral Sciences. (2004b). Examinations: Marriage and family therapist standard written examination handbook. [http://www.bbs.ca.gov/].

California Board of Behavioral Sciences. (2004c). "Examinations: Marriage and family therapist written clinical vignette handbook. [http://www.bbs.ca.gov/]."

California Board of Behavioral Sciences. (2004d). Examinations: Test plan. [http://www.bbs.ca.gov/].

Haley, Jay. (1971). A review of the family therapy field. In Jaytlaley (Ed.), *Changing families: A family therapy reader* (pp. 1–12). New York: Grune and Stratton.

Hoffman, Lynn. (2002). *Family therapy: A personal history.* New York: Norton.

Kane, M. T. (1985). Definitions and strategies for validating licensure examinations. In J. C. Fortune & Associates (Eds.), *Understanding testing in occupational licensing* (pp. 45–64). San Francisco: Jossey-Bass.

Karen, R. (1994). *Becoming Attached.* New York: Oxford University Press.

Lee, R. E. (1993). The marital and family therapy examination program. *Contemporary Family Therapy, 15*(5), 347–368.

Lee, R. E. (1998). The marital and family therapy examination program: A survey of participants. *Journal of Marital and Family Therapy, 24*(1), 127–134.

Lee, R. E. (2000). Who is getting licensed? Trends from the last five years. Unpublished Report: AMFTRB.

Lee, R. E., & Sturkie, K. (1997). The national marital and family therapy examination program. *Journal of Marital and Family Therapy, 23*(3), 255–270.

Shields, C. G., McDaniel, S. H., Wynne, L. C., & Gawinski, B. A. (1994). The marginalization of family therapy: A historical and continuing problem. *Journal of Marital and Family Therapy, 20*(1), 117–138.

Sporakowski, M., & Staniszewski, W. (1980). The regulation of marriage and family therapy: An update. *Journal of Marital and Family Therapy, 6*(3), 335–348.

Stevens-Smith, P., Hinkle, S., & Stahmann, R. (1993). A comparison of professional accreditation standards in marriage and family counseling and therapy. *Counselor Education and Supervision, 33,* 116–127.

Sturkie, K. (2001). The top ten reasons there is more professional regulation in your future. *Family Therapy News, 32*(1), 10–12.

Sturkie, K., & Bergen, L. (2001). *Professional regulation in marital and family therapy.* Needham Heights: Allyn and Bacon.

Sturkie, K., & Johnson, W. E. (1994). Recent and emerging trends in marital and family therapy regulation. *Contemporary Family Therapy, 16,* 265–290.

# 26

# Continuing Professional Development

### William C. Nichols
*Consultant*

---

## TRUTH OR FICTION?

\_\_\_ 1. The professional's privilege to practice usually is granted by his or her professional organization.

\_\_\_ 2. Most marital and family therapists are members of the American Psychological Association.

\_\_\_ 3. Teachers of marital and family therapy need to be charismatic figures.

\_\_\_ 4. More than 90% of the states license or certify MFTs for independent practice.

\_\_\_ 5. State certification is stronger than state licensure.

\_\_\_ 6. Not all states grant licenses to persons who are licensed or certified in another state.

\_\_\_ 7. Generally, one needs a business license as well as an occupational license in order to practice.

\_\_\_ 8. It is the responsibility of the professional to know how many CEUs are required by his or her licensing board.

\_\_\_ 9. The major reason for joining a professional organization is to be able to practice one's profession.

\_\_\_ 10. The International Family Therapy Association certifies individuals for practice around the world.

\_\_\_ 11. Qualitative research is concerned primarily with correlations.

\_\_\_ 12. In-depth interviews are characteristic of qualitative research.

\_\_\_ 13. Inductive reasoning is used more in qualitative research than in quantitative research.

\_\_\_ 14. Hans Selye advised us to avoid stress at all costs.

\_\_\_ 15. The best way to avoid burnout is to focus more closely on one's work.

Completion of your graduate/professional curricula, practica, internship, and other supervised clinical experience is merely the first step or set of steps through the doorway into a professional career. Ahead lie decades of practice, perhaps teaching, and service. There is a twofold task that awaits each of us: First, "unpacking and repacking" our knowledge and practice understandings and behaviors so that what we have absorbed during our basic educational and training days becomes truly ours and not merely second-hand residue from interaction with teachers and supervisors; and second, building on what we have winnowed out and made ours, adding to the base from continued observation, study, and interaction with clients and others so that we remain as fresh and up to date as we can.

## PROFESSIONAL IDENTITY AND HUMAN VALUES

What does it mean to say that we are professionals? *Professional* originally had a religious connotation; that is, one had a calling and professed to possess specialized knowledge not possessed by laypersons. This calling involved lengthy study and training and a commitment to serve one's clientele according to the ethical standards of one's professional group or organization. As a result of their knowledge, skills, and adherence to the ethics of their membership organization or association, members of the learned professions claimed a special place in society and special privileges not available to the uninitiated. The privilege to practice originally was granted by the profession itself, through either acceptance on the part of one's teacher or mentor (in an apprenticeship system) or by the organized profession (as in the case of the legal profession, where one is admitted to the bar in order to practice law). Today, with rare exceptions, professions as such do not possess the power to admit people to practice, for example, bar associations are virtually unique in their powers.

1. Professionals are characterized by:
    a. specialized knowledge.
    b. lengthy study and training.
    c. adherence to ethical standards.
    d. all of the above.

Professions carry at their core an orientation of service and values of providing essential help to fellow humans. These beliefs about the larger social values of the field constitute a sense of mission (Bucher & Stelling, 1977). Therefore, professionals typically are required to make judgments in crucial situations, strive for their clients' good, and adhere to a code of ethics. They are socialized into the values of a professional community but have some autonomy as members of that community.

The route by which we enter the field of marital and family therapy (MFT) plays a major role in the formation and development of our professional identity. If we obtain our basic educational foundation in MFT, we tend to have to deal with being identified with a field that, as a self-conscious profession, is considerably younger than other clinically related fields such as psychology, psychiatry, and social work. The oldest and largest MFT organization— the American Association for Marriage and Family Therapy (AAMFT)—developed out of the American Association of Marriage Counselors, founded in 1942. During the 1970s, what is now the AAMFT became a full-scale professional association, with a journal (now the *Journal of Marital and Family Therapy,* which emerged in 1975 under my editorship), a code of ethics which was binding on its members, and a strong, governmentally recognized program of accreditation for master's and doctoral degrees and postdegree institutes, along with annual conferences, state organizations, a somewhat unique certification of supervisors program, and other features commonly associated with professional associations (Nichols, 1992).

2. The youngest of the following professions is:
   a. marital and family therapy.
   b. psychiatry.
   c. psychology.
   d. social work.

3. The oldest and largest professional family therapy organization is the:
   a. American Family Therapy Association.
   b. American Family Therapy Academy.
   c. American Association for Marriage and Family Therapy.
   d. International Family Therapy Association.

For those of us who earn their initial graduate/professional degree in a field other than MFT and add on MFT substantive coursework and clinical training, there are three major routes that can be followed: (1) change their professional identity to that of MFT, a route that a significant number of AAMFT-Approved Supervisors have followed (Everett, 1980; Lee, Nichols, Nichols, & Odum, 2004; Nichols, Nichols, & Hardy, 1990); (2) regard oneself as a member of his or her original profession who practices MFT, rather than a professional MFT; or 3) become one who carries dual professional identities. (This is mine—I carry dual professional identities and dual licensure as an MFT and as a clinical psychologist.)

Whatever the original path in which we are socialized en route to entering into a professional field, as trainees we are faced with certain fundamental issues that significantly affect our subsequent development. What is the effect of our training program on us? It has long been recognized that there is a "programming effect," that is, "that the outcomes of socialization are, in large part, determined by the nature of the training program" (Bucher & Stelling, 1977, p. 257). The training part of professionalization, which refers to the learning of certain skills, often by imitation of our teachers and supervisors, tends to hold sway over the educational part of preparation, which refers to a process of thinking and mastering the concepts on which practice is based. (See Nichols, 1988, for a brief discussion of differences between learning in an apprenticeship approach based on the "see one, do one, teach one" model and learning through an "educere" or "leading out" from the knowledge and abilities of the student. See also Nichols & Lee, 1999, for a discussion of supervision from the perspectives of service, teaching, and learning.)

Unfortunately, one carryover from the early days of family therapy as a revolutionary approach to dealing with human problems has been reliance on charismatic figures in socializing MFTs. The results have been mixed, both within educational and training programs and in the students' subsequent functioning.. As Bucher and Stelling (1977) learned from their research on professional preparation programs: "Charismatic models . . . were on such a pedestal that the trainee did not really aspire to be like this person; they could only aspire to approximate what this person represented" (p. 271).

Furthermore, they concluded that the students constructed a composite view that represented what they would like to see themselves become by picking and choosing from what they observed in the program. If you were able to avoid getting ensnared in a "cult of personality" during your graduate program and steered a course in which you deliberately and critically sought to establish your own theoretical and clinical orientation, you are not likely to waste additional time after graduation in jumping from one novel approach to another in search of a foundation.

4. An essential part of an MFT's preparation consists of:
   a. aspiring to become like charismatic teachers.
   b. mastering the concepts on which practice is based.
   c. imitating our teachers and supervisors.
   d. following the master therapists.

## LICENSURE AND CERTIFICATIONS

Unlike the situation that prevailed a few decades ago, when almost anyone could "hang out a shingle" and offer their services as self-described experts in marriage and family counseling/guidance/therapy, it has become increasingly necessary to obtain a state **license** or to become state certified in order to practice legally. The first state MFT licensure law, in California, became effective in 1963, with Michigan following in 1968, and New Jersey in 1969 (Nichols, 1974). Forty-six states and the District of Columbia licensed or certified MFTs as of this writing. Delaware, Montana, North Dakota, and West Virginia were the only states that did not so regulate MFTs.

5. The first state to require licensure for MFTs was:
   a. California.
   b. Michigan.
   c. New Jersey.
   d. Ohio.

Some states have established full licensure for MFTs, whereas others have provided only for certification, a much weaker form of regulation. *Certification* restricts the use of a title; no one may use the restricted title (e.g., marriage and family therapist) unless he or she obtains a certificate under the provisions of the statute from the designated state board or office. *Licensure*, on the other hand, restricts function as well as title; one may not engage in the practice of a protected function such as marital and family therapy unless licensed by the state. Sections on restriction of the use of title are included in licensure laws (Nichols, 1974). (See www.AAAFT.org for information, including contact addresses, on current state regulatory requirements.) The AAMFT has supported the licensure movement primarily through its state divisions, providing some legislative grants and other forms of assistance including consultation.

Today, the simplest and most honest and ethical path for individuals to follow consists of obtaining education and training from an accredited academic institution and program in a given area and then securing state licensure or certification before attempting to practice in that area. There have been some ugly and unnecessary battles stemming from "boundary jumping" by clinicians such as MFTs who invaded areas of evaluation and practice in which they had inadequate preparation and from "professional imperialism" on the part of others such as psychiatrists or psychologists who attempted to erect fences and limit access to therapy to practitioners from their own profession.

We need to become aware of the differences in state/provincial regulations (Sturkie & Paff-Bergen, 2001), so that if we are geographically mobile and move across state/provincial lines, we can obtain appropriate licensure. We also need to stay abreast of changes in the licensing and practice regulations where we live. Each state sets its own standards and may or may not recognize your previous licensure or certification. Does the state to which you plan to move offer reciprocity or endorsement so that your current license can be used as a basis for licensure in the new state of residence? Check carefully with the regulating agency in the state to which you wish to move.

6. If you move from California to Kentucky and wish to practice independently as an MFT, you:
   a. do not need a Kentucky license because you are licensed in California.
   b. can practice because you are an AAMFT Clinical Member.
   c. are required to secure a Kentucky MFT license in order to practice.
   d. do not need a Kentucky license because you have a California psychologist's license.

7. Regarding MFT licensure, which of the following statements is correct?
   a. All states provide reciprocity with other licensing states.
   b. Each state sets its own standards.
   c. All states except Georgia license MFTs.
   d. All states provide for endorsement with other licensing states.

Professional, nongovernmental certifications may carry a considerable amount of prestige and attaining them may contribute significantly to our personal growth but they cannot be expected to grant the right to practice. Clinical membership in the AAMFT, for example, may be highly regarded but it is an "honorific" rather than a legal credential. For the last several years, licensure in one's state of residence has been the path of membership in the AAMFT.

If you are going to enter into private or independent practice, as opposed to offering your services as an employee of some kind of human services or educational agency or clinic, you typically must obtain a city and sometimes also a county business license, as well as a professional occupational license. Business licenses are not concerned with your professional qualifications but are issued to you as a permit for you to conduct a business within a given governmental jurisdiction.

8. In order to practice independently in most states, an MFT needs:
   a. an occupational and a business license.
   b. endorsement by the AAMFT.
   c. endorsement by AFTA.
   d. none of the above.

Licenses can be regarded as necessary but not sufficient conditions for gaining access to clients in some instances. Simply possessing a license does not give one access to clients and practicing therapy in a hospital, for example; the hospital will have its own criteria and procedures for granting staff privileges. Continuing developments in the health care field, such as health maintenance organizations and managed care, continue to shape and limit what one does and is able to do with clients.

## CONTINUING EDUCATION

Continuing education constitutes an established part of the MFT field. A large cottage industry has emerged in which continuing education units (**CEUs**) are offered for a variety of workshops, institutes, and conference presentations. Some states require applicants for licensure renewal to obtain specified amounts of CEUs, despite the fact that there continue to be questions about whether contemporary continuing education actually contributes to the continuing growth and development of professionals. Consequently, as professional MFTs we need to be sophisticated consumers, choosing carefully and not being seduced into becoming uncritical audiences for entertainment that is lacking in substance.

*Caveat emptor*—"let the buyer beware"—prevails as an important guideline when examining the myriad of flyers and brochures on continuing education offerings that flood our mail boxes. It is up to us to know how much and what kind of continuing education is required by our licensing board—some boards require core requirements and specify a given number of hours of CEUs in ethics, hypnosis, or other areas, and permit additional hours in associated areas—and to make certain that the program is approved by our licensing board for CEU credit. Beyond meeting those technical requirements, our continuing growth and development demands that we also look critically at what we are signing up for before we send a check or use our credit card to purchase what is being offered. What is the content? Does the program add to what I know, or is it a repetition of something with which I am already acquainted? Does it add to my knowledge and development as a professional?

As is the case with other professionals, staying up to date on developments in our field is essential if we are to be adequate practitioners who serve our clients adequately and effectively. Perhaps you can recall your reactions to professional practitioners such as physicians or dentists that you have known who became routinized and fell behind in their awareness of new knowledge and practices in their field. How did you regard them? What kind of reputation did they have among their peers? Did you have any professors in graduate school who gave the same lectures term after term, or who obviously had only a superficial or outdated grasp of the current knowledge in their field? Some of us feel that such individuals are taking money under false pretenses when they present themselves as professionals but demonstrate ignorance and incompetence.

9. Continuing education:
   a. is required by all MFT licensing boards.
   b. advertising claims can be trusted.
   c. requirements differ among states.
   d. all of the above.

Falling into the trap of confusing information with knowledge and understanding happens easily. We live in a world in which it is virtually possible to drown in the glut of stimulation and flow of information that washes over and around us. The television world with its "sound-bite" dispensing of information in an entertainment context can seduce us into being essentially passive recipients of presentations and conclusions delivered by others. We can unwittingly become passive–reactive rather than active, self-directed learners. Our current technology is wonderful in many ways, but we owe it to ourselves and to our clients to develop ourselves as proactive learners who guide our own learning.

The most productive approach to continued learning, in my judgment, is to make a continuing assessment of what you need to learn in order to keep growing and understanding and then to

**TABLE 26.1**

Some Guiding Questions for Our Continuing Education

---

- Have I acquired the ability to think critically and to examine carefully and dispassionately the data and information that I am exposed to and that I seek out, instead of merely being a collector of information?
- Have I developed the ability to integrate what I have learned in the past and what I am learning in the present?
- Have I developed a tolerance of the ambiguity that I face when I encounter two different ideas or observations that each seem valid but which are contradictory?

---

seek out the kinds of experiences that provide what you need (Table 26.1). Can you lay out an educational plan for yourself that will cover several years and will enable you to search out and deepen your understanding of significant issues, rather than falling into the trap of being spoon fed by others from what interests them?

10. Selecting sound continuing education requires development and use of our:
    a. critical thinking abilities.
    b. integrative abilities.
    c. tolerance of ambiguity.
    d. all of the above.

Continuing education would seem to serve us best when we recognize that it has two dimensions—the old and the new—that it is not merely the pursuit of the novel, the new, but also the deepening of our comprehension of what we were exposed to during our basic graduate/professional education. What did you encounter in terms of survey course information in your formal graduate education that you need to reexamine, to explore in depth? What intrigued you that you did not find time to explore adequately? What did you feel that you did not understand fully? What did you like and feel that you would benefit from by studying again, at a more leisurely, reflective pace?

Whenever we get our understandings from summaries of materials done by someone else, by summarizing authors or lecturers, we are relying on secondhand sources for our comprehension of the original work. I have required my graduate students to read as much of the pertinent material in their field as possible, to read the original sources, rather than depend on interpretations formed by others.

11. Continuing education seems to work best for us when we:
    a. seek out the newest offerings.
    b. determine for ourselves what we need.
    c. are not critical of what is offered.
    d. find no ambiguity in what we find.

Some practitioners of MFT resemble religious revivalists who seek out charismatic presenters, flocking from one highly touted person or technique to another, getting one new inoculation or charge after another in continuing education programs. Not infrequently, within a year or two, perhaps less, the recent therapeutic converts are often found disparaging the knowledge and skills of their former hero or heroine.

We are not compelled to follow such an unfortunate course. We can learn on our own. Among the other options open to us are: the use of journals, libraries, the Internet, and examining our own cases.

Broadly based, **omnibus** publications of marital and family therapy theory, research, and practice material provide one of the best resources for adding to our knowledge and understanding of our field. Four journals in the United States—the *American Journal of Family Therapy, Contemporary Family Therapy, Family Process,* and the *Journal of Marital and Family Therapy* fit into this category. Besides these, there are "niche" journals that provide information on more limited and focused aspects of marital and family therapy such as the *Journal of Family Psychotherapy, Behavior Therapy, Journal of Substance Abuse Treatment, Journal of Family Psychology, Journal of Couple and Relationship Therapy,* and others.

12. Which of the following journals is an omnibus journal publishing family therapy theory, research, and practice materials?
    a. *Journal of Family Psychotherapy*
    b. *Journal of Couple and Relationship Therapy*
    c. *Personal Relationships*
    d. *Contemporary Family Therapy*

The Internet offers a rich source of information if we are willing to spend the time exploring what is available and choosing with some degree of care. I still am amazed at what I can find as a result of entering a key word or words on the screen and pressing the "Go" or "Search" button after getting online. Add to that the Web site address for known sources of information and education, and the outcome provides enough material for a genuine ongoing education.

Learning through the use of library materials, journals, the Internet, and examination of our own cases and experiences in treating clients may not always meet the technical requirements for CEUs established by our licensing board, but can be exceedingly effective sources of development for us as professionals. Keep two sets of records, a *licensure renewal file*, containing certificates of your official CEU units to go with your applications for license renewal, and a *professional development file*, containing records on your own independent reading and study. Computer files make an excellent place to keep notes from your reading, observations, and reflections.

13. MFTs are advised to keep continuing education files to:
    a. validate their official CEUs for licensure renewal purposes.
    b. assist their professional development through independent study.
    c. both of the above.
    d. none of the above.

## AFFILIATIONS WITH PROFESSIONAL ORGANIZATIONS AND AGENCIES

Why join professional organizations today? More than once when asked why one should join professional organizations such as the AAMFT, I have replied,

*Not because it gives me any right to practice; my license to practice is granted by the state—it's represented by the piece of paper in my pocket and the certificate on my office wall. I belong*

*to the AAMFT (and to other professional organizations) because of the intellectual stimulation, contacts with fellow professionals, and general professional development opportunities that such participation brings to me.*

Significant differences exist among the major marital and family therapy associations. The AAMFT contains the largest number of members of those whose professional identity is marriage and family therapist, and can be accurately described as the closest thing to a union that exists in the field. As it has moved out of its earlier role as a quasi-credentialing organization for practitioners it has assumed a larger educational role through its annual conferences and regularly scheduled winter and summer institutes. Despite widespread state recognition of licensed MFTs as supervisors, the AAMFT's *Approved Supervisor* credential is still rather widely sought (Lee, Nichols, Nichols, & Odum, 2004); the Approved Supervisor credential, or, in some instances, its equivalent, is required in programs accredited by the Commission on Accreditation for Marriage and Family Therapy Education (COAMFTE).

14. The Approved Supervisor program and credential are offered by the:
    a. International Family Therapy Association.
    b. National Council on Family Relations.
    c. American Association for Marriage and Family Therapy.
    d. American Family Therapy Academy.

The American Family Therapy Academy (AFTA), founded in the 1970s as the American Family Therapy Association, has been a purposely size-limited organization that seeks experienced teachers and practitioners for its membership. It conducts an annual meeting and produces a newsletter.

The International Family Therapy Association (IFTA), founded in 1987, is open to family therapists from around the world. It conducts congresses (conferences) in different countries, and has met in Europe, the Middle East, and Latin America, and sponsors the *Journal of Family Psychotherapy*. (See Table 26.2 for contact information for these organizations.)

Your relationship with professional organizations and agencies is comparable to one's relationship as a citizen with voluntary associations and community agencies. What kind of professional citizen am I? Do I belong to national and state MFT organizations only for what they can do for me, for what I can get from them? What can I do for my professional field and organizations? How can I contribute and what can I give back?

Undoubtedly, there are many things one can gain from professional associations, including contact with colleagues; keeping up with current developments in the field; and assistance in obtaining licensure, in dealing collectively with problems of reimbursement and other guild issues, as well as attaining the credibility among our clients that comes from belonging to the recognized organizations for our profession.

Participation in the activities of general mental health organizations as a citizen of the community or state and serving on the board of directors or as a consultant to mental health and family service agencies should be done with a clear sense that one's role and responsibilities are those of a citizen rather than a self-serving practitioner. The professional rewards are indirect, and a strong, clear line between citizenship and professional practice needs to be maintained at all times.

Some MFTs are appointed to regulatory boards that are charged with the responsibility of licensing or certifying practitioners and disciplining those who violate the statutes, rules, and regulations under which they are privileged to practice. If you are appointed, it is likely that you may have been recommended for the appointment by your state professional organization.

**TABLE 26.2**

Contact Information for Family Therapy Associations

---

American Association for Marriage and Family Therapy
    112 South Alfred Street
    Alexandria, VA 22314
    Telephone: 703-838-9808
    Web site: www.aamft.org
American Family Therapy Academy
    2020 Pennsylvania Avenue, NW, PMB 273
    Washington, DC 20006-1846
    Telephone: 202-333-3690
    Web site: www.afta.org
    E-mail: afta@afta.org
International Family Therapy Association
    c/o Family Studies
    Purdue University Calumet
    2200 169th Street
    Hammond, IN 46323
    Telephone: 219-989-2027
    Web site: www.ifta-family therapy.org

---

We are expected to serve on the board as knowledgeable professionals who are committed to protecting citizens from improper and inadequate practice by MFTs. We are not there as representatives of a professional organization. Being named to the board does not grant us a license to enter into attacks on or power struggles with other professional or occupational groups. Rather, we are expected to behave as knowledgeable and impartial persons who are committed to administering the requirements of the relevant state regulations primarily to protect the citizenry against unauthorized and harmful practices. At the same time we strive to protect citizens, we also are expected to treat applicants for licensure in fair and appropriate ways under the statutes and regulations; applicants also are citizens who deserve equity under the law. Unfortunately, sometimes licensure board members do not treat applicants and licensees with appropriate courtesy, failing to recognize that their task is neither to admit to practice everybody who applies or to deny admission to virtually all who seek licensure. Similarly, some board members have been removed and have even been responsible for the sunsetting of the licensure law under which they were functioning and the disbanding of the licensing board as a result of their inappropriate behavior.

15. The major purpose of an MFT licensing law is to:
    a. protect MFTs from unfair competition.
    b. give the AAMFT a licensing board.
    c. keep physicians from practicing MFT.
    d. protect the public.

Some straightforward advice based on eight years of service on a state regulatory board, seven of which were as chair of the board, may be helpful. First, if you are appointed to a state regulatory board, study the law and rules and regulations carefully until you have a sound understanding of the requirements and procedures under which your board operates. Second, treat the people in staff positions serving the licensing board respectfully and be prepared to work with them on a peer level, respecting their areas of responsibility and knowledge and expecting them to acknowledge and respect yours.

## APPROPRIATE COLLABORATION AND RELATIONSHIPS WITH OTHER HEALTH PROFESSIONALS

In addition to the contacts and collaborative work with other professions that go on in relation to dealing with cases (e.g., obtaining and rendering reports, accepting and giving referrals, and communicating with other professionals), MFTs can contribute to their own growth and understanding by seeking and maintaining contacts in other settings. Respect for the general and unique knowledge and skills of other professionals and appropriate knowledge, skill, and confidence in ourselves so that our behaviors and demeanor merit respect can provide opportunity to function as peers and thus provide better and extended service to our clients and afford mutual learning between us and our peers. Those who have been in practice for an extended period of time are likely to observe the confidence other professionals have in them, and the not unimportant fact that many of the referrals they receive are more likely than otherwise to stem from impressions and evaluations formed in informal contacts and interaction, rather than from examining their vita.

For example, at the organizational level, the Michigan Interprofessional Association for Marriage, Divorce, and the Family, Inc. composed of judges, attorneys, mental health professionals, and family life educators, exercised a powerful influence for many years in Southeastern Michigan and noticeably advanced understanding and collaboration in a variety of areas through monthly luncheon meetings, periodic programs, and eventually public service courses such as a pioneering adjustment to divorce series (Nichols, 1977). Not the least of the outcomes to this interprofessional contact and collaboration was the strong support from judges and some attorneys for a state licensure law for MFTs.

Knowledge of fields that are reciprocal to marital and family therapy as well as important sharing and the formation of collegial and perhaps important personal relationships can be achieved through engaging in discussion groups with other professionals.

Collaborating with a colleague or colleagues to make presentations and to write manuscripts on theory or practice can provide a path to professional growth. This may be particularly relevant if you make good observations from your reading and contact with clients but do not feel confident in your own writing ability. Choosing a colleague who has developed writing skills and will work with you to get your and his or her ideas on paper may serve as a launching pad into the publication world for you.

16. Members of other professions are most likely to be positively influenced toward us by:
    a. sending them a copy of our curriculum vita.
    b. sending them a promotional brochure.
    c. informal contacts and interaction.
    d. reading our telephone yellow page advertisements.

17. Productive professional and interprofessional results are likely to develop from:
    a. collaboration on clinical cases.
    b. engaging in discussion groups.
    c. collaboration on presentations and writing.
    d. all of the above.

## EVALUATING RESEARCH REPORTS

Clinicians, regardless of whether they have extensive education in research methodology, can learn to evaluate research reports. The basic key to understanding and interpreting research for most clinicians resides not so much in comprehending the esoteric details of research methodology, but in understanding the logic of the research. What is the researcher studying? Are the methods he or she is using appropriate? Does it make sense to a reasonable person to draw the conclusions the researcher has drawn from the questions asked? What is the meaning of inferences drawn from the data?

Studying and evaluating research can increase your understanding of theory and help you to glean clinical implications from the work of researchers. We can also learn by acquiring the discipline to examine our case files and by training ourselves to be *participant observers* in our sessions. Going back to school for a course or two in basic statistics or perhaps in qualitative methods can have several benefits, not the least of which may be stimulation that lowers the possibility of boredom and burnout.

> 18. The basic key to understanding and comprehending research for most clinicians is understanding:
>     a. the role of sampling procedures.
>     b. the esoteric details of research methodology.
>     c. the logic of the research.
>     d. nonparametric statistics.

Becoming sufficiently proficient in interpreting research results can help us, once again, to be able to rely, to a much greater degree than many clinicians do, on ourselves in learning—and in learning what we feel is important to us in terms of families, marriage, systems, personality, and related matters.

The journals in the MFT field periodically need new referees to critique manuscripts submitted for possible publication. If you are willing to work at the task of learning how to evaluate materials in your own areas of interest and expertise, there may well be a place for you. In my judgment, the possibility of serving on an editorial review board will be greater after you have done some writing and submitted some of your own materials for consideration to some journals. Careful study and reflection on the responses received from journals on our writing can be a major contributor to our learning about how to evaluate our research.

## Quantitative Methods

Despite the fact that accredited graduate programs in MFT have included research curricula requirements, the culture of family therapy generally has not valued research, as Sprenkle (2003) has noted. This appears to be changing. Crane, Wampler, Sprenkle, Sandberg, and Hovestadt (2002), for example, recently produced a comprehensive list of suggestions for improving research training in MFT academic programs, such as recommending empirically based theses in master's programs, establishing research practica and internships, and making postdoctoral research training normative.

> 19. With regard to research, the culture of family therapy:
>     a. has traditionally valued research highly.
>     b. now values research less than in the past.

> c. appears to value research more than in the past.
> d. none of the above.

Broadly speaking, we need to understand two kinds of research, quantitative research and qualitative research. Perhaps most of us are more likely to think of quantitative methodology when research is mentioned. *Quantitative research* methods emerged from the natural sciences, where they were developed to study natural phenomena. These methods are concerned with quantification, the strength of associations between variables with causation. Statistics which express effects, such as correlations, differences between means, and relative frequencies, help determine the effect of independent variables upon dependent (outcome) variables. Researchers form hypotheses from preexisting theory that can be tested. They seek to draw inferences from the study of the sample that can be applied to the larger population of which the sample is representative. A random selection procedure provides the surest way to make certain the sample is representative of the population for which the results apply. Quantification researchers also seek results that can be replicated so that the findings can be confirmed by others or disconfirmed, and so that research can be systematic and cumulative.

> 20. Quantitative research techniques can include:
>     a. survey methods.
>     b. experimental studies.
>     c. case studies.
>     d. all of the above.
>
> 21. Quantitative research is aimed at:
>     a. the study of social and cultural phenomena.
>     b. systematic, cumulative, replicable results.
>     c. the use of inductive reasoning.
>     d. exploring hermaneutics.

Common quantitative research techniques in the mental health fields include survey methods, experimental studies, and observational (descriptive) techniques. Observational studies involve the observation of people without any other intervention. Examples include case studies, cross-sectional studies in which variables are observed and assessed at a single point in time, longitudinal or prospective studies in which variables are noted at the beginning and the outcomes noted later, and case-control or retrospective studies in which persons with particular characteristics (cases) are compared with controls (persons lacking the characteristics), the characteristics presumably resulting from identified past conditions that affected the cases but not the controls. Experimental studies include interventions with the persons studied. The well-known pattern in which participants are measured before and after a given intervention or treatment probably is most familiar to most of us. Those receiving the treatment are termed the *experimental group* and the others who do not and thus provide a basis for comparison are called the *control group*.

> 22. Which, if any, of the following is most characteristic of qualitative research?
>     a. longitudinal studies.
>     b. experimental studies.
>     c. use of control groups.
>     d. none of the above.

## Qualitative Methods

*Qualitative research methods*, sometimes called *interpretative methods*, emerged from the social sciences and were designed to study social and cultural phenomena. These methods focus on "what" and "why" questions rather than on "how many," as in quantitative research. That is, the data are collected and analyzed in nonnumerical form. The goal is to understand people from their points of view and from the social and cultural contexts in which they live. Specific qualitative methods include observations, interviews (including in-depth interviews), case studies (using ethnographic and participant observer methods), focus groups, and action research. Approaches to analysis include narrative and metaphor analysis (e.g., stories, particularly those told in the first person), semiotics (concern with the meaning of signs and symbols in language), and hermeneutics (e.g., the meaning of a text).

23. Qualitative research is primarily concerned with:
    a. the study of natural phenomena.
    b. the study of social and cultural phenomena.
    c. numerical results.
    d. correlational studies.

Whereas data in quantitative research consist of numbers, data in qualitative research generally consist of words. The data from qualitative studies are analyzed through coding, categorization, and comparison. Data analysis in quantitative studies is handled through the use of statistical inference and statistical estimation. Qualitative research, as contrasted with quantitative, relies more on inductive reasoning (using data to develop theories, concepts, and hypotheses) rather than testing hypotheses formed from preexisting theories.

24. Which, if any, of the following is most characteristic of quantitative research?
    a. the use of statistical inference.
    b. the use of deductive reasoning.
    c. testing hypotheses formed from preexisting theory.
    d. all of the above.

Increasingly, researchers are combining quantitative and qualitative research methods (Casebeer & Verhoef, 1997; Creswell, 1994; Frechtling & Westat, 1997; Mertens, 1998). When one is seeking primarily to generalize findings to larger groups than the study sample, quantitative methods are generally used in order to secure quantitative data. When the perceptions and reactions of the target population are sought, qualitative methods such as in-depth interviews or focus groups are used.

25. Researchers wishing to know the perceptions of a target population would most likely use:
    a. statistical research.
    b. qualitative methods.
    c. bibliographic research.
    d. quantitative methods.

26. Which of the following is not considered a qualitative method?
    a. experimental methods
    b. in-depth interviews
    c. focus groups
    d. hermeneutics

Today's technologies make surveying the literature on a given topic and forming a good working bibliography much easier than was the case a few decades ago. Gaining access to resources such as PsychLit and others quickly provides us with printouts of abstracts or complete articles quickly and relatively easily in comparison to past days in which one had to go through library stacks opening journals or books one by one to find out whether they contained anything on the topic we were researching. Once I start looking for material on a topic, I keep going until there are no more "squishy" areas, meaning that I seem to have a solid foundation under me. When I begin to encounter the same sources again and again and am not finding new items, I can conclude that the area has been covered adequately, that probably nothing significant has been missed. Such searches of the literature also tend to furnish us with some understanding of the ways in which what we are studying is evaluated by others and with the opportunity to raise questions of our own. What sounded so great when presented by a charismatic presenter in a workshop or conference address may or may not seem so strong and sound when we run across careful critiques in the literature. Conversely, what was originally presented in a dull manner by a speaker or teacher may come to life when we encounter it in lucid writing and in strong research results.

# THERAPIST BURNOUT

Dealing with stress and avoiding burnout are significant concerns for many persons at all occupational levels in today's complex society. Avoiding stress is not possible, since as Hans Selye (1956) pointed out, *stress* refers to the response our body makes to any demand on it. He distinguished between *eustress* ("good" stress, which is associated with good feelings such as achievement, fulfillment, and joy) and *distress* ("bad" stress, which is stress that occurs too often or lasts too long).

27. Hans Selye described *eustress* as:
    a. stress which lasts too long.
    b. stress which is harmful.
    c. the source of burnout.
    d. good stress.

*Burnout*, a concept originally applied to machines, has been widely used in reference to humans for more than a quarter century (Freudenberger, 1975, 1977; Hall, Gardner, Perl, Stickney, & Pfefferbaum, 1979; Maslach, 1982). Freudenberger (1980) has defined burnout in terms of depleting oneself, exhausting one's physical and mental resources, wearing oneself out by excessively striving to achieve some unrealistic expectation imposed by oneself or imposed by the values of society. Maslach (1982) included feelings of helplessness and hopelessness, and development of a negative self-concept and negative attitudes toward work, other people, and life.

28. Burnout is characterized by:
    a. depleting oneself.
    b. exhausting our physical and mental resources.
    c. excessive striving to achieve unrealistic expectations.
    d. all of the above.

We do not need to live through our practice and our clients but to maintain other interests and commitments. Since taking a sabbatical from practice is seldom practical for full-time practitioners, going the "dual interests" or "multiple interests" route may be the best way to try to avoid burnout. (I took two years off back in the late 1980s, serving as the executive of a state governmental family office. When I went back to practice after that hiatus, I was wonderfully energized and had the feeling of being "back home.")

If you have any question about how well you are handling stress or fear that you may be in danger of experiencing burnout, there are helpful materials available to give you some answers and guidance. Musick (1997), for example, offers a simple instrument for assessing your risk for burn-out and reproduces an Adult APGAR Test. You probably are familiar with the APGAR test for measuring wellness in newborn infants; Shay Bintliff, M.D. has created the Adult APGAR Test, for physicians to use in assessing their wellness and to recognize the indications of burnout in themselves. This self-scored test, which consists of five questions, can be used by any of us as a general, but helpful guide to our degree of wellness and possible need for assistance to achieve wellness (Musick, 1997). Bintliff (1997) also has described "The 12 Commandments of Wellness," which are well worth studying. An older and longer scale is offered by Freudenberger (1980, pp. 17–18), along with some words of caution for using the scale. If you are in burnout, you need to reduce stress in order to get things under control, which involves learning the causes of your stress and taking steps to reduce it.

The father of stress theory and study, Hans Selye (1978), suggested a more simple approach, dividing people in to two main types: *racehorses*, who thrive on stress and enjoy a fast-paced life, and *turtles*, who need peace, quiet, and an essentially tranquil environment. Furthermore, he declared that each of us is the best judge of himself or herself, and that we can, by observing ourselves, our body clues, and behavioral indicators such as irritability or insomnia, decide whether we are functioning above or below the stress level that is most suitable for us. Selye's attitudes regarding stress can be interpreted as supporting the idea that getting to know oneself and deciding what we are personally comfortable with—a "racehorse" life or a "turtle existence"—is a highly individual matter and that spotting stress is not difficult once we become self-aware.

29. The advice of Hans Selye, the "father of stress theory," to us would best be summed up as:
    a. avoid eustress at all costs.
    b. become a serene "turtle" and seek tranquility.
    c. get to know yourself and decide what you are comfortable with.
    d. read *The Power of Positive Thinking*.

Personal experience as well as the literature on burnout indicate that the wise course for a professional is to seek to achieve a balance between professional life and personal and family life. Overemphasis on the work world provides a major source of burnout. We need to take our nonwork world seriously and to plan for personal and family renewal, whether we think that we need renewal or not. Compartmentalization of life is critical for the serious professional; we need to learn to leave our work at the office as much as we practically can and find ways that we can enjoy doing productive things in the nonwork sphere on a daily basis. Many persons find that doing physical labor in the yard, woodworking, engaging in play with children or spouse, watching a bit of uncomplicated television, reading, cooking, and so on help them to erect firm fences between work and personal life and to minimize the possibility of burnout. Finding ways to "gear down" or "decompress" after leaving work constitute important steps in relaxing and making the transition between work and personal life.

Both as prevention and as prophylaxis, contacting a therapist or using the services of someone such as a life coach in dealing with real or potential burnout can be exceedingly helpful.

30. A major source of burnout is:
   a. guilt feelings from ignoring work.
   b. overemphasis on the work world.
   c. inadequate emphasis on the personal world.
   d. compartmentalization of work and family/personal life.

# KEY TERMS

**burnout:** A work-related condition in which one's expectation level is dramatically opposed to reality and the person persists in trying to reach that expectation, resulting in depletion of resources and lowering of vitality, energy, and ability to function (modeled after Freudenberger, 1980).

**CEU:** Continuing education unit. Most state licensing boards require given amounts of approved continuing education units annually for relicensing.

**distress:** Stress which lasts too long or occurs too often, called "bad stress."

**eustress:** Stress which is associated with good feelings such as achievement and joy, "good stress."

**license:** State credential restricting use of title and right to practice to those who have obtained the requisite state license. All states except Delaware, Montana, North Dakota, and West Virginia license MFTs.

**omnibus journals:** Journals that publish theory, research, and practice materials. In the United States, this includes the *American Journal of Family Therapy, Contemporary Family Therapy, Family Process,* and the *Journal of Marital and Family Therapy.*

**professional:** Occupations marked by specialized knowledge not available to laypersons, long study and training, professional organization, a binding code of ethics, and specialized treatment in the society (e.g., licensure).

**qualitative research:** Drawn from the social sciences, these approaches focus on what and why questions, rather than how many, and have the goal of understanding people from their points of view and their cultural contexts.

**quantitative research:** Traditional research methods derived from natural sciences, concerned with quantification, use statistics and draw inferences from study of a sample to be applied to the larger population of which sample is representative.

**stress:** The wear and tear caused by life (Selye, 1956, p. viii).

## DISCUSSION QUESTIONS

1. What distinguishes professions from other occupations? What are the key characteristics of a profession?
2. Describe the emergence of the American Association for Marriage and Family Therapy as a full-fledged professional organization in the 1970s. What is its current role in the field of marital and family therapy? How does it differ from the American Family Therapy Academy and the International Family Therapy Association?
3. What are the purposes of occupational licensure? Briefly delineate the differences between licensure and certification. What is the current status of MFT regulation in the United States?
4. What are the differences between organizational certification and state licensure/certification; between legal and honorific regulation and recognition?
5. You have been appointed to a state licensing board for licensing MFTs in your state. What are your responsibilities and what are the expectations held regarding your role on the board?
6. Describe how you would establish a program of professional learning for yourself after you secure your master's or doctoral degree and become licensed so that you can practice as an MFT? Distinguish between the formal continuing education you are required to secure in terms of CEU (continuing education unit) requirements of the licensing board and the professional development and learning pattern that you would establish to fulfill your personal interests and goals.
7. How do you plan to go about improving your ability to evaluate research reports? Select an article from one of the four omnibus journals listed in this chapter and critique it, noting the question(s) that the author was seeking to answer and illustrate how the author did or did not select research methods appropriate to the question(s).
8. Distinguish between quantitative and qualitative research in MFT. What is the major purpose and focus of each approach? Illustrate with case material.
9. Describe and briefly discuss the distinctive methods of qualitative and quantitative research methods.
10. How do you plan to maintain wellness and avoid burnout in your chosen profession?

## SUGGESTED FURTHER READING

Bintliff, S. (1997). Balancing act: The 12 commandments of wellness. *Family Practice Management, May*. Retrieved February 27, 2004, from http://www.aapf.org/fpm/970500fm/suite_2html.

A simple but comprehensive list of ways to cope with the major problem areas that most people face. Written for physicians but easily adaptable. Avoid burnout.

Moore, W. E. (1970). *The professions: Roles and rules*. New York: Russell Sage Foundation.

An old but excellent sociological analysis of the roles and rules associated with professions. Most of the useful materials on professions tend to come out of the 1970s and earlier.

StatSoftInc. http://www.statsoftinc.com/textbook/contents.html

Good coverage of elementary statistics with references to many other sources.

Weitzman, E. A., & Miles, M. B. (1995). *A software sourcebook: Computer programs for qualitative data analysis.* Thousand Oaks, CA: Sage.

Just what it says it is, a guide to software and computer programs for qualitative data analysis.

# REFERENCES

Bintliff, S. (1997). Balancing Act: The 12 commandments of wellness. *Family Practice Management May.* Retrieved February 27, 2004 from http://www.aapf.org/fpm/970500fm/suite_2html

Bucher, R., & Stelling, J. G. (1977). *Becoming professional.* Beverly Hills, CA: Sage.

Casebeer, A. L., & Verhoef, M. J. (1997). Combining qualitative and quantitative research methods: Considering the possibilities for enhancing the study of chronic diseases. *Chronic Diseases of Canada, 18,* 130–135.

Crane, D. R., Wampler, K. S., Sprenkle, D. H., Sandberg, J. G. , & Hovestadt, A. J. (2002). The scientist-practitioner model in marriage and family therapy doctoral programs. *Journal of Marital and Family Therapy, 28,* 75–83.

Creswell, J. W. (1994). *Research design: Qualitative and quantitative approaches.* Thousand Oaks, CA: Sage.

Everett, C. A. (1980). An analysis of AAMFT supervisors: Their identities, roles, and resources. *Journal of Marital and Family Therapy, 6,* 215–226.

Frechtling, J., & Westat, L. M. (1997). *User-friendly handbook for mixed method evaluations.* National Science Foundation. Retrieved various dates from http://ehr.nsf.gov/EHR/REC/pubs/NSF97-153/START.HTM

Freudenberger, H. J. (1975). *The staff burn-out syndrome.* Washington, DC: Drug Abuse Council.

Freudenberger, H. J. (1977). Burn-out: The organizational menace. *Training and Development Journal, July,* 27–29.

Freudenberger, H. J. (1980). *Burn-out: The high cost of high achievement.* Garden City, NY: Anchor Press, Doubleday.

Hall, R., Gardner, G., Perl, M. S., Stickney, S., & Pfefferbaum, B. (1979). The professional burn-out syndrome. *Psychiatric Opinion,* April, 12–17.

Lee, R. E., Nichols, D. P., Nichols, W. C., & Odum, T. (2004). Trends in family therapy supervision: The past 25 years and into the future. *Journal of Marital and Family Therapy, 30,* 61–69.

Maslach, C. (1982). *Burnout: The cost of caring.* Englewood Cliffs, NJ: Prentice-Hall.

Mertens, D. M. (1998). *Research methods in education and psychology: Integrating diversity with quantitative and qualitative approaches.* Thousand Oaks, CA: Sage.

Moore, W. E. (1970). *The professions: Roles and rules.* New York: Russell Sage Foundation.

Musick, J. L. (1997). How close are you to burnout? *Family Practice Management, 4*(4). Retrieved February 27, 2004, from http://www.aafp.org/fpm/9704000fr/lead.html

Nichols, W. C. (1974). *Marriage and family counseling: A legislative handbook.* Claremont, CA: American Association of Marriage and Family Counselors.

Nichols, W. C. (1977). Divorce and remarriage education. *Journal of Divorce, 1*(2), 53–61.

Nichols, W. C. (1988) . An integrative and psychodynamic approach. In H. A. Liddle, D. C. Breunlin, & R. C. Schwartz (Eds.), *Handbook of family therapy training and supervision* (pp. 110–127). New York: Brunner/Mazel.

Nichols, W. C. (1992). *The AAMFT: Fifty years of marital and family therapy.* Washington, DC: American Association for Marriage and Family Therapy.

Nichols, W. C., & Lee, R. E. (1999). Mirrors, cameras, and blackboards: Modalities of supervision. In R. E. Lee & S. Emerson (Eds.), *The eclectic trainer* (pp. 45–61). Galena, IL: Geist & Russell.

Nichols, W. C., Nichols, D. P., & Hardy, K. V. (1990). Supervision in family therapy: A decade restudy. *Journal of Marital and Family Therapy, 16,* 275–285.

Selye, H. (1956). *The stress of life.* New York: McGraw-Hill.

Selye, H. (March, 1978) Straight talk about stress. Interview by L. Cherry in *Psychology Today.*

Sprenkle, D. H. (2003). Effectiveness research in marriage and family therapy: Introduction. *Journal of Marital and Family Therapy, 29,* 85–96.

Sturkie, K., & Paff-Bergen, L. (2001). *Professional regulation in marriage and family therapy.* Boston: Allyn & Bacon.

# About the Authors

## THE EDITOR

**Robert H. Coombs, PhD, CAS,** Professor of Biobehavioral Sciences at the UCLA School of Medicine, is trained as a sociologist (Doctorate), counseling psychologist (postdoctoral Master's), family therapist (California licensed), certified addiction specialist (CAS, nationally certified) and certified group psychotherapist (CGP, nationally certified). Early in his career, he served on the Executive Committee of the National Council on Family Relations and was an invited participant at two White House conferences—the 1970 White House Conference on Children and Youth (delegate) and the 1980 White House Conference on Families. Formerly Director of the UCLA Family Learning Center, he currently serves on the International Certification Advisory Committee of the American Academy of Healthcare Providers in the Addictive Disorders. When a member of the California Commission for the Prevention of Drug Abuse, he developed the conceptual framework—a family strengthening model—that guided the Commission's activities. Author or editor of more than two hundred publications, including eighteen books, he is currently coediting a *Series on Treating Addictions* for John Wiley & Sons. He is a recipient of the Award for Excellence in Education from the UCLA School of Medicine, the Distinguished Faculty Educator Award from the UCLA Neuropsychiatric Institute and Hospital, and he was nominated for the Faculty Excellence Award from the UCLA Mortar Board Senior Honors Society.

## CONTRIBUTING AUTHORS

**James F. Alexander, PhD,** Professor of Psychology at the University of Utah, is a progenitor of Functional Family Therapy (FFT). A past director of clinical training at the University of Utah, he has received such honors as Distinguished Contributions to Family Therapy Research, American Family Therapy Academy; Family Psychologist of the Year, Division 43 of the

American Psychological Association; *Good Housekeeping* List of Top U.S. Mental Experts; Superior Teaching Award and Superior Research Award, University of Utah, College of Social and Behavioral Science; Presidential Citation for Lifetime Contribution to Family Therapy Research, Division 43 of the American Psychological Association; *Scientist Exemplar* Award, American Association for Marriage and Family Therapy Research Conference; Distinguished Alumnus Award, California State University, Long Beach; Cumulative Contribution to Family Therapy Research Award, American Association for Marriage and Family Therapy (AAMFT). Provider of more than 350 national and international clinical training workshops and conference presentations, he has received over 20 clinical research and training grants, has authored almost 100 publications (chapters, books, and journal articles), and is a past president of Division 43 of the American Psychological Association.

**Joan D. Atwood, PhD,** Director of both the Graduate Programs in Marriage and Family Therapy and the Marriage and Family Therapy Clinic at Hofstra University, has a private practice in individual, marriage, and family therapy. A past president of the New York State Association for Marriage and Family Therapists, she received the Long Island Family Therapist of the Year Award for outstanding contributions in the field. Author of seven books and more than one hundred journal articles relating to families in transition, human sexuality, and family health, she is an AAMFT Clinical Member and Approved Supervisor and she serves on the editorial boards of several journals. An American Board of Sexology diplomate and clinical supervisor, she is a certified Imago therapist. Elected to the National Academy of Social Workers, she has served on the President's Commission for Domestic Policy. She co-developed an educational program for divorcing parents, as well as the P.E.A.C.E. Program (Parent Education and Custody Effectiveness), a court-based psychoeducational program for parents obtaining a divorce.

**Dorothy S. Becvar, PhD, MSW,** is a Licensed Marital and Family Therapist and a Licensed Clinical Social Worker who is an Associate Professor in the School of Social Service at St. Louis University. She is also co-founder of The Haelan Centers, a not-for-profit corporation dedicated to promoting growth and wholeness in body, mind, and spirit. Dorothy has published extensively and is the author of the books *In the Presence of Grief: Helping Family Members Resolve Death, Dying and Bereavement Issues* (Guilford Press, 2001), *Soul Healing: A Spiritual Orientation in Counseling and Therapy* (Basic Books, 1997), as well as the editor of *The Family, Spirituality and Social Work* (Haworth, 1997). With her husband, Raphael J. Becvar, she has co-authored *Family Therapy: A Systemic Integration* (Allyn & Bacon, 1988, 1992, 1996, 2000, 2003), *Pragmatics of Human Relationships* (Geist & Russell, 1998), *Hot Chocolate for a Cold Winter's Night: Essays for Relationship Development* (Love Publishing, 1994), and *Systems Theory and Family Therapy: A Primer* (University Press of America, 1982, 1999). Recently she coedited, with William Nichols, Mary Anne Pace-Nichols, and Augustus Napier, the *Handbook of Family Development and Intervention* (Wiley, 2000). She is also a well-respected teacher and trainer who has been a member of the faculties of the University of Missouri–St. Louis, St. Louis University, Texas Tech University, Washington University, and Radford University, and she has presented workshops and taught courses, both nationally and internationally, on a wide variety of topics.

**Lee Duke Bowen, PhD,** is the director of the MFT program in the Department of Psychiatry and Behavioral Science, at the Mercer University School of Medicine. Dr. Bowen also serves as the Chair of the Composite Board of Professional Counselors, Social Workers, and Marriage and Family Therapists in the state of Georgia. His interests are in the collaborative education and training of marriage and family therapy students with medical students and the development of a culture of collaborative practice with MFTs and primary care physicians and also on the personal development of the therapist. He has presented at national and international conferences and is published in these areas.

**David G. Byrom, PhD,** Co-Director of the Family Therapy Institute of Suffolk in Smithtown, New York, is a clinical psychologist practicing in both private/community practice and public sector settings. He is also Supervising Psychologist at the Suffolk County Division of Community Mental Health Services (Mental Health and Alcohol & Drug Abuse). As President of The National Coalition of Mental Health Professionals and Consumers, Inc., he works to preserve high standards for mental health and substance abuse care.

**Carrie C. Capstick, MA,** a doctoral student in clinical psychology at the City University of New York, is Research Project Director of the Women's Health Project Research and Treatment Center of St. Luke's–Roosevelt Hospital Center, a program providing expertise in the areas of trauma and substance abuse. She received clinical and research experience in trauma at the Boston Veteran's Outpatient Clinic and McLean Hospital and completed training in trauma studies at The New York University.

**Jon Carlson, PsyD, EdD, ABPP,** Distinguished Professor of Psychology and Counseling at Governors State University in University Park, IL, is a psychologist at the Wellness Clinic in Lake Geneva, Wisconsin. He holds earned doctoral degrees in counseling and clinical psychology and a Diplomate in Family Psychology from the American Board of Professional Psychology. He is the author of twenty-five books and more than 125 professional articles. A past president of the International Association of Marriage and Family Counseling (IAMFC), he has received professional service awards from the American Psychological Association, American Counseling Association, American Board of Professional Psychology, North American Society of Adlerian Psychology, and IAMFC.

**Stephanie L. Carnes, PhD,** an adjunct faculty member at the University of San Diego and Alliant International University in San Diego, is an AAMFT Clinical Member and Approved Supervisor Candidate. Her interests include a multidisciplinary approach to healthcare, marital therapy substance abuse, sexual compulsivity, and domestic violence. A presenter at national and state conferences, she serves on the board of directors for the American Foundation for Addiction Research.

**Richard Cook, M Couns (Hons), BD, BEd, Dip. Tchg. MNZAC,** holds a Master of Counseling degree with Honours from the University of Waikato, and a Bachelor of Divinity degree from the Melbourne College of Divinity. Trained in teaching, clinical pastoral education, grief counseling, family education, narrative therapy, and clinical supervision, he is a member of the New Zealand Association of Counselors. Currently he has a private counseling practice and is Senior Lecturer at Bethlehem Institute of Education in Tauranga, New Zealand, where he lectures, coordinates the counseling and family studies faculty, and manages promotions and developments.

**Shonda M. Craft, MS,** a doctoral student in marriage and family therapy at The Ohio State University, has research interests in HIV/AIDS, domestic violence, and sexual assault. For the past $3^1/_2$ years, she has worked as a research associate with Dr. Julianne Serovich on an NIH-funded study regarding issues related to disclosure and mental health among HIV-positive women and gay men. Prior to working with Dr. Serovich, she spent one year researching adult and adolescent male sex offenders, as well as antisocial behaviors among adolescent female detainees.

**Hugh C. Crethar, PhD,** Professor of Counseling Psychology at Governors State University, directs the school counseling program. His primary scholarly interests are in the areas of family systems applications, multicultural counseling, clinical supervision, ethics, value-orientation, and clinically related public policy. He also serves as Co-Chair of the Public Policy and Legislation Committee of the American Counseling Association. He is a founding member and President of Illinois Counselors for Social Justice, whose focus is on the application of systemic models to overcome community challenges.

**Frank M. Dattilio, PhD, ABPP,** maintains a joint faculty appointment with the Department of Psychiatry at both Harvard Medical School and the University of Pennsylvania School of Medicine. A clinical psychologist who is board certified by the American Board of Professional Psychology in both behavioral and clinical psychology, he is a clinical member and AAMFT Approved Supervisor. He trained in behavior therapy under the direction of the late Joseph Wolpe, MD, and received postdoctoral training at the University of Pennsylvania under the direction of Aaron T. Beck, MD. A noted expert in cognitive–behavior therapy, he has authored more than 150 publications, including eleven books. His work has been translated into more than sixteen languages. On the editorial boards of a number of national and international journals, he has lectured in 30 countries and has won numerous awards, including Psychologist of the Year from the American Psychological Association in 2002. His books on couples and family therapy are widely referenced and utilized.

**Sarah Dauber, MA,** a doctoral student in applied developmental psychology at Fordham University, is a research assistant at Columbia University working on a NIDA-funded study investigating therapist adherence and competence in two empirically supported treatments for adolescent drug abuse. Her research interests include psychotherapy for adolescent drug abuse and the prevention and treatment of child abuse.

**John DeFrain, PhD,** Extension Professor of Family and Community Development at the University of Nebraska–Lincoln, received his doctorate from the University of Wisconsin–Madison. He has focused his professional energy on the development of strong families. Experienced as a newspaper reporter, a preschool and kindergarten teacher, a family educator, and family therapist, he has coauthored and coedited sixteen books on family issues, including *Marriage and the Family: Diversity and Strengths* (2000) and *Building Relationships* (1998).

**Patricia C. Dowds, PhD,** is a clinical psychologist who has been practicing for thirty years. She is currently a faculty and board member at The Minuchin Center for the Family, New York City, and is Co-Director of The Family Therapy Institute of Suffolk in Smithtown, New York. A teacher of interns for over twenty years, she has consulted at hospitals and clinics to establish family therapy programs. Currently she conducts research in family treatment of adolescent substance abuse and consults at New York City child welfare centers to increase family participation when treating children. She also works as a health care activist fighting to protect and expand mental health benefits for families. She serves on the executive board of the Universal Health Care Action Network (UHCAN) and is Vice President of The National Coalition of Mental Health Professionals and Consumers, Inc.

**Maureen P. Duffy, PhD,** Associate Professor, and Chair of the Counseling Department at Barry University in Miami Shores, Florida, is a licensed marriage and family therapist, a licensed mental health counselor, a Florida Supreme Court Certified Family Mediator, and an AAMFT Clinical Member and Approved Supervisor. Her research interests include neuroscience applications in systemic family therapy, teen gangs, and mothers in prison. Her recent publications have focused on family health and qualitative research.

**Elisabeth M. Dykens, PhD,** Professor of Psychology and Human Development at Peabody College of Vanderbilt University is Deputy Director of Vanderbilt's Kennedy Center on Human

Development. A clinical psychologist who has directed clinics for children with specific genetic disorders and their families, she was previously at the Yale Child Study Center and then in the Child Psychiatry Division of UCLA's Neuropsychiatric Institute (NPI). Author of more than one hundred publications on emotional–behavioral problems of children with Prader–Willi, Williams, Down, and other genitic syndromes of mental retardation, including *Genetics and Mental Retardation Syndromes* (2000), she is an associate editor of the *American Journal on Mental Retardation*, a member of the editorial board of *Mental Retardation*, and a member of the Steering Committee for the NICHD-sponsored Gatlinburg Conference on Mental Retardation and Developmental Disabilities.

**Todd M. Edwards, PhD,** is Associate Professor and Director of the Marital and Family Therapy program at the University of San Diego. An AAMFT Clinical Member and Approved Supervisor, he is licensed as a marriage and family therapist in Michigan. His primary research interests are collaboration among family therapists, family physicians and psychiatrists; medical family therapy; and medical family therapy supervision. His recent published articles focus on family therapy supervision, medical family therapy, and family therapy training in medical settings.

**Craig A. Everett, PhD,** Director of the Arizona Institute for Family Therapy, is in private practice in Tucson, Arizona. A past president of the American Association for Marriage and Family Therapy and a Fellow and Approved Supervisor with that organization, he is Editor of the *Journal of Divorce and Remarriage* and has served on the editorial boards of numerous publications. He was formerly on the faculties and Director of AAMFT-accredited Marital and Family Therapy Graduate Programs at Florida State University and Auburn University. His most recent publications include *The Integrative Family Therapy Supervisor: A Primer* (with Bob Lee, Brunner-Routledge, 2003), *Family Therapy with ADHD: Treating Children, Adolescents, and Adults* (with Sandra Volgy Everett, Guilford Press, 1999), and *Healthy Divorce* (with Sandra Volgy Everett, Wiley, 1994). He has also edited numerous works in the divorce field for Haworth Press.

**Leyla Faw, MA,** a doctoral student in applied developmental psychology at Fordham University, is currently working as a research assistant at Columbia University on a NIDA-funded project examining therapist adherence and competence in two empirically supported treatments for adolescent substance abuse. Her current research interests include measuring fidelity in program evaluation and prevention and treatment of delinquency and substance abuse in at-risk youth.

**Peter Fraenkel, PhD,** is Associate Professor of Psychology, City University of New York, Director of the Ackerman Institute's Center for Time, Work, and the Family, Clinical Assistant Professor at NYU Medical School, and is in private practice. He is coauthor of *The Relational Trauma of Incest: A Family-Based Approach to Treatment*, and author of many articles and chapters in the field of family therapy on such topics as treatment of child sexual abuse, prevention of relationship distress, work/family balance, the impact of technology, and time issues in couples and families. He is an advisory editor for *Family Process* and for the *Journal of Marital and Family Therapy* and a contributing editor for *The Psychotherapy Networker*. He is a board member of the american family therapy academy.

**Scott E. Gillig, PhD,** a counselor educator, is Professor and Coordinator of the Mental Health Counseling Specialization at Barry University in Miami Shores, Florida. He teaches both master's and doctoral courses. He is also the Council for Accreditation of Counseling and Related Educational Programs (CACREP) Liaison and Chi Sigma Iota Faculty Advisor in the Barry

University Counseling Program. A licensed mental health counselor, a certified addictions professional, and a National Certified Counselor (NCC) Approved Clinical Supervisor, his research interests include counseling outcomes, depression, chemical dependency, treatment planning, and student mentoring.

**Samuel T. Gladding, PhD,** Professor and Chair of the Department of Counseling at Wake Forest University is a National Certified Counselor (NCC), a Certified Clinical Mental Health Counselor (CCMHC), a Licensed Professional Counselor (North Carolina), and an AAMFT Approved Supervisor and Clinical Member. He is President of the American Counseling Association (ACA; 2004–2005), as well as a past president of the Association for Counselor Education and Supervision (ACES), the Association for Specialists in Group Work (ASGW), and Chi Sigma Iota (international counseling academic and professional honor society). He has received numerous awards for service, and is the author of more than one hundred publications including more than a dozen books, such as *Family Therapy: History, Theory, and Process* (2002), *Group Work: A Counseling Specialty* (2003), and *Counseling: A Comprehensive Profession* (2004).

**Gloria Gonzales-Kruger, PhD,** is Assistant Professor in the Department of Family and Consumer Sciences and the Marriage and Family Therapy Program at the University of Nebraska–Lincoln and a licensed marriage and family therapist. Also a Clinical Member and Approved Supervisor in the AAMFT, her research interests include the quality of life of underserved communities, with a focus on Latinos, their culturally based mental health, community youth programming. Her recent publications have focused on university–community based collaborations.

**Edward L. Hendrickson, MS, LMFT, LSATP,** Clinical Supervisor with the Arlington County Alcohol and Drug Treatment Program, has provided treatment, supervision, training, and consultation in substance abuse since 1971, and has specialized in the area of dual diagnosis since 1982. Author of numerous articles and reports on these topics, he is Co-Chair of the Committee on Co-Occurring Disorders of the Metropolitan Washington Council of Governments. He received an achievement award from the National Association of Counties in 1991 for work with dually diagnosed clients.

**Robert M. Hodapp, PhD,** Professor of Special Education at Peabody College of Vanderbilt University is a member of Vanderbilt's Kennedy Center on Human Development. He holds a doctoral degree from Boston University in developmental psychology and was earlier at Yale University (where he worked with Edward Zigler) and at the UCLA Graduate School of Education. His work examines issues concerning development of and family reactions to children with different genetic forms of mental retardation, how approaches to typical development can inform our knowledge of children with mental retardation, and the possibility of etiology-based educational and family interventions. Author of more than one hundred professional articles, his books include *Understanding Mental Retardation* (1986), *Issues in the Developmental Approach to Mental Retardation* (1990), *Development and Disabilities* (1998), and *Genetics and Mental Retardation Syndromes* (2000). He is also on the editorial boards of the *American Journal of Mental Retardation, Mental Retardation,* and the *McGill Journal of Education.*

**Aaron Hogue, PhD,** Senior Research Associate at the National Center on Addiction and Substance Abuse at Columbia University, is a licensed clinical psychologist. He received his doctorate from Temple University and a postdoctoral fellowship in family-based intervention research at the Center for Treatment Research on Adolescent Drug Abuse. His research interests include development of family-based interventions for adolescent drug use and delinquency, risk and resiliency in high-risk youth, and process research on family intervention models.

**Phillip M. Kleespies, PhD,** Coordinator of Emergency and Urgent Care Services for Psychology and a clinical psychologist in the Mental Health Clinic of the VA Boston Healthcare System, received his doctorate in clinical psychology from Clark University in 1971. A diplomate in clinical psychology of the American Board of Professional Psychology, he is a fellow of the American Psychological Association (Division 12—Society of Clinical Psychology) and holds an appointment as Assistant Clinical Professor of Psychiatry at Boston University School of Medicine. He is also the founding president of the Section on Clinical Emergencies and Crises (Section VII of APA Division 12). Dr. Kleespies is the Editor of *Emergencies in Mental Health Practice: Evaluation and Management* (Guilford Press, 1998) and the author of *Life and Death Decisions: Psychological and Ethical Considerations in End-of-Life Care* (APA Press, 2004).

**Edward F. Kouneski, PhD, LP, MA,** is in private practice and licensed as psychologist in Minnesota. He earned his doctorate in family social science and completed the Marriage and Family Therapy training program at the University of Minnesota–Twin Cities. As an adjunct faculty member, he taught courses in family psychology, men and masculinity in families, and parent–child relationships. He has conducted research and published on topics related to couple intimacy, fatherhood, family functioning, and child and adolescent health and development. Prior to graduate studies, he gained nearly twenty years' experience in management consulting and program management in both the private and public sectors. In addition to his work as a psychotherapist serving individuals, couples, and families, he provides research consultation, organizational training, and education seminars.

**Catherine J. Kutter, PhD,** a research project manager and clinician at the National Center for Posttraumatic Stress Disorder (PTSD) at the Jamaica Plain Campus of the VA Boston Healthcare System, where she also performs emergency evaluations and supervises psychology interns in the urgent care service, was awarded her doctoral degree in counseling psychology by the University of Kansas in 2001. A member of the American Psychological Association (Division 12—Society of Clinical Psychology and (Section VII of Division 12, Clinical Emergencies and Crises) and the International Society for Traumatic Stress Studies, she has numerous presentations and publications related to the effects of psychological trauma and PTSD.

**Jacqueline V. Lerner, PhD,** Professor of Educational Psychology at the Boston College Lynch School of Education, received her doctorate from Pennsylvania State University. Her current research and teaching interests include the study of normative child development within the school and home contexts, temperament, maternal employment and day care influences on child development, early adolescent transitions, and positive youth development. She is the author or editor of numerous books, articles, and chapters including: *Theoretical Foundations and Biological Bases of Development in Adolescence* (1999) with R. Lerner ; "Maternal Employment and Education: Predictors of Young Adolescent Career Trajectories" (1998) with D. Castellino, R. Lerner, and A. von Eye; *Working Women and Their Families* (1994); and "The Context of Infancy: Daycare and Maternal Employment in the Twenty-First Century," In H. Fitzgerald and T. Luster (Eds.), *The Ecology of Infancy* (2002). She is the Associate Editor of *Developmental Psychology* and is active in the Society for Research in Child Development, the Society for Research in Adolescence, and the International Society for the Study of Behavioral Development.

**Howard A. Liddle, EdD,** Professor of Epidemiology and Public Health, is Director of the Center for Treatment Research on Adolescent Drug Abuse at the University of Miami Medical School. A nationally recognized psychologist and expert on adolescent substance abuse and delinquency, he reviews grants and serves on expert panels addressing the problems of adolescents for many national and private funding institutes and received awards from several national associations. A faculty member at the University of Miami Medical School, he previously was at the University of California, San Francisco, and Temple University in Philadelphia. His research center at the University of Miami was the first NIH-funded center focusing on adolescent drug abuse treatment research. He and his team are currently conducting treatment studies in Miami and around the country on a comprehensive, family-based treatment for juvenile justice–involved, drug abusing adolescents.

**Steve E. Livingston, PhD,** Clinical Coordinator of the Impaired Educator Recovery Network Program for the state of Florida Department of Education, previously was Assistant Professor at Mercer University School of Medicine Department of Psychiatry and Behavioral Science, where he taught in the master's program in family therapy. A licensed marriage and family therapist and mental health counselor, he received his doctorate in marriage and family therapy from Florida State University. A Clinical Member of the AAMFT, he is also an Approved Supervisor. He has served in the past as Chair of the Continuing Education Committee for the Georgia Association for Marriage and Family Therapy.

**Joan M. Lucariello, PhD,** Associate Professor and Director of the Doctoral Program in Applied Developmental and Educational Psychology at Boston College Lynch School of Education, serves on the editorial board of the *Journal of Applied Developmental Psychology* and the consulting editorial board of *Child Development*. A member of the National Science Foundation's advisory panel for the Human Cognition and Perception Program, she is a Fellow of the American Psychological Association (APA) and has been an elected officer of the executive committee of APA's Division 7—Developmental Psychology. Currently, she is a member of the program committee for the Society for Research in Child Development and is Program Co-Chair for their biennial meeting in 2007. Her research interests and recent publications are in the area of children's cognitive development and learning.

**Eric E. McCollum, PhD,** Professor of Marriage and Family Therapy and Clinical Director of the Marriage and Family Therapy Program in The Department of Human Development at Virginia Tech's Northern Virginia Center in Falls Church, VA, is both a Licensed Clinical Social Worker and a Licensed Marriage and Family Therapist in Virginia. An AAMFT Clinical Member and Approved Supervisor, his research interests are in family therapy of substance abuse and domestic violence. With Dr. Terry Trepper, he is author of *Family Solutions for Substance Abuse*. He has published articles on substance abuse treatment and other topics in a wide range of professional journals.

**William G. McCown, PhD,** Associate Professor of Psychology at The University of Louisiana at Monroe, received his doctorate in psychology from Loyola University–Chicago as a President's Fellow specializing in clinical psychology. Prior to entering graduate school, he spent several years as a crisis worker, during which he received extensive training in family systems theory from some of its early pioneers. At Tulane University Medical Center, he subsequently completed a child and adult internship and a neurobiologically oriented postdoctorate with the V.A. Medical Center, Tulane. A research scientist at the Nathan Kline Institute, a biological psychiatric research facility affiliated with New York University and the World Health Organization, he has training in computational neuroscience. His eclectic interests are reflected in ten books, more than fifty peer-reviewed articles and chapters, and more than three hundred professional presentations.

**William C. Nichols, EdD, ABPP,** a marital and family therapist and diplomate in clinical psychology, is a Fellow, Clinical Member, and Approved Supervisor of the AAMFT; a charter member of both the American Family Therapy Academy and the International Family Therapy Association; and a Fellow of both the American Psychological Association and the American Psychological Society. He was in full-time private practice for nearly twenty-five years and taught and supervised postdoctoral, doctoral, and master's students in MFT programs and postdegree professionals for thirty-five years at the Florida State University, the Merrill–Palmer Institute, and elsewhere. Founder and first editor of the *Journal of Marital and Family Therapy,* he also edited *Family Relations,* and currently edits *Contemporary Family Therapy.* Former president of the AAMFT, IFTA, and the National Council on Family Relations, he has published eight MFT and therapy books, conceptualized and launched MFT accreditation, wrote the first model of licensing laws, co-wrote the national licensing examination, and chaired a state licensing board.

**Barbara L. Niles, PhD,** a staff psychologist at the National Center for Posttraumatic Stress Disorder at the VA Boston Healthcare System, is Assistant Professor of Clinical Psychology at the Boston University School of Medicine. Dr. Niles works with veterans with PTSD and related disorders and conducts research focusing on health psychology and the longitudinal course of PTSD. She received her PhD in clinical psychology from Rutgers University, New Jersey.

**Barbara F. Okun, PhD,** Professor of Counseling Psychology and Training Director of the Combined School and Counseling Psychology Doctoral Program at Northeastern University, formerly served on the faculty of the Harvard Medical School at the Cambridge Family Couples and Family Therapy Training Program. Maintaining a diverse clinical practice in individual, couples, and family therapy, she consults with family court judges at the National Council for Juvenile and Family Court Judges in Reno, Nevada. She has served on the board of directors of the Massachusetts Psychological Association, as Editor-in-Chief of the *MPA Quarterly,* and is currently coediting a special issue of the American Psychological Association's *Journal of Family Psychology Special Issue: entitled, Family Psychology and Family Law.* Her recent books include *Effective Helping: Interviewing and Counseling* (6th edition), *Understanding Diversity*, and *Understanding Diverse Families.*

**David H. Olson, PhD,** is Emeritus Professor of Family Social Science at the University of Minnesota where he taught for about thirty years. He is a Fellow in APA and AAMFT and a past president of the National Council on Family Relations (NCFR). He has received distinguished awards for his scholarly contributions from APA, AAMFT, AFTA, and ACA. He has written more than twenty books and one hundred journal articles in the marital and family field. Olson and colleagues have developed the Circumplex Model of Marital and Family Systems and a variety of couple and family assessments including FACES, PREPARE, ENRICH, PAIR, AWARE, and the Clinical Rating Scale. Over 1,500 published studies have been done on the Circumplex Model and the PREPARE/ENRICH Couple Inventory is used by over fifty thousand counselors. His latest books include *Empowering Couples: Building on your Strengths, Building Relationships, Developing Skills for Life, and Marriage and Family: Diversity and Strengths.* (4th ed.).

**Jo Ellen Patterson, PhD,** Professor of Marriage in Family Therapy in the marital and family therapy program at the University of San Diego, is an instructor of psychiatry in the Department of Psychiatry at the University of California, San Diego, (UCSD) and a member of the clinical faculty in the Department of Psychiatry at UCSD. An AAMFT Clinical Member and Approved Supervisor, she is licensed as a marriage and family therapist in North Carolina and California. Her primary research interests are family functioning and physical health, health care reform and mental health, and family therapy training. Her publications include articles on family systems medicine, education and training of therapists, and ethics in therapy.

**Allison N. Ponce, PhD,** a postdoctoral fellow at the Connecticut Mental Health Center of the Yale University School of Medicine, received her doctorate in clinical psychology at the University of Connecticut. Her dissertation dealt with revictimization of women in violent relationships and the effects of early childhood trauma on the acceptance of violence. She completed her predoctoral internship at the Boston Consortium in Clinical Psychology.

**Roy Resnikoff, MD,** Clinical Professor of Psychiatry at the University of California, San Diego, teaches family therapy to psychiatric residents. A Distinguished Fellow of the American Psychiatric Association, he has, since 1975, had a private family psychiatry practice in La Jolla, California. Author of the book, *Bridges for Healing: Integrating Family Therapy and Psychopharmacology*, he conducts training workshops and gives presentations regarding the integration of psychopharmacology and relational therapy. He attended medical school at the Albert Einstein College of Medicine in New York and completed his psychiatric training at the University of Colorado.

**Patricia Robey, MA,** is a counselor at Oak Lawn Family Services, a community counseling agency in Illinois. With master's degrees in both communication studies and counseling, she is a senior faculty member of The William Glasser Institute (WGI) and has served on the WGI board of directors, including two years as board chair and three years as a member of the WGI professional development committee. She has taught choice theory, reality therapy, lead management, and Glasser Quality School principles to individuals in the fields of education, social service, business, and corrections. As owner of PAR Consultants, she teaches workshops on such topics as conflict management, stress management, and mediation.

**Karen H. Rosen, EdD,** Associate Professor of Human Development in the Marriage and Family Therapy program at Virginia Tech's Northern Virginia Campus, is an AAMFT Approved Supervisor and is licensed as a marriage and family therapist in Virginia. With a primary research interest in intimate partner violence, she has authored several book chapters and journal articles and coedited a book on domestic violence, *Violence Hits Home*, with her colleague Dr. Sandra M. Stith.

**Marcy Rowland, BA,** a doctoral student in the Counseling Psychology program at Indiana University, is a project leader on several research teams at the Center for Adolescent and Family Studies. Currently, she is working on a large scale outcome study comparing Functional Family Therapy to treatment-as-usual. Her research interests include process and outcome research and adolescent identity development.

**Jaclyn N. Sagun, BA,** a research associate at the UCLA Neuropsychiatric Institute, is involved in multiple research projects in child psychiatry including a study on communication and thought disorder in children with epilepsy and another on social skills training for children with fetal alcohol syndrome. Her degree in psychology was earned at UCLA.

**Julianne M. Serovich, PhD,** Professor of Marriage and Family Therapy at The Ohio State University, is an AAMFT Clinical Member and Approved Supervisor. She received her master's degree in counseling psychology at Loyola College in Baltimore and her PhD in Marriage and Family Therapy from the University of Georgia. Her research interests include family communication and privacy as it relates to disclosure of HIV/AIDS. An associate editor of the *Journal of Marital and Family Therapy*, she has published articles in several marriage and family journals.

**Thomas L. Sexton, PhD, ABPP,** Professor of Counseling Psychology in the Department of Counseling and Educational Psychology at Indiana University, is the Director of the Clinical Training Center, Director of the Center for Adolescent and Family Studies, and teaches in the APA accredited Counseling Psychology Program. Editor of the new *Handbook of Family Therapy*, he has written on outcome research and its implications for clinical practice and training. His recent publications include major research articles in the *Handbook of Psychotherapy and Behavior Change* and the *Comprehensive Handbook of Psychotherapy*. An expert on family-based treatment interventions for at-risk adolescents, he is, with Jim Alexander, the author of the most recent theoretical presentations and developments in Functional Family Therapy (FFT). One of two national Functional Family Therapy trainers, he supervises the FFT externship program, and directs the national and international FFT implementation and dissemination projects. An AAMFT Approved Supervisor, he is Vice President of Scientific Affairs for Division 43 (Family Psychology) of the American Psychological Association, and a diplomate in Family Psychology (ABPP).

**Kim Snow, MA, LCPC,** an adjunct professor of counseling at Governors State University, is a counselor at Oak Lawn Family Services Agency in Illinois. In addition to working with Dr. Carlson on various video projects and articles, she is pursuing a doctorate in counselor education from Northern Illinois University.

**Len Sperry, MD, PhD,** Professor of Mental Health Counseling and Coordinator of the Doctoral Program at Florida Atlantic University, Boca Ratan, FL, is also Clinical Professor of Psychiatry and Behavioral Medicine at the Medical College of Wisconsin, Milwaukee, WI. Board certified by the American Board of Psychiatry and Neurology, the American Board of Preventive Medicine, and the American Board of Professional Psychology in Clinical Psychology, he is a Fellow of the American Psychiatric Association, the American Psychological Association, and the American College of Preventive Medicine. He has more than three hundred professional publications, including forty books, has given more than 150 invited presentations at national conferences, and has served on the editorial boards of the *American Journal of Family Therapy, Family Journal, Journal of Family Psychology* and the *Journals of Child Psychiatry and Human Development*.

**Sandra M. Stith, PhD,** Director of the MFT program at Virginia Tech's Falls Church Campus, is author of over forty articles and book chapters on domestic violence and coeditor of two books. Funding for her research on domestic violence has come from the National Institutes of Health, the U.S. Air Force, and the U.S. Department of Agriculture. Licensed as a marriage and family therapist in Virginia, she is an AAMFT Clinical Member and Approved Supervisor.

**Kinly Sturkie, PhD,** Professor and Chair in the Department of Sociology at Clemson University in South Carolina, is President of the university's Faculty Senate. He received his training in social work at the University of Southern California and is licensed as an MFT in South Carolina. An AAMFT, Clinical Member and Approved Supervisor, he is the former president of both his state licensing board and the Association of Marital and Family Therapy Regulatory Boards. He is coauthor (with Lois Paff Bergen) of *Professional Regulation in Marital and Family Therapy* (Allyn & Bacon, 2001).

**Alice Sydnor, MA,** a doctoral student in the Counseling Psychology program at Indiana University, is trained in Functional Family Therapy (FFT) and been involved in the implementation of FFT. The Program Director of the Indiana Family Project, she leads several research teams at the Center for Adolescent and Family Studies. Her research interests includes the organizational, individual, and community barriers involved in the implementation of FFT in multi-agency workgroups, evidence-based family interventions, and family assessments.

**Richard M. Tureen, PhD,** Assistant Professor in the Counseling Program at Barry University, received his doctorate from Nova Southeastern University in Family Therapy where he teaches master's and doctoral courses on marriage and family systems, marital and couples therapy, and counseling theories and interventions. A licensed marriage and family therapist in Florida, his interests include systems theory, complexity theory, chaos theory, and postmodernism.

# Appendix: Answer Key

## CHAPTER 1

### Truth or Fiction Answers

| | | | |
|---|---|---|---|
| 1. F | | 9. F | |
| 2. F | | 10. F | |
| 3. T | | 11. F | |
| 4. F | | 12. T | |
| 5. F | | 13. T | |
| 6. F | | 14. T | |
| 7. F | | 15. T | |
| 8. F | | | |

### Multiple Choice Answers

| | | | |
|---|---|---|---|
| 1. d | | 14. a | |
| 2. d | | 15. d | |
| 3. d | | 16. d | |
| 4. d | | 17. c | |
| 5. b | | 18. c | |
| 6. c | | 19. d | |
| 7. b | | 20. d | |
| 8. c | | 21. b | |
| 9. a | | 22. d | |
| 10. d | | 23. c | |
| 11. d | | 24. d | |
| 12. d | | 25. d | |
| 13. d | | 26. d | |

# CHAPTER 2

## Truth or Fiction Answers

1. T
2. F
3. F
4. T
5. F
6. T
7. T
8. F

9. F
10. T
11. F
12. T
13. T
14. F

## Multiple Choice Answers

1. c
2. a
3. d
4. d
5. b
6. b
7. a
8. c
9. c
10. d
11. c
12. c
13. c
14. a
15. d

16. c
17. a
18. b
19. c
20. a
21. c
22. d
23. b
24. b
25. c
26. d
27. d
28. c
29. a
30. b

# CHAPTER 3

## Truth or Fiction Answers

1. F
2. T
3. T
4. F
5. T
6. F
7. F
8. F

9. T
10. T
11. F
12. T
13. T
14. T
15. T

## Multiple Choice Answers

1. c
2. d

3. d
4. c

5. c

6. c

7. a

8. b

9. a

10. d

11. d

12. c

13. a

14. a

15. d

16. b

17. d

18. c

19. b

20. a

21. c

22. c

23. c

24. b

25. c

26. c

27. d

28. d

29. d

30. c

# CHAPTER 4

## Truth or Fiction Answers

1. T

2. F

3. F

4. T

5. F

6. T

7. T

8. F

9. T

10. T

11. F

12. F

13. F

14. T

15. F

## Multiple Choice Answers

1. c

2. c

3. d

4. d

5. d

6. d

7. b

8. c

9. c

10. c

11. b

12. a

13. a

14. a

15. b

16. b

17. d

18. b

19. a

20. d

21. c

22. a

23. c

24. d

25. b

26. c

27. b

28. d

29. c

30. a

31. a

32. d

## CHAPTER 5

### Truth or Fiction Answers

1–15 all T

### Multiple Choice Answers

| | |
|---|---|
| 1. b | 20. c |
| 2. d | 21. b |
| 3. e | 22. b |
| 4. d | 23. b |
| 5. d | 24. d |
| 6. d | 25. c |
| 7. c | 26. d |
| 8. b | 27. d |
| 9. c | 28. d |
| 10. d | 29. d |
| 11. d | 30. d |
| 12. d | |
| 13. d | |
| 14. b | |
| 15. d | |
| 16. d | |
| 17. b | |
| 18. d | |
| 19. a | |

## CHAPTER 6

### Truth or Fiction Answers

| | |
|---|---|
| 1. T | 13. T |
| 2. F | 14. T |
| 3. T | 15. F |
| 4. F | 16. T |
| 5. T | 17. F |
| 6. F | 18. T |
| 7. T | 19. F |
| 8. T | 20. F |
| 9. T | 21. T |
| 10. F | 22. F |
| 11. T | 23. T |
| 12. F | 24. F |

## Multiple Choice Answers

| | |
|---|---|
| 1. d | 14. c |
| 2. b | 15. a |
| 3. c | 16. c |
| 4. b | 17. a |
| 5. a | 18. d |
| 6. a | 19. b |
| 7. d | 20. c |
| 8. a | 21. a |
| 9. a | 22. b |
| 10. c | 23. d |
| 11. d | 24. d |
| 12. d | 25. a |
| 13. d | |

# CHAPTER 7

## Truth or Fiction Answers

| | |
|---|---|
| 1. T | 9. F |
| 2. T | 10. F |
| 3. F | 11. T |
| 4. F | 12. T |
| 5. F | 13. F |
| 6. T | 14. F |
| 7. F | 15. T |
| 8. T | |

## Multiple Choice Answers

| | |
|---|---|
| 1. a | 13. d |
| 2. d | 14. c |
| 3. d | 15. a |
| 4. b | 16. a |
| 5. c | 17. c |
| 6. c | 18. b |
| 7. a | 19. a |
| 8. b | 20. c |
| 9. d | 21. d |
| 10. c | 22. b |
| 11. d | 23. d |
| 12. d | 24. d |

## CHAPTER 8

### Truth or Fiction Answers

| | |
|---|---|
| 1. T | 9. T |
| 2. F | 10. T |
| 3. F | 11. T |
| 4. F | 12. F |
| 5. T | 13. F |
| 6. F | 14. F |
| 7. T | 15. F |
| 8. F | |

### Multiple Choice Answers

| | |
|---|---|
| 1. a | 16. c |
| 2. c | 17. b |
| 3. b | 18. d |
| 4. d | 19. a |
| 5. d | 20. c |
| 6. d | 21. c |
| 7. d | 22. d |
| 8. d | 23. d |
| 9. d | 24. b |
| 10. a | 25. c |
| 11. c | 26. d |
| 12. d | 27. b |
| 13. d | 28. a |
| 14. a | 29. d |
| 15. a | 30. a |

## CHAPTER 9

### Truth or Fiction Answers

All True

### Multiple Choice Answers

| | |
|---|---|
| 1. c | 10. d |
| 2. c | 11. d |
| 3. d | 12. a |
| 4. d | 13. d |
| 5. a | 14. d |
| 6. d | 15. d |
| 7. d | 16. c |
| 8. a | 17. d |
| 9. d | 18. c |

| | |
|---|---|
| 19. d | 25. b |
| 20. c | 26. c |
| 21. d | 27. c |
| 22. d | 28. a |
| 23. c | 29. d |
| 24. d | 30. d |

## CHAPTER 10

### Truth or Fiction Answers

| | |
|---|---|
| 1. T | 9. F |
| 2. F | 10. T |
| 3. T | 11. F |
| 4. F | 12. T |
| 5. F | 13. F |
| 6. T | 14. F |
| 7. F | 15. T |
| 8. T | |

### Multiple Choice Answers

| | |
|---|---|
| 1. c | 14. d |
| 2. b | 15. d |
| 3. d | 16. a |
| 4. c | 17. b |
| 5. d | 18. c |
| 6. a | 19. c |
| 7. a | 20. a |
| 8. d | 21. a |
| 9. b | 22. c |
| 10. b | 23. b |
| 11. a | 24. d |
| 12. c | 25. b |
| 13. d | 26. b |

## CHAPTER 11

### Truth or Fiction Answers

| | |
|---|---|
| 1. T | 9. T |
| 2. F | 10. T |
| 3. T | 11. F |
| 4. T | 12. F |
| 5. F | 13. T |
| 6. F | 14. T |
| 7. F | 15. F |
| 8. F | |

## Multiple Choice Answers

| | |
|---|---|
| 1. a | 16. b |
| 2. d | 17. a |
| 3. c | 18. d |
| 4. a | 19. c |
| 5. d | 20. d |
| 6. b | 21. b |
| 7. c | 22. d |
| 8. d | 23. a |
| 9. c | 24. a |
| 10. b | 25. b |
| 11. d | 26. c |
| 12. b | 27. d |
| 13. a | 28. a |
| 14. b | 29. c |
| 15. c | 30. b |

# CHAPTER 12

## Truth or Fiction Answers

| | |
|---|---|
| 1. T | 9. F |
| 2. T | 10. F |
| 3. F | 11. F |
| 4. F | 12. T |
| 5. T | 13. T |
| 6. T | 14. T |
| 7. F | 15. F |
| 8. T | |

## Multiple Choice Answers

| | |
|---|---|
| 1. c | 16. a |
| 2. c | 17. b |
| 3. a | 18. b |
| 4. c | 19. b |
| 5. b | 20. a |
| 6. c | 21. d |
| 7. a | 22. c |
| 8. a | 23. b |
| 9. c | 24. c |
| 10. d | 25. b |
| 11. a | 26. c |
| 12. d | 27. d |
| 13. d | 28. b |
| 14. a | 29. c |
| 15. d | |

## CHAPTER 13

### Truth or Fiction Answers

| | |
|---|---|
| 1. F | 9. F |
| 2. T | 10. F |
| 3. T | 11. F |
| 4. F | 12. F |
| 5. F | 13. T |
| 6. T | 14. T |
| 7. F | 15. T |
| 8. T | |

### Multiple Choice Answers

| | |
|---|---|
| 1. a | 16. b |
| 2. d | 17. d |
| 3. d | 18. a |
| 4. d | 19. a |
| 5. b | 20. a |
| 6. a | 21. a |
| 7. b | 22. d |
| 8. c | 23. c |
| 9. a | 24. b |
| 10. a | 25. d |
| 11. c | 26. d |
| 12. d | 27. a |
| 13. b | 28. d |
| 14. b | 29. c |
| 15. c | 30. d |

## CHAPTER 14

### Truth or Fiction Answers

| | |
|---|---|
| 1. F | 9. F |
| 2. T | 10. T |
| 3. T | 11. F |
| 4. F | 12. F |
| 5. F | 13. F |
| 6. F | 14. T |
| 7. F | 15. T |
| 8. F | 16. T |

## Multiple Choice Answers

| | |
|---|---|
| 1. b | 15. b |
| 2. d | 16. d |
| 3. d | 17. b |
| 4. d | 18. c |
| 5. a | 19. b |
| 6. d | 20. d |
| 7. d | 21. d |
| 8. b | 22. b |
| 9. d | 23. d |
| 10. a | 24. b |
| 11. a | 25. d |
| 12. c | 26. c |
| 13. c | 27. b |
| 14. a | |

## CHAPTER 15

### Truth or Fiction Answers

| | |
|---|---|
| 1. T | 9. T |
| 2. F | 10. F |
| 3. T | 11. T |
| 4. F | 12. T |
| 5. F | 13. T |
| 6. T | 14. F |
| 7. T | 15. T |
| 8. F | |

### Multiple Choice Answers

| | |
|---|---|
| 1. d | 16. c |
| 2. b | 17. a |
| 3. c | 18. d |
| 4. a | 19. c |
| 5. d | 20. d |
| 6. b | 21. b |
| 7. c | 22. c |
| 8. c | 23. a |
| 9. b | 24. d |
| 10. a | 25. b |
| 11. d | 26. c |
| 12. b | 27. c |
| 13. d | 28. d |
| 14. d | 29. c |
| 15. b | 30. a |

## CHAPTER 16

### Truth or Fiction Answers

| | |
|---|---|
| 1. T | 9. T |
| 2. F | 10. T |
| 3. F | 11. T |
| 4. T | 12. T |
| 5. F | 13. F |
| 6. T | 14. T |
| 7. F | 15. T |
| 8. F | |

### Multiple Choice Answers

| | |
|---|---|
| 1. c | 16. b |
| 2. d | 17. b |
| 3. a | 18. c |
| 4. b | 19. d |
| 5. b | 20. c |
| 6. c | 21. a |
| 7. c | 22. c |
| 8. a | 23. d |
| 9. d | 24. b |
| 10. b | 25. d |
| 11. c | 26. c |
| 12. d | 27. d |
| 13. d | 28. a |
| 14. c | 29. b |
| 15. a | |

## CHAPTER 17

### Truth or Fiction Answers

| | |
|---|---|
| 1. F | 9. T |
| 2. T | 10. T |
| 3. T | 11. T |
| 4. F | 12. T |
| 5. F | 13. F |
| 6. T | 14. T |
| 7. T | 15. F |
| 8. F | |

## Multiple Choice Answers

| | |
|---|---|
| 1. c | 16. c |
| 2. c | 17. c |
| 3. b | 18. b |
| 4. b | 19. b |
| 5. c | 20. a |
| 6. a | 21. c |
| 7. c | 22. c |
| 8. d | 23. a |
| 9. c | 24. b |
| 10. b | 25. d |
| 11. a | 26. a |
| 12. d | 27. c |
| 13. b | 28. c |
| 14. d | 29. d |
| 15. b | |

## CHAPTER 18

### Truth or Fiction Answers

| | |
|---|---|
| 1. T | 9. F |
| 2. F | 10. T |
| 3. T | 11. F |
| 4. T | 12. T |
| 5. F | 13. T |
| 6. F | 14. F |
| 7. T | 15. T |
| 8. T | |

### Multiple Choice Answers

| | |
|---|---|
| 1. c | 16. d |
| 2. b | 17. d |
| 3. c | 18. b |
| 4. a | 19. b |
| 5. c | 20. a |
| 6. d | 21. a |
| 7. d | 22. d |
| 8. c | 23. d |
| 9. c | 24. a |
| 10. b | 25. c |
| 11. d | 26. d |
| 12. b | 27. b |
| 13. b | 28. d |
| 14. c | 29. c |
| 15. a | 30. d |

# CHAPTER 19

## Truth or Fiction Answers

| | | | |
|---|---|---|---|
| 1. F | | 9. F | |
| 2. F | | 10. T | |
| 3. F | | 11. F | |
| 4. F | | 12. T | |
| 5. F | | 13. F | |
| 6. T | | 14. F | |
| 7. T | | 15. F | |
| 8. F | | | |

## Multiple Choice Answers

| | | | |
|---|---|---|---|
| 1. d | | 16. d | |
| 2. b | | 17. c | |
| 3. b | | 18. c | |
| 4. c | | 19. b | |
| 5. b | | 20. c | |
| 6. a | | 21. b | |
| 7. d | | 22. b | |
| 8. d | | 23. a | |
| 9. c | | 24. c | |
| 10. c | | 25. a | |
| 11. c | | 26. c | |
| 12. a | | 27. d | |
| 13. b | | 28. b | |
| 14. a | | 29. c | |
| 15. d | | 30. b | |

# CHAPTER 20

## Truth or Fiction Answers

| | | | |
|---|---|---|---|
| 1. F | | 9. F | |
| 2. F | | 10. F | |
| 3. T | | 11. T | |
| 4. T | | 12. F | |
| 5. F | | 13. T | |
| 6. T | | 14. F | |
| 7. F | | 15. T | |
| 8. T | | | |

## Multiple Choice Answers

| | |
|---|---|
| 1. b | 16. c |
| 2. c | 17. c |
| 3. a | 18. b |
| 4. b | 19. d |
| 5. d | 20. d |
| 6. d | 21. c |
| 7. c | 22. c |
| 8. b | 23. d |
| 9. a | 24. a |
| 10. b | 25. b |
| 11. c | 26. a |
| 12. a | 27. c |
| 13. d | 28. c |
| 14. b | 29. c |
| 15. b | 30. d |

# CHAPTER 21

## Truth or Fiction Answers

| | |
|---|---|
| 1. T | 9. F |
| 2. F | 10. T |
| 3. T | 11. T |
| 4. F | 12. T |
| 5. T | 13. T |
| 6. F | 14. T |
| 7. F | 15. T |
| 8. F | |

## Multiple Choice Answers

| | |
|---|---|
| 1. c | 15. d |
| 2. d | 16. c |
| 3. c | 17. a |
| 4. c | 18. c |
| 5. b | 19. d |
| 6. c | 20. a |
| 7. b | 21. d |
| 8. c | 22. a |
| 9. b | 23. d |
| 10. d | 24. b |
| 11. b | 25. b |
| 12. c | 26. d |
| 13. b | 27. d |
| 14. c | |

## CHAPTER 22

### Truth or Fiction Answers

1. T
2. F
3. F
4. F
5. F
6. T
7. F
8. T

9. T
10. F
11. T
12. T
13. F
14. T
15. F

### Multiple Choice Answers

1. b
2. c
3. a
4. d
5. c
6. d
7. a
8. c
9. b
10. d
11. b
12. a
13. b
14. d
15. a

16. c
17. c
18. d
19. b
20. c
21. b
22. a
23. c
24. b
25. d
26. b
27. a
28. a
29. c
30. c

## CHAPTER 23

### Truth or Fiction Answers

1. T
2. F
3. T
4. T
5. F
6. F
7. T
8. F

9. T
10. T
11. F
12. T
13. F
14. T
15. F

## Multiple Choice Answers

| | | | |
|---|---|---|---|
| 1. d | | 16. c |
| 2. c | | 17. c |
| 3. a | | 18. d |
| 4. b | | 19. a |
| 5. a | | 20. d |
| 6. c | | 21. a |
| 7. c | | 22. d |
| 8. c | | 23. c |
| 9. b | | 24. b |
| 10. b | | 25. c |
| 11. d | | 26. d |
| 12. b | | 27. b |
| 13. d | | 28. d |
| 14. d | | 29. d |
| 15. b | | 30. d |

## CHAPTER 24

### Truth or Fiction Answers

| | | | |
|---|---|---|---|
| 1. F | | 9. T |
| 2. F | | 10. F |
| 3. T | | 11. T |
| 4. T | | 12. T |
| 5. T | | 13. F |
| 6. T | | 14. F |
| 7. F | | 15. T |
| 8. T | | |

### Multiple Choice Answers

| | | | |
|---|---|---|---|
| 1. b | | 16. d |
| 2. a | | 17. b |
| 3. b | | 18. b |
| 4. d | | 19. c |
| 5. d | | 20. d |
| 6. a | | 21. a |
| 7. a | | 22. a |
| 8. c | | 23. b |
| 9. c | | 24. d |
| 10. b | | 25. b |
| 11. b | | 26. c |
| 12. c | | 27. a |
| 13. a | | 28. c |
| 14. c | | 29. b |
| 15. d | | 30. d |

## CHAPTER 25

### Truth or Fiction Answers

| | | | |
|---|---|---|---|
| 1. T | | 9. T | |
| 2. T | | 10. T | |
| 3. F | | 11. F | |
| 4. T | | 12. T | |
| 5. F | | 13. T | |
| 6. F | | 14. F | |
| 7. F | | 15. F | |
| 8. T | | | |

### Multiple Choice Answers

| | | |
|---|---|---|
| 1. b | | 16. c |
| 2. a | | 17. c |
| 3. d | | 18. a |
| 4. c | | 19. c |
| 5. a | | 20. c |
| 6. c | | 21. c |
| 7. d | | 22. c |
| 8. b | | 23. b |
| 9. d | | 24. b |
| 10. b | | 25. a |
| 11. c | | 26. d |
| 12. a | | 27. c |
| 13. a | | 28. d |
| 14. c | | 29. d |
| 15. b | | 30. d |

## CHAPTER 26

### Truth or Fiction Answers

| | | |
|---|---|---|
| 1. F | | 9. F |
| 2. F | | 10. F |
| 3. F | | 11. F |
| 4. T | | 12. T |
| 5. F | | 13. T |
| 6. T | | 14. F |
| 7. T | | 15. F |
| 8. T | | |

## Multiple Choice Answers

| | | | |
|---|---|---|---|
| 1. d | | 16. c | |
| 2. a | | 17. d | |
| 3. c | | 18. c | |
| 4. b | | 19. c | |
| 5. a | | 20. d | |
| 6. c | | 21. b | |
| 7. b | | 22. d | |
| 8. a | | 23. b | |
| 9. c | | 24. d | |
| 10. d | | 25. b | |
| 11. b | | 26. a | |
| 12. d | | 27. d | |
| 13. c | | 28. d | |
| 14. c | | 29. c | |
| 15. d | | 30. c | |

# Author Index

Note: Numbers in *italics* indicate pages with complete bibliographic information.

## A

AAMFT, *See* American Association for Marriage and Family Therapy
Aarons, G. A., 356, *367*
Abbott, D. W., 535, *547*
Abrantes, A. M., 356, *367*
ACA, *See* American Counseling Association
Acton, R. G., 404, *410*
Adair, C., *526*
Agras, S., 497, *505*
Agulnik, P. L., 497, *505*
Ahrons, C., 265, *274*
Ainsworth, M. D. S., 29, 30, *39*
Akiskal, H. S., 100, *112*
Aldarondo, E., 222, *231*, 305, 310, *319*, *321*
Aldrich, L. M., 425, *433*
Aleman, J. C., 524, *526*
Alexander, J., 363, *368*
Alexander, J. F., 350, 351, 352, 353, 354, 355, 357, 358, 359, 362, 363, *366*, *367*, *368*, *369*
Allmari, D., 221, *230*
Altepeter, T. S., 353, 354, 355, *367*
AMA, *See* American Medical Association
American Association for Marriage and Family Therapy, 267, *274*, *526*, 536, *546*
American Counseling Association, 521, *526*
American Medical Association, 520, *526*

American Psychiatric Association, *85*, 102, 104, *112*, 196, *211*, 284, *298*, 351, *367*, 377, *390*, 436, *455*, 463, *481*, 485, *505*, 550, *568*
American Society of Addiction Medicine, 440, *455*
AMFTRB, *See* Association of Marital and Family Therapy Regulatory Boards
Anderson, B. S., 539, 540, 543, *546*
Anderson, C., 284, *298*
Anderson, J., 453, *456*
Anderson, S. A., 313, *319*
Anglin, D., 308, *320*
Anglin, K., 307, *320*
Angoff, W. H., 562, *568*
Angold, A., 353, *367*
Anthony, J. C., 378, *390*
Antoni, M., 351, *368*
APA, *See* American Psychiatric Association
Arbuthnot, J., 271, *274*, 363, *367*
Arias, I., 223, *229*
Arkinson, M. K., 405, *410*
Armstrong, H. E., 221, *230*
Arnold, B., 18, *20*
Arnow, B., 88, *112*
Asai, S. G., 244, *255*
Asay, T. P., 192, *211*
Asher, S. R., 351, *368*
Ashman, T., 520, *527*

# Subject Index